AF506084

Violence Against Women

Contemporary Examination of Intimate Partner Violence

STM **Learning**, Inc.

Leading Publisher of Scientific, Technical, and Medical Educational Resources
Saint Louis
www.stmlearning.com

OUR MISSION

To become the world leader in publishing and

information services on child abuse,

maltreatment, diseases, and domestic violence.

We seek to heighten awareness of these issues,

and provide relevant information to

professionals and consumers.

A portion of our profits is contributed to nonprofit organizations
dedicated to the prevention of child abuse and the care of victims
of abuse and other children and family charities.

Violence Against Women

Contemporary Examination of Intimate Partner Violence

Paul Thomas Clements, PhD, RN
Associate Clinical Professor
Coordinator - Contemporary
Trends in Forensic
Health Care Certificate Online
Drexel University
College of Nursing and
Health Professions
Philadelphia, Pennsylvania

Jennifer Pierce-Weeks, RN, SANE-P, SANE-A
Project Director
International Association
of Forensic Nurses
Elkridge, Maryland
Forensic Nurse Examiner
Emergency Department
Memorial Hospital, University
of Colorado Health
Colorado Springs, Colorado

Karyn E. Holt, PhD, CNM, RN
Associate Clinical Professor
and Director of Online Quality
Division of Nursing
College of Nursing and Health
Professions
Drexel University
Philadelphia, Pennsylvania

Angelo P. Giardino, MD, PhD
Professor and Section Chief
Academic General Pediatrics
Baylor College of Medicine
Senior Vice President/Chief
Quality Officer
Texas Children's Hospital
Houston, Texas

Soraya Seedat, MBChB, FC Psych (SA), MMed (Psych), PhD
Executive Head of the Department of
Psychiatry
Co-Director: Medical Research Council
Unit on Anxiety and Stress Disorders
South African Research Chair in PTSD
(hosted by University of Stellenbosch, funded
by the DST, and administered by NRF)
Department of Psychiatry
Faculty of Medicine and Health Sciences
Stellenbosch University
Cape Town, South Africa

Catherine M. Mortiere, PhD
Clinical Instructor
Department of Psychiatry
New York University, College of Medicine
Licensed Psychologist
Kirby Forensic Psychiatric Center
New York, New York

STM **Learning**, Inc.

Leading Publisher of Scientific, Technical, and Medical Educational Resources
Saint Louis
www.stmlearning.com

Publishers: Glenn E. Whaley and Marianne V. Whaley

Graphic Design Director: Glenn E. Whaley

Managing Editor: Ashley Maurer

Book Design/Page Layout: Jennifer Jones / GW Graphics

Print/Production Coordinator: Jennifer Jones / GW Graphics

Cover Design: Jennifer Jones / GW Graphics

Color Prepress Specialist: Kevin Tucker

Acquisition Editor: Glenn E. Whaley

Developmental Editor: Kristen Prysmiki

Copy Editor: Ashley Maurer

Proofreader: Paul Goode / Ashley Maurer

Printed in the United States.

Publisher:

STM Learning, Inc.

55 Westport Plaza, Suite 455, Saint Louis, Missouri 63146 USA

Phone: (314) 434-2424 Fax: (314) 434-2425 Toll Free: (800) 600-0330

http://www.stmlearning.com

Library of Congress Cataloging-in-Publication Data

Violence against women (Clements)

Violence against women : a contemporary examination of intimate partner violence / [edited by] Paul Thomas Clements, Jennifer Pierce-Weeks, Karyn E. Holt, Angelo P. Giardino, Soraya Seedat, Catherine M. Mortiere.

p. ; cm.

ISBN 978-1-878060-95-2 (flexibound : alk. paper)

I. Clements, Paul T. (Paul Thomas), 1962- editor. II. Pierce-Weeks, Jennifer, editor. III. Holt, Karyn E., 1959- editor. IV. Giardino, Angelo P., editor. V. Seedat, Soraya, 1966- editor. VI. Mortiere, Catherine, editor. VII. Title.

[DNLM: 1. Battered Women--psychology. 2. Spouse Abuse--prevention & control. 3. Spouse Abuse--legislation & jurisprudence. WA 309.1]

RC569.5.F3

362.82'92--dc23

2014018824

CONTRIBUTORS

Kimberly Adams Tufts,
DNP, WHNP-BC, FAAN
Assistant Dean for Interprofessional Education
College of Health Sciences
Old Dominion University
Norfolk, Virginia

Tracie O. Afifi, PhD
Assistant Professor
Department of Community Health Sciences
University of Manitoba
Winnipeg, Manitoba

Katherine Kaby Anselmi, JD, PhD, CRNP-BC
Associate Clinical Professor
Assistant Dean of Accreditation/Regulatory Affairs
and Online Innovation
College of Nursing and Health Professions
Drexel University
Philadelphia, Pennsylvania

Megan H Bair-Merritt, MD, MSCE
Associate Professor of Pediatrics
Associate Division Chief of General Pediatrics
Fellowship Director, Academic General Pediatrics
Boston Medical Center, Department of Pediatrics
Boston, Massachusetts

Kathy Bell, MS, RN
Forensic Nursing Administrator
Tulsa Police Department
Tulsa, Oklahoma

Dr Belinda Bruwer,
MBChB(Stell), MMed(Psych), FCPsych(SA)
Senior Specialist Psychiatrist and Lecturer
Department of Psychiatry
Stellenbosch University
Cape Town, South Africa

Nancy B. Cabelus, DNP, MSN, AFN-BC
Forensic Consultant
Program on Sexual Violence in Conflict Zones
Physicians for Human Rights
New York, New York
Adjunct Faculty
College of Nursing
University of St. Francis
Joliet, Illinois

Jacquelyn C. Campbell, PhD, RN, FAAN
Professor and Anna D. Wolf Chair
Community of Public Health
Johns Hopkins University School of Nursing
National Program Director
Robert Wood Johnson Foundation Nurse Faculty
Scholars Program
Baltimore, Maryland

Mary E. Campise, LICSW
Senior Program Analyst
Military Community and Family Policy
Office of Family Policy/Children and Youth
Family Advocacy Program
Department of Defense,
Alexandria, Virginia

Linda Chamberlain, PhD, MPH
Adjunct Faculty
University of Alaska
School of Public Health
Anchorage, Alaska

Amy Carney, NP, PhD, FAAFS
Assistant Professor
School of Nursing
California State University San Marcos
San Marcos, California

Diana Faugno, MSN, NR, CPN, SANE-A, SANE-P,
FAAFS, DF-IAFN
Forensic Nurse Examiner
Emergency Department
Eisenhower Medical Center
Rancho Mirage, California

Theresa M Fay-Hillier, MSN, PMHCNS-BC,
Certified in Danger Assessment
Assistant Clinical Professor
College of Nursing and Health Professions
Drexel University
Philadelphia, Pennsylvania

Margit B. Gerardi,
PhD, WHCNP, PMHNP-BC
Center for Health Care Services
Assistant Professor
Webster University
San Antonio, Texas

Casey Gwinn (J.D.)
President
National Family Justice Center Alliance
San Diego, California

Tara Henry, MSN, FNP-C, SANE-A, SANE-P
Forensic Nurse Services
Anchorage, Alaska

Richard E. Heyman, PhD
Professor
Family Translational Research Group
New York University
New York, New York

Aaron Holt, JD
Former Assistant District Attorney
Alaniz, Schraeder, Linker, Farris & Mayes LLP
Houston, Texas

Cheryl C.D. Hughes, PhD
Associate Professor of Humanities
and Religious Studies
Liberal Arts Division
Tulsa Community College
Tulsa, Oklahoma

D. Jolene Kinley, MA
PhD Candidate
Department of Psychology
University of Manitoba
Winnipeg, Manitoba

Kathryn Laughon, PhD, RN, FAAN
Associate Professor
University of Virginia School of Nursing
Charlottesville, Virginia

Megan Lechner, MSN, RN, CNS, SANE-P, SANE-A
Forensic Nurse Examiner, Clinical Team Lead
Memorial Hospital, University of Colorado
Adjunct Professor
University of Colorado at Colorado Springs
Colorado Springs, Colorado

David W. Lloyd, J.D.
Former Director (1995-2011, retired)
Family Advocacy Program
Office of the Deputy Assistant Secretary of Defense
for Military Community and Family Policy
United States Department of Defense
Washington, DC

Jennifer Gentile Long, JD
Director
AEquitas
Washington, DC

Jill Malik, MS
Junior Research Scientist
Family Translational Research Group
New York University
New York, New York

Pamela E Marcus, RN, APRN/PMH-BC
Owner of Private Practice, Advance Practice, Nurse
Psychotherapist
Private Practice
Upper Marlboro, Maryland
Associate Professor of Nursing
Nursing
Prince George's Community College
Largo, Maryland

Jenifer Markowitz, ND, RN, WHNP-BC, SANE-A, DF-IAFN
Forensic Nursing Consultant
Alexandria, Virginia

Grace Mattern
Author and Nonprofit Advisor
www.gracemattern.com
Northwood, New Hampshire

Jill Theresa Messing, MSW, PhD
Assistant Professor
School of Social Work
Arizona State University
Phoenix, Arizona

Marie Elizabeth Mugavin, PhD, FNP-BC, SAFE-A
Adjunct Assistant Professor,
Department of Emergency Medicine
University of New Mexico, School of Medicine
Family Nurse Practitioner,
Sexual Assault Forensic Examiner
Sage Neuroscience Center, Inc.
Albuquerque, New Mexico

Carol Post
Executive Director
Delaware Coalition Against Domestic Violence
Wilmington, Delaware

Brian C. Ross, JD
Former Program Analyst (2001-2011)
Office of the Deputy Assistant
Secretary of Defense for Military
Community and Family Policy
United States Department of Defense
Washington, DC

C. Gabrielle Salfati,
MSc, PhD, C.Psychol, F.IA-IP
Professor of Psychology
Department of Psychology
John Jay College of Criminal Justice
City University of New York
New York, New York

Jitender Sareen,
MD, FRCPC
Professor
Department of Psychiatry, Psychology,
and Community Health Sciences
University of Manitoba
Winnipeg, Manitoba

Richard T. Sochor, MA
Research Coordinator/Assistant
Department of Psychiatry
Columbia University
New York State Psychiatric Institute
New York, New York

Susan Solecki,
FNP-BC, PNP-BC
Assistant Clinical Professor
College of Nursing and Health Professions
Drexel University
Philadelphia, Pennsylvania

Rae Spiwak, MSc
PhD Candidate
Department of Community Health Sciences
University of Manitoba
Winnipeg, Manitoba

Nandrie Steyn, MBChB(Stell), DMH(SA) Diploma
in Mental Health
Medical Officer
Department of Psychiatry
University of Stellenbosch
Cape Town, South Africa

Heidi Stöckl, PhD
Lecturer
Social and Mathematical Epidemiology Group Department of Global Health and Development
London School of Hygiene and Tropical Medicine
London, UK

Gael Strack, JD
CEO
National Family Justice Center Aliiance
San Diego, California

Jonathan D. Thackeray, MD
Chief, Division of Child and Family Advocacy
Medical Director, Center for Family Safety and Healing
Department of Pediatrics
Nationwide Children's Hospital
Columbus, Ohio

Jonel Thaller, MSW
PhD Candidate
School of Social Work
Arizona State University
Phoenix, Arizona

Charlotte Watts, PhD
Professor
Social and Mathematical Epidemiology Group Department of Global Health and Development
London School of Hygiene and Tropical Medicine
London, UK

Kassia Wosick, MA, PhD
Associate Professor
New Mexico State University
Department of Sociology
Las Cruces, New Mexico

Foreword

Intimate partner violence (IPV) is an entirely stoppable yet crippling epidemic in the United States and around the globe. The 2010 National Intimate Partner and Sexual Violence Survey (NISVS) from the Centers for Disease Control and Prevention report that more than 1 in 3 women and 1 in 4 men experience rape, physical violence, and/or stalking by an intimate partner in their lifetime. Moreover, the majority of both men and women experiencing IPV do so for the first time before the age of 25.[1] Many require medical and other healthcare related encounters. A study by Bonomi and colleagues found significantly higher healthcare costs for physically abused women, and greater utilization of services in emergency, hospital outpatient, primary care, pharmacy, and specialty services departments.[2] Reviewing all homicides in the US between 1980 and 2008, nearly 1 in 5 victims was killed by an intimate partner; in 2008, 45% of all female victims were killed by an intimate partner, a rate far higher than their male counterparts.[3]

IPV exists within small towns and big cities, wealthy communities and poor; on military installations, and on high school and college campuses across the nation. It would be difficult to find any community not impacted by IPV. Legislation related to IPV has improved drastically over the years. Every state has some form of anti-stalking law on the books, and as of 1993 all states and the military criminalize rape of a spouse. The Victims of Crimes Act (VOCA) as well as the Violence Against Women Act (VAWA) have done much to assist victims of crimes in meaningful ways. Felony strangulation laws have become increasingly common—a majority of states now have them—making it easier to hold offenders accountable for a frequently used and potentially lethal form of violence. However, jurisdictions differ widely in the ways they approach the investigation and prosecution of crimes related to IPV, be it in definition, level of criminal offense, or types of available punishment upon successful prosecution. Regardless, criminal justice professionals and colleagues in allied professions, including healthcare and victim advocacy, will certainly come into contact with victims of abuse. Understanding the broad spectrum of ways in which IPV can manifest itself and the ripple effect it can have on the lives of victims and their families is critical.

Violence Against Women: A Contemporary Examination of Intimate Partner Violence is a one-stop reference book. It is relevant for victim advocates, social workers, law enforcement professionals, prosecutors, judges, healthcare workers, and any other professional who desires a well-rounded understanding of the implications and impact of IPV. This book systematically examines all aspects of IPV and contains detailed and well-resourced chapters on broad issues, such as risk assessment, healthcare implications and investigation, as well as more focused examinations of IPV within specific communities. I am not aware of a more comprehensive look at IPV than Violence Against Women: A Contemporary Examination of Intimate Partner Violence. The authors, contributors, and editors are to be commended for its excellence.

Sasha N. Rutizer
Senior Attorney
National District Attorneys Association

1. Black MC, Basile KC, Breiding MJ, et al. The National Intimate Partner and Sexual Violence Survey (NISVS): 2010 Summary Report. Atlanta, GA: National Center for Injury Prevention and Control, Centers for Disease Control and Prevention; 2011.

2. Bonomi AE, Anderson ML, Rivara FP, Thompson RS. Health care utilization and costs associated with physical and nonphysical-only intimate partner violence. Health Serv Res. 2009;44(3):1052-1067.

3. Cooper A, Smith EL. Homicide Trends in the United States, 1980-2008. Washington, DC: US Department of Justice, Office of Justice Programs, Bureau of Justice Statistics; 2011.

Foreword

Over the last several decades we have come to realize that exposures to violence is in fact a major social determinant of health. Some great visionaries of our country 'got' violence way before most. One visionary was Dr. Martin Luther King, he stated:

"Violence as a way of achieving racial justice is both impractical and immoral. It is impractical because it is a descending spiral ending in destruction for all. The old law of an eye for an eye leaves everybody blind. It is immoral because it seeks to humiliate the opponent rather than win his understanding; it seeks to annihilate rather than to convert. Violence is immoral because it thrives on hatred rather than love. It destroys community and makes brotherhood impossible. It leaves society in a monologue rather than a dialogue. Violence ends by defeating itself. It creates bitterness in the survivors and brutality in the destroyers." I believe Dr. King captured the devastating effects of violence like no other before or since.

Globally, Gender Based Violence (GBV) affects millions of women (and some men). Over the last 4 decades much evidence has evolved on the health consequences of GBV, and a major focus this decade is exploring interventions and health outcomes. We know that GBV is deeply rooted in socio-political factors, inequality, racism, sexism, and poverty. Addressing these route causes is vital and inherent to preventing and intervening in cases of GBV. Our success will best be measured by the acceptance of zero tolerance for violence across our Nation and the World.

Health care professionals are in a unique and privileged position to prevent and intervene when caring for patients exposed to violence. A Trauma and Patient Informed theoretical framework offers the best opportunity to engage patients. This scholarly written book illuminates the impact of violence on individuals and provides information that is applicable to practice and policy. Worthy of note is the breath and depth of the authors- representing medicine, nursing, lawyers, researchers, academics, and advocates. Their unique and combined contributions are complimentary to each other and provide a wealth of information.

I am confident this book will serve as a beacon for those providing services to victims of GBV. I commend each and every author as surely the parts of this book equal the whole. I also want to acknowledge the patients we serve- it is an honor and a privilege to be in a position of working with them- I know I am a better provider and person for having had this opportunity in my career. In solidarity- Annie Lewis-O'Connor

Annie Lewis-O'Connor PhD, NP, MPH
Nurse Scientist & Founder and Director
Women's C.A.R.E Clinic
Coordinated Approach to Recovery and Empowerment
Brigham and Women's Hospital
Instructor- Harvard Medical School
Boston, MA

FOREWORD

Violence against women is pervasive. A pregnant woman in Pakistan is stoned to death by her family as an "honor killing," 2 girls in India are raped and hung, nearly 300 girls in Nigeria are kidnapped—all are recent examples of egregious, violent acts based on historic, cultural, social, and religious norms of gender inequality. Violence against women is a tragedy of personal, interpersonal, societal, generational, and global proportions, inflicting a vast impact, both economic and moral. Widely recognized as a fundamental human rights violation, this type of violence affects as many as 35% of women worldwide, many of whom experience the highest risk in their own home.[1]

As a newly minted emergency medicine physician in 1980, I had solidified my desire to be on the front lines in caring for people from diverse walks of life. I was prepared to render care and relieve suffering from a variety of health concerns, including forms of inflicted violence. I was given the unique privilege to provide medical direction for what was then known as the Rape Crisis Program at Saint Luke's Hospital in Kansas City, Missouri. Established in 1974, this was the first private sexual assault program in the country.[2-4] I did not realize at the time, but I was embarking on a career-altering shift into the emotionally-charged realm of combatting violence against women and helping to establish a new specialty: clinical forensic medicine. This specialty applies medical forensic knowledge to living patients.[5,6] William Smock, MD, MS, FACEP, FAAEM was the first to complete a clinical forensic medicine fellowship in the United States.[7]

The concept that violence is a public health issue, which we in the health care professions have a responsibility to address, has yet to be fully adopted. After the leading causes of death shifted mid-century from infectious diseases to violence, the Centers for Disease Control and Prevention (CDC) established the Violence Epidemiology Branch and the Division of Injury Epidemiology and Control. In 1985, one of my mentors, US Surgeon General C. Everett Koop, MD, articulated the challenge:[8]

Identifying violence as a public health issue is a relatively new idea. Traditionally, when confronted by the circumstances of violence, [we] . . . have deferred to the criminal justice system. Over the years we have tacitly and, I believe, mistakenly agreed that violence was the exclusive province of the police, the courts, and the penal system. To be sure, those agents of public safety and justice have served us well. But when we ask them to concentrate more on the prevention of violence and to provide additional service for victims, we may begin to burden the criminal justice system beyond reason. At that point, the professions of medicine, nursing, and the health-related social services must come forward and recognize violence as their issue and one that profoundly affects the public health.[9]

Historically, criminal justice professionals have borne the responsibility "to protect the public" and serve the community, primarily by removing from society persons who demonstrate violent behavior, typically after they have committed a crime. Now, doctors, nurses, and social service professionals realize that we also bear a responsibility: "to prevent harm to the public" from violent behavior or disease by implementing interventions that reduce or eliminate risk factors and increase protection. This distinction suggests a profound shift not only in roles and responsibilities but in models and tools for addressing violence. The public health approach is collaborative; it engages criminal justice, health care, education, and social services. Moreover, this approach is grounded in data. This data encompasses a 360-degree view of all types and severity levels of violence, eg, minor trauma, psychological violence, threats of violence, and neglect or deprivation. Historically, in most areas, the collection of violence-related injury data is segregated and reflects a mere tip of the injury iceberg. Victims of violence that results in fatal injury present through the criminal justice system. Victims of significant violence, both fatal and non-fatal, enter the health care system through the doors of emergency departments. The health care data, although rich regarding types of injury and circumstances, usually captures little information about perpetrators, which is necessary for prevention strategies. The emerging sub-specialty of clinical forensic medicine integrates the public health model with criminal justice practices. As emergency departments implement forensic medicine concepts, the increased use of injury surveillance tools will provide victim-perpetrator relationship insight and will yield more accurate epidemiologic data surrounding these events.

The World Health Organization[10] defines violence as "[t]he intentional use of physical force or power, threatened or actual, against oneself, another person, or against a group or community that either results in or has a high likelihood of resulting in injury, death, physiological harm, mal-development, or deprivation." Based on this definition, a typology has developed, dividing the concept of violence into 3 categories: self-directed, interpersonal, or collective.[11] Interpersonal violence, that is, violence that involves the family or community, is sub-classified into child, intimate partner, and elderly. The CDC defines the distinct sub-category of intimate partner violence (IPV) as "physical, sexual, or psychological harm by a current or former partner or spouse. This type of violence can occur among heterosexual or same-sex couples and does not require sexual intimacy."[12]

IPV affects both females and males; however, most IPV is directed against women, affecting 1.3 to 5.3 million women annually in the United States.[13] The 2010 National Intimate Partner and Sexual Violence Survey found that over their lifetimes, 24.3% of women experience severe physical violence by an intimate partner; 18.3% are raped, with 9.4% being raped by an intimate partner; nearly 17% experience non-rape sexual violence by an intimate partner; and 48% experience psychological aggression by an intimate partner.[14] The highest prevalence of physical violence, rape, and stalking occurs among multiracial groups, and Native Americans experience sexual assault and rape at a rate more than double that of other racial groups.[15] These behaviors also tend to be generational. Forty-five percent to 70% of children exposed to domestic violence become physical abuse victims,[16] and the strongest risk factor for parental violence toward children is childhood exposure to a father who abuses the child's mother.[17]

The year 2014 marks the 20-year anniversary of the Violence Against Women Act (VAWA). This landmark legislation mandates the collaboration between the criminal justice system and health care that Dr. Koop championed decades ago. Between 1993, when the VAWA was first authorized, and 2008, the rate of IPV decreased by 53%. New provisions of the VAWA 2013 now address violence against Native American women, after an Oklahoma study found that 82.7% of their 422 subjects had experienced IPV or physical violence in their lifetime.[18] Indeed, the murder rate on some reservations is more than 10 times the national average.[19] The VAWA also addresses lesbian, gay, bisexual, transgender, and queer (LGBTQ) issues, being as studies find that nearly 44% of lesbian women and 61% of bisexual women report IPV, compared to 35% of women who identify as heterosexual.[20]

Offering a comprehensive review, this book seeks to sharpen the reader's focus on and understanding of violence against women and illuminate the multifaceted issues of IPV. The target audiences are health care professionals, law enforcement officials, advocacy personnel, those teaching at the university level, and those beginning their journey into this domain. The authors and contributors—physicians, nurses, district attorneys and lawyers, professors, psychiatric researchers, and domestic violence program directors and board members—are subject matter experts, sharing their considerable knowledge from diverse disciplines. The content is well-organized. The initial chapters discuss IPV assessment, risk factors, effects on women's health, and risk reduction. Subsequent chapters examine criminal justice aspects, including orders of protection; aspects of prosecution; and promising practices to decrease the incidences of IPV, including safety planning. The closing chapters explore specific areas of IPV, such as strangulation, stalking, sex-related homicide, child maltreatment, pregnancy, LGBTQ, and military aspects. Each chapter begins with well-referenced key points, and the text incorporates multiple tables, graphs, and figures to visually convey key concepts, some of which are also explored through case studies.

This excellent book reflects in its construct the public health collaborative model that Dr. Koop envisioned. Similarly, Saint Luke's Hospital has become one of the first programs to expand this model beyond sexual assault to address general trauma, domestic violence, and child and elder abuse.

In an increasingly global society, we in the health care professions have a moral obligation to break the cycle of violence against women whenever and wherever it occurs; to bring to bear those tools that fundamentally change the way in which women are viewed, valued, and treated; and to embrace the energies and benefits that women bring to humanity. Those of you who are engaged and dedicated to this work are to be commended, and you will find this book a powerful tool and an essential resource to carry with you as you face the challenges ahead in decreasing the incidence and prevalence of IPV in the US and throughout the world.

Michael L. Weaver, MD, FACEP, FCC, CDM
Associate Clinical Professor, UMKC School of Medicine
Medical Director, Clinical Forensic Medicine Program
Vice President, Clinical Diversity
Saint Luke's Health System
Kansas City, MO

---

1. *World Health Organization, London School of Hygiene and Tropical Medicine, South African Medical Research Council. Global and Regional Estimates of Violence Against Women: Prevalence and Health Effects of Intimate Partner Violence and Non-Partner Sexual Violence. Geneva, Switzerland: World Health Organization; 2013:2.*
2. *Morgan J. Rape treatment center opens at St. Luke's. Johnson County Sun. August 3, 1974.*   *(continued)*

(continued)

3. Sexual assault center unique in area. *Johnson County Herald.* December 10, 1976.

4. SART toolkit—learn about SARTs: history of SARTs. *Office for Victims of Crime Web site.* http://ovc.ncjrs.gov/sartkit/about/about-evolve-hs-a.html. Published March 2011. Accessed June 29, 2014.

5. Stark MM. *A Physician's Guide to Clinical Forensic Medicine.* Totowa, NJ: Humana Press; 2000:1.

6. Lynch VA, Duval JB. *Forensic Nursing Science.* St Louis, MO: Elsevier; 2011:3.

7. Aaron B. Body of work: Louisville's Dr. Smock leads country in living forensics. *Louisville Med.* 2014;62(1):13-15.

8. United States Department of Health and Human Services, United States Department of Justice. *Surgeon General's Workshop on Violence and Public Health Report.* Washington, DC: Health Resources and Services Administration; 1986.

9. Koop CE. Foreword. In: Rosenberg ML, Fenley MA, eds. *Violence in America: A Public Health Approach.* New York, NY: Oxford University Press; 1991:v.

10. World Health Organization Global Consultation on Violence and Health. *Violence: A Public Health Priority.* Geneva, Switzerland: World Health Organization; 1996:2-3 (WHO/EHA/SPI.POA.2).

11. Violence: A global public health problem. In: Krug EG, Dahlberg LL, Mercy JA, et al, eds. *World Report on Violence and Health.* Geneva, Switzerland: World Health Organization; 2002:1-21.

12. Injury prevention and control: intimate partner violence. *Centers for Disease Control and Prevention Web site.* http://www.cdc.gov/ViolencePrevention/intimatepartnerviolence/index.html?s_cid=fb_vv487. Updated May 5, 2014. Accessed June 29, 2014.

13. Nelson HD, Bougatsos C, Blazina I. Screening women for intimate partner violence: a systematic review to update the US Preventive Services Task Force recommendation. *Ann Intern Med.* 2012:156(11):796-808.

14. Black MC, Basile KC, Breiding MJ, et al. *The National Intimate Partner and Sexual Violence Survey: 2010 Summary Report.* Atlanta, GA: Centers for Disease Control and Prevention; 2011.

15. Perry SW. *American Indians and Crime -- A BJS Statistical Profile, 1992–2002.* Washington, DC: United States Department of Justice, Office of Justice Programs, Bureau of Justice Statistics; 2004.

16. Margolin G. Effects of domestic violence on children. In: Trickett PK, Schellenbach CJ, eds. *Violence Against Children and Family in the Community.* Washington, DC: American Psychological Association; 1998:4.

17. *Violence and the Family: Report of the American Psychological Association Presidential Task Force on Violence and the Family.* Washington, DC: American Psychological Association; 1996.

18. Malcoe LH, Duran BM. Intimate partner violence and injury in the lives of low-income Native American women. In: Fisher BS, ed. *Violence Against Women and Family Violence. Developments in Research, Practice, and Policy Conference Proceedings.* Washington, DC: US Department of Justice, National Institute of Justice; 2004: I-2-1 to I-2-16.

19. Statement of associate attorney general Thomas J. Perrelli before the committee on indian affairs on violence against Native American Women. *The United State Department of Justice Web site.* http://www.justice.gov/iso/opa/asg/speeches/2011/asg-speech-110714.html. Published July 14, 2011. Accessed July 1, 2014.

20. Walters ML, Chen J, Breiding MJ. *The National Intimate Partner and Sexual Violence Survey (NISVS): 2010 Findings on Victimization by Sexual Orientation.* Atlanta, GA: National Center for Injury Prevention and Control, Centers for Disease Control and Prevention; 2010.

PREFACE

Significant advances have been made in understanding violence and developing effective prevention and treatment methods. However, addressing interpersonal violence effectively demands involvement from many players, from healthcare professionals, victims, perpetrators, families, educators, community leaders, law enforcement officials, legislators, faith-based organizations, and the media.

Intimate partner violence (IPV) is manifested by four types of behaviors: physical violence, sexual violence, threats of physical or sexual violence, and emotional abuse.

Oftentimes, psychological and emotional violence is the beginning of a continuum of behaviors that commence with relational tensing progressing to emotional mistreatment, escalating to battering, and further progress to violence. This book was compiled from well known worldwide experts in violence and abuse and is intended to be used as a reference and handbook for hospital providers, the law enforcement team, media, educators, and legislators.

Intimate partner violence is the most common cause of nonfatal injury to women.

The Center for Disease Prevention and Control reports that about 4.8 million women experienced physical assault or rape related to IPV in 2009, while 2.9 million men experienced IPV. The related death rate in women is 78%, while in men it is only 22%. Within the United States, one in three female homicides is a result of intimate partner violence, while only one in twenty male homicides is a result of IPV. Clearly, intimate partner violence is a problem that needs to be eradicated, and this is possible through partnerships between educators, health care professionals, law enforcement, and the media using the best assessments and treatments. It is our hope that you will find this book helpful in your fight against intimate partner violence.

Karyn Holt, RN, CNM

REVIEWS

Violence Against Women: A Contemporary Examination of Intimate Partner Violence is a comprehensive overview of violence perpetrated against women. Experts share their knowledge, from understanding the scope of the problem, to assessment and treatment while including a review of multifaceted legal issues. Emphasized is the need for cross training and cooperation among professionals of different disciplines. The text discusses that the distinctly different intervention systems for child abuse and intimate partner violence can make it very difficult for victims to navigate. An integrated approach that may include co-located services to provide better support for victims of intimate partner violence and their children is suggested. Child abuse professionals will benefit by gaining a better understanding of intimate partner violence, the significant impact on children, and the need for professionals to employ a collaborative approach.

Dan Powers, ACSW, LCSW
Sr. Vice President, Clinical Services
Children's Advocacy Center of Collin County
Plano, Texas

Violence Against Women is a critical and comprehensive tool for anyone in the field of social work or mental health. The text provides a clear understanding of the complex and often overlapping factors that contribute to both victimization and perpetration of violence. It is applicable for a broad audience and provides valuable tools for the multi-disciplinary team approach needed to address this issue. The text educates the reader on the lasting effects of violence against women from a global standpoint and also provides valuable insight into effective therapeutic responses across cultures and victim populations. Specific chapters which address child maltreatment and the commercial sexual exploitation of women and children offer new perspectives for systemic responses to both parents and children in the child protection system. While social workers and mental health professionals will utilize the theoretical and clinical approaches recommended within the text, law enforcement professionals will gain valuable investigation insights, medical professionals will benefit from assessment techniques and victim dynamics identified, and prosecutors will gain tools to successfully maneuver through the unique legal components of these types of crimes. This is truly a must read for anyone who advocates for the vulnerable in our society.

Sally Howard
Court Appointed Special Advocates Collin County, Texas
Child Welfare Specialist and Educator

Intimate Partner Violence is on the rise in today's society. This book, Violence Against Women, is a well-articulated and comprehensive view of Intimate Partner Violence (IPV) and provides a detailed roadmap of how Law Enforcement, Social Services, Health Care, and other advocates must rise up and attack this growing problem. Breaking the cycle of violence takes a team, and these professionals provide knowledge and experience that should be studied by those charged with assisting victims in these times of need. In cases of IPV, victims are not always obvious, children and relatives also suffer. This book, written by professionals in the field of IPV, not only covers many aspects of this violation, but also provides methods and ideology that will help to empower providers to help victims survive and escape this terror.

Jeff Rich, Detective
Sexual Assault/Family Violence Investigator
Family Violence Unit
Criminal Investigations Division
Plano Police Department
Plano, Texas

Contents in Brief

CONTENTS IN DETAIL

Chapter 27: Violence on the Streets: The What, the Who, and the Why of Abuse, Assault & Murder of Sex Workers

Chapter 28: The Co-occurrence of Intimate Partner Violence and Human Immunodeficiency Virus

Violence Against Women

Contemporary Examination of Intimate Partner Violence

STM **Learning**, Inc.

Leading Publisher of Scientific, Technical, and Medical Educational Resources
Saint Louis
www.stmlearning.com

Chapter 1

Risk and Protective Factors for Intimate Partner Violence

Heidi Stöckl, PhD
Charlotte Watts, PhD

Key Points

1. Studying the risk and protective factors for intimate partner violence (IPV) will help in understanding the causes of IPV, and inform interventions to address and prevent its occurrence.

2. There was a high correlation between alcohol abuse by a violent partner and experiencing intimate partner violence.

3. Exposure to abuse during childhood was cited in most studies as a risk factor for IPV, both for perpetrators and women who experience IPV. This may be because children model the behavior of their parents.

4. IPV is correlated with having a low income, high levels of unemployment, and poor education. In some areas, studies found that abuse was more prevalent in relationships where the female partner earned more or was better educated than the male partner.

5. Other factors, such as race, rigid gender roles, permissive attitudes towards violence, infidelity, unmarried cohabitation, and number of children have been identified as possible risk factors for IPV.

Introduction

Intimate partner violence is one of the most widespread human rights violations and a public health problem in need of urgent attention. This chapter provides an overview of factors associated with an increase or decrease in women's likelihood of experiencing IPV, which is important both to understanding pathways leading to IPV and to informing interventions to prevent and address its occurrence.

This chapter presents the findings of detailed reviews based on current global evidence of factors associated with IPV in different settings. This evidence comes from multi-country studies; single-country population-based analyses; and previous reviews. This chapter focuses primarily on factors supported by strong evidence from most multi-country and individual population-based studies. Theoretical explanations for these risk factors are discussed alongside the evidence.

Methodology

The sources used in this review consist of 4 multi-country studies, 9 risk and protective factor analyses from African countries, 15 analyses from Asia and Australia, 11 analyses from Europe and North America, and 4 analyses from Latin America.

The 4 multi-country studies that explored risk factors for IPV each used comparable survey data from more than 1 country and more than 1 continent. These studies are: (1) the WHO Multi-Country Study, consisting of population-based surveys in 15 rural and urban sites in 10 countries[1] and surveying 24 097 women across all sites; (2) an analysis of 10 countries of the Demographic and Health Surveys, (referred to as DHS analysis),[2] that surveyed 7000 to 23 000 women per country; (3) the World Safe Study, a collection of small population-based surveys of 3975 women in different sites in four different countries[3]; and (4) a macro analysis by Kaya and Cook of more than 50 countries, using different survey estimates.[4]

In addition to evidence from multi-country studies, risk and protective factor analyses of population-based surveys from individual countries across the world are also used if they identified factors that put women at risk for IPV, while controlling for the effect of other known risk factors. The 9 African studies under review include an analysis of 8 Southern African countries,[5] as well as individual studies from Egypt,[6] Ethiopia,[7,8] Lesotho,[9] South Africa,[10] Uganda,[11,12] and Zambia.[13] The 15 analyses from Asia and Australia used in this chapter include studies from Australia,[14] Bangladesh,[15,16,17] China,[18] India,[19-23] Iran,[24] Mongolia,[25] Philippines,[26] Thailand,[27] and Vietnam.[28] European and North American studies under consideration consist of nationally representative studies from Canada,[29] Denmark,[30] Germany,[31] Norway,[32] the UK,[33] and the US,[34,35] as well as population-based studies of capital or major cities in Albania,[36] Greece,[37] Spain,[38] and Turkey.[39] Population-based studies from Haiti,[40] Mexico,[41] Nicaragua,[42] and Peru[43] provided insight into the risk factors for IPV in Latin America.

Three important methodological issues have to be considered when interpreting the risk and protective factors for IPV described in this chapter: reverse causality, their probabilistic nature, and the influence of third variables. The issue of reverse causality acknowledges that studies investigating risk factors for IPV using cross-sectional data are often unable to distinguish if certain associations are outcomes or causes of IPV. The terms "risk" and "protective factors" are therefore only used loosely in this chapter, because the cited evidence mainly draws on cross-sectional studies. Furthermore, the outlined risk and protective factors are probabilistic and not deterministic, which means that a person with a specific risk factor is more likely to experience IPV than a person who does not share that risk factor, but not that every person with a specific risk factor necessarily experiences IPV. The influence of third-factor variables cannot be ignored, and may impact the risk factors in the results, being as it suggests that the correlation between IPV and a risk factor may be due to their association with an unmeasured and unknown third factor.

RESULTS

The review of risk and protective factors in these studies showed strong evidence for associations between women's experiences of IPV and alcohol abuse, childhood experiences of violence, and issues of women's empowerment. The reviewed studies also gave substantial support to the identification of certain other risk factors, such as attitudes towards violence and gender, male abusers with multiple partners, non-marital cohabitation, low-quality relationships, several children, and social and geographic disadvantages. Each risk factor is discussed below along with an outline of its supporting evidence and theoretical grounding.

ALCOHOL ABUSE

Both the WHO Multi-Country Study[1] and the DHS analysis[2] found in all sites that women who reported experiencing IPV were more likely to report alcohol abuse by their partners. The World Safe Study found similar results in all sites, but El-Sheik Zayed and Santa Rosa.[3] The WHO Multi-Country Study further showed that the odds of IPV were even higher in more than five sites if both partners or if only the woman had an alcohol problem.[1] Further evidence for the association between alcohol abuse and IPV comes from three systematic reviews,[44-46] population-based studies from individual countries around the world, (including China,[18] Denmark,[30] Germany,[31] Haiti,[40] Mongolia,[25] Mexico,[41] Peru,[43] South Africa,[10] and Uganda[12]), and a prospective, longitudinal study from New Zealand.[47] The latter showed that a partner's reliance on alcohol often precedes his violence.

At least three different models explain the association between alcohol abuse and IPV, as can be seen in **Figure 1-1**.[48] The spurious model suggests that alcohol abuse is associated with IPV due to other factors related to alcohol abuse and IPV, such as youth and low socio-economic status. The indirect effects model claims that alcohol abuse slowly destroys relationship quality by generating counterproductive argumentation styles that elevate the likelihood of aggressive or violent responses.[49] The proximal effects model argues that alcohol abuse is a direct causal agent of IPV since it heightens aggression, interferes with cognitive abilities, and disrupts their channels of communication.[48,49]

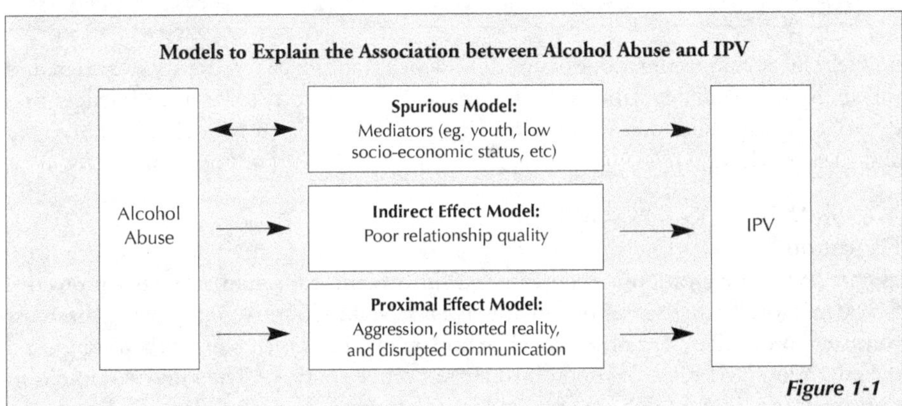

Figure 1-1.
Models to explain the association between alcohol abuse and IPV.

CHILDHOOD EXPERIENCES OF VIOLENCE

The WHO Multi-country Study[1] and the DHS analysis[2] both found evidence in most sites that childhood abuse, including physical punishment of women or their partners during childhood; childhood sexual abuse; or witnessing violence between parents significantly increased women's likelihood of experiencing IPV. In more than 10 sites, the WHO Multi-country Study determined that the risk for IPV was especially high when both a woman and her partner were abused in childhood.[1] Intergenerational transmission of violence as a risk factor of IPV also received empirical support from longitudinal and review studies[46,50-54] and from population-based surveys in Germany,[31] Greece,[37] Haiti,[40] India,[21] Mexico,[41] Nicaragua,[55] Peru,[43] South Africa,[10] and Turkey.[39]

Social Learning Theory

The social learning theory, with its key assumption being that children tend to emulate their parents' behavior, is most commonly used to explain why childhood exposure to violence is a risk factor for IPV.[46,56] The underlying pathways, as shown in **Figure 1-2**, are that children who grow up in violent families may be more likely to perceive violence as a conflict-solving strategy and may lack alternative models of conflict resolution.[57,58] In addition, witnessing and experiencing violence in childhood can disrupt children's attachment processes, hinder their ability to properly distinguish between love and violence,[59] and influence their partner choice later in life by tainting their perception of unhealthy and dangerous relationships.[60,61] Childhood sexual abuse in particular can distort children's cognitive and emotional orientation through stigmatization, portrayal,

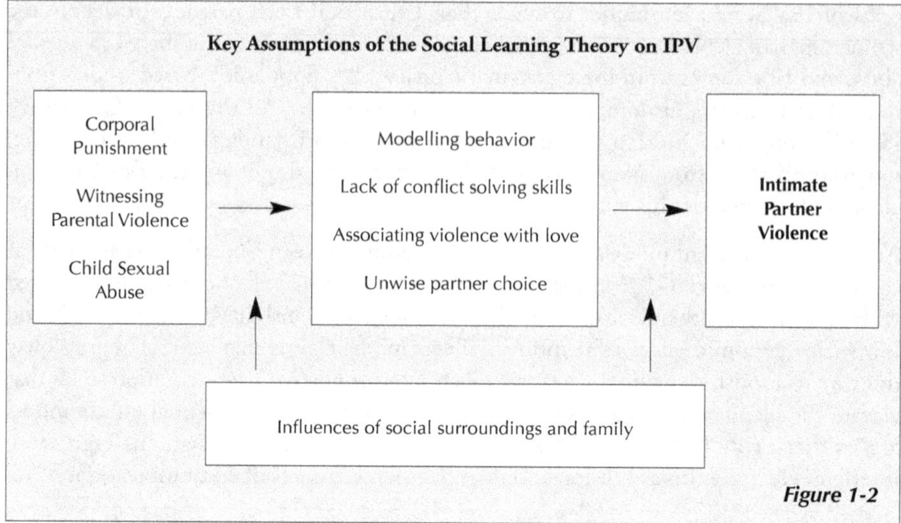

powerlessness, and traumatic sexualization, which may adversely affect self-esteem and the ability to negotiate relationship boundaries.[62,63] **Figure 1-2** also acknowledges that the influence of childhood violence on IPV may be mediated by a child's upbringing and social environment.[54]

SOCIAL AND ECONOMIC FACTORS

Education

Higher levels of education in women versus little or no education acted as a protective factor in more than 8 countries in the WHO Multi-Country Study, with the most consistent protective effect observed when both women and their partners had completed the education level most common in their respective country.[1] The same was found in some countries in the DHS analysis[2] and in Trivandrum, India and Paco, Philippines in the World Safe Study.[3] Kaye et al found that countries with low female secondary school enrollment among females had higher rates of last-year physical IPV.[4]

The patterns are more complex, however. An analysis of risk factors for physical IPV in 8 southern African countries, using nationally representative survey data, found that the average person who had not completed primary school was more likely to report physical IPV.[5] Also, while lack of education was a risk factor for IPV in Australia,[14] Bangladesh,[15-17] Haiti,[40] India,[19,20,23] Iran,[24] Mexico,[41] Norway,[32] Peru,[43] Turkey,[39] and Vietnam,[28] no association was found in China,[18,64] Mongolia,[25] Philippines,[26] or Thailand.[27] Furthermore, the association was reversed in some European countries, such as Albania[36] and Germany,[31] where a high level of education increased women's risk of experiencing IPV.

In-depth analysis on the effect of education in Egypt showed that women's education reduced the incidence of physical partner violence only if the partner also enjoyed a similar or higher level of education.[6] An Ethiopian study reinforced this finding, showing that rural women are more likely to report IPV if they are illiterate, but their odds of experiencing IPV are even higher if they are literate and their partner is illiterate.[8]

Employment, Income, and Poverty

Like education, women's employment has been significantly associated with IPV across most studies. Kaya and Cook's macro analysis showed that countries with a low percentage of women in non-agricultural labor forces also had lower levels of last-year physical IPV.[4] In contrast, the DHS analysis found that women's employment is protective in at least 5 of 10 countries,[2] a finding replicated in Germany,[31] India,[22] Iran,[24] Madrid,[38] Norway,[32] and the UK.[33] A low income was found to be a risk factor for IPV in 8 of the 14 sites in the WHO Multi-Country Study[1] as well as in Canada,[29] Turkey,[39] and the USA.[34,35] Low socio-economic status and poverty emerged as risk factors for IPV in India,[19] Mexico,[41] Mongolia,[25] Nicaragua,[55] Norway,[32] Thailand,[27] the UK,[33] and Vietnam.[28] Mixed evidence regarding the relationship between saving schemes and IPV emerged in Bangladesh, with some studies showing that saving increases women's risk of IPV,[15,17] while others show that saving reduces this risk.[16]

Resource Theory and Relative Resource Theory

The influence of education, employment, and socio-economic status on prevalence of IPV was first explained by Goode's resource theory (see **Figure 1-3**). It claims that partners may employ physical force or threats of physical force to exercise influence in their relationships if other resources are unavailable or fail to obtain a desired response.[65] These other resources are education, job prestige, income, community standing, interpersonal skills, or similar abilities. Violence is the 'ultimate' resource that partners utilize because its costs are high and may result in loss of affection and respect.[65] This means that the more resources a person commands and the more dominance a person maintains in a relationship, the less likely they are to deploy violence.[65]

The mechanisms that link a scarcity of resources to IPV are lack of prestige, money, and decision-making power, leading to a sense of frustration and bitterness. Receiving less respect outside the home during the day and working long hours may diminish the ability to withstand hurt and frustration at home. It may also diminish the ability to deal with domestic and relationship difficulties and to mediate problems, which can lead to stress and, consequently, violence.[50,65] A low level of education in particular may become a risk factor for IPV because it reduces opportunities for gainful and secure employment and influences position and prestige.

For men, unemployment, low job prestige, and low income can be difficult to handle if their status and identity are closely tied to their role as breadwinners. If status is at stake in one part of their lives, men may attempt to reinstate it at home by physically abusing their wives.[66] In contrast, women with high levels of resources may sufficiently strengthen their position in their relationships to prevent violence and deal with stressful situations and problems, because these resources provide them with access to a wider social network, to information, and to support. It may also put them in a better bargaining position in their relationships and give them more confidence from contributing to the family's income.[67]

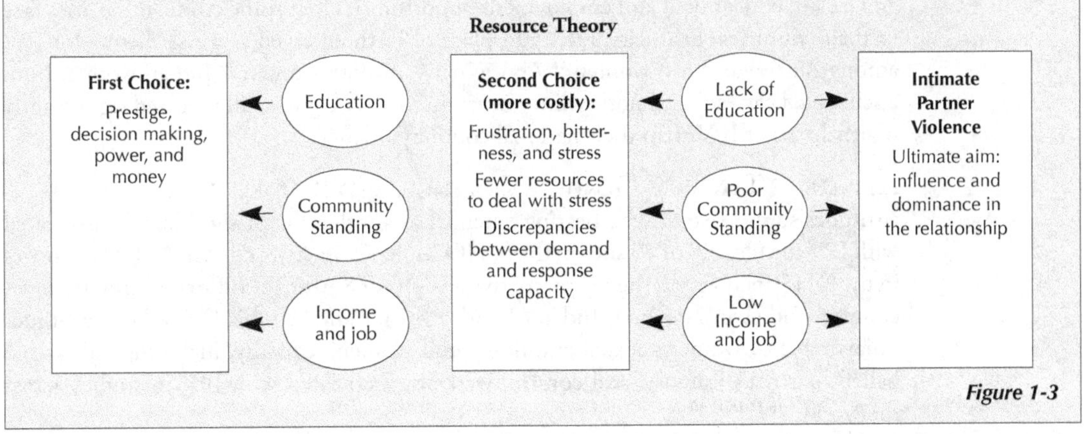

Figure 1-3.
Resource theory

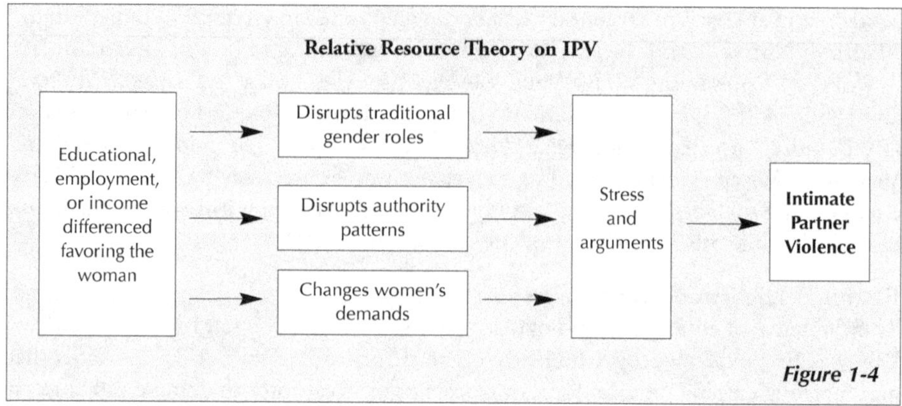

The relative resource theory is equally important in explaining IPV, especially given findings of increased IPV among couples with educational, employment, or income differences favoring the woman (see **Figure 1-4**). The theory incorporates feminist claims that IPV is deeply gendered into Goode's resource theory. When male partners identify themselves as the breadwinners in their relationships, an inequality favoring women might cause feelings of inferiority and they may resort to violence to regain dominance in their relationships.[27,49,68,69] This may be partly because in couples with educational discrepancies favoring the women, women are likely to have very different expectations about decision making, housework, and intimacy than in relationships with traditional gender roles.[70] The income gap between spouses was observed as a major predictor for IPV in an analysis of nationally representative surveys of 8 sub-Saharan African countries.[5]

Age and Ethnicity

In at least 8 of the 15 WHO Multi-Country Study sites[1] and 5 of 10 DHS countries,[2] youth increased women's risk of IPV, with similar findings in Albania,[36] Bangladesh,[16,17] Denmark,[30] Canada,[29] Ethiopia,[7] India,[19,20,22] Iran,[24] Mongolia,[25] Turkey,[39] the UK,[33] and in 18 US States.[35] Similarly, in Latin America, studies found that first sexual experience or marriage at a young age significantly increased women's likelihood to report IPV in Mexico[41] and Peru.[43] The association between youth and IPV can also be explained by the resource theory, because couples who form a union early are more likely to have early pregnancies, more children, employment instability, and financial difficulties, all stressors that may promote violence and may lead to low resource levels in the long term.[49]

One can argue that race and ethnicity lead to increased levels of IPV due to discrimination and lack of educational and employment opportunities that some ethnic minorities face in their countries. Ethnicity, race, and place of birth emerged as a risk factors for IPV among Australian-born women,[14] Aboriginal Canadian women,[29] Indian women from a scheduled castes,[20] and non-white women in the USA,[34] who all reported significantly higher levels of IPV than their national counterparts.

ATTITUDES TOWARDS GENDER, VIOLENCE, AND INFIDELITY

Attitudes supportive of wife-beating emerged as another factor significantly associated with IPV in at least 8 of 15 sites in the WHO Multi-Country Study,[1] in 5 of 10 countries in the DHS analysis,[2] in the representative analysis of 8 African countries,[5] and in single-country studies in Northern India,[19] South Africa,[10] and Zambia.[13] Similarly, attitudes unfavorable to women's sexual autonomy and women's equality, including patriarchal beliefs, partner's jealousy, and control, were also associated with IPV in studies across the world.[5,10,13,18,19,40,64]

On a related issue, in at least 8 of the 15 sites in the WHO Multi-Country Study, male partners' infidelity was found to be a major risk factor for IPV,[1] which was also found in other studies in sub-Saharan Africa.[5]

Gender Role Theories

The association between IPV and unfavorable attitudes towards gender, violence, and male infidelity can be explained by gender role theories, which have their theoretical underpinning in feminist theory. **Figure 1-5** displays the different strands of feminist theory that provide explanations for IPV, some of which have been incorporated into theories discussed above, such as the social learning theory and the resource theory. The most commonly used feminist theory to explain IPV is the radical feminist theory, which maintains that the patriarchal nature of society promotes violence against women.[71]

Gender role theory builds on claims in radical feminism. Proponents of radical feminism claim that women's socialization focuses primarily on being good wives and mothers, at the expense of personal achievements in other spheres of life, while men are socialized to be professionally successful in order to become the main breadwinners in their families. These identifications have direct implications for men's and women's sense of autonomy and how they shape relationships.[72] For example, this gendered socialization prescribes a set of male behaviors associated with power and domination that places men in opposition to one another.[72] This type of behavior may sanction use of violence between men, and, as a result, seldom challenges the use of violence within relationships.[73]

Gender role theory can explain the occurrence of IPV when men feel threatened by their partners' demands for gains of more equality if they believe this reduces their authority, shames their masculinity, or destroys their sense of control.[74] Gender role theorists may, therefore, assume that couples with strong patriarchal beliefs have higher rates of partner violence.[75] Empowerment and liberal ideas may, however, endanger women if their surroundings consider these ideas or behaviors deviant and punishable, which may especially be the case in societies undergoing changes in gender norms or in which women have a higher status.[75,76] Pallitto and O'Campo argue that until full equality is achieved, women who behave traditionally are in less danger of IPV, because they do not challenge masculine identities.[77] Under these conditions, traditional women may be less likely to experience IPV because their partners may be less likely to employ the use of force to maintain control over them; however, they are not entirely safe because their partners may use perceived deficits in household chores as a reason for IPV.[76,77]

Figure 1-5. *Feminist theories*

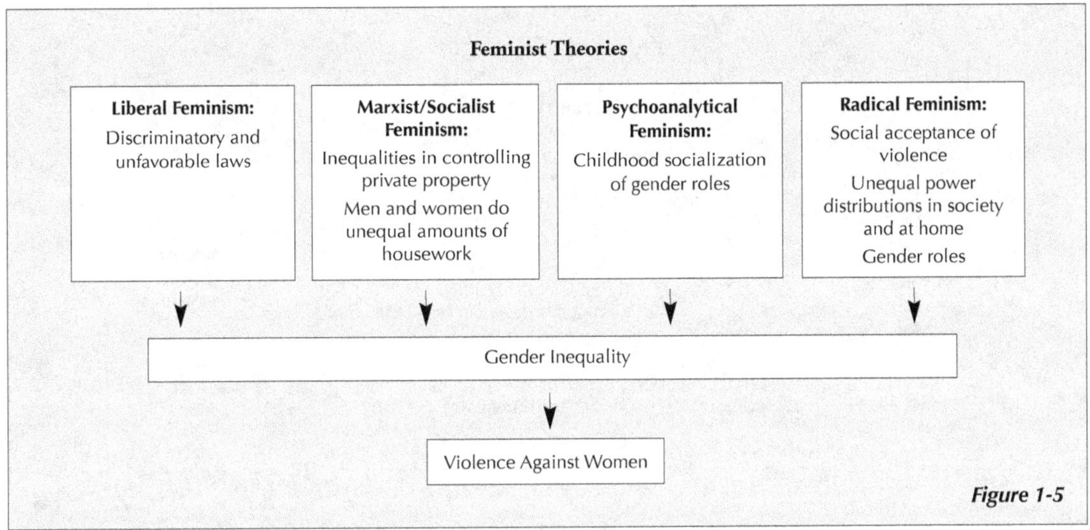

Figure 1-5

Marital Status, Relationship Quality, and Number of Children

Non-marital relationships and cohabitation emerged as significant risk factors for IPV in a few, but not all, sites in the WHO Multi-Country Study[1] and in population-based surveys in Canada,[29] Denmark,[30] Lesotho,[9] Madrid,[38] Norway,[32] Peru,[43] Uganda,[12] the UK,[33] and the USA.[34] Similarly, population-based surveys from Germany,[31] Greece,[37] Mexico,[41] and 18 US States[35] found that recently started relationships increase women's risk for IPV. Marital dissatisfaction was found to be a risk factor for IPV in Uganda,[11] as was frequent quarrelling in the Philippines[26] and Thailand,[27] and dowry-related controversies in Bangladesh.[15,17]

Number of children and pregnancies was found to be a risk factor for IPV in Canada,[29] Germany,[31] Mexico,[41] Nicaragua,[55] Peru,[43] Turkey,[39] and the UK,[33] while a population-based survey in Norway[32] suggested that having no children can also put a woman at risk of IPV. Kaya and Cook, in their macro analysis of data from 50 countries, further found that countries with a high total fertility rate had higher levels for IPV.[4] The WHO Multi-Country Study found that children from previous relationships significantly increased women's risk of IPV in a few sites.[1]

Social Exchange Theory

The association between marital status, relationship quality, children, and IPV are best explained by social exchange theory (**Figure 1-6**). Its main argument is that partners become violent if they believe the cost of abuse is less than its rewards.[78,79] The assumption is that social behavior consists of a series of exchanges in which individuals are willing to accept certain costs in exchange for rewards and vice versa.[80,81] Potential costs of IPV include the abused hitting back, calling the police, or ending the relationship, although the risk of these costs are smaller the more sure an abusive partner is of his dominant physical, psychological, and economic position in the relationship. The exchange theory claims that these costs are further reduced if the couple is not married, because an abuser might be less committed to the relationship and therefore less interested in its quality and duration. Furthermore, the social costs of IPV are lower among cohabiting couples who experience less social control by neighbors, family, and friends, who might detect the violence and shame the abuser.[79] Finally, cohabiting couples are more likely to have arguments about the boundaries of their relationships, which can lead to stress and trigger violence.[79]

Figure 1-6.
Exchange theory and IPV

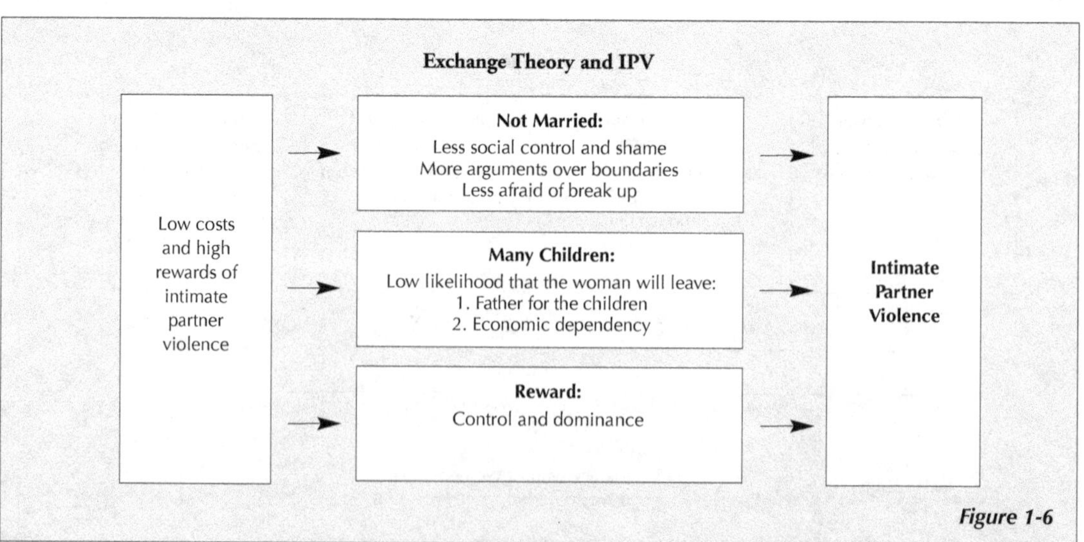

Children can also reduce the cost of violence when abusive partners believe their female partners are unlikely to leave because of their children. This is especially true of women experiencing IPV who are economically dependent on their abusers and prioritize keeping their families together.[66] Furthermore, children may act as a risk factor for violence if they are the focus of arguments about discipline, methods of upbringing, supervision, financial resources, or the amount of time a couple can spend together.[27]

Nevertheless, children may also act as protective factors against IPV, because they may tie a relationship together and prevent aggressive arguments, being as parents are normally more reluctant to fight in front of their children. Children may also reduce isolation by connecting parents with schools, neighbors, and broader social networks. Such connections increases the potential to receive support in stressful situations and increase social control.[66]

Women's Social and Geographical Surroundings

Risk factors for IPV related to social and geographical surroundings examined in different studies include living in rural areas, social isolation, and experiences of non-partner violence.

Living in an urban or rural area has been associated with IPV in the studies reviewed. Whether risk for IPV is higher for women living rural areas or women living in urban areas varies from country to country. In Albania,[36] Australia,[14] Ethiopia,[8] India,[22] and Uganda,[11] women had an increased risk for IPV if they lived in a rural area, while their risk was lower in Nicaragua,[55] the Philippines,[26] and Peru.[43] Studies also found that in China,[18] South Africa,[10] and the USA, risk of IPV may depend on the state or province in which a woman lives.[34]

An association between high crime levels and IPV was found in several studies. For example, the WHO Multi-Country Study found in at least 8 of 15 sites that a woman's experience of non-partner violence and her partner's involvement in fights with other men both increased her likelihood of reporting IPV.[1] These findings were supported by a study in Mexico that established a link between IPV and women's history of rape[41] and a study in Germany that found an association between IPV and women's experiences of physical and sexual non-partner violence.[31]

Social Disorganization Theory

Social disorganization theory, as seen in **Figure 1-7**, provides an explanation for the association of IPV and factors related to social and geographical surroundings by explaining why some poor neighborhoods have higher crime rates and more incidents of interpersonal violence than others.[82] Neighborhoods with structural features that support a positive sense of community and encourage social networks, community involvement, and friendships between neighbors have lower rates of IPV, because residents share common values and exert social control on one another.[83] Surveillance by neighbors limits physical aggression in the household by forcing couples to conform to socially-approved forms of behavior. Close neighborhood networks can support couples by providing third parties to help prevent or resolve disputes within relationships and by raising the cost of IPV by threatening to diminish the reputations of abusers.[49] Neighborhood surveillance and social cohesion also reduces stress and dissatisfaction by lowering crime rates and discouraging anti-social behavior in the neighborhood.[49] Whether or not IPV occurs more often in rural and urban areas therefore depends on the societal structure.

Two studies that examined social isolation as a risk factor for IPV, a study in Germany[31] and a study of 18 US States,[35] both found that limited contact with others and feelings of social exclusion increased women's risk for IPV. Social disorganization theory offers an explanation. Women without strong social networks lack social control over their relationships, as well as comfort, encouragement, and financial assistance.

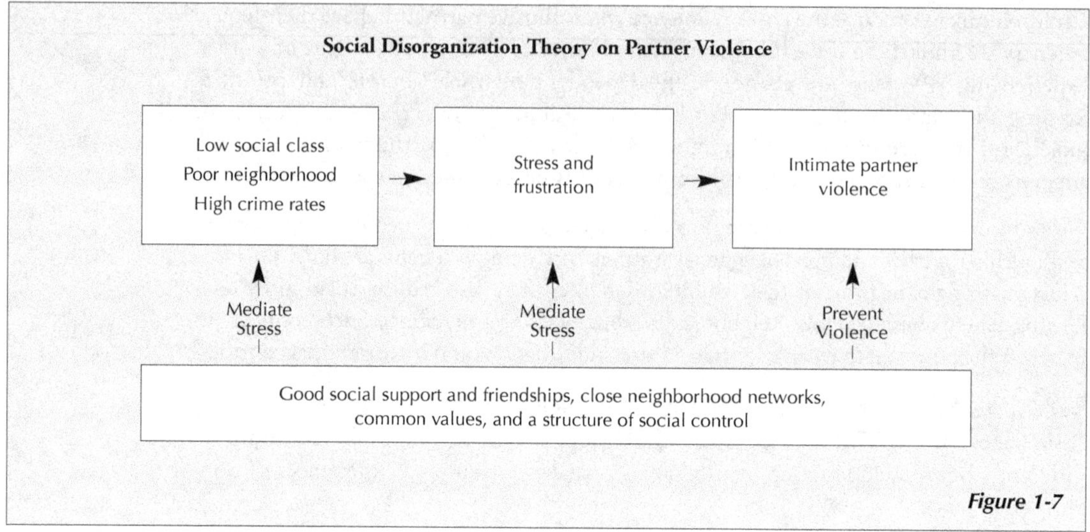

Figure 1-7. Social disorganization theory on partner violence

CONCLUSION

Multi-country and single-country analyses have identified associations between IPV and alcohol abuse, childhood violence, and issues related to women's empowerment. Other risk factors for IPV, such as unfavorable attitudes towards violence and gender, male partners engaging in multiple relationships, non-marital cohabitation, poor relationship quality, many children, and women's disadvantaged social surroundings. Because the evidence for these risk factors differed across studies and sometimes conflicted, further evidence and more in-depth analyses are still needed. Nevertheless, theoretical underpinnings emphasize the importance of these factors in occurrences of IPV.

The interpretation of the risk factors' relative importance made in this chapter must be tempered by several limitations, including reverse causality and third factor influences and their probabilistic nature. While this chapter lists risk and protective factors according to the amount of evidence reported in studies cited, it needs to be acknowledged that not all studies considered in this review measured the same factors. Some factors were only examined in 1 or 2 countries and, therefore, lack broad support. For example, disability and social isolation were only investigated in the German[31] and the UK[33] analyses.

There are several additional limitations to this chapter. The evidence is not fully conclusive because the risk factors were not compared to other risk factors to indicate relative importance. Some risk factors, such as communication between couples, might have been omitted because of measurement difficulties, while other factors have only been measured in some of the studies. In addition, this chapter only focuses on population-based survey data and does not include clinical studies or qualitative evidence on risk factors for IPV. Neither does it consider risk factors specific to certain types of women, such as pregnant women, disabled women, or adolescents. While many of the risk factors for IPV in these groups are probably similar to those observed in the general population, some factors, such as unwanted pregnancy or dependence on a partner who is also a primary caregiver, may be specific to these groups.

Nevertheless, this chapter provides a comprehensive overview of risk and, to some extent, protective factors for IPV with important implications for the development of interventions to prevent and address IPV. While issues related to women's education, employment, and household income contribution will not be resolved quickly, the impact of these factors on the prevalence of IPV should not be neglected when designing interventions. Similarly, alcohol consumption should not be neglected in interventions addressing IPV. Knowledge of the links between alcohol abuse and IPV should be incorporated into alcohol programming to help reduce the effect of excessive drinking on violence in relationships.[48] Prevention measures should include efforts to curb physical and sexual abuse in childhood, such as programs to support disclosure, punish perpetrators, change social norms, and intervene in violent homes. Overall, the risk factors discussed in this chapter suggest a need to develop interventions that may holistically address these factors to reduce the prevalence of IPV.

REFERENCES

1. Abramsky T, Watts CH, Garcia-Moreno C, et al. What factors are associated with recent intimate partner violence? findings from the WHO multi-country study on women's health and domestic violence. *BMC Public Health.* 2011;11(1):109.

2. Hindin MJ, Kishor S, Ansara DL. *DHS Analytical Studies No. 18: Intimate Partner Violence Among Couples in 10 DHS Countries: Predictors and Health Outcomes.* Calverton, MD: Macro International Inc; 2008.

3. Jeyaseelan L, Sadowski LS, Kumar S, Hassan F, Ramiro L, Vizcarra B. World studies of abuse in the family environment—risk factors for physical intimate partner violence. *Int J Inj Control Safety Promotion.* 2004;11(2):117-124.

4. Kaya Y, Cook KJ. A cross-national analysis of physical intimate partner violence against women. *Int J Comp Sociol.* 2010;51(6):423-444.

5. Andersson N, Ho-Foster A, Mitchell S, Scheepers E, Goldstein S. Risk factors for domestic physical violence: national cross-sectional household surveys in eight southern African countries. *BMC Womens Health.* 2007;7(11).

6. Akmatov MK, Mikolajczyk RT, Labeeb S, Dhaher E, Khan MM. Factors associated with wife beating in Egypt: analysis of two surveys (1995 and 2005). *BMC Womens Health.* 2008;8:15.

7. Deyessa N, Berhane Y, Alem A, et al. Intimate partner violence and depression among women in rural Ethiopia: a cross-sectional study. *Clin Pract Epidemiol Ment Health.* 2009;5:8.

8. Deyessa N, Berhane Y, Ellsberg M, Emmelin M, Kullgren G, Högberg U. Violence against women in relation to literacy and area of residence in Ethiopia. *Global Health Action.* 2010;3.

9. Brown L, Thurman T, Bloem J, Kendall C. Sexual violence in Lesotho. *Stud Fam Plann.* 2006;37(4):269-280.

10. Jewkes R, Levin J, Penn-Kekana L. Risk factors for domestic violence: findings from a South African cross-sectional study. *Soc Sci Med.* 2002;55(9):1603-1617.

11. Karamagi CA, Tumwine JK, Tylleskar T, Heggenhougen K. Intimate partner violence against women in eastern Uganda: implications for HIV prevention. *BMC Public Health.* 2006;6:284.

12. Koenig MA, Lutalo T, Zhao F, et al. Domestic violence in rural Uganda: evidence from a community-based study. *Bull World Health Organ.* 2003;81(1):53-60.

13. Okenwa L, Lawoko S. Social indicators and physical abuse of women by intimate partners: a study of women in Zambia. *Violence Vict.* 2010;25(2):278-288.

14. Taft AJ, Watson LF, Lee C. Violence against young Australian women and association with reproductive events: a cross-sectional analysis of a national population sample. *Aust N Z J Public Health*. 2004;28(4):324-329.

15. Naved RT, Persson LA. Factors associated with spousal physical violence against women in Bangladesh. *Stud Fam Plann*. 2005;36(4):289-300.

16. Koenig MA, Ahmed S, Hossain MB, Mozumder ABMKA. Women's status and domestic violence in rural Bangladesh: individual-and community-level effects. *Demography*. 2003;40(2):269-288.

17. Bates LM, Schuler SR, Islam F, Islam MK. Socioeconomic factors and processes associated with domestic violence in rural Bangladesh. *Int Fam Plann Perspect*. 2004;30(4):190-200.

18. Parish WL, Wang T, Laumann EO, Pan S, Luo Y. Intimate partner violence in China: national prevalence, risk factors and associated health problems. *Int Fam Plann Perspect*. 2004;30(4):174-181.

19. Martin SL, Tsui AO, Maitra K, Marinshaw R. Domestic violence in northern India. *Am J Epidemiol*. 1999;150(4):417.

20. Dalal K, Lindqvist K. A National study of the prevalence and correlates of domestic violence among women in India. *Asia Pac J Public Health*. 2012;24(2):265-277.

21. Martin SL, Moracco KE, Garro J, et al. Domestic violence across generations: findings from northern India. *Int J Epidemiol*. 2002;31(3):560.

22. Babu BV, Kar SK. Domestic violence against women in eastern India: a population-based study on prevalence and related issues. *BMC Public Health*. 2009;9:129.

23. Ackerson LK, Kawachi I, Barbeau EM, Subramanian S. Effects of individual and proximate educational context on intimate partner violence: a population-based study of women in India. *Am J Public Health*. 2008;98(3):507-514.

24. Ghazizadeh A. Domestic violence: a cross-sectional study in an Iranian city. *East Mediterr Health J*. 2005;11(5-6):880-887.

25. Oyunbileg S, Sumberzul N, Udval N, Wang JD, Janes CR. Prevalence and risk factors of domestic violence among Mongolian women. *J Womens Health*. 2009;18(11):1873-1880.

26. Hindin MJ, Adair LS. Who's at risk? factors associated with intimate partner violence in the Philippines. *Soc Sci Med*. 2002;55(8):1385-1399.

27. Hoffman KL, Demo DH, Edwards JN. Physical wife abuse in a non-western society: an integrated theoretical approach. *J Marriage Fam*. 1994;56(1):131-146.

28. Dang Vung N, Ostergren PO, Krantz G. Intimate partner violence against women in rural Vietnam - different socio-demographic factors are associated with different forms of violence: need for new intervention guidelines? *BMC Public Health*. 2008;8:55.

29. Romans S, Forte T, Cohen MM, Du Mont J, Hyman I. Who is most at risk for intimate partner violence? *J Interpers Violence*. 2007;22(12):1495-1514.

30. Helweg-Larsen K, Sørensen J, Brønnum-Hansen H, Kruse M. Risk factors for violence exposure and attributable healthcare costs: results from the Danish national health interview surveys. *Scan J Public Health*. 2011;39(1):10-16.

31. Stöckl H, Heise L, Watts C. Factors associated with violence by a current partner in a nationally representative sample of German women. *Soc Health Illness.* 2011;33(5):694-709.

32. Nerøien AI, Schei B. Partner violence and health: Results from the first national study on violence against women in Norway. *Scan J Public Health.* 2008;36(2):161-168.

33. Finney A. Domestic violence, sexual assault and stalking: findings from the 2004/05 British Crime Survey. British National Archives Web site. http://webarchive.nation-alarchives.gov.uk/20110220105210/rds.homeoffice.gov.uk/rds/pdfs06/rdsolr1206. pdf. Published 2006. Accessed February 18, 2013.

34. Van Wyk JA, Benson ML, Fox GL, DeMaris A. Detangling individual-, partner-, and community-level correlates of partner violence. *Crime Delinquency.* 2003;49(3):412-438.

35. Breiding MJ, Black MC, Ryan GW. Prevalence and risk factors of intimate partner violence in eighteen US states/territories, 2005. *Am J Prev Med.* 2008;34(2):112-118.

36. Burazeri G, Roshi E, Jewkes R, Jordan S, Bjegovic V, Laaser U. Factors associated with spousal physical violence in Albania: cross-sectional study. *BMJ.* 2005;331(7510):197–201.

37. Papadakaki M, Tzamalouka GS, Chatzifotiou S, Chliaoutakis J. Seeking for risk factors of intimate partner violence (IPV) in a Greek national sample: the role of self-esteem. *J Interpers Violence.* 2009;24(5):732-750.

38. Zorrilla B, Pires M, Lasheras L, et al. Intimate partner violence: last year prevalence and association with socio-economic factors among women in Madrid, Spain. *Eur J Public Health.* 2010;20(2):169-175.

39. Kocacık F, Kutlar A, Erselcan F. Domestic violence against women: a field study in Turkey. *Soc Sci J.* 2007;44(4):698-720.

40. Gage AJ. Women's experience of intimate partner violence in Haiti. *Soc Sci Med.* 2005;61(2):342-264.

41. Rivera-Rivera L, Lazcano-Ponce E, Salmerón-Castro J, Salazar-Martínez E, Castro R, Hernández-Avila M. Prevalence and determinants of male partner violence against Mexican women: a population-based study. *Salud Pública de México.* 2004;46(2):113-122.

42. Ellsberg MC, Peña R, Herrera A, Liljestrand J, Winkvist A. Wife abuse among women of childbearing age in Nicaragua. *Am J Public Health.* 1999;89(2):241-244.

43. Flake DF. Individual, family, and community risk factors for domestic violence in Peru. *Violence Against Women.* 2005;11(3):353-373.

44. Foran HM, O'Leary KD. Alcohol and intimate partner violence: a meta-analytic review. *Clinical Psychology Review.* 2008;28(7):1222-1234.

45. Gil-Gonzalez D, Vives-Cases C, Alvarez-Dardet C, Latour-Pérez J. Alcohol and intimate partner violence: do we have enough information to act? *Eur J Public Health.* 2006;16(3):278-284.

46. Stith SM, Smith DB, Penn CE, Ward DB, Tritt D. Intimate partner physical abuse perpetration and victimization risk factors: a meta-analytic review. *Aggression Violent Behav.* 2004;10:65-98.

47. Magdol L, Moffitt TE, Caspi A, Silva PA. Developmental antecedents of partner abuse: a prospective-longitudinal study. *J Abnorm Psychol.* 1998;107(3):375-389.

48. Klostermann KC, Fals-Stewart W. Intimate partner violence and alcohol use: exploring the role of drinking in partner violence and its implications for intervention. *Aggression Violent Behav.* 2006;11(6):587–597.

49. DeMaris A, Benson ML, Fox GL, Hill T, Van Wyk J. Distal and proximal factors in domestic violence: a test of an integrated model. *J Marriage Fam.* 2003;65(3):652-667.

50. Holtzworth-Munroe A, Smutzler N, Bates L. A brief review of the research on husband violence part 3: sociodemographic factors, relationship factors, and differing consequences of husband and wife violence. *Aggression Violent Behav.* 1997;2(3):285-307.

51. Capaldi DM, Clark S. Prospective family predictors of aggression toward female partners for at-risk young men. *Dev Psychol.* 1998;34(6):1175-1188.

52. Fergusson DM, Horwood LJ. Exposure to interparental violence in childhood and psychosocial adjustment in young adulthood. *Child Abuse Negl.* 1998;22(5):339-357.

53. Moffitt TE, Caspi A. *Findings About Partner Violence From the Dunedin Multidisciplinary Health and Development Study.* Washington DC: US Department of Justice; 1999.

54. Fergusson DM, Boden JM, Horwood LJ. Examining the intergenerational transmission of violence in a New Zealand birth cohort. *Child Abuse Negl.* 2006;30(2):89-108.

55. Ellsberg M, Peña R, Herrera A, Liljestrand J, Winkvist A. Candies in hell: women's experiences of violence in Nicaragua. *Social Sci Med.* 2000;51(11):1595-1610.

56. Murrell AR, Christoff KA, Henning KR. Characteristics of domestic violence offenders: associations with childhood exposure to violence. *J Fam Violence.* 2007;22(7):523-532.

57. Renner LM, Slack KS. Intimate partner violence and child maltreatment: understanding intra- and intergenerational connections. *Child Abuse Negl.* 2006;30(6):599-617.

58. Dodge KA, Bates JE, Pettit GS. Mechanisms in the cycle of violence. *Science.* 1990;250(4988):1678-1683.

59. Aldarondo E, Sugarman DB. Risk marker analysis of the cessation and persistence of wife assault. *J Consult Clin Psychol.* 1996;64(5):1010-1019.

60. Riggs DS, Caulfield MB, Street AE. Risk for domestic violence: factors associated with perpetration and victimization. *J Clin Psychol.* 2000;56(10):1289-1316.

61. Tolan P, Gorman-Smith D, Henry D. Family violence. *Ann Rev Physiol.* 2006;57:557-583.

62. Romito P, Saurel-Cubizolles M-J, Crisma M. The relationship between parents' violence against daughters and violence by other perpetrators: an Italian study. *Violence Against Women.* 2001;7(12):1429-1463.

63. Grauerholz L. An ecological approach to understanding sexual revictimization: linking personal, interpersonal, and sociocultural factors and processes. *Child Maltreat.* 2005;5(1):5-17.

64. Xu X, Zhu F, O'Campo P, Koenig MA, Mock V, Campbell J. Prevalence of and risk factors for intimate partner violence in China. *Am J Public Health*. 2005;95(1):78-85.

65. Goode WJ. Force and Violence in the Family. *J Marriage Fam*. Nov 1971;33(4):624-636.

66. Johnson H. Rethinking survey research on violence against women. In: Dobash RE, Dobash RP, eds. *Rethinking Violence Against Women*. Thousand Oaks, CA: Sage 1998:23-51.

67. McMullan EC. Education as a risk factor for domestic violence. In: Jackson NA, ed. *Encyclopedia of Domestic Violence*. New York, London: Routledge; 2007:267-270.

68. Atkinson MP, Greenstein TN, Lang MM. For women, breadwinning can be dangerous: gendered resource theory and wife abuse. *J Marriage Fam*. Dec 2005;67(5):1137-1148.

69. Kaukinen C. Status compatibility, physical violence, and emotional abuse in intimate relationships. *J Marriage Fam*. May 2004;66(2):452-471.

70. Anderson KL. Gender, status, and domestic violence: an integration of feminist and family violence approaches. *J Marriage Fam*. 1997;59(3):655-669.

71. Basile KC. Rape by acquiescence: the ways in which women 'give in' to unwanted sex with their husbands. *Violence Against Women*. 1999;5(9):1036-1058.

72. Fernandez M. Cultural beliefs and domestic violence. *Ann N Y Acad Sci*. 2006;1087:250-260.

73. Sugarman DB, Frankel SL. Patriarchal ideology and wife-assault: a meta-analytic review. *J Fam Violence*. 1996;11(1):13-40.

74. Jewkes RK, Levin JB, Penn-Kekana LA. Gender inequalities, intimate partner violence and HIV preventive practices: findings of a South African cross-sectional study. *Soc Sci Med*. 2003;56(1):125-134.

75. Yllo KA. Through a feminist lens: gender, power, and violence. In: Gelles RJ, Loseke DR, eds. *Current Controversies on Family Violence*. Newbury Park, CA: Sage Publications; 1993:47-62.

76. Jewkes R. Intimate partner violence: causes and prevention. *Lancet*. 2002;359(9315):1423-1429.

77. Pallitto CC, O'Campo P. Community level effects of gender inequality on intimate partner violence and unintended pregnancy in Colombia: testing the feminist perspective. *Soc Sci Med*. May 2005;60(10):2205-2216.

78. Williams KR. Social sources of marital violence and deterrence: testing an integrated theory of assaults between partners. *J Marriage Fam*. 1992;54(3):620-629.

79. Gelles RJ. Exchange theory. In: Jackson NA, ed. *Encyclopedia of Domestic Violence*. New York, London: Routledge; 2007:302-305.

80. Homans GC. Social Behavior as Exchange. *Am J Soc*. 1958;63(6):597-606.

81. Blau PM. *Exchange and Power in Social Life*. New York, NY: John Wiley & Son; 1964.

82. Almgren G. The ecological context of interpersonal violence: from culture to collective efficacy. *J Interpers Violence*. 2005;20(2):218-224.

83. Cunradi CB. Drinking level, neighborhood social disorder, and mutual intimate partner violence. *Alcohol Clin Exp Res*. 2007;31(6):1012-1019.

Chapter 2

ASSESSING FOR INTIMATE PARTNER VIOLENCE

Amy Carney, NP, PhD, FAAFS

KEY POINTS

1. A large number of cases of intimate partner violence go undetected by health care professionals, often due to lack of training. Clinicians often also find it difficult to broach the subject of IPV with patients.

2. Intimate partner violence is prevalent among both men and women in the US and globally. Some studies have shown that in up to 50% of cases, men are the victims of IPV.

3. Early indicators of intimate partner violence perpetration include substance abuse and childhood exposure to abuse.

4. Re-victimization is a serious risk for those who have experienced IPV. Women are more at risk immediately following separation from their partner. A study has shown that in about two-thirds of cases, women are able to accurately predict their risk for repeat abuse.

5. Questionnaires and other assessment tools are available for clinicians to guide assessment of IPV. In 2006, the Centers for Disease Control and Prevention published a list of over 20 such tools.

INTRODUCTION

Intimate partner violence occurs across all cultural and socioeconomic levels and age brackets; it is both global and local. Assessing for possible interpersonal violence can be intimidating for even the most seasoned professional, but knowing what questions to ask and when can make the difference in getting the best care for a victim of violence. The diversity in types of violence and type of aggressor make assessing for intimate partner violence (IPV) challenging. This chapter will address assessment for interpersonal violence, examine behavioral indicators of violence in personal relationships, and offer suggestions on reaching out to victims of interpersonal violence.

BACKGROUND AND SCOPE OF IPV

A large number of cases of IPV go undetected and unreported by clinicians and other professionals. Barriers include lack of education on what to look for and how to convey those findings to the appropriate agency. Experiencing discomfort while asking a possible victim of violence questions, is a hurdle for many.[1] Another difficulty is understanding what constitutes "screening" and what is meant by "assessment." While screening someone for IPV might include general questions at a routine visit, identification of possible signs of abuse warrant a thorough assessment. Knowing these signs and their consequences can aid in asking sensitive and relevant questions, evaluating the victim's physical and emotional needs, and moving them to a place of safety.[2]

It is evident that intimate partner violence is a serious problem in the United States. The National Center for Injury Prevention and Control at the Centers for Disease Control has stated that each year more than 12 million women and men are victims of rape, physical violence, and stalking. In 2007, IPV resulted in 2340 deaths, most of whom were female. The number of cases is estimated to be much higher as IPV often goes unreported for fear of not being believed or fear that law enforcement cannot help.[3] The impact of IPV can also be seen globally: the World Health Organization (WHO) reported in a study of over 24 000 women in 10 countries with both urban and rural settings that up to 71% reported physical and sexual abuse by a partner.[4] Costs for mental health services, medical treatment, and lost productivity associated with IPV continue to rise. The ability to detect and assess for IPV is necessary for both the immediate safety of the victim of violence and to prevent future recurrence.

Many organizations, including the American Nurses Association (ANA) and the American Medical Association (AMA), have taken strong stands in the fight against intimate partner violence. In 'Social Causes and Health Care' the ANA says, "There is a critical need for attention to and increased awareness of the problems of violence against women by all healthcare providers in order to reduce immediate and long term physical and psychological injuries associated with this crime."[5] The AMA notes that "Interpersonal violence and abuse were once thought to primarily affect specific high-risk patient populations, but it is now understood that all patients may be at risk."[6] The Academy on Violence and Abuse has developed a set of interdisciplinary competencies arranged in three levels of responsibility: health system competencies, institutional competencies for academic institutions and training programs, and individual learner competencies. The authors note that these are meant to be a common starting point for both professional societies and academic institutions in various disciplines to develop specific criteria concerning the skills, knowledge and attitudes needed to deal with violence and abuse.[7]

Multiple approaches to assessment can be found in the literature on IPV. In 2006, the California Department of Health Services issued the paper California Statewide Policy Recommendations for the Prevention of Violence Against Women. This document detailed an approach to IPV that advocated making violence against women a community responsibility rather than a "woman's problem." By approaching IPV as a human rights issue, a wider range of approaches can be used, broadening the focus from solely the victim to a public health basis across multiple fields and inter-disciplinary groups. Recommendations included a state-wide campaign to shift social norms to reflect that violence against women is not tolerated in this society; to articulate violence against women as a threat to public safety; to establish programs in school to support a violence-free society; and to identify and institute core competencies and resources across disciplines to sustain identification, prevention, and intervention on violence against women and girls. Assessment needs to be addressed as a coordinated effort across the spectrum of services with education and training for all levels of staff as well as lay people who may be the first to see signs of abuse.[8]

Violence against men by female partners is receiving more attention since it was first noted in the 1970s (see **Table 2-1**). Studies have indicated that at least 12% of men are the targets of physical aggression from female partners, with many being victims of severe violence. Population-based studies show up to 50% of victims of interpersonal violence are men. Psychological aggression, such as being threatened, being sworn at, or being insulted, affects a large percentage of men. While men are more likely to use more violent means of aggression, such as physically restraining or strangling their

Table 2-1. Interpersonal Violence Legislation: A Brief Timeline

1874	The New York Society for the Prevention of Cruelty to Children is founded–world's first child protection agency
1909	First White House Conference on the Care of Dependent Children
1911	First Family Court created in Buffalo, New York
1919	19th Amendment to the U.S. Constitution is passed, giving American women the right to vote.
1940s	In response to World War II, women move out of the home and into the workforce.
1960s-1970s	The Feminist Movement grows and takes shape, giving rise to the Battered Women's Movement.
1965	Congress begins passing laws prohibiting discrimination against women in the workplace and requiring equal pay for equal work.
1981	Duluth, Minnesota: the Duluth Model: The Duluth Domestic Abuse Intervention Project becomes the first multi-disciplinary program designed to address the issue of domestic violence.
1990	Stalking identified as a crime
1994	Congress passes the Violence Against Women Act.
2000	Congress re-authorizes the Violence Against Women Act.
2002	The Institute of Medicine issues the report *Confronting Chronic Neglect* citing the lack of adequate training of health care professionals who it states have an ethical responsibility to recognize and address exposure to abuse in patients.
2005	The Violence Against Women Act again re-authorized by Congress
2011	The Family Violence Prevention Fund, founded in 1980, changes its name to Futures Without Violence.

partners, no gender differences were shown when the perpetrator slapped, punched, or stabbed the victim. Injury rates were also consistent for abrasions, broken bones, and broken teeth. Social service and criminal justice agencies are often unsure how to proceed when the victim is male.[9] One of the problems in assessing the prevalence of male victims includes men being unwilling to admit they are being abused and to seek professional help. In some cases, men who reported being physically assaulted were arrested or threatened with arrest, in effect blaming the victim.[10] Further complicating the assessment picture is the unfortunate fact that, although there are multiple tools for assessment of violence, most have been developed and tested for evaluation of violence against women and only with heterosexual samples.[11]

Early Indicators of Potential to Abuse

Many studies have been conducted in order to evaluate whether future violence can be predicted, giving teachers, professionals, and parents signs to look for when evaluating for potential abuse. A number of these studies center on the concept of modeling, in which behavior that modeled by a parent is later seen in his or her grown child. Men who use or have used violence in their own relationships have described growing up in families with a culture of violence and how these early experiences of trauma shaped their mental health. Wei and Brackley found that assessing these relationships in violent men could assist nurses with intervening and preventing violence against women. Interviews were conducted with participants from a batterers' intervention program. The participants described growing up in a family culture that promoted and supported a violent lifestyle; none of the participants reported treatment for the abuse they experienced. These authors stated that before interventions can be developed, the context of IPV must be understood.[12]

Assessing for violence in childhood can lead to conflict resolution strategies and intervention in IPV. It is estimated that male survivors of family violence are up to 10 times more likely to be violent in an intimate relationship than men without a history of childhood violence.[13] Less is known about female perpetrators of IPV. Although studies have shown that female abusers share many of the personality and psychological traits of male abusers, most studies still focus on women as victims of abuse. Witnessing violence in childhood is not as closely correlated with female abusers.[11]

Recent research on bullying may show links to domestic violence. Aggression towards peers at a young age may carry over into adolescence in the form of teen dating violence and into adult IPV.[14] In a study of children 6 to 13 years of age exposed to domestic violence who reported being bullied, the participants had a higher likelihood of internalizing behaviors and physical aggression but were not more likely to engage in relational bullying.[15] Education of preteens on bullying and inappropriate behavior toward girls could have a lasting impact on promoting healthy relationships.[16] Evaluation of bullying may offer an opportunity for early intervention, and assessment of adult perpetrators of IPV can help the evaluator understand early indications of violent behavior.

Substance Abuse in Interpersonal Violence

Substance abuse has been shown to play a role in interpersonal violence. Co-morbidities of depression and substance abuse, common among victims of IPV, may interfere with recovery and lead to vulnerability in revictimization. Substance use can also result in sensory and cognitive impairment restricting the person's ability to recognize risk and to take measures to protect themselves. It has been theorized that offenders can detect a potential victim's social or psychological vulnerabilities, leading to increased likelihood of acting aggressively toward a potential victim with mental health or substance abuse problems.[17]

Substance abuse in either partner has been shown to increase risk of IPV. Approximately 44% of men entering treatment for alcohol abuse report being violent toward a partner in the preceding year. While reports to law enforcement generally show the female partner as victim and the male partner as aggressor, evaluation of incidents of IPV not reported to law enforcement show that IPV perpetration may occur equally between the sexes. Drug and alcohol use have been reported by survivors of IPV in about 42% of cases reported to police. Among those who relapse to alcohol after treatment, the odds of male-to-female violence was 6 times greater than those who did not relapse.[18] In a study of 1197 university students it was found that substance abuse was common for both victim and perpetrator in incidents of interpersonal victimization, such as sexual assault or rape.[19] Failure to evaluate for substance abuse can lead to further abuse and post-abuse mental and physical health problems.

ASSESSING FOR RE-VICTIMIZATION

Assessing for risk of re-victimization often involves input from the victims themselves to assess danger. This is important for a variety of reasons: victims will choose a course of action based on how much danger they think they are in, and these assessments are often the key component of counseling victims of IPV and making system-related decisions. Early studies indicated that victims were moderately accurate but imperfect in their perception of risk and that the victim's state of mental health is likely to have an effect on his or her perceived level of risk. Emotional responses to traumatic stress may change over time, which can alter the mental health symptomatology. Both post-traumatic stress disorder (PTSD) and substance abuse may influence a victim's selectivity in processing and remembering threatening cues and information. Substance abuse could be used as a coping strategy to put distance between a victim and violent acts and to impair risk assessment. Shock or numbness after IPV may likewise blunt the ability to correctly assess danger in a given situation. In a study of 246 women seeking help for IPV, 66% were accurate in their assessment of risk for repeat abuse. Those who reported higher levels of substance abuse were more likely to underestimate their risk for re-abuse, while participants who reported more symptoms of PTSD were correct when they predicted they would be re-abused.[20]

The timing of repeat abuse has also been found to be a factor in IPV. Multiple studies over 30 years have shown that women are at risk for both lethal and non-lethal violence immediately after separation.[21] Research also indicates that separated women have the highest risk of post-relationship IPV, followed by divorced women; both of these groups show a higher number of incidents than married women.[22] Opportunity for contact between offender and victim has also been shown to have an effect on repeat incidents of IPV. ***Opportunity theories*** include lifestyle and routine activity theories which take into account how daily activities and lifestyle put individuals at risk for victimization and re-victimization. ***Lifestyle theory*** describes participation in daily activities such as attending work or school as a determinant of whether a person might be victimized through associations or exposure. ***Routine activity theory*** describes the occasion of the motivated offender and the target being together at a certain place and time without the presence of a guardian; together this set of circumstances facilitates crime, such as IPV. In the presence of a motivated abuser, any length of time a victim spends offers the opportunity for violence. Situational factors, such as victim unemployment or dependent children, increase the chance for offender-victim contact. Opportunity theory emphasizes the importance of situational factors that help create opportunities for victimization. It has also been noted that for certain predictive factors for IPV (eg, having obtained a restraining order) the period between attacks decreases while the frequency of attacks increases. Other factors may also contribute to opportunistic victimization, such as cohabitation of victim and offender.[23]

Interpersonal violence between a victim and an offender often occurs in the presence of other forms of abuse. In households where one form of abuse is seen, such as spousal IPV, co-occurrence of other forms of familial violence may also take place. This may include child abuse, violence between siblings, or violence by or against other family members, such as grandparents. Often, children attacked by siblings are not seen as victims of violence. Arguments and conflict between multiple family members can escalate into physical confrontation. Variables which may contribute to co-occurring family violence include larger household size (eg, those with a greater number of children or multi-generational family members) and households including members with less than a high-school education. Focusing on a single type of victim may lead to missing the assessment of multiple types of co-occurring family violence.[24]

Re-victimization in sexual assault is also well documented in the literature. In a study of more than 8000 college-age women who experienced violence, those who had experienced sexual violence reported more re-victimization than those who reported violence of other types, such as simple assault.[25] However, repeat victimization does not occur only with women; in a Danish study of 1027 victims of repeated IPV, 72% were male.[26]

ASSESSMENT OF INTIMATE PARTNER VIOLENCE IN SPECIAL POPULATIONS

Barriers such as fear or shame may make victims of IPV less likely to report incidents of violence. Similarly, health care providers may be reluctant to screen for interpersonal violence due to lack of training, skills, or awareness in addition to personal discomfort. Social stigma and stereotypes may make victims from diverse racial and ethnic backgrounds even more reluctant to report. The inability to access culturally sensitive services keeps the victim of IPV in a cycle of violence affecting both physical and mental health.[27]

Victims of IPV with mental disabilities may communicate differently than victims without disabilities. Often dependent on a caregiver, persons with mental disabilities may be exposed to violent conditions. A lower capacity for abstract thought and reduced function of memory may alter the way they perceive the surrounding world. Messages and communication might be conveyed with the whole body or body movements rather than understandable words.[28] People with developmental disabilities (DD) may express physical symptoms to show loss and fear or may demonstrate negative behaviors such as self-injury, aggression, or apathy. Ascribing these symptoms to pathology or to the developmental disability itself may lead to the underlying cause being ignored. People with DD whose loss or fear is not recognized may show higher levels of complicated trauma. While persons with developmental disabilities experience the same symptoms and reactions to IPV as others, they may interpret the experience and express symptoms differently, requiring the assessing professional to develop a creative approach involving a variety of techniques and adapting to the victim's disability.[29]

Certain geographic populations may also require an assessor to adapt their approach to evaluating IPV. While the majority of research in interpersonal violence has been concentrated on urban settings, about 25% of the population of the United States lives in rural areas. Victims of IPV in rural settings may experience differences in economic and social conditions as well as accessibility compared to urban victims of IPV. Rural communities tend to be isolated, with homes set farther back from roads and farther from each other. Residents may have longer commutes to services like hospitals or women's shelters. Cell phone service may be poor or absent. Fewer public services may be available; police or sheriff coverage may be spread over larger rural areas. In addition to physical characteristics, culture may be different in small towns, making confidentiality challenging in a close-knit community. A professional evaluating IPV in this setting needs to be aware of the limitations on resources in these communities as well as to their unique characteristics, such as the likelihood of rural families having a weapon in the home, in order to adapt his or her assessment to effectively evaluate the rural victim of IPV.[30]

The elderly may also require an adaptation in assessment of IPV. Aging brings differences in health, cognitive abilities, and activity levels. Compared to younger survivors, older women are more likely to stay in violent relationships, experience chronic violence, and report physical and mental health problems. Re-victimization across the lifespan is common and has been shown to be a predictor of PTSD. Older victims also report substance abuse, nervousness, and low energy levels at higher rates.[31] Evaluation of IPV in older persons needs to include an evaluation of the victim's current level of cognitive function, underlying health status, and functional ability to remain in a safe environment.

ASSESSMENT MODALITIES IN INTIMATE PARTNER VIOLENCE: SCREENING, QUESTIONNAIRES, AND TOOLS

In the 2 1/2 decades since intimate partner violence studies were first published, many tools and questionnaires were developed to aid in the assessment for potential and actual IPV. Screening for potential victims of domestic violence began to take place in medical clinics and emergency rooms, often in the form of simply asking if the victim was in an abusive relationship while eliciting a medical history. Short questionnaires were also used.[32] Early barriers to assessment were overcome when domestic violence began to be discussed as a health issue instead of a "private family matter." Clinicians and health providers started to identify actual victims as well as at-risk individuals in need of intervention. Interviews with individuals and couples who sought marital counseling identified high rates of physical aggression. Self-report rating scales and questionnaires were developed, which had both advantages and disadvantages. Advantages included ease of use and confidentiality; typically these scales did not require specialized training for the evaluator and were inexpensive. Disadvantages included the untrustworthy nature of a self-administered scale: battered women were likely to minimize violence out of shame or fear, while batterers were likely to respond to questionnaires in a way that made them look more socially acceptable.[33]

Routine screening as a method for detection and early intervention became prominent in the literature starting in the 1980s and early 1990s. The multi-faceted nature of interpersonal violence was beginning to be identified, and tools for evaluation were being developed, but which professionals should use those tools was under debate. Specialists who ultimately assisted victims of IPV typically were not the first to see them in the professional setting; often the first contact was by a general healthcare provider, such as a nurse or physician, who may or may not have been trained to identify abused clients.[34]

One of the first widely used tools in interpersonal violence was the Conflict Tactic Scale (CTS), Form N. This self-reporting 18-item test was designed for face-to face interviews with both men and women currently or previously in an intimate relationship. Form R, a 19-item test, was used in the 1985 National Family Violence Survey. The CTS was noted to be brief, simple, and easy to administer, and has been widely used since its inception. It has also been adapted for use in a variety of relationships such as child-to-parent and sibling-to-sibling.[33]

Following the wide use of the CTS, two more self-report measures based on it were developed: the Modified Conflict Tactics Scale (MCTS), with 23 items, and the Adapted Conflict Tactic Scale (ACTS), with 29 items. The MCTS differentiated between mild and severe physical aggression. The original CTS was restructured into the MCTS in order to reduce redundancy, provide greater content validity, and balance items in each domain. The Adapted Conflict Tactics Scale, expanded from the CTS and MCTS, assesses the frequency with which either partner engaged in conflict tactics in the previous year and the impact, allocation of blame, and any injuries resulting from aggressive acts. The ACTS added to the CTS by assessing partner aggression in the form of injury and impact of violence while retaining the short self-report format.[33]

The Revised Conflict Tactics Scale (CTS2) was developed in the mid-1990s and contains five scales: negotiation, psychological aggression, physical assault, injury, and sexual coercion. A sample emotional negotiation item is "I showed my partner I cared even though we disagreed;" a sexual coercion item is "insisted on sex when my partner did not want to" and could include either minor sexual coercion ("did not use physical force") or severe sexual coercion ("used force to make my partner have sex"). Among the changes in this version of the CTS were the addition of two new scales; the addition of new items to the preexisting scales; and the improvement of item wording, replacing 'him' for abusers and 'her' for victims with 'my partner.'[36] A short form of the CTS2 was published in 2004.[35]

Several other assessment tools were also being developed during the 1980s and 1990s. The Index of Spousal Abuse (ISA) was developed in the late 1970s and consists of 30 items on a self-report scale. Items included statements such as, "My partner tells me I am ugly or unattractive," "My partner belittles me intellectually," "My partner treats me like a dunce," and "My partner acts like he would like to kill me." The person completing the form is asked to rate them on a 1-to-5 scale, with 1 being "never" and 5 being "very frequently." It was estimated that the form took about 5 minutes to complete. The items were noted to include some very serious and less serious types of abuse, therefore two different scores were given on each completed test: an ISA-P score for severity of physical abuse and an ISA-NP score representing the severity of nonphysical abuse. Each score ranged from 1 to 100, with lower scores indicative of a relative absence of abuse and higher scores a greater degree of abuse. Detailed instructions were given for scoring the ISA. Three studies showed that the ISA was a highly reliable and valid measure of the degree of abuse that a female victim received from a male spouse or partner. It was noted that due to the way the individual items on the tool were weighted strict attention needed to be placed on the scoring system. As with other self-report measures, the possibility for under-reporting the degree or severity of abuse existed.[36]

The Spousal Assault Risk Assessment (SARA) was developed to utilize both quantitative and clinical data. Designed to assist professionals in evaluating risk for re-abuse by domestic violence offenders, it scores 20 items in areas such as childhood abuse and neglect experiences, relationship history, substance abuse, spousal assault, and criminal history. It is not used as a psychological evaluation but as a tool to augment professional judgment regarding risk. Assessment areas are scored on a 0 to 3 scale: absent, subthreshold, and present. The SARA also has the evaluator make use of critical items that can stand alone in their indication of risk; these items include stalking or possession of a firearm. In addition to assessing future violence against a spouse, it can be used in judicial proceedings such as pretrial assessment and presentencing and in correctional intake and discharge.[37]

The Abuse Assessment Screen (AAS) was designed by the Nursing Research Consortium on Violence and Abuse. Intended to be direct and straight-forward, it consists of questions to evaluate the severity, frequency, perpetrator, and body site of injury that has occurred within a given period of time. Used with both pregnant and non-pregnant women, it includes a short questionnaire and a body map for detailing the locations of injuries. The victim of violence self-administers the test and notes injuries on the body map, although a protocol that accompanies the tool recommends the questions be read to the woman. The questions cover physical and emotional abuse, forced sexual activity, presence of a weapon and wound from a weapon, and presence or absence of fear. This tool was used only to identify presence or absence of IPV in women and did not evaluate for future risk of re-injury.[38]

The Propensity for Abusiveness Scale (PAS) was developed by assessing items that were given as a comprehensive evaluation to a group of convicted batterers. The 29 item self-report tool includes questions about the respondent's background, such as parental treatment (eg, punishment or scolding), questions about themselves (eg, stability of self-concept and anger response), and more recent events, such as restless sleep and feelings of tension. Used mainly for evaluation of emotional abuse and the risk of physical abuse, it was shown to correlate well with female partners' reports of abusiveness by men.[33,37]

Instruments for assessment of IPV continue to be developed and revised. A collaboration between the Colorado Department of Probation Services, domestic violence researchers, and community involvement lead to the development of the Domestic Violence Screening Instrument (DVSI). Using data collected from 9000 domestic violence cases sentenced to probation in the mid-1990s, the Colorado Domestic Violence Risk Reduction Project chose items for inclusion based on a clinical assessment tool previously used in Colorado. Evaluation of perpetrators with a history of repeated IPV showed the most common social and behavioral characteristics in this group. Behavioral items included imposition of court orders, arrests for family and non-family violence, convictions, and non-compliance with court and probation orders. Social characteristics were limited to recent victim and perpetrator separation and employment status. Items were reviewed by focus groups consisting of judges, prosecutors, probation officers, and community members, resulting in a 12-item tool. Intended for use by probations officers, prosecutors, and judges after an offender is arrested, a higher score on the DVSI indicates risk for re-offending, non-compliance with the courts and probation orders, and, ultimately, higher risk to victims of IPV. Evaluation items include prior domestic violence treatment; prior arrests for assault, harassment, or menacing behavior; presence of children during the IPV incident; and prior drug or alcohol treatment.[39]

A revision of the DVSI was undertaken by the Family Violence Risk Assessment Project in Connecticut. Modifications included re-wording some of the items found to be confusing, such as "a history of having a protection order" versus "a history of violating a protection order." The result was the DVSI-R with 11 items; 7 items evaluated the behavioral history of the perpetrators (eg, frequency and escalation of violence in the last 6 months and family assaults, arrests, or convictions), while the remaining 4 items examined substance abuse, presence of children, use of weapons, and employment status. Family relations counselors using the tool could also provide their own assessment of imminent risk of violence to the victim of the current IPV incident and imminent risk to another person known by the perpetrator. The purpose of the revision was to include perpetrator demographics in the risk assessment process and to examine the effect of multiple victims on risk scores, which was ultimately found to be associated with recidivistic violence.[40]

In order to provide front-line police officers with a tool for use in predicting repeated wife assault, the Ontario Provincial Police (OPP) developed the Ontario Domestic Assault Risk assessment (ODARA). During a domestic violence investigation, OPP officers are required to complete a Domestic Violence Supplementary Report, a 22-item review pertaining to the perpetrator's history including stalking, threats, violence towards pets, disobeying court orders, and mental illness. The accuracy of these scores was determined and perpetrator cases involving forceful physical contact between a man a woman in an intimate, cohabiting relationship evaluated. Cases were scored for substance abuse, prior criminal history, injury to the victim(s), including total prior injury to partners and injury to non-domestic victims, and victim barriers to support. Additionally, each case was evaluated using the CTS for severe violence. The result of these case reviews, the evaluation of other variables like correctional sentences and reports of sexual jealousy, and the calculation of the link between all of these components and recidivism was the ODARA. It was anticipated that this assessment would be used by officers immediately after completing a domestic violence investigation. The ODARA was found to have a large prediction effect on repeating wife assault as well as its frequency and severity and, as an additional benefit, could be scored by officers with no statistical training.[41]

The evaluation of ongoing IPV through a brief assessment was addressed by the Ongoing Abuse Screen (OAS). It was noted that other tools were less practical and more cumbersome to use in acute clinical settings or asked about IPV that had occurred in the past year (eg, the AAS) or throughout a person's lifetime. The 5 questions on the OAS screen for abuse that occurs in the present, at the time of contact between evaluator and respondent. The scale includes questions about present physical and emotional abuse, being forced into sexual activities, fear of a partner, and abuse during a current pregnancy. While the OAS was shown to be accurate in assessing current IPV and was more accurate than the AAS in detecting ongoing intimate partner violence, questions were added to the scale to increase its sensitivity; the resulting tool became the Ongoing Violence Assessment Tool (OVAT).[42] This new tool was then validated against the ISA. It was noted that the 4-question OVAT took about 1 minute to complete compared to about 5 minutes for the 30 questions contained in the ISA. The Ongoing Violence Assessment Tool was shown to be both sensitive and accurate in assessing IPV with a short form questionnaire.[43]

The Risk Assessment Validation Evaluation (RAVE) was the basis for the development of another short-form tool for use in Emergency Departments. The RAVE study compared the victim's evaluation of the likelihood of future assault and serious harm by a current or former partner against 4 IPV risk assessment methods: the Danger Assessment, the DV-Mosaic, the Domestic Violence Screening Instrument, and the Kingston Screening Instrument for Domestic Violence. It was noted that the length of screening questionnaires was a barrier to their use in an Emergency Department setting, coupled with over-crowding and discomfort on the part of the interviewer regarding IPV. Five questions found to independently predict potentially lethal assault or serious injury were selected from the 20-question Q&A. Examples of the questions used in the brief screen included asking if the physical violence had increased in frequency or severity in the past 6 months and if the victim believed the perpetrator was capable of killing her. Three "yes" answers were established as the threshold for high risk. To be used when a woman has already been identified as a victim of IPV, this screen should alert Emergency Department personnel that this patient is at high risk for serious injury or lethal assault.[44]

Two tools mentioned previously, while not specifically used to assess for IPV, are important in the discussion of serious risk lethality in intimate partner violence. The Danger Assessment, meant to be used as a collaborative exercise between the abused victim of IPV and a health care practitioner, criminal justice professional, or domestic violence advocate has been shown to accurately identify women who are at risk of murder at the hands of their intimate partners, is discussed elsewhere in this book.[33] The DV-Mosaic is a computer-assisted method for evaluating a domestic violence situation for danger and escalated risk factors. This assessment was not developed as a tool for screening in the traditional sense; it was originally used as a system to assist law enforcement in evaluating threat assessment in domestic violence.[45]

Some instruments not specifically designed to evaluate IPV but to evaluate other violent crime have been utilized to predict violence among men who assault their wives. The Violence Risk Appraisal Guide (VRAG) was constructed using information gathered from male patients at a maximum security psychiatric facility who were receiving pretrial or presentencing evaluations after a violent offense. The 12-item instrument includes demographic information, childhood and criminal history, and psychiatric assessment variables. VRAG was shown to be accurate in predicting violence in forensic patients, sex offenders, and incarcerated offenders. A study of 88 wife assaulters was done to assess the accuracy of the VRAG in predicting recidivism in incarcerated men. While it was shown that this tool performed well at predicting violent recidivism in serious wife assaulters, the study population was not considered to represent wife assaulters in general; however, it was noted that most of the risk factors identified as predictors of repeat wife assault were also predictors of criminal violence in general and may be useful in the prediction of risk for serious IPV.[46]

Another instrument used in the evaluation of the victim of IPV is the Domestic Violence Survivor Assessment (DVSA). This tool, which measures IPV survivor movement toward a violence-free life over time, examines 12 personal and relationship issues common to domestic violence survivors. Examples of personal issues include self-identity and seeking medical care for injuries and stress, while examples of relationship issues include triggers of abusive incidents and attachment to the relationship. The DVSA follows survivors through levels of change, from committed to continuing the relationship with the abusive partner through establishing a new life, apart or together. The model focuses on the individual survivor and the non-linear path of change while guiding counselors in their support of IPV survivors through the change process.[47]

A short, 3-question tool called "STaT" was developed for rapid evaluation of lifetime IPV. The 3 questions were "Have you ever been in a relationship where your partner pushed or slapped you?", "Have you been in a relationship where your partner threatened you with violence?", and "Have you ever been in a relationship where your partner has thrown, broken, or punched things?" An affirmative answer to any one of the 3 questions is followed by assessment questions for current incidents of abuse.[48]

In 2006, the Centers for Disease Control (CDC) published "Measuring Intimate Partner Violence Victimization and Perpetration: A Compendium of Assessment Tools." Noting that the ability to accurately measure intimate partner violence is critical for the success of intervention and research activities, it includes over 20 scales for assessing IPV. Some are intended to evaluate 1 type of violence, such as psychological or sexual, while others assess more than 1 type. Researchers choosing a scale are encouraged to take into account how an intimate partner is defined, the culture in which the scale is being used, and the age of the victim of violence, such as adult or adolescent.[49]

ASSESSMENT OF INTIMATE PARTNER VIOLENCE

Ultimately the most appropriate tool to assess IPV is the one the health care professional or interviewer feels is the right one to use at that moment. Whether it is a short routine questionnaire or a longer, more formal tool will depend on the circumstances of the interview and the rapport established between the participants. Some studies have shown that brief, 1-sentence questions, such as "Do you feel safe in your current relationship?' or "Are you in a relationship where you feel threatened?", may elicit information to start a dialog on IPV. Leaving out words that might seem intimidating, such as 'abusive" or "violent" can make the question less frightening. Using just 1 of the 3 STaT questions could be an opening for discussion. Sometimes simply asking "If there was one thing you could change in your relationship, what would it be?" is the simplest and most direct route to talking with a victim of IPV.

THE FUTURE OF IPV ASSESSMENT

Assessment in intimate partner violence continues to evolve. A computerized safety decision aid has been developed for use by survivors in assessing their own risk for lethal violence and options for safety and in setting priorities for safety. After answering demographic questions, the user is asked about safety-seeking behaviors, resources, and if they have a safe place to go. Following these questions, the participant completes a low-literacy version of the Decisional Conflict Scale. The computerized aid then provides an activity which helps the user set priorities for safety as related to the abusive relationship. In the final step, the user completes the Danger Assessment and a message is generated regarding the participant's priorities and the estimated level of danger he or she faces. An opportunity is provided for changing answers in order to reprioritize for safety, and contact information for local advocates is provided.[2]

An assessment tool for providers who use Palm-based technology was developed by the Family Violence Prevention Fund, now called "Futures without Violence." "Intimate Partner Violence: An Assessment Tool for Providers – PALM Version" was available in two formats and included facts and web links for IPV[50] but was not widely used. Many electronic medical record formats have tools for collecting and documenting IPV as well.

CONCLUSION

Assessing for IPV is a dynamic and interactive process. As this chapter has shown, multiple factors must be taken into account, from early indicators of abuse through risk for re-abuse. While many approaches to assessment exist, the priorities of safety and client-centered evaluation remain. The tool that the assessor uses must be chosen for the specific patient and circumstances at the time. These approaches will continue to evolve as research and practice in IPV advances.

REFERENCES

1. Halphen JM, Varas GM, Sadowsky JM. Recognizing and reporting elder abuse and neglect. *Geriatrics*. 2009;64(7):13-18.

2. Glass N, Eden KB, Bloom T, Perrin N. Computerized aid improves safety decision process for survivors of intimate partner violence. *J Interpers Violence*. 2010;25 (11):1947-1964.

3. Centers for Disease Control and Prevention. Understanding intimate partner violence. Centers for Disease Control and Prevention Web site. http://www.cdc. gov/violenceprevention/pdf/ipv_factsheet-a.pdf. Accessed January 24, 2013.

4. World Health Organization. *Preventing Intimate Partner and Sexual Violence Against Women: Taking Action and Generating Evidence*. Geneva, Switzerland: World Health Organization; 2010.

5. American Nurses Association. Violence against women: ANA position statement - 3/24/00. American Nurses Association Web site. http://www.nursingworld. org/MainMenuCategories/Policy-Advocacy/Positions-and-Resolutions/ANA PositionStatements/Position-Statements-Alphabetically/Violence-Against-Women.html. Accessed July 25, 2013.

6. American Medical Association. Opinion 2.02 - Physicians' obligations in preventing, identifying, and treating violence and abuse. American Medical Association Web site. http://www.ama-assn.org/ama/pub/physician-resources/medical-ethics/code-medical-ethics/opinion202.page?. Accessed July 25, 2013.

7. Ambuel B, Trent K, Lenahan P, et al. Competencies needed by health professionals for addressing exposure to violence and abuse in patient care. Academy on Violence and Abuse; April 2011. Nation Sexual Violence Resource Center Web site. http://www.ns vrc.org/publications/competencies-needed-health-professionals-addressing-exposure-violence-and-abuse-patient.PublishedApril2011. Accessed January 24, 2013.

8. California Department of Health Services: Epidemiology and Prevention for Injury Control Branch: Violence Against Women Statewide Prevention Project. California statewide policy recommendations for the prevention of violence against women. Sacramento, CA: California Department of Health Services; 2006.

9. Hines DA, Douglas EM. Women's use of intimate partner violence against men: prevalence, implications, and consequences. *J Aggress Maltreat Trauma*. 2009;18(6):527-586.

10. Barber CF. Domestic violence against men. *Nurs Stand*. 2008;22(51):35-39.

11. Gilfus ME, Trabold N, O'Brien P, Fleck-Henderson A. Gender and intimate partner violence: evaluating the evidence. *J Soc Work Educ*. 2010;46(2):256.

12. Wei C, Brackley M. Men who experienced violence or trauma as children or adolescents and who used violence in their intimate relationships. *Issues Ment Health Nurs*. 2010;31(8):498-506.

13. Godbout N, Dutton DG, Lussier Y, Sabourin S. Early exposure to violence, domestic violence, attachment representation, and marital adjustment. *Pers Relatsh*. 2009;16(3):365-384.

14. Corvo K, DeLara E. Towards an integrated theory of relational violence: is bullying a risk factor for domestic violence? *Aggress Violent Behav*. 2010;15(3):181-190.

15. Bauer NS, Herrenkohl TI, Lozano P, Rivara FP, Hill K G, Hawkins JD. Childhood bullying involvement and exposure to intimate partner violence. *Pediatrics*. 2006;118(2):e235-e242.

16. Barclay H, Mulligan D. Tackling violence against women-lessons for efforts to tackle other forms of targeted violence. *Safer Communities*. 2009;8(4):43-50.

17. Hedtke KA, Ruggiero KJ, FitzGerald MM, et al. A longitudinal investigation of interpersonal violence in relation to mental health and substance use. *J Consult Clin Psychol*. 2008;76(4):633-647.

18. Brackley MH, Williams GB, Wei CC. Substance abuse interface with intimate partner violence: what treatment programs need to know. *Nurs Clin North Am*. 2010;45(4):581-589.

19. Reed E, Amaro H, Matsumoto A, Kaysen D. The relation between interpersonal violence and substance use among a sample of university students: examination of the role of victim and perpetrator substance use. *Addict Behav*. 2009;34(3):316-318.

20. Cattaneo LB, Bell ME, Goodman LA, Dutton MA. Intimate partner violence victims' accuracy in assessing their risk of re-abuse. *J Fam Violence*. 2007;22(6):429-440.

21. Brownridge DA. Violence against women post-separation. *Aggress Violent Behav*. 2006;11 (5):514-530.

22. Brownridge DA, Chan KL, Hiebert-Murphy D, et al.The elevated risk for non-lethal post-separation violence in Canada: a comparison of separated, divorced, and married women. *J Interpers Violence*. 2008;23(3):117-135.

23. Mele M. The time course of repeat intimate partner violence. *J Fam Violence.* 2009;24(8):619-624.

24. Goodlin WE, Dunn CS. Three patterns of domestic violence in households: single victimization, repeat victimization, and co-occurring victimization. *J Fam Violence.* 2010;25(2):107-122.

25. Daigle LE, Fisher BS, Cullen FT. The violent and sexual victimization of college women: is repeat victimization a problem? *J Interpers Violence.* 2008;23(9):1296-1313.

26. Faergemann C, Lauritsen JM, Brink O, Mortensen PB. Do repeat victims of interpersonal violence have different demographic and socioeconomic characters from non-repeat victims of interpersonal violence and the general population? A population-based case-control study. *Scand J Public Health.* 2010;38(5):524-532.

27. Anderson TR, Aviles AM. Diverse faces of domestic violence. *ABNF J.* 2006;17(4):129-132.

28. Strand M, Benzein E, Savemann B. Violence in the care of adult persons with intellectual disabilities. *J Clin Nurs.* 2004;13(4):506-514.

29. Focht-New G, Clements PT, Barol B, Faulkner MJ, Service KP. Persons with developmental disabilities exposed to interpersonal violence and crime: strategies and guidance for assessment. *Perspect Psychiatr Care.* 2008;44(1):3-13.

30. Annan S. Intimate partner violence in rural environments. *Annu Rev of Nurs Res.* 2008;26:85-113.

31. Bright CL, Bowland SE. Assessing interpersonal trauma in older adult women. *J Loss Trauma.* 2008;13(4):373-393.

32. Yonaka L, Yoder MK, Darrow JB, Sherck JP. Barriers to screening for domestic violence in the emergency department. *J Contin Educ Nurs.* 2007;38(1):37-45.

33. Rathus JH, Feindler, EL. *Assessment of Partner Violence: A Handbook for Researchers and Practitioners.* Washington, DC: American Psychological Association; 2004.

34. Hoff LA, Rosenbaum L. A victimization assessment tool: instrument development and clinical implications. *J Adv Nurs.* 1994;20(4):627-634.

35. Strauss MA, Douglas EM. A short form of the revised conflict tactics scales, and typologies for severity and mutuality. *Violence Vict.* 2004;19(5):507-520.

36. Hudson WW, McIntosh SR. The assessment of spouse abuse: two quantifiable dimensions. *J Marriage Fam.* 1981;43(4):873-885, 888.

37. Dutton DG, Kropp PR. A review of domestic violence instruments. *Trauma Violence Abuse.* 2000;1(2):171-181.

38. Soeken KL, McFarlane J, Parker B, Lominack MC. The abuse assessment screen a clinical instrument to measure frequency, severity, and perpetrator of abuse against women. In: Campbell JC, ed. *Empowering Survivors of Abuse: Health Care for Battered Women and Their Children.* Thousand Oaks, CA: Sage Publications; 1998:195-203.

39. Williams KR, Houghton AB. Assessing the risk of domestic violence reoffending: a validation study. *Law Hum Behav.* 2004;28(4):437-455.

40. Williams KR, Grant SR. Empirically examining the risk of intimate partner violence: the revised domestic violence screening instrument (DVSI-R). *Public Health Rep.* 2006;121(4):400-408.

41. Hilton NZ, Harris GT, Rice ME, Lang C, Cormier CA, Lines KJ. A brief actuarial assessment for the prediction of wife assault recidivism: the Ontario domestic assault risk assessment. *Psychol Assess*. 2004;16(3):267-275.

42. Weiss SJ, Ernst AA, Cham E, Nick TG. Development of a screen for ongoing intimate partner violence. *Violence Vict*. 2003;18(2):131-141.

43. Ernst AA, Weiss SJ, Cham E, Hall L, Nick TG. Detecting ongoing intimate partner violence in the emergency department using a simple 4-question screen: The OVAT. *Violence Vict*. 2004;19(3):375-384.

44. Snider C, Webster D, O'Sullivan CS, Campbell J. Intimate partner violence: development of a brief risk assessment for the emergency department. *Acad Emerg Med*. 2009;16(11):1208-1216.

45. Campbell JC. Commentary on Websdale: lethality assessment approaches: reflections on their use and ways forward. *Violence Against Women*. 2005;11(9):1206-1213.

46. Hilton NZ, Harris GT, Rice ME. Predicting violence by serious wife assaulters. *J Interpers Violence*. 2001;16(5):408-423.

47. Dienemann J, Glass N, Hanson G, Lunsford K. The domestic violence survivor assessment (DVSA): a tool for individual counseling with women experiencing intimate partner violence. *Issues Ment Health Nurs*. 2007; 28(8):913-925.

48. Paranjape A, Liebschutz J. STaT: A three question screen for intimate partner violence. *J Womens Health*. 2003;12(3):233-239.

49. Thompson MP, Basile KC, Hertz MF Sitterle D. *Measuring Intimate Partner Violence Victimization and Perpetration: A Compendium of Assessment Tools*. Atlanta, GA: Centers for Disease Control and Prevention, National Center for Injury Prevention and Control; 2006.

50. Family Violence Prevention Fund. Electronic palm domestic violence assessment tool. Family Violence Prevention Fund Web site. http://www.endabuse.org/section/programs/health_care/_electronic_dv. Accessed January 24, 2013.

Chapter 3

RISK ASSESSMENT IN INTIMATE PARTNER VIOLENCE

Catherine Mortiere, PhD

KEY POINTS

1. The high prevalence of intimate partner violence (IPV) underlines the need for a valid and systematic means of evaluating domestic violence cases. It is critical that we identify those cases most likely to escalate, ultimately to lethality.

2. The Danger Assessment (DA) tool is an effective tool used to assess the level of danger being experienced in IPV. This instrument has been revised since its original development. There are various other screening tools that are also viewed as effective.

3. Risk assessment is performed by many people in the justice, advocacy, and healthcare sectors. Such people include law enforcement officers, probation officers, parole officers, psychiatrists and psychologists, social workers, and emergency room employees. Competent risk assessment requires education and training, although many who perform risk assessments lack such training.

4. The use of standard assessment instruments in combination with clinical interviewing is necessary for optimal risk assessment.

5. Law enforcement officers have adapted the DA for a more rapid response in domestic violence situations they encounter. This tool is known as the Lethality Assessment (LA).

INTRODUCTION

The United States Department of Justice's Bureau of Justice Statistics (BJS) reported that between 2001 and 2005, females were more likely than males to experience nonfatal intimate partner violence (IPV).[1] The annual average was 510 970 incidents for non-fatal female victims of IPV. This represented 22% of the total non-fatal, violent victimizations against females. During the same period, there was an average of 104 820 male victims of IPV, representing 4% of total non-fatal, violent victimization. Of the victims, 96% of females were victimized by their male partners and 82% of males by their female partners. Thirty percent of all female homicides (femicides) committed by intimate partners, as reported by BJS.[1] From 2001 to 2005 the number of these homicides remained relatively constant, with statistics for 2005 showing 1100 murdered females. Male intimate partner homicides were relatively low at 5%. What is no surprise is the rate of male IPV which goes unreported. The BJS study indicated that 40% of male and 22% of female victims stated that their reason for not reporting the violence was "private" or "a personal matter." These statistics emphasize the need for valid, systematic means of evaluating domestic violence cases and identifying those most likely to escalate, ultimately to lethality.

Using a combination of research-based standardized instruments and clinical judgment, experts attempt to predict a level of risk in IPV. In order to prevent IPV, risk assessments are performed in a variety of settings. Professionals, including police, probation and parole officers, healthcare providers and emergency room staff, social workers, judges, and shelter workers, estimate the level of risk that an abuser will commit further acts of violence against a partner. In some settings this may be done through a brief screening process, such as when a police officer responds to a domestic disturbance call and asks key questions before deciding how to proceed. In other settings, experts in the area of risk assessment conduct comprehensive risk analyses. This is accomplished by lengthy interviewing, careful administration of risk assessment instruments, and reviewing documentation before offering an opinion as to a particular level of risk, within a reasonable degree of medical or psychological certainty. Determining the level of risk may also dictate what course of action is appropriate, for example that discharge to the community is or is not consistent with the safety and protection of the public, that treatment is necessary, or that supervision should be mandatory.

In IPV murder cases, most victims had contact with agencies that may have been able to predict and prevent those tragedies.[2] When taking a retrospective look at cases, professionals often are able to see some kind of a sign that was either ignored, not seen in context, or misunderstood at the time. There are also times when the victims themselves refuse to be persuaded to take action in order to escape a dangerous situation.

Inherent in risk assessment is a profound responsibility on the part of an evaluator. If one underestimates the level of dangerousness of an IPV perpetrator, it is possible that a victim may be hurt, or possibly killed. On the other hand, if one errs too much on the side of caution, the rights of accused perpetrators may be violated and a false-positive result may also have an adverse effect on the family. Furthermore, a disproportionate response may make a victim reluctant to seek help in the future. Many times, victims of IPV fail to realize the level of danger in their situation. Throughout the process of interviewing during risk assessment, victims may also be able to view their situation more clearly, and possibly become convinced that they need to leave their home or relationship and seek shelter.[3,4]

It is a matter of tremendous importance that professionals perform risk assessments with great care. The choice of risk assessment instruments, those with the highest degree of validity and reliability, is vital to accurately identifying high-risk offenders. Furthermore, researchers must continue to study and refine the process of risk assessment, in order to improve its predictability.

HISTORY OF ASSESSING FOR RISK OF VIOLENCE IN IPV

Public attitudes towards IPV have changed drastically over the past few decades. In the past, domestic violence was viewed as a family problem. Police responding to calls for help from victims often hesitated to make an arrest, even when there was evidence of abuse. The only risk assessment performed was the result of the subjective judgment of a police officer or social worker responding to the scene. He or she would decide whether or not the abuse warranted arrest, or if the abuser was likely to hurt the victim again.

In 1986, nurse and researcher Jacquelyn Campbell, working with battered women, shelter workers, police, and psychologists, developed the Danger Assessment (DA), to help determine the likelihood that a woman will be killed by her intimate partner.[5] Since that time, the DA has been revised, and several other risk assessment instruments have been developed by other researchers. That was one of the first research projects that actually had an impact on educating the public, mostly the victims of IPV, about the seriousness of this issue.

Among the factors contributing to the evolution of both public attitudes and the official response to IPV was the OJ Simpson murder trial in 1994. Nicole Brown Simpson was found murdered in her home, along with her friend Ronald Goldman. Several times prior to the murder, Nicole had told both friends and police that she believed her ex-husband, former football star OJ Simpson, would kill her. Her sister had even taken pictures of bruises she allegedly incurred during beatings by her husband. Although at trial Simpson was acquitted, the case drew public attention to the fact that domestic violence is a serious crime, not merely a family problem.

The Simpson case also served as a turning point for police response to domestic violence calls. Since that time, police officers' discretionary assessment has been restricted when responding to domestic violence scenes. Previously, an officer would assess the risk of IPV, and decide whether or not to arrest the accused perpetrator, often asking the aggressor to leave the home for a cooling-off period. After the Simpson trial, it became standard practice for police to arrest perpetrators of alleged domestic violence even if the victim recants her or his story or asks the police not to make an arrest. Prosecutors will charge the perpetrator even if the victim changes her (or his) story or does not wish to prosecute.[6]

The response to IPV has changed in a number of areas since the early 1990s, including the criminal justice system, social services, and health care. Law enforcement and officers of the court now receive training in domestic violence, special domestic violence courts have been set up to hear IPV cases, and hospital emergency departments routinely screen patients for IPV. The prevalence of this form of violence has necessitated some sort of triage, especially in the criminal justice system, and this need has driven the development of risk assessment tools specific to this problem. Although the combination of scores on a risk assessment instrument, in addition to clinicians' judgment, yield a more accurate evaluation of risk than was possible twenty years ago, risk assessment remains an inexact science.

Victims of IPV often have the information experts need to formulate a risk profile. Such information includes specific things the perpetrator has said and done in the past that led to previous violence, indications of the perpetrator's current state of mind and things the perpetrator has said or done which may be threatening in the present, but the victims are not always able or willing to access or provide such information. There are psychological reasons why a victim of IPV may or may not have the ability to communicate this information to appropriate parties, including trauma, shock, fear, denial, privacy concerns, and resistance to outside help. Therefore, one of the most important tools used in risk analysis is sound clinical interviewing; in other words, asking the questions that take into account a victim's limitations. This requires skill and experience in getting the information necessary to form an opinion on the risk of violence.

WHO PERFORMS RISK ASSESSMENT?

As outlined in **Table 3-1**, a variety of people in different roles and settings are put in the position of performing some type of assessment for risk of violence. Competent risk assessment requires specialized expertise combining the use of standardized instruments with clinical interviews, as well as information gathered from collateral sources. Unfortunately, not everyone who performs risk assessment has been adequately trained to do so. In particular, the proper and proficient use of standardized instruments in risk analysis requires education and training. A layman cannot be expected to fill out a questionnaire or administer a psychological test and reach an expert, clinical opinion on level of risk. These sources were meant to be used by trained examiners. Scores from these sources are meant to be a guide for experts in addition to clinical interviewing and information from collateral sources. Adequate training is required in order to reach level of expertise similar to an expert professional.

Table 3-1. Assessors and Calls for Assessment

WHO PERFORMS RISK ASSESSMENT?	WHEN IS RISK ASSESSMENT PERFORMED?
Law enforcement officers	When responding to reports of domestic violence, officers must decide what course of action is appropriate, taking into account their departmental policies, once they have assessed the level of risk for violence from information available at the scene.
Probation officers	When designating terms of probation, such as where probation will be served, what restrictions will be placed on the defendant, with whom the perpetrator will be allowed contact throughout the duration of probation, and boundaries of reporting.
Parole officers	When supervising incarcerated offenders released prior to serving their full sentences.
Psychologists and psychiatrists	When determining whether someone poses a risk to him- or herself, or others. This is standard throughout the United States when committing a person to in-patient psychiatric treatment, and in some states when an offender is soon to be released to the community.
Social workers	When monitoring troubled families. Monitoring by social workers can be mandated by courts and Child Protective Services.
Shelter workers	When a woman living in a shelter considers going home or integrating back into a relationship with her aggressor. Shelter employees assume responsibility to discuss risk factors with those willing to re-join their families or move back into the family home.
Colleges and other educational settings	When a student exhibits threatening or violent behavior.
Emergency room employees	When treating victims for injuries sustained in domestic conflicts. Where a minor or other incapacitated person is involved, a determination must be made whether or not there is further risk for harm, and if the health care workers perceive a risk, they must report it to legal authorities.

(continued)

Table 3-1. Assessors and Calls for Assessment *(continued)*

WHO PERFORMS RISK ASSESSMENT?	WHEN IS RISK ASSESSMENT PERFORMED?
Judges who preside over domestic violence and family court cases	Judges are often in a good position to determine whether a particular situation is dangerous or volatile and act on that determination. They have the authority to mandate psychiatric evaluations, psychological testing, or comprehensive risk assessment, under threat of contempt, if necessary. Judges rely on experts to advise the court as to the level of risk in the case at hand before taking appropriate action.
Prosecutors	When deciding whether or not to ask a judge for an Order of Protection. Sometimes, judges themselves have to make educated decisions based on the information presented to them by prosecutors. These court hearings usually take place with short notice, in emergency situations where victims or potential victims fear for their safety.

Effective clinical interviewing also requires specialized skill derived from years of education and experience, particularly in the field of forensics. Comprehensive risk assessment utilizes all of these tools in order to arrive at a sound, expert clinical opinion that can be used to protect potential victims of IPV.

Unfortunately, many of the settings described above do not employ experts in risk analysis. Many of those charged with the responsibility of determining level of risk do not have the level of education and training necessary to render an expert opinion in risk analysis. Obviously, it would be ideal to employ experts in risk assessment for all settings related to IPV, but it is not always possible given limited financial resources available in some of these settings. The bright side of this less-than-ideal reality is that in addition to education and training, experience can be an excellent teacher. Personnel in some of the settings listed above regularly deal with victims of IPV and develop keen instincts for issues relating to both victims and perpetrators.

Mandatory Risk Assessment for IPV

Due to overcrowded courts, lack of funding, and lack of trained personnel, risk assessment does not happen as a matter of course, or with uniform rigor, in all of these settings. There are several situations in which full-fledged, mandatory risk assessment would significantly improve the safety of victims. Some of these situations include:

— Whenever someone seeks a court order of protection from IPV

— When a person is released from incarceration, after serving time for a domestic violence conviction

— When a defendant is sentenced to probation, after being found guilty of a domestic violence charge

— When psychiatric patients are discharged from civil commitment, and the danger they previously posed to others was related to IPV

In certain states, such as Colorado, risk assessment is mandatory in all domestic violence cases that reach the criminal justice system.[7] This practice serves to protect victims from further acts of violence, and given the prevalence of IPV, mandating risk assessment has the potential to reduce the incidence of violence.

ASSESSING PERPETRATORS AND VICTIMS

Multiple sources of information are necessary in comprehensive risk analysis. Ideally, risk assessments for IPV should employ in-depth interviews with both victims and perpetrators. Most of the time, however, those performing the assessment only have access to one of the two parties. Risk assessment instruments have been developed specifically for use with either the victim or the perpetrator.

Most perpetrators are not in custody, and many refuse to voluntarily undergo risk assessment. In such cases, where the victim is the primary source of information, those performing the risk assessment may only have access to the perpetrator's prior criminal history and record of orders of protection. In cases where an examiner does not have access to the perpetrator, or the perpetrator refuses to participate in the assessment, there are standardized actuarial instruments one can use in order to evaluate the salient risk factors. These instruments mostly gather information from prior criminal history, collateral sources, and court records. When a perpetrator is in custody in a forensic setting or a civil hospital setting and refuses to be interviewed, pertinent records are made available by the entity seeking risk assessment and used for court purposes.

THE USE OF STANDARDIZED INSTRUMENTS
AND CLINICAL INTERVIEWING IN EXPERT OPINION

There has been continuous debate as to whether standardized "actuarial" instruments are more valid than clinical judgment.[8,9] The ***actuarial method*** can be defined as the use of an instrument that provides empirically-based scores related to variables considered predictors of violence in representative samples.[10,11] When assessing risk of violence, an actuarial instrument is one that has been formally and independently tested and shown to predict violent outcomes based on samples with similar risk factors. In addition to actuarial instruments, evaluators utilize structured, clinical guides that only ensure important risk factors are considered when assessing risk but also suggest ways to score the results.

In practice, optimal risk assessment should use standardized instruments and clinical judgment. Actuarial risk assessment instruments in combination with the clinical interview yields a more reliable risk analysis than either method can provide by itself. Actuarial instruments provide a guide to the expert and prompt the gathering of specific information organized in such a way as to indicate a "range" of risk (ie, low, medium, or high risk). This is the objective portion of the examination. Through the clinical interview, the examiner can gain more insight into various factors that help determine level of risk. First-hand observations made during the clinical interview, such as body language and demeanor; information and insight gained about previously known details; and collateral information used to clarify facts may contradict some of the statements a perpetrator or victim has made in response to an objective questionnaire.

Using the 2 methods in tandem yields a comprehensive analysis of level of risk; however, practitioners must exercise caution when using assessment instruments that rely solely on self-reporting. Here, evaluators often find that perpetrators tend to minimize the violence they have used toward a victim. Even the victims themselves do not always answer questions accurately and, at times, tend to minimize conflicts and previous instances of violence.[12] Fear, denial, repressed memory, the impulse to protect a beloved partner (even an abuser), and battered partner syndrome may render a victim's responses unreliable.

Many victims are found to be poor historians when it comes to situations related to IPV. This can be challenging to clinicians attempting to gain information for use in assessment. One benefit of standardized instruments is that they assist victims and other interviewees in recalling incidents and details they may otherwise have forgotten, and help them report violence they might otherwise have minimized. They also help to structure the information given, which makes it easier to identify inconsistencies in their narratives.

It is important to understand that victims sometimes become desensitized to violence. Serious incidents of IPV do not usually occur without a history of smaller, seemingly less serious occurrences. What may begin as pushing or slapping often ends as punching, kicking, stabbing, or shooting. Especially after a severely violent incident, the victim may dismiss less serious physical episodes as unimportant when speaking with an examiner. It is crucial to overcome this tendency, however, because the pattern of escalation of violence is a vital piece of evidence when analyzing levels of dangerousness and risk. The evaluator must convey to interviewees that even seemingly unimportant details should be included in their descriptions of incidents and interpersonal relationships.

RISK ASSESSMENT INSTRUMENTS COMMONLY USED IN IPV

There are actuarial instruments and structured clinical guides that have been developed specifically for use with IPV in different settings. There are others not designed specifically for use in relation to IPV but target general risk for violence. The following are descriptions of some of the tools most commonly used.

THE DANGER ASSESSMENT (DA)

The examiner performing the DA (usually a victim advocate) reviews the past year of the perpetrator's behavior with a victim, and documents the frequency and severity of violent episodes. By creating this record, interviewers assist victims in getting beyond some of the psychological reactions typical to victims of abuse. For example, victims often minimize the abuse they have suffered. This is often an unconscious mechanism of defense against a number of negative feelings that victims suffer. Research has been dedicated to such reactions in victims of IPV. Campbell et al[13] conducted a multi-site national study of risk factors for femicide by intimate partners. She compared women who were victims of femicide or attempted femicide, to other women from the same cities, some of whom had been battered, and some of whom had not. Findings indicated that only 47% of the femicide victims and 53% of the attempted victims believed that the perpetrator was capable of killing him.[13]

The DA is a short yes/no instrument developed in 1985 to assist women in assessing the risk of lethality in abusive intimate partner relationships. Since its creation, it has been used in many domestic violence programs by shelter advocates, criminal justice practitioners, and health care professionals as well as in prior research.[4,14] There is a shorter four-question version named the Lethality Assessment created for police responding to domestic violence calls, in order to quickly gauge the need to protect a victim from potential violence.[15]

The DA is an instrument that includes 20 yes-or-no questions regarding risk factors; the more 'yes' responses, the higher the risk of deadly violence in the future. Campbell also found that 84% of the women who were later killed by their intimate partners had answered 'yes' to eight or more of the questions. Among those who answered affirmatively to 12 or more questions, 94% were either killed or nearly killed by their partners.[13]

A secondary benefit of the DA, beyond estimating risk, is to increase victims' awareness of the dangers they face and to help them form a plan of action that will keep them safe.[15]

Domestic Violence-Method of Selecting Areas of Inquiry Consistently (DV-MOSAIC)

The DV-MOSAIC, which is virtually always referred to by its acronym, was designed for use by police officers investigating domestic violence cases. It was developed by Gavin de Becker[16] using over 24 000 cases originating from the Los Angeles Police Department. The instrument was intended to guide officers to an appropriate response in domestic violence cases; however, it is now widely used by victim advocates, social workers, psychologists, and others involved with safety planning for victims and potential victims of IPV.

Roehl et al[7] commented on the DV-MOSAIC manual, stating that dangerousness is not only determined by an individual's psychological profile, but is situational; it is not a permanent or stable trait. Certain situations have been linked to domestic violence, and the DV-MOSAIC calculates the level of danger based on these situational risk factors. Using the DV-MOSAIC, a police investigator gathers answers to 48 questions, based on interviews with the victim, and at times, the perpetrator as well as criminal records and police reports. The resulting score, rated on a 1-10 scale, is based on calculations of risk that the perpetrator will severely or lethally assault the victim in the near future. This instrument includes a software package that produces a report from raw scores that describes, among other things, the similarity of each case profile to others that have ended in murder.

Domestic Violence Screening Instrument—Revised (DVSI-R)

The DVSI-R measures the risk of re-assault by use of 11 items covering the perpetrator's behavioral history, including assaults, convictions, violence, violation of court orders, verbal and emotional abuse, frequency and escalation of violence, substance abuse, employment, and other factors. Probation or parole officers can complete the instrument using the perpetrator's record and an interview process.[17]

The DVSI-R is intended to be used as a screening tool. There is a cutoff score which indicates that a more in-depth assessment is warranted. If the cutoff score is reached, further assessment is recommended with the Spousal Assault Risk Assessment, or SARA.[7] Authors of the DVSI-R suggest gaining information from 5 other sources to supplement evidence indicating the presence and intensity of the items on the DVSI-R: the defendant, victim, police report, criminal history record, and protective order registry.

Kingston Screening Instrument for Domestic Violence (K-SID)

The K-SID was designed to assist criminal justice professionals in measuring the risk of re-assault to set conditions for release, conditions of probation, and limitations of protective orders. It consists of 3 parts: a poverty chart, an index of abuse and injuries, and a 10-question section related to risk factors. The instrument is completed based on interviews with the victim and the offender and a review of police reports. It rates risk of re-assault as low, moderate, high, or very high.[18]

Spousal Assault Risk Assessment Guide (SARA)

The SARA measures risk of future violence in men arrested for or suspected of assaulting their wives or children. It is based on 20 risk factors, organized under 4 headings: criminal history, psychological adjustment, spousal assault history, and alleged current offense.[19] The SARA is meant to be used as part of an in-depth assessment, for sentencing, probation and parole. The SARA requires a combination of clinical opinion from a trained, experienced examiner and psychological assessment of the perpetrator. The SARA recommends that evaluators draw upon as many sources of information as possible, including interviews with victim and perpetrator; criminal justice records; and the Hare Psychopathy Checklist (PCL-R), an actuarial instrument that indicates a range of psychopathy.[7]

HISTORY, CLINICAL, RISK MANAGEMENT-20 SCALE (HCR-20)

The HCR-20 was created to assist in determining risk for violence in criminal defendants, prisoners, forensic patients, and civil psychiatric patients. It is used with a wide range of subjects and not specifically tailored to perpetrators of IPV. It is considered a reliable instrument in dangerousness and risk assessment and is frequently used in courts of law. It was designed by the authors to serve as a guide for risk assessment.[20]

The instrument includes 10 historical factors, 5 clinical factors, and 5 risk management factors. There is also an item derived from the total score on the Hare Psychopathy Checklist that addresses psychopathy. Psychopathy, as measured by the PCL-R, is significantly related to violent behavior. Therefore, on those uncommon occasions when a subject's score reaches the level of psychopathy, it must be included in the overall appraisal of violence risk potential. . The HCR-20 was recently updated to a new version, HCR-20V3. The HCR-20V3 follows Versions 1 and 2, but does not require the use of the PCL-R or PCL:SV. The Historical, Clinical, and Risk management sections remained the same, though some of the terminology changed to reflect greater relevance of the 20 key violence risk factors and some sub items were added to the more complex risk factors.[21]

One advantage of the HCR-20 (all versions) is that it can be used without the cooperation of the subject. Information can be gathered from other records, such as arrest, court, and hospitalization. Version 2 of the HCR-20 has been adopted or evaluated in 35 countries and is widely used in the United States, Canada, Europe, Asia, Australia, and New Zealand.[21]

KEY RISK FACTORS

Different assessment instruments organize available information in different ways. Though the instruments' questions may vary, and the scoring system may differ with regard to risk factors and amount of weight given to a particular factor or group of factors, many key markers overlap. Research studies have identified the risk factors most predictive of repeated IPV. Among the factors most closely correlated with IPV are:

— Alcohol use, daily or near-daily

— Recent relationship termination, especially termination initiated by the victim

— A controlling relationship in which the perpetrator controls most or all of the victim's activities, including friendships and spending

— Unemployment

— Previous threats, or previous use of a weapon in IPV

— Stalking behavior

Other important risk factors appearing on most risk assessment instruments include:[22]

— Increased violence in recent months

— Threats to kill the victim

— Gun ownership

— A history of violent behavior

— Children in the household who are not the perpetrator's biological children

— A history of forced sex

— Drug use

— Childhood abuse suffered by the perpetrator

— Violated restraining orders

Although victims' predictions of violent behavior are not considered risk factors, Weisz, Tolman, and Saunders found that "the addition of survivors' predictions to risk factors significantly improved the accuracy of prediction of severe re-assault."[23] Further, Gondolf's 2002 study[24] concluded that women's predictions were as useful as all the batterer characteristics combined.

STATIC VS. DYNAMIC FACTORS

Certain risk factors are considered static. These factors must be considered when assessing risk; however, an examiner must not solely consider historical factors when assessing for level of risk. If that were the case, a subject with high risk for violence in his history could never be considered a lower risk, because historical factors do not change. Other factors are considered dynamic. An examiner must consider dynamic factors that may compound or mitigate the level of risk for violence. As evidenced in **Table 3-2**, comprehensive risk analysis requires consideration of risk factors empirically supported in the literature, including both static and dynamic risk factors.

THE ACCURACY OF RISK ASSESSMENT

Even research-based risk assessment methods do not yield perfect results. Although many victims who were subsequently killed or re-assaulted initially presented with many key risk factors for IPV, or a particularly troubling score on a risk assessment instrument, these factors and scores cannot necessarily predict violence. Many perpetrators who seem to be at a high risk for repeated violence do not re-assault their partners, while some who do commit

Table 3-2. Contributing Factors to the Risk of Violence	
Static Factors	— Psychological history
	— Criminal history
	— Gender
	— Nature of past relationship between victim and perpetrator
	— Previous history of violence toward a particular victim pool, such as women
	— Substance use involved in previous violent episodes
	— Previous protective orders and violations of protective orders
Dynamic Factors	— Stress
	— Age
	— Mental health
	— Attitude, criminal or anti-criminal
	— Feelings of hostility, aggression, and anger
	— Desire for domination and control
	— System of support
	— Social adjustment
	— Psychological treatment since the last incident of IPV

violence have been assessed as low-risk.[24] A study of 4 risk assessment instruments commonly used by law enforcement, probation, and victim assistance programs concluded that "none of the instruments or methods was impressive in predicting re-assault."[7] This study ranked the DA as the strongest of the instruments studied, but found that victims' perception of risk predicted re-assault more accurately than the DA; however, Roehl et al[7] commented that even victims' predictions "left much of the re-assault unanticipated." In an 11-city study of femicide "only 47% of the actual femicide victims and 54% of the victims of attempted femicide accurately assessed that their perpetrator was capable of killing them."[7] Heckert and Gondolf[25] found that the best method of predicting violence was a combination of the DA and victims' perceptions of risk. It has not yet been documented by research that risk assessment instruments perform better than the judgment of experienced practitioners in the field of IPV; however, in cases involving sexual assault and mental health, research has found the use of instruments more accurate than expert judgment, and combining the two is considered the optimal method for risk assessment.[26,27]

This is not to suggest that risk assessment for IPV is pointless; the safety and survival of victims will often depend on the intervention of professionals who see likelihood of future violence in the evidence. What the imperfection of current methods tells us is that we need to keep refining the risk assessment tools now available. It is especially important to note that each component added to a risk assessment improves the accuracy of predictions. Even without the use of an instrument, an assessment based on the clinical opinion of a trained expert in IPV will yield a more accurate estimate of risk than the opinion of a judge or police officer without training to assess risk of IPV. Adding a research-based instrument further improves the estimate, and adding other sources of information, such as interviews with victims and perpetrators, and criminal justice records, yields the best possible results.[7]

ORDERS OF PROTECTION AND RISK ASSESSMENT

When a court order of protection is granted in a case of IPV, it means that a judge feels that the information presented by the prosecutor on behalf of the petitioner is such that protection of the respondent is required. When a court issues such an order, it makes sense that a comprehensive assessment for dangerousness and risk should also be performed by a qualified professional as soon as possible. According to a study by Holt et al,[28] "Permanent, but not temporary, protection orders are associated with a significant decrease in risk of police-reported violence against women by their male intimate partners." A review of the literature by Benitez, McNiel and Binder[29] found protection order violations so common that risk assessment would seem to be especially important when granting a protection order.

MOVING FORWARD IN ASSESSMENT OF RISK

Trained experts have abundant opportunities in the United States to identify individuals at high risk of perpetrating or suffering IPV but, at present, do not often enough utilized these opportunities. Many victims murdered by intimate partners and the partners themselves are seen in the health care or criminal justice system prior:

— "In 65% of the cases of femicide or attempted femicide studies, either the victim or the perpetrator had been seen by a criminal justice or health care professional before the event.

— The majority (55%) of victims of actual or attempted femicides had called the police before they were killed.

— 58% of the abusive perpetrators had been arrested before they killed their partners, and 22% had been seen in the mental health care system."[12]

These statistics present important information indicating a need to further protect victims and potential victims of IPV when opportunities present themselves. Police, courts, shelters, and emergency rooms could all assist in reducing rates of IPV by assessing risk as a matter of course when carefully-defined signs of danger suggest a need for intervention. For example, researchers have defined certain key questions in the Danger Assessment that can be used as a quick screening tool by police. In 60 Maryland police departments, officers use the Lethality Assessment Checklist when responding to domestic violence calls.[30] First, the officers ask the victim 3 questions:

1. Has your partner ever used a weapon against you or threatened you with a weapon?

2. Has he or she ever threatened to kill you or your children?

3. Do you think he or she might try to kill you?

If the answer to any of these questions is 'yes,' the officers have a domestic abuse counselor confer with the victim immediately. If the answers are 'no,' additional questions are asked in order to assess for risk of violence. This approach seems efficient, and could prevent many incidents of violence and murder if it were more widely applied. Eventually, American criminal justice, health, and victim advocacy systems will recognize the need for mandated, structured risk assessment and its potential to pre-empt IPV. In the future, comprehensive risk assessment, performed by qualified experts, will hopefully become standard procedure in these situations (see **Table 3-3**).

Table 3-3. When Structured Comprehensive Risk Assessment Is Necessary

— When a judge grants an order of protection. If there is cause for a protective order, there is cause for a risk assessment by a qualified examiner.

— When a defendant violates the terms of a protective order.

— When a judge decides whether or not to incarcerate an abuser. A score of 12 on the Danger Assessment might serve as the threshold for imprisonment.[12]

— When a parole officer considers terms of release. In many states, risk analyses are already performed to educate parole boards.

— When a probation officer determines terms of probation.

— When police respond to domestic violence call.

— When an emergency room patient shows signs of injury that is suspected to be the result of IPV.

— When social workers find evidence of domestic violence.

— When shelter workers counsel a client returning home or integrating back into a relationship with an aggressor.

There are some arguments against increased use of risk assessment. Some argue that there have been many cases in which intervention resulted in increased violence as outraged perpetrators lashed out at their partners.[31] Others contend that because risk assessment does not conclusively predict future violence, it should not be used more often.[24] In answer to these objections, one might suggest that further acts of violence in retaliation for risk analyses should be swiftly and strictly dealt with in the courts and that the present imperfection in risk assessment as a predictive tool does not mean it has no value. When combined with expert clinical judgment, the instruments already in use can prevent re-assault and even death. If evaluation fails to prevent some incidents of IPV and if some families are separated unnecessarily, those failures may be outweighed by the many tragedies averted due, in part, to risk analysis. Every failure should inspire continued research and refining of methods. It is imperative that professionals who come in contact with victims and perpetrators of IPV err on the side of caution and demand comprehensive risk assessment when warranted. Victims' rights groups and women's organizations should advocate strenuously to make risk assessment standard procedure in the settings mentioned above. There are few systemic changes with such potential to protect victims of intimate partner violence.

REFERENCES

1. United States Department of Justice, Office of Justice Programs, Bureau of Justice. *Intimate Partner Violence in the United States, 2001-2005.* Washington, DC: Bureau of Justice Statistics; 2007.

2. Sharps PW, Koziol-McLain J, Campbell JC, McFarlane J, Sachs CJ, Xu X. Health care providers' missed opportunities for preventing femicide. *Prev Med.* 2001;33(5):373-380.

3. Humphreys JC, Campbell JC. *Family Violence in Nursing Practice.* Philadelphia, PA: Lippincott Williams & Wilkins; 2004.

4. Campbell JC. Prediction of homicide of and by battered women. In: Campbell JC, ed. *Assessing the Risk of Dangerousness: Potential for Further Violence of Sexual Offenders, Batterers and Child Abusers.* Newbury Park, CA: Sage; 1995:96-113.

5. Campbell JC. Nursing assessment of risk of homicide for battered women. *Adv Nurs Sci.* 1986;8(4):36-51.

6. Grimes DM. OJ Simpson and the evolution of domestic violence cases. Grimes & Warwick Web site. http://www.grimesandwarwick.com/o-j-simpson-and-the-evolution-of-domestic-violence-cases/. Accessed April 2012.

7. Roehl J, O'Sullivan C, Webster D, Campbell J. *Intimate Partner Violence Risk Assessment Validation Study, Final Report.* Baltimore, MD: Johns Hopkins University; 2005.

8. Quinsey V, Harris GT, Rice ME, Cormier C. *Violent Offenders: Appraising and Managing Risk.* Washington, DC: American Psychological Association; 1998.

9. Litwack TR, Schlesinger LB. Dangerousness risk assessments: research, legal, and clinical considerations. In: Hess A, Weiner I, eds. *The Handbook of Forensic Psychology.* New York, NY: John Wiley & Sons; 1999:171-217.

10. Hilton NZ, Harris GT, Rice ME, Lang C, Cormier CA, Lines KJ. A brief actuarial assessment for the prediction of wife assault recidivism: the ontario domestic assault risk assessment. *Psychol Assess.* 2004;16(3):267-275.

11. Webster CD, Harris GT, Rice ME, Cormier C, Quinsey VL. *The Violence Prediction Scheme: Assessing Dangerousness in High Risk Men.* Toronto, ON: Centre of Criminology, University of Toronto; 1994.

12. Pence E. Risk and lethality assessment in the field of intimate partner violence. In: *Safety Evaluation for Battered Women: A Resource Packet for Advocates, Practitioners and Policymakers.* Duluth: Praxis International; 2004.

13. Campbell JC, Webster D, Koziol-McLain J, et al. Risk factors for femicide in abusive relationships: results from a multi-site case control study. *Am J Public Health*. 2003;93(7):1089-1097.

14. Campbell JC, Sharps P, Glass NE. Risk Assessment for IPV. In: Pinard GF, Pagani I, eds. *Clinical Assessment of Dangerousness: Empirical Contributions*. New York, NY: Cambridge University Press; 2000:136-157.

15. Campbell JC, Webster D, Koziol-McLain J, Block CR, Campbell D, Curry MA, Gary F, Sachs C, Sharps P, Ulrich Y, Wilt SA. Assessing risk factors for intimate partner homicide. *Natl Inst Justice J*. 2003;250:14-19.

16. De Becker G. *The Gift of Fear & Other Survival Signals That Protect Us From Harm*. New York, NY: Dell Publishing; 1997.

17. Williams KR, Grant SR. Empirically examining the risk of intimate partner violence: the Revised Domestic Violence Screening Instrument (DVSI-R). *Public Health Reports*. 2006;121(4):400-408.

18. Gelles R, Tolman R. *The Kingston Screening Instrument for Domestic Violence (K-SID)*. Providence, RI: University of Rhode Island: 1998.

19. Kropp P, Hart S, Webster C, Eaves D. *Manual for the Spousal Assault Risk Assessment Guide*. 2nd ed. Vancouver, BC: British Columbia Institute on Family Violence; 1995.

20. Webster CD, Douglas KS, Eaves D, Hart SD. HCR-20: assessing risk for violence (version 2). Burnaby, BC: Mental Health, Law, and Policy Institute, Simon Fraser University; 1997.

21. Douglas KS, Hart SD, Webster CD, Belfrage H. HCR-20V3: Assessing Risk of Violence – User Guide. Burnaby, Canada: Mental Health, Law, and Policy Institute, Simon Fraser University; 2013.

22. Snider C, Webster D, O'Sullivan C, Campbell J. Intimate partner violence: development of a brief risk assessment for the emergency department. *Acad Emerg Med*. 2009;16(11):1208-1216.

23. Weisz AN, Tolman RM, Saunders DG. Assessing the risk of severe domestic violence: the importance of survivors' predictions. *J Interpers Violence*. 2000;15(1):75-90.

24. Gondof EW. *Batterer Intervention Systems: Issues, Outcomes and Recommendations*. Thousand Oaks, CA: Sage Publications; 2002.

25. Heckert DA, Gondolf EW. Battered women's perceptions of risk versus risk factors and instruments in predicting repeat assault. *J Interpers Violence*. 2004;19(7)778-800.

26. Pinard GF, Pagani L. *Clinical Assessment of Dangerousness: Empirical Contributions*. New York, NY: Cambridge University Press; 2004.

27. Hanson RK, Morton-Bourgon KE. *Predictors of Sexual Recidivism: An Updated Meta-Analysis*. Ottawa, ON: Public Safety and Emergency Preparedness Canada; 2004.

28. Holt VL, Kernic MA, Lumley T, Wolf ME, Rivara FP. Civil protection orders and risk of subsequent police-reported violence. *JAMA*. 2002;288(5):589-594.

29. Benitez CT, McNiel DE, Binder RL. Do protection orders protect? *J Am Acad Psychiatry Law*. 2010;38(3):376-385.

30. Remsberg C. "Lethality assessment" helps gauge danger from domestic disputes. PoliceOneWebsite.http://www.policeone.com/patrol-issues/articles/1638964-Lethality-Assessment-helps-gauge-danger-from-domestic-disputes/. Accessed April 2012.

31. Rhodes KV, Iwashyna TJ. Male perpetrators of intimate partner violence: support for health care interventions targeted at level of risk. *Behav Change*. 2009;26(3):174-189.

GENERAL INDICATORS OF IPV IN WOMEN'S HEALTH

Karyn E. Holt, PhD, RN, CNM
Margit B. Gerardi, PhD, RN, WHNP

KEY POINTS:

1. Intimate partner violence is a serious public health problem, concerning all of us and affecting many of us, which is preventable.

2. The goal is to stop IPV before it begins. This chapter identifies numerous identifiers and risk factors to assist.

3. Identify physical, emotional, and psychological violence and their impact on relationships.

4. Recognize risk factors for and consequences of IPV in women.

5. Identify evidence-based screening tools in use as medical screening.

INTRODUCTION

Intimate partner violence manifests as four types of behaviors: physical violence, sexual violence, threats of physical or sexual violence, and emotional abuse. The Centers for Disease Control and Prevention (CDC)[1] uses the following definitions for these behaviors, and, in an effort to standardize definitions, this chapter will use those CDC definitions:

— *Physical violence* is the intentional use of physical force with the potential for causing death, disability, injury, or harm.

— *Sexual violence* is defined as a deliberate or threatened action or behavior of sexual aggression directed toward a person by another individual with an intention to control, humiliate, or harm. Threats of physical or sexual violence use words, gestures, or weapons to communicate the intent to cause death, disability, injury, or physical harm.[1]

— *Psychological/emotional violence* involves trauma to the victim caused by acts, threats of acts, or coercive tactics.[1]

Oftentimes, psychological or emotional violence is the beginning of a continuum of behaviors that commence with relational tensing progressing to emotional mistreatment, escalating to battering, and further progressing to violence. The absence of caring and respectful partner behaviors is just as powerful in creating an emotionally abusive experience as openly abusive behaviors.[2] Emotional abuse is a dynamic event, encompassing multiple culminations, secondary physical and mental health symptoms, and quality of life issues that extended well beyond the immediate abuse experience. Cooley-Strickland et al[2] found that those who have experienced or witnessed IPV are more likely rather than reject to accept IPV, because of its familiarity.[2]

Those who provide health care services in hospital and outpatient settings commonly see women in their practices who have experienced or are currently experiencing intimate partner violence (IPV). The World Health Organization (WHO) Multi-Country Study of Women's Health and Domestic Violence Against Women reports a lifetime prevalence of IPV in the United States of 25-60%.[3,4] The Department of Justice[5] estimates there are 960 000 to 3 million incidents of violence per year including physical abuse from husbands or boyfriends to violence against current or former spouses, boyfriends, and girlfriends. Intimate partner violence crosses socioeconomic strata, ethnic groups, and opposite as well as same-sex relationships. It occurs in every culture, race, and nation, regardless of economic and social status, education, or religious preference. According to Gunter,[6] IPV is the most common cause of nonfatal injury to women.

The CDC reports that about 4.8 million women experienced physical assault or rape related to IPV in 2009, while only 2.9 million men experienced IPV.[4] Intimate partner homicide victims are 78% female and only 22% male.[5] Puzone et al[7] reports that in the US, 1 in 3 female homicides are a result of intimate partner violence, while only 1 in 20 male homicides are a result of intimate partner violence. Oregon reports that between 1997 and 2001, 50% of in-state female homicides (151) were murdered by intimate partners, whereas only 4% of in-state male homicides were murdered by intimate partners between 1997 and 2001.[8] Homicides are the second leading cause of death in 15-24 year olds and the third leading cause of death in 25-34 year olds in the United States.[1] Women aged 20-24 are at highest risk for nonfatal intimate partner violence.[9,10] While these figures are significant, it is even more alarming to realize these rates may be underestimated, as many victims do not report incidences of IPV to the police, to family, or even to health care providers.[4]

Stalking is often included among types of IPV. Stalking generally refers to "harassing or threatening behavior that an individual engages in repeatedly, such as following a person, appearing at a person's home or place of business, making harassing phone calls, leaving written messages or objects, or vandalizing a person's property."[11,12] In the United States 503 485 women are stalked annually by intimate partners.[4] IPV takes many forms and familiarity with each one is necessary in order to identify and assess the violence and assist the victims.

Both women and men suffer and perpetrate IPV; however, 85% of victims of IPV are women, while men make up the other 15% of victims.[5] Women who perpetrate violence as teens or young adults often have childhood experiences of violence. DiNapoli[13] notes that for some girls, the strongest predictor of committing future violence is their experience of past victimization and violence. In essence, victimized girls may perpetuate the cycle of abuse. When women engage in IPV, it often occurs as a reciprocal event in an argument or self-protection in the context of victimization.[14] Furthermore, Kelly and Johnson[15] note female IPV usually manifests in *situational couple violence* versus *coercive controlling violence* more commonly exhibited by male abusers. This chapter will address women as victims of IPV, not as perpetrators.

PRACTITIONER IMPACT ON IPV

Health care practitioners, such as nurses, nurse practitioners, physicians' assistants, and physicians, specifically providing care to women can make a difference through early assessment of and intervention on behalf of patients and families affected by intimate partner violence. Often a woman's only visit for health services may be for her yearly well-woman examination and periodic screening. These visits offer opportunities for assessment and individualized discussion about IPV; however, almost half of the victims of intimate partner femicide were seen in health care settings in the year preceding their death[16] but went undetected as victims of abuse. Two hundred and ninety women in prenatal health care clinics were asked if they were assessed for IPV at their last prenatal visit and they unanimously reported they had not been assessed. Within this group, 36% had been battered with slaps, kicks, punches, and choking.[17] Health care providers need to increase their comfort level with assessment of IPV and their ability to safely advise and appropriately refer in such situations.

IPV assessment can be defined as assessing clients for harm or risk for harm in their intimate relationships.[18] Health care practitioners must be vigilant, ready to pick up on both subtle and overt cues of victimization, and take advantage of identification and assessment instruments to help target those in need. Two common tools for assessment and intervention easily incorporated into clinic visits are the RACE tool for identification and assessment and Campbell's Danger Assessment.[19]

THEORETICAL FRAMEWORK

The *socio-ecological model* offers health care practitioners and others a means to see the "gestalt" when considering important individual aspects that influence violence in the lives of women and their families (see **Figure 4-1**). The Centers for Disease Control (CDC) and many other organizations and individuals have adopted the socio-ecological model as the framework to understand and target interventions toward preventing violence in the United States.[20,21] The framework consists of multiple, interacting levels to understand the relationship between violence and potential prevention strategies.[22]

The first level of the socio-ecological model is personal or individual risk factors for violence, including an individual's unique psychological characteristics; physical factors, such as age, income, education, and substance abuse; and immediate physical setting, such as one's home (see **Figure 4-1**).[21] The second level examines close relationships that may also increase the risk for becoming either a perpetrator or a victim of IPV. These relationships may be with close friends, partners, or family members. Prevention strategies would be aimed at mentoring and peer prevention programs. The third level identifies neighborhoods, schools, or workplaces, locations where social relationships occur outside of family and close friendships. This could include interaction with health care, education, and social service providers.[23] Societal norms, strategies, and policies are affected at this level of impact. The fourth and last level is the societal level. Looking with a broader perspective, societal factors can create a climate that either repels or encourages intimate partner violence. Other factors evaluated at this level include educational, health, economic, and societal policies.

PERSONAL RISK FACTORS FOR INTIMATE PARTNER VIOLENCE

Many women in a partner relationship can be at risk for intimate partner violence, as the above statistics reveal. Risk factors for IPV are multifactorial. Although risk factors have been segregated into categories in this chapter, it is important to remember that factors from one level influence on all remaining levels in this conceptualization. When risk increases in one part of a woman's life, it can impact frequency and severity of intimate partner violence.

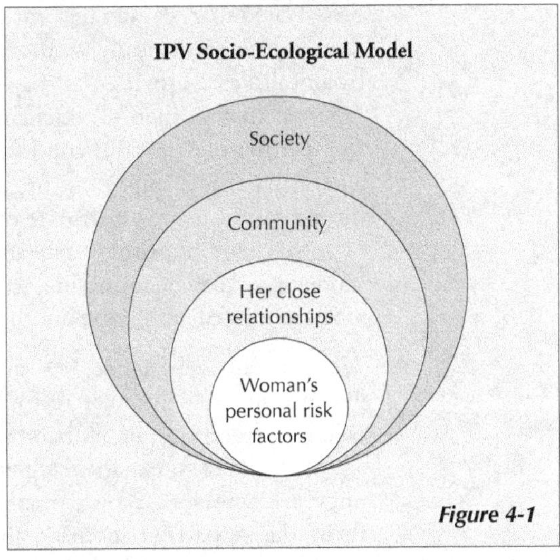

Figure 4-1.
Gerardi model of intimate partner violence (adapted from Bronfenbrenner's Ecological Systems Theory).

Personal factors associated with risk[24] are listed in **Figure 4-2**. There are five risk factors that bear special consideration and reflection by health care providers and may increase risk for IPV. These risk factors include young age, senescence, pregnancy, chronic diseases and conditions, and disability. Perhaps women in these vulnerable populations experience increased risk of IPV because of the additional financial burden, social isolation, and emotional dependency they commonly bear.[25,26] Screening for these at-risk groups should be individualized to each practice setting.

PREGNANCY

Pregnancy deserves special consideration as a period of time placing particular medical, psychological, emotional, and financial burdens on an otherwise healthy female. A pregnant woman spends a good deal of time attending to medical appointments where attention is given to her and to her unborn child. This focus diverts her attention and her health care provider's attention from her partner. In some partner relationships, this change in balance is enough to begin a cycle of abuse.

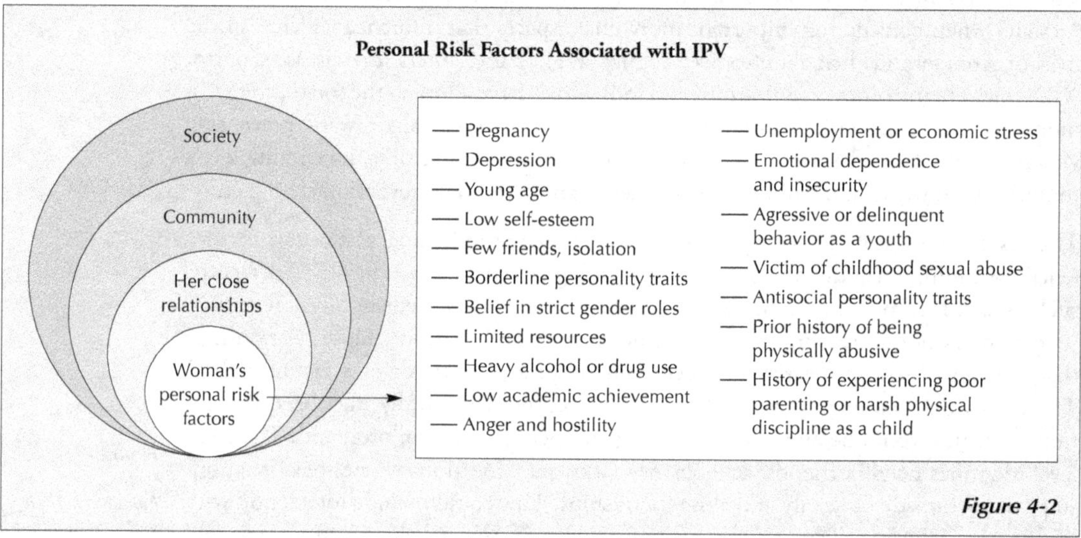

Figure 4-2. *Factors associated with risk for IPV.*

Women in abusive relationships may lose much of their ability to make contraceptive choices and engage in proactive family planning activities. *The WHO Multi-Country Study*[3] cited that women become pregnant out of fear of implied violence, fear of asking their partners to comply with contraceptive needs, and even fear of violence discovery by a health care provider, so they do not seek prenatal care or contraception. Gee et al[27] reported that women experiencing IPV were more likely to agree with the statement "my partner makes it difficult to use birth control." Abusive partners may also sabotage a woman's efforts to prevent pregnancy. This can take the form of removing a condom during coitus, using a perforate condom, or hiding a woman's birth control medication or apparatus.[28] In primary care and family planning settings, a major marker to identify hidden IPV may be found in a woman's acknowledgement of her partner's refusal to use a condom or to let her use another form of contraception.[29]

Women who experience IPV are more likely than women who do not experience violence in their intimate relationships to have unprotected coitus and to seek post-coital contraception or abortion services.[27,30] When women seek abortion services, they are more likely to experience greater severity of IPV as the number of abortions they undergo increases.[31] Approximately 1 out of 5 women experiencing IPV will not tell their abusive partner about an abortion.[32] Non-disclosure to the abuse partner (father of the pregnancy) is related to closed or difficult communication patterns or subsequent lack of contact. Clinical services and intervention needs are thus heightened for women experiencing both an abortion and IPV. Furthermore, women who have abortions are more likely to experience greater severity of physical and sexual assaults from former partners than current partners. It is important to encourage patients in practice settings to reconsider safety plans during and after this procedure.

Forced pregnancy is a means to force control women, especially teens, to stay in violent relationships. Some women who are raped by their partners do become pregnant. These pregnancies provide abusers a continued means to be involved in the victim's life, perpetuating the cycle of violence. Clinicians should be able to tell their patients about medical counseling on pregnancy options, legal counseling about protective orders, and psychological counseling about IPV.

IPV during pregnancy can be lethal and femicide is the most common cause of injury-related maternal deaths in the United States.[6] Ten percent of all assault-related injuries to women of reproductive age occurred during pregnancy, and women assaulted during pregnancy are 3 times more likely to be hospitalized as a result[33] and 3 times more likely than their nonpregnant counterparts to be the victim of a successful or attempted femicide.[34] 45% of pregnant women report a history of IPV, while the incidence of IPV during pregnancy ranges from 6% to 22%.[3,35] Pregnancy-associated homicides are most often committed by current or former intimate partners, usually during the first trimester.[36]

Women who experience physical and sexual abuse during pregnancy may sustain additional trauma to the body or fetus related to multiple factors. Women experiencing IPV may start care at a later gestational age and come more often for antenatal visits than women not experiencing IPV.[37] Women experiencing IPV may also be at increased risk for substance abuse. Pregnant women who abuse substances are at risk for intentional overdose and hospitalization. Injuries seen in clinics from physical abuse during pregnancy are diverse. Maternal effects of trauma may include preterm labor. Uterine rupture from a direct blow to the abdomen may result in fetal death.[38] Indirect fetal injury may result from placental abruption and fetomaternal hemorrhage. Fetal injury may also arise from gunshot wounds or stabbing injury to the abdomen. Lastly, IPV has been associated with low birth weight infants, fetal head trauma, and bone fractures.

Depression and posttraumatic stress disorder are more common among women experiencing IPV during pregnancy. Abuse during pregnancy has been associated with significantly higher rates of depression and suicide attempts.[39,40] Pregnancy-related depression has been linked to increased risk for low birth weight infants (<2500g) and preterm delivery (<37wk).[41] Maternal depression during pregnancy is also linked with increased irritability, decreased attentiveness, inactivity, and fewer facial expressions in infants. When new mothers experience IPV and depression, they may have difficulty with adequate bonding and attachment with their newborns.

Violence does not end with the delivery of the baby. A woman's experiences of IPV in the first year after delivery may be equal to or greater than experiences of violence during pregnancy.[42] The postpartum period often pressures relationships. This is especially true if unexpected outcomes, such as premature delivery, a serious medical condition, or a congenital anomaly, occur. The financial burdens of a healthy and medically uncompromised infant is great, but the expense of an unhealthy or compromised infant is even greater. Many families who struggled to make ends meet before pregnancy will be further taxed by loss of income related to work absences due to pregnancy.

It is important to use culturally sensitive and reliable tools to identify postpartum IPV, especially in women with a past history of childhood or spousal abuse. Many women in postpartum visits will not identify their partners' behavior as abusive when, in fact, IPV is present.[43] Resistance to identifying spousal abuse may present due to economic, familial, or cultural pressures to sustain spousal relationships and the perpetuation of violence as a "routine" part of a victim's worlds.

Very Young Women

Due to youth and inexperience, very young women are a vulnerable population. Their age alone is a risk factor for intimate partner violence and pregnancy, and as statistics show, the two combined can be lethal. Rennison[44] reports that between the ages of 15 and 19, 25% of teens report physical abuse, 14% report sexual abuse, and 90% report verbal abuse. Femicide, most often perpetrated by an intimate partner, is the primary cause of death in African American women aged 15 to 24 years and the secondary cause of death in white women in the same age group.[44-46]

Young women may experience abuse when entering new romantic relationships. Teens may lack the skills to create or negotiate healthy boundaries when meeting potential romantic partners, and even if they possess these social and relationship building skills, abusers may still target teens for opportunistic sexual gratification and dominance. Dating violence and rape are increasingly common among teens and involves either overt or covert manifestations of abuse. Several commonly used drugs may render a young woman unable to refuse sex and may cloud or eliminate her memory of the event. Common date rape drugs include GHB (gamma hydroxybutyric acid), ketamine (ketamine hydrochloride), or rohypnol (flunitrazepam).[47] Perpetrators may easily use these drugs because they lack color, odor, or taste and can be easily mixed into a beverage at parties or other social gatherings.

Teens have limited skills to navigate complex relationships, especially those involving controlling and abusive partners. For female adolescents, sexual behavior is most often linked with a desire for emotional commitment, while males typically view their early experimentation as more casual and directly fulfilling of sexual needs. For females attempting to enhance perceived relationship intimacy, the disparity between gender-based meanings of sexual behaviors may lead to greater sexual risk taking and vulnerability.

Research investigating young women's reasons for staying in abusive relationships is sparse, but it has been hypothesized to be related to that their reasons may need for social acceptance and peer approval.[48] It is concerning to note that most teens will stay in relationships with physically abusive males. Furthermore, over half of young women experiencing sexual violence will remain in abusive relationships. Teens in sexual relationships with abusive partners are also at risk for unplanned pregnancy. It is estimated that in the majority of teen pregnancies, the male partner is much older.[49] In age-discordant relationships, disproportionate control by an older partner may perpetuate cycles of violence.

Teenage females experiencing or having experienced IPV are much less likely to disclose abuse to health care providers and other care professionals. Professionals in health care settings or service agencies need to create environments conducive to safe disclosure and discussion of teen sexual experiences. Disclosure may enhance the likelihood of a more positive outcomes for teen IPV victims. Safe disclosure may allow for reframing of traumatic life events in a manner fostering decreased shame and stigmatization and may also reduce sexual risk behavior.

AGING

Older women in abusive relationships are commonly considered "hidden victims." IPV is often viewed by health care practitioners and the public as a problem of younger adulthood. One may encounter women who have been in abusive relationships for years before they disclose their experiences or seek assistance. Women may have attempted to leave an abusive spouse several decades ago when conversation about spousal abuse was taboo, often secret, and met resistance on several fronts. These women may be the group least likely to report abuse to law enforcement or legal professionals.

As they may have endured years of abusive maltreatment, many internal barriers may be present in older victims of IPV. Feelings of hopelessness, powerlessness, emotional gridlock, secrecy, and self-blame may reduce older women's ability to access help and disclose experiences of violence.[50] They may have stayed in abusive relationships for years, unable to leave for a variety of reasons, ranging from economic to an internalized belief that staying was better for the sake of their children.

When caring for older women in clinical settings, it is important to give them time, compassion, and a private setting to discuss their present relationship. Repeatedly, women describe health care practitioners' responses to abuse disclosures as less than supportive.[51] When women have chosen to stay with abusers, practitioners have often dismissed them and failed to discuss options to help them stay safer within their relationships. Although getting a woman out of a dangerous relationship is often a clinician's first response, an older woman may not feel comfortable leaving a partner of several decades. Women assisted with counseling at this point may be better able to break the cycle of violence later.

DISABILITIES AND IPV

Women with disabilities are at a higher risk for IPV. Estimates based on the 2011 American Community Survey (ACS) reported that 3% (16.3 million) of women in the United States, regardless of age, education, race, or ethnicity, experienced visual, hearing, or ambulatory disability.[52] Disabilities increase risk for all types of IPV in a dose-dependent manner, and this association has been frequently reported.[53,54] Physically disabled women are less likely to seek help or disclose abuse in health care settings for a variety of reasons, ranging from fear of retribution to heightened vulnerability due to isolation.[55] Many centers providing services for women with disabilities may overlook screening for IPV and resources and care facilities for such cases.

There are very few studies exploring the nature of IPV in the lives of women with intellectual disability (ID). It is estimated that 6 761 100, or slightly over 4.7%, of non-institutionalized women experience cognitive or intellectual disability of some form.[52] Taggert and colleagues reported that women with ID were at a much higher risk of IPV than those without ID.[56] It was also noted that women with ID were 1.5 times more likely to have experienced any form of violence in their childhood. These women then continue to experience violence with an abusive partner, and the cycle of violence continues. Health and social services for those experiencing ID are often not gender focused and, similar to physically disabled people experiencing IPV, opportunities to identify and intervene in cases of IPV are often missed. In some cases, women's physical and/or psychological disabilities are a direct result of trauma from IPV.

HIV

HIV infection is a global health care and societal concern. In 2008, it was estimated that there were 15.7 million women living with HIV/AIDS globally.[57] Rates for new infections in women, primarily from heterosexual transmission, are highest in Eastern

Europe, Central Asia, and Sub-Saharan Africa. Many new infections to children are thought to be acquired from *in utero*, delivery, or postpartum transmission from HIV-infected mothers. HIV intersects in the lives of women experiencing IPV in 2 major ways.[58] First, a woman may be exposed to infection from sexual coercion or IPV. Second, a woman who has HIV may be at additional risk to be victimized in an intimate relationship.

IPV may increase a woman's risk to be exposed to unsafe sexual practices, leading to the acquisition of HIV through direct transmission.[59] Women often have reduced protective powers as they lack control over sexual activities in abusive relationships with men who are HIV/AIDS-positive and frequently feel victimized by their male partners who infect them.[60] Risk of viral infection is greatest with repeated exposure to HIV, as is commonly experienced by women in relationships marked by physical and sexual IPV. Additionally, their partners may be more controlling and violent and more likely to have additional sexually transmitted infections.

Substance abuse, HIV/ STI risk, and IPV are entwined in the lives of many women. Transmission of HIV may come from partnering with an HIV-positive substance abuser. In a recent study examining these relationships in India, Berg et al[61] reported that physical and sexual IPV with a substance-abusing male partner was associated with an increased risk for HIV infection for a female partner. While under the influence of alcohol and other substances, male partners may be less tolerant of their partners' perceived shortcomings and engage in additional IPV.[61] Furthermore, male inhibitions to perpetrate IPV against female partners may be lowered under the influence of alcohol and other substances.

It is posited that living with an HIV infection poses several challenges in intimate relationships for women.[62] Often, HIV-positive women have limited resources and may be dependent on a romantic partner for shelter and food. Very early on in the HIV epidemic, Rothenberg and Paskey[63] reported that disclosure of infection to an abusive partner, regardless of his HIV status, could result in escalated IPV. Women in new relationships may be reluctant to disclose their HIV status, fearing this information will trigger the onset of IPV. HIV-positive women may experience a range of abusive behaviors by partners, including sexual slavery, confinement, stalking, threatening behaviors, physical assault, and sexual assault.[60] Often, IPV catalyzes declining health in women experiencing hopelessness, depression, and a decrease in health-related activities. These women may not go for HIV-related care, or they may miss appointments or stop antiretroviral therapy initiated earlier in the course of their disease.

PSYCHIATRIC CO-MORBIDITY

Problem behaviors in childhood and adolescence may signal risk conditions that enable future violence in the lives of women. Early behavioral problems, especially conduct disorder in childhood, were identified by Mason et al[64] as the strongest predictor for future violence risk in early adulthood. Seimer[65] comments that personality characteristics such as aggression, coercion, and dominance coupled with poor interpersonal skills may increase the risk of violence in intimate relationships. Daane[66] also links aggressive and acting-out behavior in young children as causally associated with adolescent violence risk.

Substance-abusing women may not have the power to negotiate safer sex and are at increased risk for violence in their intimate relationships.[67] Often times, women rely on male partners for drugs or support both of their habits by bartering sex for money. They may also engage in higher-risk activities while intoxicated or high. Because women are often "second on the needle," their continued use increases risk for HIV, hepatitis, and other sexually transmitted infections." If women try to stop using drugs, their partners may retaliate with escalating acts of violence.

In the literature, psychiatric patient status has been associated with violence risk.[68] Rice et al[69] noted that a diagnosis of schizophrenia or psychotic symptomatology was, in fact, negatively associated with violence risk. Appelbaum, Robbins, and Monahan[68] further explored these relationships by using data gathered from the MacArthur Violence Risk Assessment Study to examine whether delusional thought disorder was associated with increased risk for violence in recently discharged psychiatric patients. Their study did not support that relationship.

CLOSE RELATIONSHIPS

An intimate relationship may be loving, respectful, and trusting, but it may become violent as 1 partner tries to control the other. (**Figure 4-3** lists common relational risk factors.) In a case of IPV, factors that created or defined a relationship are no longer based on mutual trust and respect.

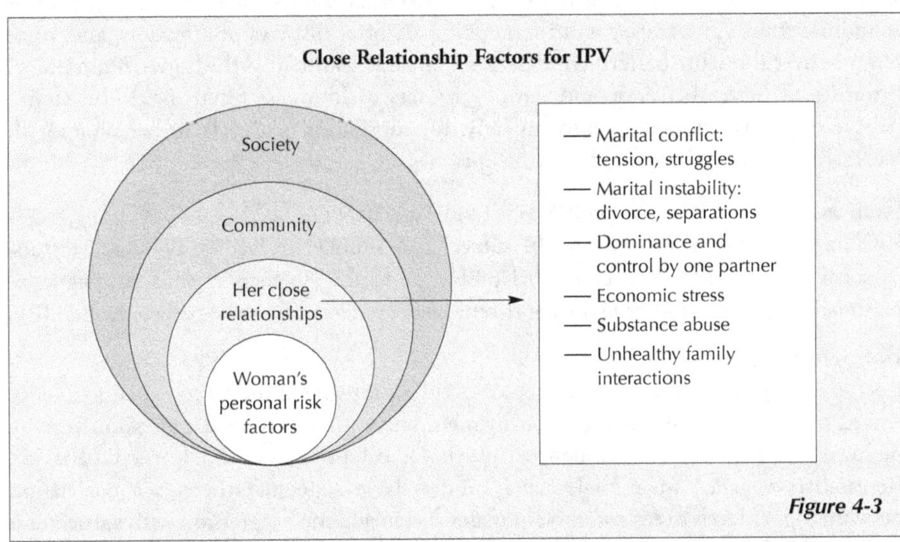

Figure 4-3.
Close relationship factors for IPV.

MARITAL OR RELATIONSHIP INSTABILITY AND BREAKDOWN

IPV may be sparked by 1 partner forcing the other to take actions not of their own choosing and are often physically or emotionally harmful. Early in the relationship, this may result in marital conflict and tension, and quickly escalate to unhealthy family relationships and interactions. Perpetrators may take power and control (the Duluth Model) by "using coercion and threats, intimidation, emotional abuse, isolation, minimizing, denying, blaming, and male privilege."[70] The perpetrator may also threaten children, threaten flight with them, or use them to spread misinformation. Further degradation of the familial relationship results in marital instability and ultimately separation and divorce adding economic stress to already strained marital and family relationships. It is during these times of stress that emotional and physical violence may surface for the first time. The slow and insidious nature of this development anchors the abused partner in the degrading relationship as they believe it will not happen again and/or that they "deserved" the violence because of their behavior.

Health care providers are often at a loss to understand why women remain in violent relationships, and thinking their patients are unwilling to take action, they often terminate counseling and related services when a woman does not immediately leave abusive partners. The stigma of a failed relationship and the degradation of single, female head of households[71,72] are two reasons that victims choose to stay in abusive relationship; however, when psychological abuse enters a victim's circle of influence, including friends and acquaintances, a victim is more likely to leave.[72] Knowing that and being a part of their patients' circles of influence, health care providers have a duty to provide safe environments and education to those in abusive relationships.

Lenore Walker[73] portrayed the progressive and cyclic nature of the abusive intimate partner relationships as *battered wife syndrome.* In her classic description, early in a relationship, conflict begins with escalating acts of intimidation, poor communication, verbal put-downs, and blaming. Out of fear, the victim may try to calm the perpetrator by staying out of his or her way and becoming passive, to avoid additional confrontation. The abuser becomes more possessive, cruel, and aggressive. Tension and stress continue to build over time, leading to an overt act of violence. The acute battering involves the acting out of domination and aggression in the form of physical, sexual, and psychological abuse. The abuser and even the victim may initially rationalize the event as being caused by behavior of the victim or external factors, such as work conflict or economic stress. The abuser will then apologize, offer displays of affection, and voice remorse over the acute battering incident(s), in what is known as the honeymoon phase. Promises of better behavior and temporary acts of kindness often make the victim believe the abuse will end. Unfortunately, for most, this is a cycle of behaviors with increasingly destructive acute battering episodes.

RISK FACTORS ASSOCIATED WITH PERPETRATION OF IPV

Risk for morbidity from IPV may be subject to a number of factors. Biological factors, personal traits or behaviors, emotional problems, family violence, psychiatric diagnoses, personality disorders, and drug use contribute to the potential for male perpetration of IPV.

Biological Factors

Boettcher[74] recommended the incorporation of an integrated model to explain violence risk as a multi-factorial phenomenon in men, encompassing innate aggression (drive), biological factors, societal influences, psychological processes, and learned behavior. Researchers engaged in animal analog studies have suggested there is a correlation between higher levels of testosterone in males and heightened aggression with subsequent violence.[75-77] Researchers have also investigated 4 other potential neurobehavioral aspects of violence involving frontal lobe and amygdala dysfunction, low cortisol reactivity, altered neurotransmitter metabolism (primarily serotonin), and hereditary predisposition.[75,78-80] There is controversy in the literature about potential associations between mental disorders and increased risk for violence.[69] In non-psychiatric patient adults, antisocial personality disorder of a male partner was noted by Rice et al[69] as a predicting factor associated with increased violence risk for women.

Higher levels of anger and hostility are present in men who engage in IPV versus men who do not.[81] It is thought that high levels of anger in some males may decrease inhibitions against IPV, either by justifying the abusive response or interrupting a more normative cognitive response that would suppress such violence. When assessing a male's potential for violence, the past may hold clues to future behavior. Men with significant criminal history or a history of violence may be more likely to commit violence in an intimate relationship. Difficulty with past interpersonal relationships may also identify males at heightened risk for IPV. If a male has a history of severe or frequent violence toward partners, troubled or no friendships, and dysfunctional family dynamics, he is more likely to have problematic intimate relationships in the future.

Substance Abuse

If a male is a heavy drug or alcohol abuser, he presents a heightened risk for IPV in an intimate relationship, especially if he uses daily. Substance abuse and addiction as a moderating variable is readily supported in the literature as a factor associated with violence risk in both male adolescents and adults. Daane[66] and Seimer[65] cited multiple sources that strongly suggest positive associations between the use of cigarettes, alcohol, marijuana, and other illegal drugs with violence risk, especially in school settings. Substance abuse has also been associated with risk of violence in adulthood, especially in male-female intimate relationships.[82,83] Additionally, prior drug abuse and addiction history have been associated with teenage and adult female victimization.[84,85]

Ownership of Weapons

It is always important to ask about access weapons, especially firearms, in abusive relationships and to ask patients experiencing IPV about this concern. The presence of weapons in a couple's residence or with an abuser may signal increased risk and potential for femicide. Male IPV perpetrators are more likely to have weapons in their homes than non-violent males.[86] According to Sorenson and Wiebe,[86] approximately 65% of abused women reported that their abusers used weapons to perpetrate emotional IPV in the form of threats of harm when firearms were present in their homes. The majority of those women noted that the threat was to kill or harm them. Threats with weapons are also made against those whom victims may care for; children, friends, and pets are common targets for abusive partners.[87]

SAME-SEX RELATIONSHIPS

Intimate partner violence can also occur in same-sex relationships. Although it has been generally believed that rates of same sex intimate partner violence (SSIPV) are comparable to rates in heterosexual relationships,[88,89] findings from a more contemporary study suggest this often hidden group may be at greater risk. Messinger[90] analyzed data from the National Violence Against Women Survey and reported that women in same-sex relationships are more likely to experience verbal, physical, and sexual IPV than women in heterosexual relationships. This is thought to be because members of this victim group have experienced IPV at the hands of both male and female perpetrators. Tjaden et al[91] found that male partners pose a greater risk for IPV than female partners in same-sex relationships. In their study, 30.4% of victims were raped or physically abused by male partners while only 11.4% were raped or physically abused by female partners. It may be difficult for a woman in a health care setting to talk about her same-sex relationship, even in a general fashion. Many women in same-sex relationships have experienced hostility and stigma when disclosing their sexual orientation and fear even greater negativity if they try to access services to cope with experiences of violence in their lives.[92] If they report IPV, they may have difficulty receiving the same type of services offered to heterosexual victims by law enforcement, prosecutors, and the judicial system.[93,94] Some health care providers who provide services to same-sex victims of IPV may be inexperienced or lack the necessary training to provide effective services to this special population.[92] There are few agencies dedicated to same-sex victims of IPV, and most domestic violence services do not offer programs to meet the unique needs of this group.[95]

CHILDREN

Children are affected by IPV in multiple ways as both witnesses and casualties. Often, children are used by perpetrators to hurt their partners. This is done by denying access to the child by means of flight from the city, state, or even the country with the child. A perpetrator may also use a child to emotionally and psychologically control a victim. A perpetrator may try to emotionally manipulate a child or children to make them believe the victim is the source of familial distress or use them to relay hurtful information or comments. If a child recognizes that the mother is the victim of IPV, family roles can become distorted as the child tries to shield or protect the victim in cases of physical or sexual violence.[96] This dynamic gives them a sense of responsibility and obligation to stop the abuse cycle, often at an age at which they are not emotionally, physically, or developmentally ready to intervene. Living in a home with IPV will be evident in subsequent behavioral and emotional problems as well as difficulties in forming future relationships.[97,98] Children may also be injured by physical and sexual abuse.[99] Physical abuse by a perpetrator could include hitting the face, punching the body, kicking, or hitting with a variety of objects. Oftentimes, sexual and physical abuse concur and may involve multiple occurrences over time.

COMMUNITY/SOCIETAL FACTORS

Swanger and Petcosky[100] differentiate women's risk for experiencing violence by macro-level analysis of the nature of socially-structured variables. Patients in today's health care settings come from many different cultural backgrounds. Patients and their families may have a different worldview and set of experiences related to the role of women in intimate relationship and the value of women in society.

This is especially problematic in regions of the world ravaged by warfare. Women are often traumatized by societal violence and rape by invading aggressors and devalued by their partners and communities upon their perpetrators' departure. Collective violence is rooted in competitive behavior between groups. Goldstein[101] writes that an "us versus them" mind-set may escalate aggression and violence toward another racial, ethnic, economic, or religious group identified as "other." Stewart[102] commented, in regard to the "group motivation hypothesis," that scapegoating and group resentment may lead to violence, as evidenced in last century's genocides. Oftentimes, this violence is directed toward women. He also stated in the "green war" hypothesis that groups will engage in violence for access to scarce resources. Using resource control acquisition as a causal theory of violence risk may be supported by violence in nations experiencing economic inequity and increased population density.[82,83,103]

Barzelatto asserts that violence stems from power imbalance, injustice, and a lack of democracy in society as a whole. On a micro-system level, gender-based violence against women is thought to share macro-system causes, as described.[83,84] Special groups of concern for violence risk include female adolescents and sex workers, who are deemed more vulnerable due to both to their limited resources and power base.[66,84,85]

Members of groups, cultures, and societies with positive attitudes toward male dominance are more likely to tolerate or accept IPV.[104] Acceptance of violence against women is also related rigid gender roles and inequity between men and women.[105] Commonly, women are given less financially productive activities in the workforce and have less economic independence when compared with males, leading to economic inequity.[106] Higher rates of IPV are found in urban communities with lower residential mobility, pronounced social isolation, and low income.[107] These and other factors associated with increased risk for IPV, are maintained by social control of prevalent religious or ethical codes and established legal systems.[108] **Figure 4-4** depicts the community and societal factors beyond individuals and individual relationships that can encourage or discourage intimate partner violence.

Community-level analysis of violence risk also involves examining person-to-person violence from a socio-psychological perspective.[100] Bandura[109] and others have suggested that violence is learned and repeated by observation and modeling of individuals displaying aggressive behavior and committing acts of violence.[75,110,111] Seimer[65] suggests

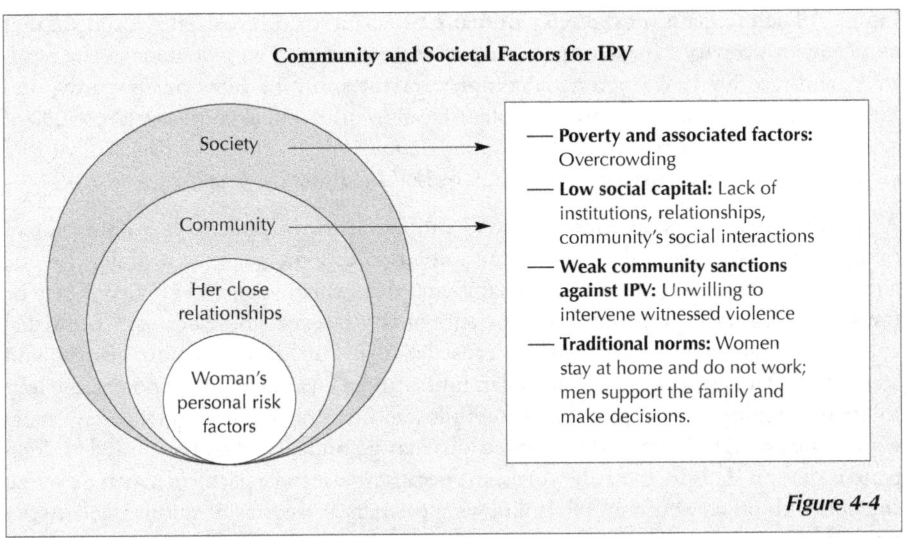

Figure 4-4.
Community and societal factors for IPV

that children who watch their parents use violence to resolve conflict will be more likely to engage in or see violence as acceptable in future relationships.

Risk for violence has also been associated with environmental factors. Although school violence receives a great deal of press and media attention, Daane[66] notes that children and teens are more likely to exhibit, witness, or be victimized by violence in their home or community. Childhood exposure to a dysfunctional family unit may also be associated in other ways with the development of violent tendencies in adolescence and adulthood.[112,113] Tarter and colleagues associated future risk for violence with childhood exposure to parents who are substance abusers, have psychiatric disorders, and provide inadequate supervision. Family instability, maternal rejection, marital conflict, and an absent or rejecting father have also been associated with a greater potential for male children to later engage in violence or female children to experience IPV in future relationships.[83,114]

CONSEQUENCES OF IPV

FINANCIAL CONSEQUENCES

The financial cost of intimate partner violence to women in the United States exceeded $5.8 billion in 1995, according to the CDC in a survey performed in 2003.[115] 1.8 billion dollars was the indirect cost related to lost productivity, and victims of severe IPV lost close to 8 million days of work productivity. Direct medical costs were 4.8 billion.[115] These costs increased most dramatically with physical abuse; however, costs also increased with emotional and sexual abuse. Lloyd and Tulac[117] report that women and children whose lives are threatened or who are not allowed to continue school are more likely to be unemployed, be on public assistance, and have health problems.

PHYSICAL CONSEQUENCES

The physical consequences of IPV most often thought of are injury, specifically trauma, to the victim. As the number of times a person is on the receiving end of IPV increases, the encounters are associated with increasingly severe injury.[118,119] The cycle of violence escalates in severity as time passes.[120] What might have started as emotional abuse progresses to physical abuse. Physical violence that in the beginning may be a shove or a slap progresses to a hitting, punching, and kicking. Eventually, IPV may result in death.

It is important to recognize patterns of acute trauma related to IPV in order to identify and intervene in cases of covert IPV. Most traumas to women will be inflicted by abusers slapping with their hands or striking with their fists and most will involve soft tissue injury.[121] Their target is most often a woman's face. Saddki and colleagues[122] suggest that clinicians in primary care settings should assess any woman with trauma to the head, neck, and face for IPV. Zygomatic complex fractures, orbital blow-out fractures, and intracranial injuries are the most prevalent facial injuries and account for over 50% of severe trauma associated with IPV.[123] Strangulation is experienced by over half of IPV victims, yet often remains a covert marker of IPV in clinical settings.[121]

A second type of physical consequence of intimate partner violence is a result not of injury but of disease. All sexually transmitted infections, such as syphilis, herpes, gonorrhea, bacterial vaginosis, human papilloma virus, chlamydia, and HIV,[120,124] may be transmitted from the perpetrator to the victim of IPV if sexual abuse occurs. Chlamydial and gonococcal cervical infections can cause fallopian tube inflammation, abscess, and scarring.[125] Damage to a female's fallopian tubes can be lifelong and may potentially lead to life-threatening ectopic pregnancy, infertility, and chronic pain. Unfortunately, many women are asymptomatic, and such infections may go undetected and untreated for long periods of time. This is especially worrisome because abuse male partners may hide sexual contacts with others and put their unknowing partners at risk for infection. Lag between time of infection to time of treatment leads to greater rates of disease transmission and increased health risks. The most common consequences are listed in **Table 4-1**.

Table 4-1. Health Consequences of Intimate Partner Violence

PHYSICAL	PSYCHOLOGICAL AND BEHAVIORAL
— Abdominal/thoracic injuries	— Alcohol and drug abuse
— Bruises and welts	— Depression and anxiety
— Chronic pain syndromes	— Eating and sleep disorders
— Disability	— Feelings of shame and guilt
— Fibromyalgia	— Phobias and panic disorder
— Fractures	— Physical inactivity
— Gastrointestinal disorders	— Poor self-esteem
— Irritable bowel syndrome	— Post-traumatic stress disorder
— Lacerations and abrasions	— Psychosomatic disorders
— Ocular damage	— Smoking
— Reduced physical functioning	— Suicidal behavior and self-harm
— Sexual and reproductive	— Unsafe sexual behavior
— Gynecological disorders	— Fatal health consequences
— Infertility	— AIDS-related mortality
— Pelvic inflammatory disease	— Maternal mortality
— Pregnancy complications/miscarriage	— Homicide
— Sexual dysfunction	— Suicide
— Sexually transmitted diseases, including HIV/AIDS	
— Unsafe abortion	

Adapted from Heise L, Garcia Moreno C.[126]

Victims of IPV have higher rates of cervical cancer than non-victims.[124,127] Human papilloma virus (HPV) is now considered the most prevalent viral sexually transmitted infection.[128] Over 30 types of HPV virus withan affinity for reproductive tract surface epithelia (basal layer) and mucous membranes have been identified and classified by number. Among these viruses, the risks differ between those considered low-risk (eg, Types 6 and 11), moderate-risk (eg, Types 31 and 33), and high-risk (eg, Types 16 and 18) due to their increased potential as cancer-causing agents. Females are biologically at a greater risk from HPV. Because the virus targets rapidly dividing epithelial basal cells found in the cervix transformation zone, adolescent females are particularly vulnerable.[129] HPV is commonly found in areas prone to micro trauma during sexual activity, such as the female introitus. This region may be more vulnerable to infection when unwanted sexual contact or sexual IPV occurs. Rogers and colleagues[130] reported that anogential trauma was detected in 68% of the women they examined after forced coitus. Over one third of those experiencing anogential injuries had multiple sites of trauma. The pregnancy-related immuno-suppression mechanism also increases risk of viral infection in females.

There are also indirect effects of physical violence and sexual assault, some short lived, others long lasting. These often hidden consequences include suicidal thoughts and suicide attempts, depression, anxiety, pregnancy, and resultant adverse effects on maternal and neonatal outcomes.[127,131-133] The chronic stress experienced by IPV victims affects the endocrine and immune systems.[134,135] Resulting consequences may include: fibromyalgia, gynecological disorders, irritable bowel syndrome, central nervous system disorders, sexually transmitted diseases, gastrointestinal disorders, and heart and circulatory disorders.

Morbidity related to abused pregnant women must take into account 2 victims, the mother and her baby. Oftentimes, the gravid abdomen is kicked, punched, or hit, which may result in spontaneous loss of the pregnancy, abruption, late entry into prenatal care, stillbirth, premature labor, delivery, and of course, femicide.[131-133,136]

Psychological Consequences

The experience of IPV commonly results in psychological consequences for its victims.[137] It is often difficult to identify whether psychological dysfunction or stressors were present prior to abuse or whether the experience of violence was the etiologic factor in the development of mental health problems. It has been well established that there is a significant difference in the experience of negative psychological sequela between women experiencing IPV and those who have not experienced violence.[138-140] Common psychological consequences include: depression; suicidal behavior; anxiety disorders including PTSD; and substance abuse.[141,142] When abuse occurs in intimate relationships, emotional and affective changes of personality and psychological milieu may arise from victimization.[143] These changes may include lowered self-esteem, inability to trust romantic partners or others, fear of intimacy, anger, shame, feelings of helplessness, emotional detachment, and the intrusive and recurrent remembrances of degrading experiences in the victim's mind.[144]

Long-Term Health Consequences

Women with a history of IPV have more chronic health concerns, and more frequently report poor health, and unhealthy lifestyle choices than women who have not been exposed to IPV.[133] Relationships marked by months or years of IPV may lead to activation of the HPA axis and dysregulation of normal cortisol production, which has been linked to cardiovascular disease and other disease states, such as diabetes.[145] Furthermore, stressors experienced in IPV may also initiate immune dysregulation across a wide range of immune responses, especially when this stress is chronic. In a recent national study,[146] the CDC included questions about both general health status and IPV experiences.[147] Not surprisingly, when women experienced IPV, their number of unhealthy behaviors and long-term, serious health consequences were significantly greater. Increased cardiovascular risk was demonstrated in higher adjusted odds ratios for women experiencing IPV, 1.1 aOR for elevated cholesterol, 1.4 aOR for heart disease, and 1.4 aOR for stroke versus risk for women who did not experience violence. Similarly, rates of joint disease and asthma were also higher in abused women. The more severe the violence, the stronger the correlation with negative health behaviors by victims.[119,126,148,149]

ASSESSMENT, IDENTIFICATION, AND INTERVENTION FOR IPV IN THE WOMEN'S HEALTH CARE SETTING

Women entering health care settings may be reluctant to disclose their experiences of IPV to a health care practitioner due to uncertainty.[150] They may be uncertain whether their stories will be believed, what can be done, and if they can truly break free from their abuser. Having posters and pamphlets openly displayed about IPV may send a signal to women that the practice setting they are in and the practitioners who will care for them are responsive and supportive of IPV disclosure. Health care professionals in clinical settings also need tools and support to effectively screen and provide services for at-risk adolescents and women in order to decrease the risk of harmful sequela related to experiences of IPV.

By examining these issues, health care professionals (HCPs) may better understand how to talk with women about their relationships in ways that encourages open communication. This dialogue can lead to the design and implementation of medical, psychological, and legal interventions intended to reduce violence in the lives of women. Early recognition of the need for identification and assessment of IPV to every woman was noted by both the American Nurses Association (ANA) and the American Medical Association (AMA) recommending health care providers routinely assess for intimate partner violence.[151,152]

Unfortunately, some health care providers in women's health care settings may be reluctant to screen for IPV. The Agency for Health care Research and Quality (AHRQ)[153] reported that providers may omit identification and assessment due to lack of training; limited confidence in their ability to ask the right questions to identify abuse; and uncertainty about what to do after identifying IPV where to refer, or how to counsel clients. HCPs may be worried that asking questions about violence will offend their patients. They may also fear for their own safety should identifying IPV lead to abuser retaliation. Lastly, some HCPs are unsure whether intervening will make a difference.

When considering a screening tool or questions for screening in your practice, defining IPV, measuring its severity, and noting the length/temporal aspects of IPV is key. It is important to compare screening tools because some focus on physical and sexual aspects of violence without exploring elements of emotional and psychological violence.[154] Several good instruments with adequate internal consistency are available to implement as aids in assessing and intervening in cases of IPV. Commonly used IPV tools include the Hurt, Insult, Threaten, and Scream (HITS), the Danger Assessment (DA), the Woman Abuse Screening Tool/Woman Abuse Screening Tool-Short Form (WAST/WAST-SF), the Partner Violence Screen (PVS), and the Abuse Assessment Screen (AAS)[15,155] and RACE tools. These instruments vary from 3 to 20 questions in length, have documented reliability and validity, and have been extensively used for identification and assessment of IPV.

It is essential to select the tool that best matches your practice needs. Some tools can be effectively modified; for example, the AAS has been widely used to screen for women's past and current history of IPV in pregnancy but is commonly modified to be used with non-pregnant patients as well.[156] Some may be used without modification or cost. The Danger Assessment[15] measures episodes and severity of IPV in the past year, rates risk for victim homicide by the perpetrator, and is available in Spanish, French, and Portuguese language versions.

After identifying that a client is currently experiencing IPV, identifying available options for action is appropriate. It is up the the client to decide whether or not to take action and when any action is to take place. Available programs and services, such as alternative housing, follow-up services, safety plans, legal actions and assistance, advocate assistance escape plans, and future education and training, are just possible referrals and should be offered to the victim. It has been well established that the time during and immediately following an attempt to leave an abusive partner is the most dangerous time for life threatening injury and femicide related to IPV.[157] Patients may not be able to leave their relationships immediately, so it is important to establish a safety plans before they leave the practice setting. Safety plans may enable patients to plan for contingencies and future escapes in a way that reduces harm to them and their children. In many larger cities, agencies dedicated to assisting victims of IPV are available for patient care. In smaller cities and rural areas, it is important to gather contact information from social work service agencies, local women's shelters, and legal aid in advance of anticipated need. Hot line numbers for telephone crisis intervention and information may be useful. Lastly, as victims' rights and legal protection vary widely from state to state, it is imperative to know what your city and state can do to protect your patient.

CONCLUSION

Although focusing on the aftermath of IPV has been important in clinical practice to intervene for the well being of survivors, examining why IPV arises and what makes individuals vulnerable to harm could, in the long term, be a more effective and preventative approach. If all health care practitioners design assessments and interventions based on solid research to intervene with those at risk for engaging in aggression and violence as well as build resistance and resiliency skills in those who may be vulnerable, perhaps the cycle of IPV could be circumvented. While risk factors for those most at risk for IPV in both the perpetrator and victim role are identified in this chapter, so also is the current identification and screening of those affected within the women's healthcare setting. The Agency for Healthcare Research and Quality[158] indicates the need for universal, evidence-based screening, detection, and identification of IPV. More detailed research on screening for IPV, more effective treatments for IPV victims, and improved methods for identifying, treating, and prosecuting IPV perpetrators are absolutely essential.

APPENDIX 4-1: RESOURCES

Appendix 4-1: Resources
An Abuse, Rape, and Domestic Violence Aid and Resource Collection www.aardvarc.org A website for victims of violence, their families and friends, and the a public and private agencies and programs that serve them. *(continued)*

<table><tr><td>

Appendix 4-1: Resources *(continued)*

The American Congress of Obstetricians and Gynecologists (ACOG)
www.acog.org/About_ACOG/ACOG_Departments/Violence_Against_Women
Information on state coalitions, screening tools (English and Spanish), fact
sheets, and materials for practice.

Alianza- National Latino Alliance for the Elimination of Domestic Violence
www.dvalianza.org
An alliance established as one of three domestic violence "cultural institutes"
to address needs and concerns of communities of color experiencing family
violence. Alianza works in 4 main areas: community education, policy advocacy,
research, and training and technical assistance.

The Americans Overseas Domestic Violence Crisis Center
www.866uswomen.org
A crisis center that can be reached internationally toll-free from 175 countries
that serves Americans overseas by providing domestic violence advocacy, safety
planning, case management and assisting with relocation, and funds for housing,
childcare, and legal fees.

Centers for Disease Control and Prevention – Intimate Partner Violence
www.cdc.gov/ViolencePrevention/intimatepartnerviolence/index.html
Resources include a program activities guide on prevention initiatives,
handbooks with intimate partner violence and sexual violence assessment tools,
risk factors lists, and prevention strategies.

Danger Assessment
www.dangerassessment.org
Site with resources, training opportunities, and a link to Dr. J. Campbell's
Danger Assessment tool.

Domestic Violence Brochures
voices.yahoo.com/download-free-domestic-violence-brochures-these-6937488.html
A site with links to a number of free domestic violence brochures for use in the
clinic and community.

Faith Trust Institute
www.faithtrustinstitute.org/resources
Training and educational resources for faith-based communities to address sexual
and domestic violence.

The National Netowrk to End Domestic Violence (NNEDV)
http://www.nnedv.org/about.html
Dedicated to ending violence against women by promoting social change, both
communal and political.

LEAP- Look to End Abuse Permanently
www.leapsf.org
An organization of health care providers and volunteers dedicated to ending intimate
partner violence and family violence by establishing screening, treatment, and preven-
tion programs in the health care setting. Incudes resources for practitioners
and patients.

(continued)

</td></tr></table>

Appendix 4-1: Resources *(continued)*

National Center on Elder Abuse
www.ncea.aoa.gov/
Resource topics include potential abusers, causation theories, cultural considerations, prevalence and incidence, and relationships.

National Clearinghouse on Abuse in Later Life (NCALL)
(608) 255-0539 or www.ncall.us
Nationally recognized leader on program development, policy, and technical assistance and training that addresses the nexus between domestic violence, sexual assault, and elder abuse.

National Coalition Against Domestic Violence
www.ncadv.org
A national information and referral center for the general public, media, battered women and their children, and allied agencies and organizations.

National Domestic Violence Hotline
800-787-3224 or www.thehotline.org
A nonprofit organization that provides crisis intervention, information and referral to victims and perpetrators of domestic violence as well as their friends and families. They will provide phone numbers of local domestic violence shelters and other resources.

National Online Resource Center on Violence Against Women
www.vawnet.org
A resource library with thousands of materials on violence against women and related issues, particularly the intersections between violence against women and various forms of oppression.

National Sexual Assault Hotline
800-656-4673 or www.rainn.org/get-help/national-sexual-assault-online-hotline
A hotline connecting victims with counselors in their area. The hotline may be accessed online through the Rape, Abuse and Incest National Network Web site.

National Sexual Violence Resource Center
www.nsvrc.org
The NSVRC's Mission is to provide leadership in preventing and responding to sexual violence through collaboration, sharing and creating resources, and promoting research.

Rape, Abuse and Incest National Network (RAINN)
1-800-656-4673 or www.rainn.org
RAINN operates the National Sexual Assault Hotline and Online Hotline; publicizes the hotline's free, confidential services; educates the public about sexual assault; and leads national efforts to prevent sexual assault, improve services to victims, and ensure that rapists are brought to justice.

Women's Aid
www.womensaid.org.uk
A UK site offering 24-hour hotline, advocacy, and support services for women and children.

REFERENCES

1. Centers for Disease Control and Prevention. *Intimate Partner Violence Definitions.* Atlanta, GA: Centers for Disease Control; 2013. Centers for Disease Control Web site. http://www.cdc.gov/ViolencePrevention/intimatepartnerviolence/index.html. Accessed April 23, 2013.

2. Cooley-Strickland M, Quille T, Griffin RS, et al. Community violence and youth: affect, behavior, substance use, and academics. *Clin Child Fam Psychol Rev.* 2009;12(2):127-156.

3. World Health Organization. *The WHO Multi-country Study of Women's Health and Domestic Violence Against Women. Summary of Initial Reports on Prevalence, Outcomes and Women's Responses.* Geneva, Switzerland: World Health Organization; 2005. http://www.who.int/gender/violence/who_multicountry_study/summary_report/en/index.html. Accessed August 27, 2013.

4. Tjaden P, Thoennes N. *Extent, Nature, And Consequences Of Intimate Partner Violence: Findings From The National Violence Against Women Survey.* Washington, DC: US Department of Justice; 2000. Publication No. NCJ 181867. www.ojp.usdoj.gov/nij/pubs-sum/181867.htm. Accessed August 27, 2013.

5. Rennison CM. *Intimate Partner Violence,* 1993-2001. Washington, DC: United States Department of Justice; 2003. NCJ 197838. Bureau of Justice Statistics Web site. http://www.bjs.gov/content/pub/pdf/ipv01.pdf. Accessed August 30, 2013.

6. Gunter J. Intimate partner violence. *Obstet Gynecol Clin North Am.* 2007;34:367-388.

7. Puzone CA, Saltzman LE, Kresnow MM, Thompson MP, Mercy JA. National trends in intimate partner homicide. *Violence Against Women.* 2000;6:409-426.

8. Drach L. *Intimate Partner Homicide In Oregon 1997-2003.* Portland, OR: Oregon Department of Human Services, Office of Disease Prevention and Epidemiology; 2004.Oregon Health Authority Web site. oregon.gov/DHS/ph/ipv/docs/IPV_Homocide97-03.pdf. Accessed September 17, 2013.

9. National Center for Injury Prevention and Control. *Costs of Intimate Partner Violence Against Women in the United States.* Atlanta, GA: Centers for Disease Control and Prevention; 2003. Centers for Disease Control Web site. http://www.cdc.gov/violenceprevention/pdf/ipvbook-a.pdf. Accessed on August 30, 2013.

10. Catalano S; Bureau of Justice Statistics. Intimate partner violence in the United States. Bureau of Justice Statistics Web site. http://www.bjs.gov/content/pub/pdf/ipvus.pdf. Published December 2006. Accessed August 27, 2013.

11. Black MC, Basile KC, Breiding MJ, et al. *The National Intimate Partner and Sexual Violence Survey (NISVS): 2010 Summary Report.* Atlanta, GA: National Center for Injury Prevention and Control, Centers for Disease Control and Prevention; 2011.

12. Saltzman LE, Fanslow JL, McMahon PM, Shelley GA. *Intimate Partner Violence Surveillance: Uniform Definitions And Recommended Data Elements, Version 1.0.* Atlanta, GA: Centers for Disease Control and Prevention, National Center for Injury Prevention and Control; 2002. Centers for Disease Control and Prevention Web site. http://www.cdc.gov/ncipc/pub-res/ipv_surveillance/Intimate%20Partner%20Violence.pdf. Accessed August 27, 2013.

13. DiNapoli PP. Guns and dolls: an exploration of violent behavior in girls. *Adv Nurs Sci.* 2003;18(1):140-148.

14. Rhatigan DL, Moore TM, Stuart GL. An investment model analysis of relationship stability among women court-mandated to violence interventions. *Psychol Women Q.* 2005;29:313–322.

15. Kelly J, Johnson M. Differentiation among types of intimate partner violence: research update and implications for interventions. *Fam Court Rev.* 2008;46:476-499.

16. Campbell J. Helping women to understand their risk in situations of intimate partner violence. *J Interpers Violence.* 2004;19:1464-1477.

17. Helton A, McFarlane J, Anderson E. Prevention of battering during pregnancy: focus on behavioral change. *Public Health Nurs.* 2007;4(3):166-174.

18. Nelson H, Nygren P, McInerney Y, Klein J; US Preventive Services Task Force. Screening women and elderly adults for family and intimate partner violence: a review of the evidence for the United States Preventive Services Task Force. *Ann Intern Med.* 2004;140(5):387-396.

19. Clements PT, Holt KE, Fay-Hillier T, Hasson CM. Enhancing assessment of interpersonal violence (IPV) for pregnancy-related homicide risk within nursing curricula. *J Forensic Nurs.* 2011;7(4):195-202.

20. Bronfenbrenner U. *The Ecology of Human Development: Experiments by Nature and Design.* Cambridge, MA: Harvard University Press; 1979.

21. Bronfenbrenner U. Interacting systems in human development. Research paradigms: present and future. In: Bronfenbrenner U, ed. *Making Human Beings Human: Bioecological Perspectives on Human Processes.* New York, NY: Cambridge University Press; 2005: 67-93.

22. Dahlberg LL, Krug EG. Violence—a global public health problem. In: Krug E, Dahlberg LL, Mercy JA, Zwi AB, Lozano R, eds. *World Report on Violence and Health.* Geneva, Switzerland: World Health Organization; 2002: 1–56.

23. Corcoran J. Ecological factors associated with adolescent pregnancy: a review of the literature. *Adolescence.* 1999;32:603-619.

24. World Health Organization. Intimate partner violence. In: *World Report on Violence and Health.* Geneva, Switzerland: World Health Organization; 2004:89-113.

25. Cherniak D, Grant L, Mason R, Moore B, Pellizzari R; IPV Working Group, Society of Obstetricians and Gynaecologists of Canada. Intimate partner violence consensus statement. *J Obstet Gynaecol Can.* 2005;27(4):365-418. Google Docs Web site. https://docs.google.com/viewer?url=http://sogc.org/wp-content/uploads/2013/01/157E-CPG-April2005.pdf&chrome=true. Accessed August 27, 2013.

26. Bornstein RF. The complex relationship between dependency and domestic violence. *Am Psychol.* 2006;61:595-606

27. Gee RE, Mitra N, Wan F, Chavkin DE, Long JA. Power over parity: intimate partner violence and issues of fertility control. *Am J Obstet Gynecol.* 2009;201(2):148.e1-7.

28. Miller E, Decker MR, McCauley HL, et al. Pregnancy coercion, intimate partner violence and unintended pregnancy. *Contraception.* 2010;81(4):316-322.

29. Fanslow J, Whitehead A, Silva M, Robinson E. Contraceptive use and associations with intimate partner violence among a population-based sample of New Zealand women. *Aus N Z J Obstet Gynaecol.* 2008;48(1):83-89.

30. Prager SW, Steinauer JE, Foster DG, Darney PD, Drey EA. Risk factors for repeat elective abortion. *Am J Obstet Gynecol.* 2007;197(6):575.e1-6.

31. Saftlas AF, Wallis AB, Shochet T, et al. Prevalence of intimate partner violence among an abortion clinic population. *Am J Public Health*. 2010;100(8):1412-1415.

32. Woo J, Fine P, Goetzl L. Abortion disclosure and the association with domestic violence. Obstet Gynecol. 2005;105(6):1329-1334.

33. Weiss HB, Lawrence BA, Miller TR. Pregnancy-associated assault hospitalizations. *Obstet Gynecol*. 2002;100:773–80.

34. McFarlane J, Campbell JC, Sharps P, Watson K. Abuse during pregnancy and femicide: urgent implications for women's health. *Obstet Gynecol*. 2002;100:27–36.

35. Martin SL, Mackie L, Kupper LL, Buescher PA, Moracco KE. Physical abuse of women before, during, and after pregnancy. *JAMA*. 2001;285:1581–1584.

36. Cheng D, Horon IL. Intimate-partner homicide among pregnant and postpartum women. *Obstet Gynecol*. 2010;115(6):1181-1186.

37. Chambliss LR. Intimate partner violence and it's implication for pregnancy. *Clin Obstet Gynecol*. 2008;51:385-397.

38. Chames M, Pearlman M. Trauma during pregnancy: outcomes and clinical management. *Clin Obstet Gynecol*. 2008;51:398-408.

39. Ellis KK, Chang C, Bhandari S, et al. Rural mothers experiencing the stress of intimate partner violence or not: their newborn health concerns. *J Midwifery Womens Health*. 2008;53:556-562.

40. Gomez-Beloz AW, Michelle A, Sanchez SE, Lam N. Intimate partner violence and risk for depression among postpartum women in Lima, Peru. *Violence Vict*. 2009;24:380-398.

41. Yonkers KA, Wisner KL, Stewart DE, et al. The management of depression during pregnancy: a report from the American Psychiatric Association and the American College of Obstetricians and Gynecologists. *Obstet Gynecol*. 2009;114(3):703-713.

42. Bowen E, Heron J, Waylen A, Wolke D, Team AS. Domestic violence risk during and after pregnancy: findings from a British longitudinal study. *Br J Obstet Gynecol*. 2005;112:1083–1089.

43. Ulrich YC, McKenna LS, King C, et al. Postpartum mothers' disclosure of abuse, role, and conflict. *Health Care Women Int*. 2006;27(4):324-343.

44. Rennison CM. *Intimate Partner Violence and Age of Victim, 1993-99*. Washington, DC: US Department of Justice; 2001. http://www.bjs.gov/content/pub/pdf/ipva 99.pdf. Accessed August 27, 2013.

45. Bhandari M, Dosanjh S, Tornetta P, et al. Musculoskeletal manifestations of physical abuse after intimate partner violence. *J Trauma*. 2006;61:473–479.

46. Heron MP, Smith BL. Deaths: leading causes for 2003. *Natl Vital Stat Rep*. 2007;55(10):1-92. Centers for Disease Control Web site. http://www.cdc.gov/nchs/ data/nvsr/nvsr55/nvsr55_10.pdf. Accessed August 27, 2013.

47. Olszewski D. Sexual assaults facilitated by drugs or alcohol. *Drug Educ Prev Policy*. 2009;16(1):39-52.

48. Barter C. In the name of love: partner abuse and violence in teenage relationships. *Br J Soc Work*. 2009;39(2):211-233.

49. Harner HM. Domestic violence and trauma care in teenage pregnancy: does paternal age make a difference? *J Obstet Gynecol Neonatal Nurs.* 2004;33(3):312-319.

50. Beaulaurier RL, Seff LR, Newman FL. Barriers to help-seeking for older women who experience intimate partner violence: a descriptive model. *J Women Aging.* 2008;20:231-248.

51. Zinc T, Jacobson J, Regan S, Pabst S. Hidden victims: the healthcare needs and experiences of older women in abusive relationships. *J Womens Health.* 2004;13:898-908.

52. Erickson W, Lee C, von Schrader S. *2011 Disability Status Report: United States.* Ithaca, NY: Cornell University Rehabilitation Research and Training Center on Disability Demographics and Statistics; 2012. Disability Statistics Web site. http://www.disabilitystatistics.org/reports/2011/English/HTML/report2011.cfm?html_year=2011&fips=2000000&subButton=Get+HTML.

53. Coker A, Smith P, Fadden M. Intimate partner violence and disabilities among women attendong family practice clinics. *J Womens Health.* 2005;14:829-838.

54. Cohen MM, Forte T, Du Mont J, Hyman I, Romans S. Adding insult to injury: intimate partner violence among women and men reporting activity limitations. *Ann Epidemiol.* 2006;16(8):644-651.

55. Rosen DB. Violence and exploitation against women and girls with disability. *Ann N Y Acad Sci.* 2006;1087:170-177.

56. Taggart L, McMillan R, Lawson A. Staffs' knowledge and perceptions of working with women with intellectual disabilities and mental health problems. *J Intellect Disabil Res.* 2010;54(1):90-100.

57. United Nations Programme on HIV/AIDS and World Health Organization. *AIDS Epidemic Update.* UNAIDS Publication No. UNAIDS/09.36E / JC1700E. Geneva: World Health Organization; 2009.

58. Tufts KA, Clements PT, Wessell J. When intimate partner violence against women and HIV collide: challenges for healthcare assessment and intervention. *J Forensic Nurs.* 2010;6:66-73.

59. Jewkes RK, Dunkle K, Nduna M, Shai N. Intimate partner violence, relationship power inequity, and incidence of HIV infection in young women in South Africa: a cohort study. *Lancet.* 2010;376(9734):41-48.

60. Lichtenstein B. Domestic violence, sexual ownership, and HIV risk in women in the American Deep South. *Soc Sci Med.* 2005;60(4):701-714.

61. Berg MJ, Kremelberg D, Dwivedi P, et al. The effects of husband's alcohol consumption on married women in three low-income areas of Greater Mumbai. *AIDS Behav.* 2010;14(suppl 1):S126-135.

62. Galvan F, Collins R, Kanouse DE, et al. Abuse in the close relationships of people with HIV. *AIDS Behav.* 2004;8(4):441-451.

63. Rothenberg KH, Paskey SJ. The risk of domestic violence and women with HIV infection: implications for partner notification, public policy, and the law. *Am J Public Health.* 1995;85:1569–1576.

64. Mason WA, Kosterman R, Hawkins JD, et al. Predicting depression, social phobia, and violence in early adulthood from childhood behavior problems. *J Am Acad Child Adolesc Psychiatry.* 2004;43(3):307-315.

65. Seimer BS. Intimate violence in adolescent relationships: recognizing and intervening. *MCN Am J Matern Child Nurs*. 2004;29(2):117-121.

66. Daane DM. Child and adolescent violence. *Orthop Nurs*. 2003;22(1):23-29.

67. El-Bassel N, Terlikbaeva A, Pinkham S. HIV and women who use drugs: double neglect, double risk. *Lancet*. 2010;376(9738):312-314.

68. Appelbaum PS, Robbins PC, Monahan J. Violence and delusions: data from the MacArthur Violence Risk Assessment Study. *Am J Psychiatry*. 2000;157(4):566-572.

69. Rice ME, Harris GT, Quinsey VL. The appraisal of violence risk. *Curr Opinions Psychiatry*. 2002;15(6):589-593.

70. Domestic Abuse Intervention Programs. What is the Duluth Model? Domestic Abuse Intervention Programs Web site. http://www.theduluthmodel.org/about/index.html. Accessed August 27, 2013.

71. West CM. "My soul looks back and wonders how I made it over": battered black women's healing journey. *J Aggression Maltreat Trauma*. In press.

72. Lacey KK. When is it enough for me to leave?: Black and Hispanic women's response to violent relationships. *J Fam Violence*. 2010;25:669-677.

73. Walker LE. *The Battered Woman*. New York: Harper and Row; 1979.

74. Boettcher EG. Preventing violent behavior: an integrated theoretical model for nursing. *Perspect Psychiatr Care*. 1983;32(2):54-58.

75. Brennan W. Aggression and violence: examining the theories. *Nurs Stand*. 1998;12(27):36-38.

76. Olweus D, Mattsson A, Schalling D, Low H. Testosterone, aggression, physical, and personality dimensions in normal adolescent males. *Psychosom Med*. 1980;42:253-269.

77. Orengo CA, Kunik ME, Ghusn H, Yudofsky SC. Correlation of testosterone with aggression in demented elderly men. *J Nerv Ment Dis*. 1997;185(5):349-351.

78. Davidson RJ, Putnam KM, Larson CL. Dysfunction in the neural circuitry of emotional regulation--a possible prelude to violence. *Science*. 2000;289:591-594.

79. Filley C, Price BH, Nell VD, et al. Toward an understanding of violence: neurobehavioral aspects of unwarranted physical aggression: Aspen Neurobehavioral Conference consensus statement. *Neuropsychiatry Neuropsychol Behav Neurol*. 2001;14(1):1-14.

80. Volavka J. The neurobiology of violence. *J Neuropsychiatry Clin Neurosci*. 1999;11:307-314.

81. Norlander B, Eckhardt C. Anger, hostility, and male perpetrators of intimate partner violence: a meta-analytic review. *Clin Psychol Rev*. 2005;25(2):119-152.

82. Buvinic M, Morrison AR. Living in a more violent world. *Foreign Policy* 2000;118:58-72.

83. Barzelatto J. Understanding sexual and reproductive violence: An overview. *Intl J Gynecol Obstet*. 1998;63:S13-S18.

84. Moore M. Reproductive health and intimate partner violence. *Fam Plann Perspect*. 1999;31(6):302-312.

85. Williamson C, Folaron G. Violence, risk, and survival strategies of street prostitution. *West J Nurs Res.* 2001;23(5):463-475.

86. Sorenson S, Wiebe D. Weapons in the lives of battered women. *Am J Public Health.* 2004;94:1412-1417.

87. Ascione FR, Weber CV, Thompson TM, Heath J, Maruyama M, Hayashi K. Battered pets and domestic violence: animal abuse reported by women experiencing intimate violence and by nonabused women. *Violence Against Women.* 2007;13(4):354-373.

88. Balsam KF, Rothblum ED, Beauchaine TD. Victimization over the lifespan: a comparison of lesbian, gay, bisexual, and heterosexual siblings. *J Consult Clin Psychol.* 2005;73:477-487.

89. Burke LK, Follingstad DR. Violence in lesbian and gay relationships: theory, prevalence, and correlational factors. *Clin Psychol Rev.* 1999;19(5):487-512.

90. Messinger AM. Invisible victims: same-sex IPV in the National Violence Against Women Survey. *J Interpers Violence.* 2011;26(11):2228-2243.

91. Tjaden P, Thoennes N, Allison CJ. Comparing violence over the lifespan in samples of same-sex and opposite sex cohabitants. *Violence Vict.*1999;14(4):413-425.

92. Freedberg P. Health care barriers and same-sex intimate partner violence: a review of the literature. *J Forensic Nurs.* 2006;2(1):15-41.

93. Burke TW, Jordan ML, Owen SS. A cross-national comparison of gay and lesbian domestic violence. *J Contemp Crim Justice.* 2002;18(3):231-257.

94. Pattavina A, Hirschel D, Buzawa E, Faggiani D, Bentley H. A comparison of the police response to heterosexual versus same-sex intimate partner violence. *Violence Against Women.* 2007;13:374-394.

95. National Resource Center on Domestic Violence. *Lesbian, Gay, Bisexual and Trans (LGBT) Communities and Domestic Violence: Information and Resources.* Harrisburg, PA: National Resource Center on Domestic Violence; 2007. National Online Resource Center on Violence Against Women Web site. http://www.vawnet.org/Assoc_Files_VAWnet/NRC_LGBTDV-Full.pdf. Accessed August 27, 2013.

96. Goldblatt H, Eisikovits Z. Role taking of youths in a family context: adolescents exposed to interparental violence. *Am J Orthopsychiatry.* 2005;74(4):644-657.

97. Ernst A, Weiss S, Enright-Smith S. Child witnesses and victims in homes with adult intimate partner violence. *Acad Emerg Med.* 2006;13:696-699.

98. Owen A, Thompson M, Kaslow N. The mediating role of parenting stress in the relation between intimate partner violence and child adjustment. *J Fam Psychol.* 2006;20:505-513.

99. Kellogg ND, Menard SW. Violence among family members of children and adolescents evaluated for sexual abuse. *Child Abuse Negl.* 2003;27(12):1367-1376.

100. Swanger K, Petcosky J. *Violence in the Home: Multidisciplinary Perspectives.* New York, NY: Oxford University Press; 2003.

101. Goldstein AP. *Violence in America: Lessons on Understanding the Aggression in our Lives.* Palo Alto, CA: Davies-Black Publishing; 1996.

102. Stewart F. Root causes of violent conflict in developing countries. *Br J Med*. 2002;324:342-345.

103. Kleinman A. Social violence: research questions on local experiences and global responses. *Arch Gen Psychiatry*. 1999;56(11):978-979.

104. Faramarzi M, Esmailzadeh S, Mosavi S. A comparison of abused and non-abused women's definitions of domestic violence and attitudes to acceptance of male dominance. *Eur J Obstet Gynecol Reprod Biol*. 2005;122:225-231.

105. Hadi A. Women's productive role and marital violence in Bangladesh. *J Interpers Violence*. 2005;20(3):181-189.

106. Vyas S, Watts C. How does economic empowerment affect women's risk of intimate partner violence in low and middle income countries? A systematic review of published evidence. *J Int Dev*. 2009;2:577-602.

107. Li Q, Kirby R, Sigler R, et al. A multilevel analysis of individual, household, and neighborhood correlates of intimate partner violence among low-income pregnant women in Jefferson County, AL. *Am J Public Health*. 2010;100(3):531-539.

108. Sabol W, Coulton C, Korbin J. Building community capacity for violence prevention. *J Interpers Violence*. 2004;19:322-340.

109. Bandura A, Ross D, Ross SA. Imitation of film-mediated aggressive models. *J Abnorm Soc Psychol*. 1963;66:3-11.

110. Johnson RM, Kotch JB, Catellier DJ, et al. Adverse behavioral and emotional outcomes from child abuse and witnessed violence. *Child Maltreat*. 2002;7(3):179-186.

111. Singer MI, Anglin TM, Song Y, Longhofer L. Adolescents' exposure to violence and associated symptoms of psychological trauma. *JAMA*. 1995;273:477-482.

112. Osofsky HJ, Osofsky JD. Violent and aggressive behaviors in youth: a mental health perspective. *Psychiatry*. 2001;64(4):285-295.

113. Tarter RE, Kirisci L, Vanyukov M, et al. Predicting adolescent violence: impact of family history, substance abuse, psychiatric history, and social adjustment. *Am J Psychiatry*. 2002;159(9):1541-1547.

114. Raine A, Brennan P, Mednick B, Mednick S. High rates of violence, crime, academic problems, and behavioral problems in males with both early neuromotor deficits and unstable family environments. *Arch Gen Psychiatry*. 1996;53(6):544-549.

115. Rivara FP, Anderson ML, Fishman P, et al. Healthcare utilization and costs for women with a history of intimate partner violence. *Am J Prev Med*. 2007;32(2):89-96.

116. Jones AS, Dienemann J, Schollenberger J, et al. Long-term costs of intimate partner violence in a sample of female HMNO enrollees. Womens Health Issues, 2006;16:252–262.

117. Lloyd S, Taluc N. The effects of male violence on female employment. *Violence Against Women*. 1999;5:370–392.

118. Johnson MP, Leone JM. The differential effects of intimate terrorism and situational couple violence. *J Fam Issues*. 2005;26(3):322–349.

119. Plichta SB. Intimate partner violence and physical health consequences: policy and practice implications. *J Interpers Violence*. 2004 ;19(11) :1296–1323.

120. Campbell J, Baty M, Ghandour R, et al. The intersection of intimate partner violence against women and HIV/AIDS: a review. *Int J Inj Contr Saf Promot.* 2008;15(4):221-231.

121. Sheridan D, Nash K. Acute injury patterns of intimate partner violence victims. *Trauma Violence Abuse.* 2007;8:281-289.

122. Saddki N, Suhaimi AA, Daud R. Maxillofacial injuries associated with intimate partner violence in women. *BMC Public Health.* 2010;10:268.

123. Arosarena OA, Fritsch TA, Hsueh Y, Aynehchi B, Haug R. Maxillofacial injuries and violence against women. *Arch Facial Plast Surg.* 2009;11(1):48-52.

124. Coker AL, Hopenhayn C, DeSimone C, Bush HM, Crofford L. Violence against women raises risk of cervical cancer. *J Womens Health (Larchmt).* 2009;18(8):1179-1185.

125. Eckert L, Lentz GM. Infections of the upper genital tract. In: Katz VL, Lentz GM, Lobo RA, Gershenson DM, eds. *Comprehensive Gynecology.* 5th ed. Philadelphia, PA: Mosby Elsevier; 2007: 607-632.

126. Heise L, Garcia-Moreno C. Violence by intimate partners. In: Krug E, Dahlberg LL, Mercy JA, Zwi AB, Lozano R, eds. *World Report on Violence and Health.* Geneva, Switzerland: World Health Organization; 2002: 87-121.

127. Coker AL, Smith PH, Bethea L, King MR, McKeown RE. Physical health consequences of physical and psychological intimate partner violence. *Arch Fam Med.* 2000;9(5):451-457.

128. Centers for Disease Control and Prevention. Sexually transmitted diseases treatment guidelines, 2006. *MMWR.* 2006;55(No. RR-11):62-69.

129. Moscicki A. Impact of HPV infection in adolescent populations. *J Adolesc Health.* 2005;37(suppl 6):S3-S9.

130. Rogers AJ, McIntyre SL, Rossman L, Bacon-Baguley T, Jones JS. The forensic rape examination: is colposcopy really necessary? *Ann Emerg Med.* 2008;52(suppl 4):S63.

131. Silverman JG, Decker MR, Reed E, Raj A. Intimate partner violence victimization prior to and during pregnancy among women residing in 26 U.S. States: associations with maternal and neonatal health. *Am J Obstet Gynecol.* 2006;19:140–148.

132. Cripe S, Sanchez S, Perales M, et al. Association of intimate partner physical and sexual violence with unintended pregnancy among pregnant women in Peru. *Int J Gynaecol Obstet.* 2008;100(2):104-108.

133. Ellsberg M, Jansen H, Heise L, Watts CH, Garcio-Moreno C; WHO Multi-country Study on Women's Health and Domestic Violence Against Women Study Team. Intimate partner violence and women's physical and mental health in the WHO multi-country study on women's health and domestic violence: an observational study. *Lancet.* 2008;371(9619):1165-1172.

134. Crofford LJ. Violence, stress, and somatic syndromes. *Trauma Violence Abuse.* 2007;8:299–313.

135. Leserman J, Drossman DA. Relationship of abuse history to functional gastrointestinal disorders and symptoms. *Trauma Violence Abuse.* 2007;8:331–343.

136. Silverman J, Decker M, McCauley H, et al. Male perpetration of intimate partner violence and involvement in abortions and abortion-related conflict. *Am J Public Health.* 2010;100(8):1415-1417.

137. Roberts TA, Klein JD, Fisher S. Longitudinal effect of intimate partner abuse on high-risk behavior among adolescents. *Arch Pediatr Adolesc Med.* 2003;157(9):875–981.

138. Dorahy MJ, Lewis C, Wolfe FAM. Psychological distress associated with domestic violence in Northern Ireland. *Curr Psychol.* 2007;25(4):295-305.

139. Gelles RJ, Harrop JW. Violence, battering and psychological distress among women. *J Interpers Violence.* 1989;4:400-420.

140. Kim J, Park S, Emery Cr. The incidence and impact of family violence on mental health among South Korean Women: results of a national survey. *J Fam Violence.* 2009;24(3):193-202.

141. McFarlane J, Malecha A, Watson K, et al. Intimate partner sexual assault against women: Frequency, health consequences, and treatment outcomes. *Obstet Gynecol.* 2005;105(1):99-108.

142. Tiwari A, Chan K, Fong D, et al. The impact of psychological abuse by an intimate partner on the mental health of pregnant women. *BJOG.* 2008;115:377–384.

143. McGarry J, Simpson C, Mansour M. How domestic abuse affects the wellbeing of older women. *Nurs Older People.* 2010;22(5):33-37.

144. Hurwitz E, Gupta J, Liu R, Silverman JG, Raj A. Intimate partner violence associated with poor health outcomes in U.S. South Asian Women. *J Immigr Minor Health.* 2006;8(3):251-261.

145. Tosevski DL, Milovancevic MP. Stressful life events and physical health. *Curr Opinion Psychiatry.* 2006;19(2):184-189.

146. Division of Behavioral Surveillance, Public Health Surveillance and Informatics Program. BRFSS 2005 survey data and documentation. Centers for Disease Control and Prevention website. http://www.cdc.gov/brfss/annual_data/annual_2005.htm. Published 2005. Accessed September 24, 2013.

147. Centers for Disease Control and Prevention. *Intimate Partner Violence Definitions.* Atlanta, GA: Centers for Disease Control; 2013. Centers for Disease Control and Prevention Web site. http://www.cdc.gov/violenceprevention/intimatepartnerviolence/definitions.html. Accessed April 23, 2013.

148. Roberts TA, Auinger P, Klein JD. Intimate partner abuse and the reproductive health of sexually active female adolescents. *J Adolesc Health.* 2005; 36(5):380-385.

149. Silverman JG, Raj A, Mucci L, Hathaway J. Dating violence against adolescent girls and associated substance use, unhealthy weight control, sexual risk behavior, pregnancy, and suicidality. *JAMA.* 2001;286(5):572–579.

150. Rovi S, Olson E, Miller S, et al; New Jersey Domestic Violence Fatality and Near-Fatality Review Board. "Let me see tomorrow:" a report based on interviews with women who were nearly killed by their intimate partners. State of New Jersey Web site. http://www.nj.gov/dcf/news/reportsnewsletters/taskforce/LetMeSee TomorrowOct2010.pdf. Published October 2010. Accessed August 27, 2013.

151. American Nurses Association. *Position Statement on Physical Violence Against Women*. Washington, DC: American Nurses Association; 1994.

152. Coble YD, Eisenbrey AB, Estes EH, et al. Violence against women: relevance for medical practitioners. *JAMA*. 1992;267(23):3184-3189.

153. Agency for Healthcare Research and Quality. Women and domestic violence: programs and tools to improve care for victims. *Res Action*. 2004;15:1-12. Agency for Healthcare Research and Quality Web site. http://archive.ahrq.gov/research/domviolria/domviolria.pdf. Accessed August 27, 2013.

154. Queen J, Brackley MH, Nurse A, Williams GB. Being emotionally abused: a phenomenological study of adult women's experiences of emotionally abusive intimate partner relationships. *Issues Ment Health Nurs*. 2009;30(4):237-245.

155. Rabin RF, Jennings JM, Campbell JC, Bair-Merritt MH. Intimate partner violence screening tools: a systematic review. *Am J Prev Med*. 2009;36(5):439-445.

156. McFarlane J, Parker B. Preventing abuse during pregnancy: an assessment and intervention protocol. *MCN Am J Matern Child Nurs*. 1994;19:321-324.

157. Campbell J, Webster D, Koziol-McLain J, et al. Risk factors for femicide in abusive relationships: results from a multisite case control study. *Am J Public Health*. 2003;93(7):1089-1097.

158. US Preventive Services Task Force. Screening for intimate partner violence and abuse of elderly and vulnerable adults. US Preventive Services Task Force Web site. http://www.uspreventiveservicestaskforce.org/uspstf/uspsipv.htm. Published 2012. Accessed September 25, 2013.

Chapter 5

Protective Orders and Economic Abuse in Domestic Violence: A Case Study

*Katherine Kaby Anselmi, JD, PhD, CRNP-BC

Key Points

1. Domestic violence law is a combination of civil, family, and criminal law, and any other area of the law where a victim's rights have been violated.

2. Attorneys who represent victims are often in public interest law centers.

3. Legal Advocates are trained in the area of domestic violence, sexual assault, and stalking to support victims of intimate partner violence (IPV).

4. In 1994 Congress enacted the Violence Against Women Act (VAWA), recognizing that "violence against women is a crime with far-reaching, harmful consequences for families, children and society."

5. VAWA legislation empowered the federal government, which traditionally lacked jurisdiction over many domestic violence (DV) offenses, to have greater involvement in prosecution of DV offenders in interstate travel or activity.

6. A victim of DV or IPV may obtain a protective order through any courthouse and without an attorney. There is a website for domestic violence services in each state.

7. The effects of DV often reach into the area of finances and income tax. Victims who have filed joint tax returns need to notify the IRS if they have not filed jointly.

8. It is not uncommon for an abuser to commit tax fraud by using the victim's tax return to understate owed taxes and/or forge a signature. This occurs with such frequency that the IRS established the Innocent Spouse Relief provision by which a spouse may seek relief from erroneous tax liability.

Introduction

"There was a judge in a certain city," he said, "who was a godless man with great contempt for everyone. A widow of that city came to him repeatedly, appealing for justice against someone who had harmed her. The judge ignored her for a while, but eventually she wore him out. 'I fear neither God nor man,' he said to himself, 'but this woman is driving me crazy. I'm going to see that she gets justice, because she is wearing me out with her constant requests!'" Then the Lord said, "learn a lesson from this evil judge. Even he rendered a just decision in the end, so don't you think God will surely give justice to his chosen people who plead with him day and night? Will he keep putting them off? I tell you, he will grant justice to them quickly! But when I the Son of Man, return, how many will I find who have faith?"

Luke 18:2-8[1]

Associate Clinical Professor & Assistant Dean of Accreditation/Regulatory Affairs & Online Innovation, College of Nursing & Health Professions, Drexel University, Philadelphia, PA.

The history of legal relief to right a wrong goes back to Biblical origins. Whether an act is a breach in an agreement (contract), a trespass upon the land of another (property), a civil wrong for which relief may be obtained through damages (tort), or a harm upon society for which there is punishment (crime),[2] the law offers a remedy to the victim and society. Victims must have faith in the legal system that justice will prevail. Persistence increases the probability of obtaining a desired result. Legal recourse for domestic violence victims is especially challenging due to judicial and social attitudes regarding domestic violence as a private family matter. This is reflected in 'The Rule of Thumb.' Some argue that the origins of the phrase lie with agriculture and building and that The Rule of Thumb does not refer to wife beating.[3] Nevertheless, common law references that combine wife beating, its effects, and the 'Rule of Thumb' are so numerous as to establish tacit understanding of its meaning as a rule for physical discipline.[4] In modern times, a common obstacle that plaintiff victims encounter as a barrier to obtaining relief is not lack of evidence but the circles of influence of defendant abusers. Abusers often control of flow of money, and they may be influential in their communities or neighborhoods, or leading figures with the criminal justice system (ie, friends of local police forces). A common issue seen by justice centers offering free legal representation to victims and documented by feminist websites, is that some women who experience IPV are fearful of calling the police because their partners are friends with neighborhood police and the womens' calls are ignored.[5] Moreover, there is a generalized stigma pervasive throughout society that views domestic disputes as private matters, unimportant or trivial, and not worthy of attention by law enforcement. Although not all law enforcement turns a blind eye to domestic violence, there is enough concern that, even in times of economic duress, Congress continues to fund training for police officers and other parties concerned with in matters regarding domestic violence.[6]

One compelling example of this stigma can be found in the Virginia Tech slayings of 2007. As quoted in the New York Times the day after the shootings:

Chief Flinchum said that initially officials thought that the shooting was 'domestic,' suggesting that it was between individuals who knew each other, and isolated to the dormitory. The first attack started as students were getting ready for classes or were on their way there. The university did not evacuate the campus or notify students of that attack until several hours later.[7]

The first attack would have been categorized as non-domestic, and triggered an immediate police response, which may have lead to the shooter's interception and possibly prevented the loss of 32 lives.

As a former staff attorney representing victims of domestic violence, sexual assault, and stalking in civil court, the web of legal issues triggered by domestic violence was surprising. Domestic violence can pull an innocent victim into a myriad of civil and criminal offenses perpetrated by an abuser, many of which impact finances and related tax consequences. Survivors of domestic violence often deal with multiple tax issues, such as joint returns, tax liability, and erroneous or fraudulent joint returns, after departing from an abusive relationship.[8]

This chapter examines domestic violence vis-à-vis physical abuse and tax fraud. The chapter begins with a definition of protective orders with discussion about what the court considers and how an order is issued. The next section of the chapter concerns the Violence Against Women Act of 1994 (VAWA) and its subsequent renewals and expansion of coverage. An actual case study of domestic violence (DV) illustrates how tax fraud may be used to perpetrate economic abuse after years of physical violence. The case study shows that there are no parameters or limitations to the far-reaching consequences of DV. A discussion of some of the legal issues that are raised by the fact pattern within the case study is presented, with analysis of the criminal violation of the tax code. At the end of the chapter, there is a sample of a protection from abuse court order followed by a table listing websites for every state in the US where information about domestic violence victim assistance programs, laws, and legislation can be found.

DOMESTIC VIOLENCE AND ABUSE: THE PROTECTIVE ORDER

The protective order, protection from abuse order, or PFA has different names in different jurisdictions. In some state jurisdictions it is called a temporary restraining order (TRO), restraining order, or protective order. Regardless of the name, the PFA may be used as a "sword" by a plaintiff victim; as a "shield" by a victim accused of assault; or both, to protect a victim from further assault and abuse. Every state has its own procedure for obtaining a PFA order. In fact, in Pennsylvania, each county has its own process.[9] **Table 5-1** provides a list of domestic violence centers in each state with state-specific information. A PFA can be obtained against an intimate partner or a family member only. Several different relationships are considered within this category, such as spouse or ex-spouse, current or former sexual or intimate partner, same-sex partners, parents, and children. The PFA Act does not include protection from a stranger or roommate. A final protective order may be issued by a judge; however, the temporary protective order may be issued by anyone authorized by the law, such as a PFA office, local magistrate, hearing master, or judge. Each jurisdiction has local statutes or common law that dictate the procedure. For example, in Pennsylvania, the easiest way to obtain a PFA is to petition at the local county courthouse by going to the PFA office; however, limited to business hours. Some states, such as Arizona, permit filing a petition for an order of protection online.[10] Victims filing online should use secure computers that are not available to their abusers.

Table 5-1. 50 State PFA Assessment Table

STATE	WEBSITE FOR STATUTE	STATUTE	SECTION	MAXIMUM DURATION OF PFA	WHERE TO FIND HELP
Alabama	http://alisondb. legislature.state. al.us/acas/ACAS LoginFire.asp	Title 30. Marital and Domestic Relations Chapter 5. Protection From Abuse	§30-5-6	Up to 1 year	www.acadv.org/
Alaska	http://touchngo. com/lglcntr/ akstats/ statutes.htm	Title 18. Health, Safety, and Housing Chapter 66. Domestic Violence and Sexual Assault	§18.66. 100	1 year	www.andvsa.org
Arizona	http://www.azleg. gov/Arizona Revised Statutes.asp	Title 13. Criminal Code Chapter 36. Family Offenses Sec. 02	§13-3602	1 year	www.azcadv.org/

(continued)

Table 5-1. 50 State PFA Assessment Table *(continued)*

STATE	WEBSITE FOR STATUTE	STATUTE	SECTION	MAXIMUM DURATION OF PFA	WHERE TO FIND HELP
Arkansas	http://www. arkleg.state.ar. us/assembly/ 2011/2011R/ Pages/Home.aspx	Title 9. Family Law Chapter 15. Domestic Abuse Subchapter 2. Judicial Proceedings	A.C.A. § 9-15-204	Up to 2 years	www.domestic peace.com/
California	http://leginfo. legislature.ca. gov/faces/codes. xhtml	Family Code Division 10. Prevention of Domestic Violence	§6340-6346	Up to 3 years	www.cpedv.org/
Colorado	http://www. lexisnexis.com/ hottopics/ colorado/	Title 13. Courts and Court Procedure Article 14. Civil Protection Orders	§13-14-102	Indefinite	www.ccadv.org
Connecti-cut	http://www. cga.ct.gov/lco/ statutes-index.asp	Title 46b. Family Law Chapter 815a. Family Matters	§46b-15	Up to 6 months, may be extended	www.ctcadv.org/
Delaware	http://delcode. delaware.gov/ index.shtml	Title 10. Courts and Judicial Procedures Chapter 9. The Family Court of the State of Delaware Subchapter III. Procedure	§1045	Up to 2 years	www.dcadv.org
Florida	http://www. leg.state.fl.us/ Welcome/index. cfm?CFID=1922 57703&CFTOK EN=72970553	Title XLIII. Domestic Relations Chapter 741. Marriage; Domestic Violence Section 741.30	§741.30	Indefinite	www.fcadv.org
Georgia	http://www.legis. ga.gov/en-US/ default.aspx	Title 19. Domestic Relations Chapter 13. Family Violence	§19-13-3	Up to 1 year, can be extended	www.gadfcs.org/ familyviolence/ index.php
Hawaii	http://www. capitol.hawaii. gov/hrscurrent/	Division 3. Property; Family Chapter 586. Domestic Abuse Protective Orders	§586-3	Indefinite	www.hscadv.org

(continued)

Table 5-1. 50 State PFA Assessment Table *(continued)*

STATE	WEBSITE FOR STATUTE	STATUTE	SECTION	MAXIMUM DURATION OF PFA	WHERE TO FIND HELP
Idaho	http://www.legislature.idaho.gov/idstat/TOC/IDStatutesTOC.htm	Title 39: Health & Safety Chapter 63. Domestic Violence Crime Prevention	§39-6306	3 months, may be extended	www.idvsa.org
Illinois	http://www.ilga.gov/legislation/ilcs/ilcs.asp	Chapter 725. Criminal Procedure Act 5. Code of Criminal Procedure of 1963; Title IV Proceedings to Commence Prosecution Article 112A. Domestic Violence: Order of Protection	§112A-2	Up to 2 years, may be renewed	www.ilcadv.org/
Indiana	http://www.in.gov/legislative/index.htm	Title 34. Civil Procedure Article 26. Special Proceedings: Injunctions and Restraining Orders Chapter 5. Indiana Civil Protection Order Act	§34-26-5-10	Up to 2 years, may be extended	www.icadvinc.org/
Iowa	https://www.legis.iowa.gov/law/statutory	Title VI. Human Services Subtitle 6. Children and Families Chapter 236. Domestic Abuse	§236.4	Up to 1 year, may be extended	www.icadv.org/
Kansas	http://www.kslegislature.org/li/statute/	Chapter 60. Procedure, Civil Article 31. Protection from Abuse Act	§60-3106	Up to 1 year, may be extended	www.kcsdv.org
Kentucky	http://162.114.4.13/KRS/403-00/CHAPTER.HTM	Title XXXV. Domestic Relations Chapter 403. Dissolution of Marriage; Child Custody Domestic Violence and Abuse	§403.745	3 years, may be extended	www.kdva.org

(continued)

Table 5-1. 50 State PFA Assessment Table *(continued)*

State	Website for Statute	Statute	Section	Maximum Duration of PFA	Where to Find Help
Louisiana	http://www.legis. state.la.us/	Title 46. Public Welfare and Assistance Chapter 28. Protection From Family Violence Act	§2136	Up to 18 months, may be extended	www.lcadv.org
Maine	http://www. mainelegislature. org/legis/ statutes/	Title 19-A. Domestic Relations Part 4. Protection From Abuse Chapter 101: Protection From Abuse	§4006	Up to 2 years	www.mcedv.org
Maryland	http://www. lexisnexis.com/ hottopics/ mdcode/	Family Law Title 4. Spouses Subtitle 5. Domestic Violence	§4506	Up to 1 year	www.mnadv.org
Massachusetts	https:// malegislature. gov/Laws/ GeneralLaws/ Search	Part II. Real and Personal Property and Domestic Relations Title III. Domestic Relations chapter 209A. Abuse Prevention	§7	Up to 1 year	www.janedoe.org
Michigan	http://www. legislature.mi.gov /%28S%28q0rlu d45kupr3h45x5 e4qtfk%29%29/ mileg.aspx?page =Home	Chapter 600. Revised Judicature Act of 1961 Chapter 29. Provisions Concerning Specific Actions	§600. 2950		www.mcadsv.org/
Minnesota	https://www. revisor.mn.gov/ index.php	Chapter 518B.01 Domestic Abuse Act	§518B.01	Up to 1 year, may be extended	www.mcbw.org
Mississippi	http://www. lexisnexis.com/ hottopics/ mscode/	Title 93. Domestic Relations Chapter 21. Protection From Domestic Abuse	§93-21-15	Up to the court's discretion	www.mcadv.org

(continued)

Table 5-1. 50 State PFA Assessment Table *(continued)*

STATE	WEBSITE FOR STATUTE	STATUTE	SECTION	MAXIMUM DURATION OF PFA	WHERE TO FIND HELP
Missouri	http://www.moga.mo.gov/statutes/statutes.htm	Title XXX. Domestic Relations Chapter 455. Abuse - Adults and children - Shelters and Protective Orders	§455.040	Up to 1 year, may be extended	www.mocadsv.org
Montana	http://data.opi.mt.gov/bills/mca_toc/index.htm	Title 40. Family Law Chapter 15. Partner And Family Member Assault, Sexual Assault, and Stalking - Safety and Protection of Victims	§40-15-202	Subject to judge's discretion	www.mcadsv.com
Nebraska	http://nebraskalegislature.gov/laws/browse-statutes.php	Chapter 42. Husband and Wife Article 9. Domestic Violence (A) Protection From Abuse Act	§42-924	Up to 1 year	www.ndvsac.org
Nevada	http://www.leg.state.nv.us/NRS/	Title 3. Remedies; Special Actions and Proceedings Chapter 33. Injunctions Orders for Protection Against Domestic Violence	§33.020	1 year	www.nnadv.org
New Hampshire	http://gencourt.state.nh.us/rsa/html/indexes/default.html	Title XII. Public Safety and Welfare Chapter 173-B. Protection of Persons From Domestic Violence	§173-B:3	1 year	www.nhcadsv.org
New Jersey	http://www.njleg.state.nj.us/	Title 2C. The New Jersey Code of Criminal Justice Chapter 25. Domestic Violence	§2C:25-29	Indefinitely	www.njcbw.org/

(continued)

Table 5-1. 50 State PFA Assessment Table *(continued)*

State	Website for Statute	Statute	Section	Maximum Duration of PFA	Where to Find Help
New Mexico	http://www.nmonesource.com/nmnxtadmin/NMPublic.aspx	Chapter 40. Domestic Affairs Article 13. Family Violence Protection	§40-13-4	Up to six months	www.nmcadv.org
New York	http://public.leginfo.state.ny.us/frmload.cgi?MENU-39932209	Article 8. Family Offenses Proceedings Part 4. Orders Section 842. Order of Protection	§842	Up to 5 years	www.nyscadv.org/
North Carolina	http://www.ncga.state.nc.us/gascripts/Statutes/StatutesTOC.pl	Chapter 50C. Civil No-Contact Orders	§50C-3	Up to 1 year, may be extended	www.nccadv.org/default.htm
North Dakota	http://www.legis.nd.gov/information/statutes/cent-code.html	Title 14. Domestic Relations and Persons Chapter 14-07. Domestic Violence	§14-07.1-02	Subject to judge's discretion	www.ndcaws.org
Ohio	http://codes.ohio.gov/orc	Chapter 2919.26 Temporary Protection Order	§2919.26	Up to 5 years	www.odvn.org/
Oklahoma	http://www.oscn.net/applications/oscn/Index.asp?ftdb=STOKST&level=1	Title 22. Criminal Procedure Chapter 2.	§60.4	Up to 3 years, may be extended	www.ocadvsa.org
Oregon	http://www.leg.state.or.us/ors/	Title 11: Domestic Relations Chapter 107. Marital Dissolution, Annulment and Separation; Mediation and Conciliation Services; Family Abuse Prevention	§107.718	Up to 1 year, may be extended	www.ocadsv.com/

(continued)

Table 5-1. 50 State PFA Assessment Table *(continued)*

State	Website for Statute	Statute	Section	Maximum Duration of PFA	Where to Find Help
Pennsylvania		Title 23. Domestic Relations Part VII. Abuse of Family Chapter 61. Protection from Abuse	§6107	Up to 3 years, may be extended	www.pcadv.org
Rhode Island	http://www.rilin. state.ri.us/ Statutes/ Statutes.html	Title 15. Domestic Relations Chapter 15-15. Domestic Abuse Prevention	§15-15-3	Subject to judge's discretion	www.ricadv.org/
South Carolina	http://www. scstatehouse.gov/	Title 20 - Domestic Relations Chapter 4 - Protection from Domestic Abuse	§20-4-40	Up to 1 year	www.sccadvasa.org/
South Dakota	http://legis.state. sd.us/statutes/ index.aspx	Title 25. Domestic Relations Chapter 10 - Protection from Domestic Abuse	§25-10-3	Up to 5 years	http://www.sdcedsv. org/
Tennessee	http://www. lexisnexis.com/ hottopics/ tncode/	Part 6. Domestic Abuse 36-3-605 Protection orders; hearing; extension; modification	§36-3-605	Up to 1 year, may be extended	www.tcadsv.org
Texas	http://www. statutes.legis.state. tx.us/Index.aspx	Title 4. Protective Orders and Family Violence Subtitle B. Protective Orders Chapter 84. Hearings	§84.001	Up to 2 years	www.tcfv.org
Utah	http://www. le.state. ut.us/~code/ code.htm	Title 78B. Judicial Code; Chapter 7. Protective Orders Section 106. Protective orders - Exparte protective orders - Modification of orders - Service of process - Duties of the court	§78B-7-106	Subject to judge's discretion	www.udvac.org

(continued)

Table 5-1. 50 State PFA Assessment Table *(continued)*

State	Website for Statute	Statute	Section	Maximum Duration of PFA	Where to Find Help
Vermont	http://www.leg.state.vt.us/statutes/chapters.cfm?Title=15	Title 15. Domestic Relations Chapter 21: Abuse Prevention	§1103	Up to 1 year	www.vtnetwork.org
Virginia	https://leg1.state.va.us/cgi-bin/legp504.exe?000+cod+TOC	Title 16.1. Courts Not of Record Chapter 11. Juvenile and Domestic Relations District Courts	§16.1-253.1	Up to 2 years	http://www.vsdvalliance.org/
Washington	http://apps.leg.wa.gov/RCW/	Title 26. Domestic Relations	§2008 c287	Subject to judge's discretion	www.wscadv.org/
West Virginia	http://www.legis.state.wv.us/WVCODE/Code.cfm	Chapter 48. Domestic Relations Article 27. Prevention and Treatment of Domestic Violence Part 5. Protective Orders, Visitation Orders	§48-27-501	Up to 1 year	www.wvcadv.org
Wisconsin	http://legis.wisconsin.gov/statutes/Stat0813.pdf	Chapter 813. Injunctions, NE Exeat and Receivers 813.12. Domestic Abuse Restraining Orders and Injunctions	§813.123	Up to 4 years	http://endabusewi.org/
Wyoming	http://legisweb.state.wy.us/statutes/statutes.aspx	Title 35. Public Health and Safety Chapter 21. Domestic Violence Protection	§35-21-101	Up to 1 year	http://www.wyomingdvsa.org/

A compilation of websites and information of nation-wide resources and organizations for professionals and survivors of domestic violence. It includes the state statute for domestic relations and protective orders, section number, maximum duration of time for the protective order, and a website for where to find help. The National Coalition against Domestic Violence has an affiliate in almost every state. The state websites provide information on DV legislation and state laws and the best place to find assistance. This table should not be relied upon or replace legal advice from an attorney.

A temporary PFA is granted before a final PFA order. A victim must commence proceedings by filing a petition for temporary protection that will be in effect until such time as a hearing can be held before a judge. The filing process can take up to 2 hours. The petition includes: any request for the judge's consideration, such as to evict an abuser from a joint domiciliary; cease threatening, stalking, or harassing; temporary custody; maintain confidential new address; abuser to turn over weapons; no touch, no contact with victim, children, or family; other relief such as support, return of a pet, or legal papers.[9] If a victim wishes his or her address to remain confidential, it should not be listed on the petition. In addition, the petition will include an area to explain why protection is sought and a description of the abuse or other crime. A judge decides whether to grant a temporary PFA. In either case, a hearing date will be set to review the allegations on the petition. The hearing date must occur within 10 business days or as soon as can be scheduled. A signed temporary PFA is filed with the prothonotary and copies given to the local police department and sheriff who will serve a copy of the petition upon the defendant perpetrator. The victim should make copies of the temporary order so that other entities or parties that need to know , such as the victim's home, place of work, and children's school, may have a copy.

A temporary PFA will remain in effect until the hearing date that is scheduled through the PFA office or by the court administrator. (See **Figure 5-1** for a sample PFA order.) At a hearing, both parties may have legal representation, an opportunity to be heard via plaintiff and defendant testimony, opportunity for witness testimony, and may present other relevant evidence. Should a victim be unable to hire an attorney, she may appear pro se, or with a legal advocate. Legal advocates are available in many counties throughout the country to help victims navigate the civil and criminal justice system, such as the Aurora Center at the University of Minnesota that trains such volunteers.[11] Legal advocates are not attorneys or licensed to practice law, but rather trained to provide support and education to the victim about her legal options, rights, and planning for safety.

At the end of the hearing the judge will rule one of three ways: grant a PFA for any length of time up to the maximum permitted by law, deny the PFA, or extend the temporary PFA until a final order is issued. Sometimes during a particularly long hearing where hours of testimony are heard and a large number of exhibits are entered into evidence, a judge will take all of the evidence under advisement until such time as a decision may be rendered. This could be as long as 6 months in some jurisdictions, an outcome that could be a detriment or benefit to the victim. It could be detrimental to the victim because a temporary restraining order (TRO) does not carry the weight of a permanent order among law enforcement and may also leave a great degree of uncertainty for a victim. On the other hand, a TRO may benefit a victim if a judge can issue the maximum time in addition to the TRO time, thus extending the duration of total protection. Most of the time an order will be forthcoming minutes after the hearing. A PFA may include the names of protected parties, such as children and intimate partners, all of the addresses the defendant is to avoid, custody, support, the relinquishment of firearms, payment of fees associated with the PFA hearing, and any other appropriate relief sought by the plaintiff (see **Figure 5-1**).

The PFA may be extended beyond the maximum duration; however, the laws vary in each jurisdiction. In some states a judge will only extend the PFA if there have been threats from the defendant against the protected parties. On the other some hand jurisdictions, such as New York, will permit an extension of a PFA without necessitating overt abuse:

Extension of Order of Protection – A.6195-A Weinstein / S. 2972-A Sampson

Authorize Family Court to extend a current order of protection for a reasonable period of time, upon a showing of good cause or consent of the parties. The fact that abuse has not occurred while the order has been in effect cannot, in itself, constitute sufficient ground for denying, or failing to extend, the order. The new law requires the court to state the basis for its decision on the record.[12]

The Violence Against Women Act, discussed below, significantly expanded the laws extending protection and support services for victims. The law also allowed for victims to share confidential and privileged information with legal advocates trained in domestic violence law and social services, thus informing victims of their legal rights and facilitating access to the legal system.

VIOLENCE AGAINST WOMEN ACT

The Violence Against Women Act (VAWA) became law in 1994 with the purpose of changing the criminal justice system's "…response to domestic violence, stalking, and sexual assault."[13] The program was intended to toughen the laws and penalties for domestic violence and create programs to assist victims, as well as prevention activities.

Figure 5-1.
Sample PFA Order.

2012 Kansas Statutes

60-3104. Commencement of proceedings; persons seeking relief on behalf of minor child; forms; no docket fee; confidentiality of certain matters, exceptions. (a) An intimate partner or household member may seek relief under the protection from abuse act by filing a verified petition with any district judge or with the clerk of the court alleging abuse by another intimate partner or household member.

(b) A parent of or an adult residing with a minor child may seek relief under the protection from abuse act on behalf of the minor child by filing a verified petition with any district judge or with the clerk of the court alleging abuse by another intimate partner or household member.

(c) The clerk of the court shall supply the forms for the petition and orders, which shall be prescribed by the judicial council.

(d) Service of process served under this section shall be by personal service and not by certified mail return receipt requested. No docket fee shall be required for proceedings under the protection from abuse act.

(e) If the court finds that the plaintiff's address or telephone number, or both, needs to remain confidential for the protection of the plaintiff, plaintiff's minor children or minor children residing with the plaintiff, such information shall not be disclosed to the public, but only to authorized court or law enforcement personnel and to the commission on judicial performance in the discharge of the commission's duties pursuant to article 32 of chapter 20 of the Kansas Statutes Annotated, and amendments thereto.

History: L. 1979, ch. 92, § 4; L. 1980, ch. 177, § 3; L. 1983, ch. 201, § 3; L. 1986, ch. 115, § 96; L. 1987, ch. 228, § 3; L. 1990, ch. 202, § 25; L. 1996, ch. 208, § 6; L. 1998, ch. 94, § 2; L. 2002, ch. 142, § 2; L. 2008, ch. 145, § 11; L. 2012, ch. 138, § 3; July 1.

Revisor's Note:

Section was not amended in the 2012 session.

Figure 5-1

The goal was to help communities establish a collaborative response to DV by training a variety of community constituencies. Over $4 billion has been provided to states since the inception of the act to offer services and support to victims of these crimes; train law enforcement units in VAWA; encourage prosecution of perpetrators; and educate professionals, such as legal advocates, counselors, attorneys, judges, police officers, corrections officers, health care professionals, and clergy, about the nuances of domestic violence and sexual assault.[13] Although VAWA has enabled the development of many innovative strategies in communities across the country, alarming statistics surrounding domestic violence and sexual assault still estimate 3 deaths per day in the United States as a direct result of DV. The National Coalition Against Domestic Violence (NCADV) website provides regular updates on state laws and statistical tracking of DV-related incidents.[14] Since 1994, VAWA has been reauthorized 4 times by Congress, most recently in March 2013. This latest reauthorization of the law added additional services and justice in 6 areas where previously there were gaps in protection for Native American women, survivor housing, college campuses, grant programs, LGBT survivors, and immigrant survivors.[15]

In 2000 Congress reauthorized VAWA, expanding and strengthening the 1994 law. The added provisions included protections for immigrants, enabling them to seek asylum on the basis of abuse and gain their own legal status in the US separate from their spouse. The Act penetrated state and tribal lines by increasing enforcement of protection across these barriers. The 2000 reauthorization also included protection for elderly victims and the disabled and a new emphasis on dating violence, after a survey found that 10% of teens reported being slapped, hit, or hurt by a boyfriend or girlfriend.[6]

The Violence Against Women and Department of Justice Reauthorization Act of 2005[16] includes a full faith and credit clause for PFA orders throughout the United States. This means that a PFA order is enforceable across state lines in all 50 states, Washington DC, tribal lands, territories, and Puerto Rico. The 2005 reauthorization increased access to services for underserved and vulnerable groups, including "sexual assault survivors, teenagers, children exposed to violence, and American Indian and Alaska Native women."[6] New resources to support victims of sexual assault and stalking were also implemented to assist communities in furthering coordinated response to these serious offenses. The Office of Violence Against Women (OVW) provides leadership and administers VAWA legislation.[6]

For a comprehensive overview of the history and provisions of VAWA and the Office on Violence Against Women, refer to "The Increased Importance of the Violence Against Women Act in Times of Economic Crisis" submitted to the Committee on the Judiciary of the United States Senate.[6]

A CASE STUDY OF DOMESTIC VIOLENCE AND ECONOMIC ABUSE

All cases of intimate partner violence (IPV), domestic violence, and abuse involve common elements: victims, abusers, outcomes and consequences, and legal remedies. **Case Study 5-1** involves a woman who endured years of abuse by her husband. Abuse occurs in many forms, including physical and mental; however, one form of abuse not often mentioned is economic abuse. Financial survival, fear of losing one's home, and fear of losing children and family are major reasons why women remain in hostile situations.[17] The case study below is an actual occurrence. All identifying information, such as names, ages, jurisdiction, have been omitted or altered to ensure anonymity. The woman in the case study stayed in the relationship for a very long time, leaving and returning multiple times.

Case Study 5-1

Wife was married to Husband. Together they had 2 children: Daughter, age 17, and Son, age 12. Wife was in the process of divorcing her husband after surviving years of domestic abuse in the form of physical beatings, harassment, and fraud perpetrated against her by Husband. Wife filed for a restraining order/PFA 2 years ago. The PFA was granted for the maximum term of 3 years.

Three years ago, Husband received a settlement from a lawsuit. Husband told Wife that he was filing his tax return separately. Due to the small amount she earned, Wife did not need to file a federal tax return. Husband filed the tax return; however, he included Wife's name, unbeknownst to her, making it a joint return. Husband went to a local office of a national tax preparation outfit, which he had used previously, and told them that he would be filing a joint tax return. The tax preparation company had Wife's signature authorization on file from a previous year and used it on the joint tax return that Husband presented. There was no current authorization form that Wife signed for each year's tax return in her own hand, as was required by law.

After processing the tax return, Husband presented to the tax preparation company a joint application for a refund loan on which Wife's signature was forged by Husband. Wife was not present nor had any prior knowledge that Husband was applying for the loan or had filed a joint tax return.

Since the filing of the joint tax return two years ago, Husband was incarcerated for contempt of the PFA order. He was arrested for violating the PFA that was in place because he physically attacked his wife and threatened to kill her and the children several months after filing the above-mentioned tax return. The attack was of such severity that Wife had to be taken to the hospital and admitted for multiple injuries.

Because of Husband's violent control over the marriage, marital home, and his wife, Husband also controlled all finances, bank accounts, checking accounts, and bookkeeping. He had control over all family information and would not permit Wife access. Husband's prison term ends in 4 months. Wife is appealing taxes owed on the joint tax return with her forged signature. All documentation showing the PFA order, violation of PFA, incarceration order, forged signature form, and tax return were available to accompany the appeal to the Internal Revenue Service.

CASE STUDY LEGAL ISSUES

The above case raises several legal issues within and external to domestic violence law, including restraining order, contempt of restraining order, economic abuse, forgery, fraud, and defrauding the IRS. Other dimensions to DV subsumed in family law and include divorce, custody, and support. There are tax consequences to each of these legal actions. As **Figure 5-1** shows, whether or not minor children are named as protected parties in the PFA order, their physical and legal custody must be ordered by the court. Physical custody is the visitation time with each parent. Legal custody is the responsibility of making important decisions regarding the child's welfare, such as medical, educational, and religious decisions. A parent may have legal custody but not physical custody or vice versa. It is well known that child custody and support are used by abusers as a negotiating tool to leverage their position. Abusers who have had little contact with their children will assert custody rights before PFA hearing to continue the cycle of power and control over their victims.[18] The legal implications of domestic violence reach beyond immediate physical and psychological abuse. Two legal issues are detailed below. The protection from abuse order (PFA) and contempt order were presented above. The Internal Revenue Service (IRS) appeal for relief of tax liability is discussed below.

CRIMINAL VIOLATION OF THE IRS CODE

Additional issues raised by the case study involve forgery, fraud, and fraud against the IRS. Forgery and fraud are criminal offenses outlined in the penal codes of each state. The penal codes provide a crime classification, such as misdemeanor or felony, for each infraction and the parameters of punishment. The crimes of fraud and forgery can violate both state and federal laws and are not discussed in detail here. Because the IRS is a federal agency, federal law prevails and applies to any person earning income from United States sources, regardless of his or her domiciliary or residence. The IRS Code states:

Any Person who… (1) Declaration under penalties of perjury - Willfully makes and subscribes any return, statement, or other document, which contains or is verified by a written declaration that is made under the penalties of perjury, and which he does not believe to be true and correct as to every material matter; shall be guilty of a felony and, upon conviction thereof;

— Shall be imprisoned not more than 3 years

— Or fined not more than $250 000 for individuals ($500 000 for corporations)

— Or both, together with cost of prosecution[19]

The IRS requires extensive documentation to appeal and resolve a tax dispute. The IRS has a provision called Innocent Spouse Relief provides that a spouse may be relieved of tax liability by appealing the tax, penalty, and interest of a former spouse. The innocent spouse must meet certain conditions for eligibility of relief sought. The package of documentation that is submitted to the IRS should include a cover letter explaining the circumstances, as the Statement of Disagreement, the tax returns, the electronic signature page (form 8879 for the purposes of this case), the PFA order, the PFA contempt order, and any other document that can be admitted into evidence to show that the innocent spouse had no knowledge of the fraud and that the abusing spouse had motive and means by which to perpetrate the fraud.

The Department of Treasury Internal Revenue Service Publication 971 (revised February 2011) states:

You must meet all of the following conditions to qualify for innocent spouse relief.

1. You filed a joint return.

2. There is an understated tax on the return that is due to erroneous items (defined later) of your spouse (or former spouse).

3. You can show that when you signed the joint return you did not know, and had no reason to know, that the understated tax existed (or the extent to which the understated tax existed). See Actual Knowledge or Reason To Know, later.

4. Taking into account all the facts and circumstances, it would be unfair to hold you liable for the understated tax. See Indications of Unfairness for Innocent Spouse Relief, later.[20]

In **Case Study 5-1**, Wife unknowingly filed a joint return; there was an understated tax due to an erroneous item; when the return was signed, the spouse did not know that the understated tax existed; and taking into account all of the facts and circumstances, as explicated in the cover letter with the explanation of the sequence of events, it would be unfair to hold Wife liable for the understated tax. When the IRS appeal under Innocent Spouse Relief is granted, an IRS will pursue the fraud and forgery matter. In **Case Study 5-1**, the IRS did grant the appeal and did not hold Wife liable for the understated tax. Evidence supporting all of the requirements was provided, and moreover, it was clear that the defendant had motive to commit this crime.

CONCLUSION

Domestic violence or intimate partner violence is a legal subspecialty and a synthesis of family law, criminal law, civil law, and any components therein. An abuser's intent is to assert power and control over a victim by all available means. Abuse may manifest in any branch of the law, such as intellectual property, trusts and wills, estates, contracts, personal injury, federal tax, constitutional law, property, and immigration. Each of these areas of the law has nuances determined by jurisdiction, statutes of limitation, and other statutes and rules. Any assault upon the victim's life may have a legal ramifications, thus the professional working in DV must have a working knowledge of many areas of the law and/or a well-developed network of legal colleagues to consult and refer. The Violence Against Women Act 2013 has created funding to open centers and hire and train professionals who have honed expertise in the legalities surrounding domestic violence and who work with communities to elevate and coordinate their response and intervention to this important social issue.

REFERENCES

1. Luke 18:2-8. *Holy Bible*. New Living Translation, 2011.

2. Garner BA, et al. *Black's Law Dictionary*. 9th ed. Eagen, MN: West; 2009

3. Kelly HA. "Rule of thumb" and the folklaw of the husband's stick. *J Legal Education*. 1994;44(3):341-365.

4. Amussen SD. "Being stirred to much unquietness:" violence and domestic violence in early modern England. *J Women's History*. 1994;6(2):70-89.

5. Police family violence fact sheet. National Center for Women and Policing Web site. http://www.womenandpolicing.org/violenceFS.asp. Accessed May 21, 2014.

6. Carbon, SB. *The Increased Importance of the Violence Against Women Act in Times of Economic Crisis*. Washington, DC: United States Department of Justice; 2010. United States Department of Justice Web site. http://www.ovw.usdoj.gov/docs/statement-impt-economic-crisis.pdf. Accessed May 21, 2014.

7. Hauser C, O'Connor A. Virginia Tech shooting leaves 33 dead. *New York Times*. April 16, 2007.

8. The National Consumer Law Center. *Guide to Consumer Rights for Domestic Violence Survivors*. Boston, MA: National Consumer Law Center; 2006.

9. Pennsylvania Coalition Against Domestic Violence. Domestic violence and victim resources nationwide. Pennsylvania Coalition Against Domestic Violence Web site. http://www.pcadv.org/Find-Help/Victim-Resources-National/. Accessed May 21, 2014.

10. Arizona Judicial Branch. Domestic violence information. Arizona Judicial Branch Web site. http://www.azcourts.gov/domesticviolencelaw/VirtualCourtTour.aspx. Accessed May 21, 2014.

11. The Aurora Center, University of Minnesota. Office advocate. University of Minnesota Web site. http://www1.umn.edu/aurora/involved/legal.html. Accessed May 21, 2014.

12. NY Fam Ct ch 325, § 842. Office for the Prevention of Domestic Violence Web site. http://www.opdv.ny.gov/law/summ_year/sum10.html. Accessed May 21, 2014.

13. Rosenthal L. Sixteen years of the Violence Against Women Act. White House Blog Web site. http://www.whitehouse.gov/blog/2010/09/23/sixteen-years-violence-against-women-act. Accessed May 21, 2014.

14. National Coalition Against Domestic Violence Web site. http://www.ncadv.org. Accessed May 21, 2014.

15. National Network to End Domestic Violence. The Violence Against Women Reauthorization Ace of 2013: safely and effectively meeting the needs of more victims. National Network to End Domestic Violence Web site. http://www.nnedv.org/downloads/Policy/VAWAReauthorization_Summary_2013.pdf. Accessed May 21, 2014.

16. The Violence Against Women and Department of Justice Reauthorization Act of 2005 VAWA 2005, P.L. 109-162.

17. Why women stay in abusive relationships? McHenry County Turning Point Web site. http://www.mchenrycountyturningpoint.org/powerandcontrol.html. Accessed May 21, 2014.

18. American Psychological Association. *Violence and the Family: Report of the APA Presidential Task Force on Violence and the Family.* Washington, DC: American Psychological Association; 2005. The Liz Library Web site. http://www.nnflp.org/apa/APA_task_force.htm. Accessed May 21, 2014.

19. 26 USC § 7206(1). Fraud and false statements. Internal Revenue Service Web site. http://www.irs.gov/compliance/enforcement/article/0,,id=106790,00.html. Accessed May 21, 2014.

20. Internal Revenue Service. *Publication 971: Innocent Spouse Relief.* Washington, DC: Internal Revenue Service; 2011. Internal Revenue Service Web site. http://www.irs.gov/pub/irs-pdf/p971.pdf. Accessed May 21, 2014.

Chapter 6

INVESTIGATING IPV: THE LEGAL RESPONSE

Catherine Mortiere, PhD

KEY POINTS

1. Intimate partner violence (IPV) is a term that covers physical, sexual, and psychological violence perpetrated by an intimate partner, such as a spouse, ex-spouse, or a current/former boyfriend or girlfriend. IPV also includes stalking.

2. Throughout history, laws have frequently given husbands the right to physically abuse their wives. Laws criminalizing such behavior were only introduced in the 1960s in the US.

3. Since the 1990s, domestic abuse legislation has greatly progressed. Laws against stalking have been enacted in all 50 states, and in most states against marital rape. The Violence Against Women Act of 1994, provided a federal civil remedy to victims of gender-based violence.

4. Several landmark cases have changed both popular perceptions of domestic violence as well as law enforcement practices throughout the US. In many jurisdictions there are now mandatory arrest policies in place regarding cases of IPV, although the criteria for mandatory arrest differs from state to state.

5. Since the 1970s, awareness of IPV among the general population has been growing as victim advocate groups have mobilized to advocate for legal and community protections for battered women.

INTRODUCTION

Intimate partner violence (IPV) is a growing challenge to all communities. The way in which this problem is approached by all branches of government has improved over time and continues to improve moving forward. This chapter will define IPV and provide historical perspectives on how it has been addressed by the various branches of government. Additionally, some landmark cases will be discussed in relations to their impact on this pernicious and pervasive sociological entity. The chapter will conclude with a discussion of the need for increased awareness and recommendations for future progress.

DEFINITION OF INTIMATE PARTNER VIOLENCE

Intimate partner violence (IPV) has historically been defined as the abuse of a partner or spouse through physical, sexual, or psychological violence.[1] Each case of violence is generally defined by the following parameters:

— Physical violence: The classification of physical harm may include, but is not limited to, scratching, pushing, shoving, throwing, grabbing, biting, burning, use of a weapon, and use of restraint against an intimate partner or another person.

— Sexual violence: The classification of sexual harm may include, but is not limited to, deliberate , direct or indirect touching of another individual's genitalia, buttocks, groin, breast, or inner thigh of a person against his or her own will. Congruently, this abuse is defined as the use of physical force to gain sexual control over another person.

— Psychological violence: The classification of psychological harm may include, but is not limited to, humiliating a victim, controlling what a victim can or cannot do, withholding information from a victim, and disregarding a victim's wants or basic needs.[1]

One should keep in mind that regardless of the classification, whether the violence is physical, sexual, or psychological, there is an underlying component of power and control on the part of the offender. Power and control are central recurrent themes in IPV relationships, though emotion dysregulation is also thought to be at the root of IPV.[2]

Intimate Partner Violence, Domestic Violence, and Stalking

IPV can more succinctly be defined as an act of abuse committed within a relationship between partners or spouses. The term ***domestic violence*** incorporates a broader range of abuse, usually defined as violence against members within a particular household or family. In this chapter, the terms "domestic violence" and "domestic abuse" are used specifically to refer to intimate partner violence (IPV). Domestic violence in the broader sense and IPV are 2 types of abuse that differ from what is commonly known as stalking.

The National Center for Victims of Crime define ***stalking*** as "virtually any unwanted contact between 2 people that directly or indirectly communicates a threat or places the victim in fear."[3] It is also defined as "the willful, malicious and repeated following and harassing of another person."[4]

Stalking may be, but is not limited to, following a person, appearing at a person's home or place of business, making harassing phone calls, leaving written messages or objects in or near another's vicinity, and vandalizing a person's property.[3] The largest number of stalking victims are between the ages of 18 and 39 and are predominately stalked by a former partner or an ex-spouse.[3]

An estimated 70% to 80% of stalking occurs in the context of a relationship, in which generally an individual is stalked following the separation of a romantic or sexual relationship.[5] This can usually lead to violent outbursts or acts and, in extreme cases, death. Due to the serious nature and effects of stalking, certain legislation serves to restrict and punish such behavior as a preventative measure against future acts of violent domestic aggression.[5] Actions associated with stalking that may lead to violence include harassment, violating restraining orders, defying custody or visitation orders, threats, and sexual assault.[5] The concept of stalking will be discussed in Chapter 15.

Male vs Female IPV Statistics

It is important to note the statistical difference between male and female victims of IPV. Recent studies reviewed by the National Institute of Justice (NIJ) reveal that 90% of all reported domestic abuse involves a male perpetrator and a female victim.[6] In reports of female homicide, 30% are related to domestic violence, whereas only 5% of male homicide victims are killed as the result of IPV.[6] It is important not to minimize the growing number of male victims of domestic violence, but to draw the distinction that for most domestic abuse studies and legislation, the concern for female victims' accounts for the majority of research and legislative action.

Drawing upon the information specified above, the focus of this chapter will be on IPV as defined as acts of physical, sexual, or psychological violence committed by a spouse or partner from a close emotional or physical relationship.

HISTORY OF LAW AND IPV

Until the end of the nineteenth century, IPV was perpetrated primarily against women. In some cases, women were afforded certain rights to personal property and safety; however, as a general rule, societal norms afforded women few privileges. Throughout much of history, men were not questioned and were even applauded for beating and harshly punishing their wives or partners, sometimes for doing so if the woman committed an act considered to be 'out of line' domestically.[2] Authorities in most areas, however, generally disapproved of beatings motivated by anger. Their disapproval stemmed not from concern for the woman herself, but from their view that the husband's conduct was an abuse of his status.

In 753 BC, the Romans adopted the 'laws of chastisement.' These laws ostensibly accepted and condoned the practice of spousal abuse and reiterated the commonly held sentiment that the husband was the sole head of the household, and his power in a marriage was absolute.[7] A wife was merely considered the inseparable property of her husband, and as such, he could be held guilty for any crime she committed. Because of this, it became common practice to beat a wife in order to "teach" her to follow the law and serve her husband. A husband, under Roman law, was permitted to beat his wife with a rod or stick no greater than the width of a man's right thumb. The 'Rule of Thumb,' as the law became more commonly known, set a precedent that carried throughout most of Europe and later became indoctrinated into English common law.[2]

Some theorists argue that the 'Rule of Thumb' was used more as a threat than a common practice in daily affairs; however, academics still debate the actual extent of the law, as it still allowed men leeway to beat their wives as they saw fit. Many historians have insisted that the laws of chastisement, when extrapolated, allowed husbands the right to beat, divorce, or in very rare cases, even murder their wives for offenses deemed to have affected their honor or jeopardized their property rights. There are other academics, however, who have challenged the existence of a husband's legal right, under Roman law, to inflict permanent injury or death.

Although the Roman 'laws of chastisement' further hampered the progress of women's rights in society initially, they also eventually led to a few positive outcomes. Six hundred years after the instigation of the 'laws of chastisement,' Rome underwent significant changes in the family structure. During this revolution, women became entitled to property rights. While chastisement was not prohibited during this time, women did gain the right to sue their husbands if the beatings were perceived as unjustified.[7]

However, this particular rise in women's rights was not permanent. As the Christian religion broadened, women experienced a reduction of legal domestic protection. Church leaders sought to reinstate the husband's patriarchal authority in the home. The early interpretations of the Roman 'laws of chastisement' appealed to church leaders, and they moved to a more ambivalent stance on domestic abuse. There were instances when the church would encourage husbands to be more compassionate with their wives and less strict with punishments, but the pendulum would eventually swing back in favor of domestic corporal punishment toward spouses.[2]

These church teachings found their way into law throughout Europe and continued well into the nineteenth century. The United States (US) followed suit with legislation regarding woman's rights. In 1824, the Supreme Court of Mississippi decided the country's first landmark court decision recognizing a husband's right to chastise his wife.[2] The court upheld that a man could moderately chastise his wife in an instance of emergency without being subjected to prosecution for assault and battery.

In the early 1800s, American women did not enjoy the same rights as men. A husband maintained the right to chastise his wife as he saw fit, and the law did little to protect women from such punishments. Under Anglo-American law, a woman forfeited her rights as a person, the earnings she made at any employment, and the property she may have owned prior to marriage. Like ancient Roman law, prior to the nineteenth century in the US, husbands were responsible for their wives' conduct, and wives in turn were expected to obey and serve their husbands.[2]

The evolution of women's rights progressed at a sluggish pace in the western world until the end of the nineteenth century. With the ascension of Queen Victoria, the British Parliament enacted reforms that would change the landscape for women's rights permanently. Consequent to these reforms in England, husbands could no longer hold their wives under lock and key, and any life-threatening beatings became justifiable cause for divorce.

The twentieth century heralded an era of new feminist reform and women's rights. Even with new attention being directed to the plight of women, nearly a century had passed before domestic abuse was aggressively prosecuted in England and the US. Husbands still retained the right to chastise and physically punish their wives in the US until the 1960s. The inherent privacy of a family unit as well as an emphasis on domestic harmony detracted lawmakers from passing any legitimate protection for women up until the middle of the twentieth century.[2]

Culture and tradition in the US stunted the progress of women's rights far into the twentieth century. Even with previous in-roads for women's rights, wives were still subjected to domestic violence, sexual assault, and stalking with few repercussions for their assailants. For example, California state law continued to give men complete legal control over all of their wives' earnings as recently as 1951.

The 1960s ushered in a new era of women's rights. For the first time in the history of the world, lawmakers passed standardized legislation in the US, which protected women from domestic abuse and stalking. These laws were enforced in the US and used as an example to create similar laws in other parts of the world. Since the 1960s, the US Supreme Court, congress, and state courts and legislatures have progressed toward a series of criminal, tort, and family laws that universally condemn domestic violence and protect both women and men from abuse by their intimate partners.[2]

Though there has been great improvement in the way law enforcement and the court system have treated domestic violence victims and perpetrators in the US over time, the challenges continue throughout the world. Efforts made to secure a safe environment both in the home and community are slow-moving in many countries; however, there continues to be some progress toward these goals with help of international organizations geared toward safety and autonomy of women.

THE ROLE OF THE LEGISLATIVE BRANCH IN IPV

As outlined in the previous section, legislation on IPV has not come without great effort. Laws protecting women from domestic abuse and intimate partner violence are relatively new concepts when considering the vast history of civilization. Since the 1980s, national and state lawmakers have made monumental strides to modernize domestic abuse statutes and advance them to an acceptable standard. While the current legal treatment of IPV may have room for improvement, progress in partner rights has come a long way since the days of the archaic 'Rule of Thumb.'

Laws in many states now criminalize acts that were once widely viewed as acceptable domestic behavior.[8] Since the 1990s, domestic abuse legislation, both at the state and federal level, has progressed in 3 significant ways:

— All 50 states have now adopted anti-stalking laws;

— Most states now have repealed laws that previously protected a spouse from being charged with rape within the relationship;

— Updated domestic battery laws now include unique penalties for family related cases.[8]

As with any major shift in law processes, there are key differences between the way individual states and the federal government have implemented domestic abuse and intimate partner violence laws. States' laws are subject to federal standards, but federal laws generally concentrate on issues that have a more national influence. In some instances, federal statutes are created in support of commonalities in several states' policies. In other cases, federal policies are developed as flagship rulings meant to motivate states in their individual legislation.[9] Some examples of these precedent-setting federal rulings include the Victims Of Crimes Act (VOCA) of 1984, the Family Violence Prevention and Services Act of 1992, the Violence Against Women Act of 1995, and the Victims of Trafficking and Violence Protection Act of 2000.

The Victims of Crimes Act (VOCA) of 1984 provided the victims of criminal actions with some sort of compensatory help outside of the punishment of offenders. A federal victim's compensation account was created, and provisions were given to aid state programs for the victims of crimes. The compensation system still exists and has distributed over $1 billion in funds since 1984.[10]

In 1994, the United States Congress passed the Violence Against Women Act[11] (VAWA) which provided a federal civil remedy to victims of gender-based violence, even when no criminal charges were filed. Congress enacted this private civil remedy because of what some called a mountain of data suggesting that states did not prosecute crimes against women as often as crimes against men. VAWA provided state and local law enforcement $1.6 billion to aid in the investigation and prosecution of violent crimes perpetrated against women. It also extended the time spent in jail by accused offenders prior to the trial and instigated mandatory restitution from those convicted.

United States v. Morrison[12] is a US Supreme Court case involving Virginia Tech freshman, Christy Brzonkala. Brzonkala was allegedly assaulted and raped repeatedly by Antonio Morrison and James Crawford, members of the school's football team. During the school-conducted hearing on her complaint, Morrison admitted having sexual contact with her despite the fact that she had twice told him "no." College proceedings failed to punish Crawford, but initially punished Morrison with a suspension, later struck down by the administration. A state grand jury did not find sufficient evidence to charge either man with a crime. Brzonkala then filed suit under VAWA and the US Supreme Court decision held that parts of VAWA were unconstitutional because they exceeded congressional power. In a 5:4 decision, US v. Morrison invalidated the sections of VAWA that gave victims of gender-motivated violence the right to sue their attackers in federal court. They opined that violent acts covered by VAWA are more appropriately dealt with under state branches of government and should not be made a federal case.

These landmark federal cases affected the way states created and implemented their own laws regarding domestic violence and IPV. States continue to create domestic abuse laws and statutes that influence the conduct of each state's residents and organizations. Additionally, state policies are generally more varied and region-specific than federal laws and are reliant on demographics and local needs.[9]

State policies often revolve around the following issues:

— Protective orders

— The protection of victims

— Weapon restrictions

— Availability of services for victims and abusers

— Funding for victim services

— Police practices and arrest policies, ie, mandatory arrests

— Definitions of what constitutes a domestic case

— Child support and custody

— Employment policies

— Criminal penalties and procedures, ie, "No-drop policies," wherein prosecution would continue even over the victim's objection

— The role of civil and criminal courts[9]

In addition to the variation of state and federal laws there is a marked difference in the way domestic violence and stalking laws are created, implemented, and categorized (see section "Role of Criminal Court in IPV"). Stalking and domestic abuse laws are typically charged as different crimes, dependent upon in which state it occurs and the intensity of the committed crime. For example, the state of California was the first to enact concrete stalking laws (1990). Since that time, every state has created some form of anti-stalking legislation.[8] Thirty-eight states consider a first stalking offense as a felony; however, in 24 of those states, stalking could be charged as a misdemeanor, depending on the circumstances and elements surrounding the offense.[8] Out of the remaining 12 states, 9 consider stalking a felony on the second offense and 3 on the third offense,[8] as shown in **Table 6-1**.

Table 6-1. Criminal Stalking Laws: Felonies or Misdemeanor Penalties

PENALTIES	STATE
Felony: 1st Offense	AL, AR, AZ, CO, DE, IL, IN, KS, MD, MA, RI, TX, UT, VT
Felony or Misdemeanor: 1st Offense	AK, CA, CT, FL, GA, ID, IA, KY, LA, MN, MO, NV, NJ, NM, NY, ND, OH, OK, PA, SC, SD, WA, WI, WY
Misdemeanor: 1st Offense	DC, HI, ME, MS, MT, NE, NH, NC, OR, TN, VA, WV
Felony: 2nd Offense	DC, GA, HI, ID, LA, MS, MO, MT, NE, NV, NH, NJ, NM, NC, ND, OH, OK, OR, PA, SC, SD, TN, WA, WI, WY
Felony: 3rd Offense	ME, VA, WV

Adapted from Miller N.[8]

THE ROLE OF THE JUDICIAL BRANCH IN IPV

Similar to the history of legislation regarding legal intervention for domestic abuse, the judicial branch has been slow-moving in regard to effective rulings intended to deter or stop instances of IPV in the United States. Up until recent years, the only landmark US Supreme Court cases dealing with domestic issues upheld traditions such as the 'Rule of Thumb' law and social acceptability for a husband's "right" to chastise his wife.

The first major ruling in favor of victims' rights occurred in 1874, in the state of North Carolina. The case (State v. Oliver) refuted the 'Rule of Thumb' and condemned spousal battery, as well as any violence committed against a wife.[2] Unfortunately, it was not until the middle to late twentieth century that any of these ruling were fully implemented (see **Table 6-2**).

The courts now offer legal protection, commonly referred to as orders of protection, or restraining orders. These are orders issued by a judge that prohibit the subject from making contact, be it in-person, by phone or text message, by email or other electronic communication, or by mail, with the potential victim, or petitioner. It is important to bear in mind that a restraining order does not guarantee one's safety. Further help from police, courts, or domestic violence advocates may be needed if one is concerned about future attacks.[9] There are also community outreach programs, such as legal aid services or other institutions that offer free counseling and legal assistance to victims of domestic violence; however, it should be noted that programs which facilitate these services are grossly underfunded.

Table 6-2. History of IPV Landmark Court Cases in the United States

YEAR	CASE (LOCATION)	DETAILS
1825	Bradley vs. State (Mississippi)	Verdict allowed husbands legal leniency when chastising and punishing his wife.
1864	State vs. Black (North Carolina)	Condoned "use of force as is necessary to control an unruly temper," but did not give a man the right to beat his wife in a manner that would leave permanent damage to her person.
1874	State vs. Oliver (North Carolina)	Renounced the ancient 'Rule of Thumb' practice and deemed any brutal chastisement by a husband to his wife as "barbarism."
1894	Harris vs. State (Mississippi)	Refuted statutes propagated in the case of Bradley (1825), including a man's absolute privilege to beat his wife according to his judgment.
1964	Heart of Atlanta Motel, Inc. vs. United States (Federal)	Gave more power to US Congress to legislate and enforce domestic abuse laws over state statutes.
1978	Hisquierdo vs. Hisquierdo (Federal)	Recognized that the U.S. Federal courts, rather than state courts, might better address the issues of family law.

Adapted from Ross L.[2]

With contemporary legal advances in IPV prevention, victims have numerous resources at their disposal when an instance of violence occurs. If an alleged victim seeks to pursue legal action against an individual who is accused of IPV, the case will either be heard in a civil court or a criminal court, and in some instances, it may be heard in both. The court primarily responsible for hearing domestic violence issues is usually referred to as "family court."

Recently, various cities throughout the US have created courts to manage both the civil and criminal aspects of a domestic violence case simultaneously. These specialized courts have improved the legal process for those seeking retribution in cases of IPV, and are inclusive enough to cover issues such as child custody, protection for the victim, and child support disputes.

CIVIL COURT AND IPV

A domestic abuse civil trial is sought by victims primarily to resolve monetary issues between the victim and a single individual. This type of court does not require as high of a standard of evidence as a criminal court and may try cases that may not meet the requirements for criminal prosecution. Results of a civil court may include:

— Issuance of orders of protection

— Issuance of custody, visitation, and child support orders

— Issuance of orders mandating counseling or treatment for the abuser

— Divorce proceedings

— Issuance of orders of spousal support[9]

Individuals who may benefit the most from a civil court are those who are legally married to the male abuser while pregnant with his child or someone seeking child support after a restraining order has been issued. A civil trial may be the easiest way for a woman to gain financial assistance from her partner. The purpose of these civil trials is not necessarily to prove guilt or innocence, but to prove defendants financially or otherwise liable for crimes committed.

In a civil trial, the defendant may be found liable for a crime, while the same case tried in a criminal court may find the defendant not guilty for the same offense. An infamous example of such a ruling is that of the O.J. Simpson murder trial (discussed in more detail in subsequent sections). Mr. Simpson was found not guilty in the criminal trial for the murder of Nicole Brown-Simpson and Ronald Goldman in 1995, but a later civil trial held him financially liable for their deaths and mandated that he pay the families of the deceased individuals several million dollars.

CRIMINAL COURT AND IPV

A domestic crime tried in criminal court differs on some key issues from one tried in a civil court. First, a criminal court case is heard when the police make an arrest or issue a warrant for an arrest or court appearance. Once an arrest is made, the district attorney decides whether or not to prosecute the case. On felony cases, a grand jury must convene to decide whether or not there is enough evidence to go to trial. Differing from a civil case, a criminal offense is considered to be an offense against the state, not just a crime against a victim. It is the role of the district attorney to represent the people, not just the victim, and seek retribution for a crime against the state. A criminal case requires more substantial evidence than a civil one and is set on a higher standard of proof. The term "beyond a reasonable doubt" must be applied to the verdict.

A defendant in a criminal case will receive a charge falling under 1 of 3 categories: a felony, misdemeanor, or civil infraction or violation. Each case carries with it a certain level of severity, and depending on the type of charge, the court determines level of punishment within specific guidelines. For example, a felony is considered the most serious type of charge. Should a defendant be convicted of a felony, these crimes carry a considerably longer sentence that that of misdemeanors which are typically crimes of less severity and carry shorter sentencing terms.

As in a civil court case, there are distinct benefits for victims of IPV that result from a criminal case:

— A clear message to the defendant that abusive behavior is illegal and these laws will be enforced

— The result of a conviction for domestic violence is a formal sanction, jail, prison, fine, or probation

— A criminal case holds the state, not the victim, responsible for pressing charges and trying cases

— The victim is not required to hire an attorney

— The court process and decision allows for orders of protection

— Any person convicted of IPV cannot possess a firearm

— The legal decision can include an order that the defendant attend specialized programs related to IPV[9]

LANDMARK CASES

A criminal domestic abuse case reviewed before a Connecticut court in 1983 changed the way domestic violence cases were handled throughout the county. Tracy Thurman, the plaintiff, presented overwhelming evidence to the court in the case of Thurman v. City of Torrington, which proved that the Torrington City police department did virtually nothing to protect her from her mentally unstable and abusive husband. Her husband, Charles Thurman, had a history of abuse and violence. At one point, the court issued a restraining order against Charles Thurman, but Thurman violated the order on numerous occasions.[13] Tracy Thurman called the police each time her husband violated the court order, but little or no action was taken to either arrest him or further protect her. Finally, on June 10, 1983, Charles Thurman again visited the house where his wife lived and repeatedly stabbed her in the chest and neck. After the brutal assault, she was able to call the police, but the responding officers took 20 minutes to arrive. Once the officers arrived to Tracy's residence, they did little to dissuade the enraged Charles Thurman, who took the couple's infant son and threw him on top of his mother, after stabbing her a few more times in the presence of police. He was allowed to wander around the scene and was not arrested until he lunged at Tracy as she was being taken away on a stretcher.[13]

Tracy Thurman survived the attack by her husband. She sued the police department and the City of Torrington and was awarded $2.3 million in compensatory damages. Immediately following the court's ruling, the state of Connecticut changed their existing laws to require police departments to arrest spouses and partners suspected of violence or abuse. In the year following the newly implemented law, the number of arrests for domestic assault in the state of Connecticut almost doubled, going from 12 400 to 23 830.[13]

The Equal Protection Clause of the Fourteenth Amendment influenced the outcome of the Thurman case. This clause states that no state shall "deny to any person within its jurisdiction the equal protection of the law," and prohibits states from classifying individuals by any sort of group membership. Traditionally police departments are barred from refusing help to anyone based on gender, race, or any other demographically defining trait. During the course of the trial, Tracy Thurman claimed the police department did not respond quickly to her calls for help due to the fact that she was a woman. The Equal Protection Clause supported many points brought forth in Tracy's case. Thurman v. City of Torrington has since been considered a landmark case in the progression of victims' rights in the US. It sparked a nationwide debate over what role law enforcement should play in preventing domestic abuse and protecting victims from potentially dangerous situations. Since the enactment of the verdict, the national legal framework for trying and sentencing those who impeded protection in domestic abuse cases has progressed further in the direction of victims' rights.

Other cases of note that have influenced the country's legal handling of domestic abuse are Santobello v. New York and Macias v. IHDE. In the Santobello case, the US Supreme Court ruled that plea-bargaining may and should be used if possible to speed up the trials and serve a quicker verdict.[14] This controversial decision led some to argue that encouraging plea bargains in domestic abuse cases could, in fact, act against the courts and offer more leniency to defendants. Prolonged trials and a slower speed of justice, critics argued, work better to deter potential assailants from committing acts of violence. Other individuals argue that plea-bargaining saves taxpayers millions of dollars every year in court costs and legal fees.[14]

Macias v. IHDE was similar to the Thurman case. Maria Macias was shot and killed by her estranged husband after she repeatedly called and filed complaints with the police department regarding his violent behavior. It was determined that the city's law enforcement did not take reasonable precautions to protect Maria. Her family was awarded $1 million by Sonoma County, California.[15] Maria's family claimed the police did little to protect Maria due to her race and sex: she was both Hispanic and a woman. Again, the Equal Protection Clause was used effectively in this case.

Landmark legal cases set a precedent for future cases, which is their intent. Victims of domestic abuse and families of domestic homicide victims who have been a part of any significant IPV court proceedings usually gain a sense of gratification in knowing that the court trial may have a positive impact on future rulings. There are, of course, instances where the courts are manipulated by victims and by individuals claiming to be victims of domestic abuse. Obviously, the decision is in the hands of the judges, jurors, and lawyers; they are required to determine if the presented evidence in a case is of substantial merit to warrant a conviction.

THE ROLE OF THE EXECUTIVE BRANCH IN IPV

Once domestic abuse laws have been passed, it is the responsibility of local and federal law enforcement agencies and departments to ensure they are enforced. When a domestic violence call is made, the police are dispatched to the location to assess the situation, protect the victim or victims, and ensure that the assailant is arrested and later brought before the courts for trial. The manner in which law enforcement handles domestic abuse situations differs from state to state and precinct to precinct, but each police department is subject to the laws enacted by the state and federal legislature. What is common to all law enforcement officials handling domestic disturbance calls is that they face significant safety hazards. These are among the least popular types of calls that officers respond to during their careers.

A recent report titled "Police Officer Perceptions of Intimate Partner Violence: An Analysis of Observational Data" (POPIPV) addresses issues concerning police responses to IPV disputes and explains reasons some officers may be reluctant to respond to 911 calls related to domestic violence.[16] The researchers found that officers were sometimes slow to react to domestic violence issues because it is often difficult to determine the victim and assailant. The complex nature of family makes it difficult, at times, for officers to discern who is at fault. The study found that 2 in 3, or 63%, of IPV conflicts involving law enforcement were for minor verbal disputes. One out of every 5 calls involved issues that made it difficult to determine if violence occurred during the dispute. Richard Davis, a leading sociologist who studied the POPIPV in depth, observed that one of the best ways to ease an officer's hesitancy to take action when dealing with domestic disputes may be found in education. He writes that talking with officers "may provide understanding that could introduce important and detailed comprehension about law enforcement and its intersection with IPV."[17]

DISCRETION IN POLICE ARRESTS FOR IPV

The percentage of arrests made by police officers when called to an IPV domestic situation varies from state to state. Most states have adopted a set of standardized policies and procedures for officers to follow which serves to clarify when an arrest is mandatory. These standardizations are referred to as pro-arrest policies. These policies endow the officers with more clear guidelines in order to assist them in making the decision on whether or not to make an arrest. There are still a few states that leave the decision whether or not to make an arrest for IPV to the discretion of the officers on the scene. In all 50 states, legislation currently exists to permit officers to make an arrest without a warrant if there is probable cause to believe that domestic offense has occurred.[9]

Albert and Beverly Roberts wrote on domestic violence in their book Ending Intimate Abuse[9] and found the following to be a list of likely requirements, which are used for arrest when confronted with IPV:

— A police officer has probable cause to believe that a domestic offense has
   occurred. That determination may include visible harm, ie, cuts, bruises,
   swelling, torn clothing, damage to personal property, threatening messages
   on voicemail, witness statements, the presence of weapons, etc.

— A police officer witnesses the domestic offense

— A protective order has been violated

— A victim is willing to sign a formal complaint for an arrest to take place

— A determination is made that the crime alleged to have been committed
   is a felony and not a misdemeanor

— When a crime is a felony most states require police officers to make an arrest
   regardless of the victim's wish to press charges or not

— When both parties appear to have been involved in IPV, police officers need
   to make the determination of who the primary physical aggressor is and make
   the arrest. If both persons involved have been injured, some police departments
   mandate that they arrest both parties.[9]

THE O. J. SIMPSON CASE

The O. J. Simpson murder case is considered to be one of the most publicized court cases in the history of the US. Officially called People v. Simpson, this case changed the way this country's law enforcement officials handle domestic abuse cases. Prior to the Simpson case, police officers received wide discretionary latitude when called to a domestic violence scene. A victim could dismiss the police once they arrived, ask that the assailant be removed from the scene and state that he or she does not wish to press charges, or recant her or his original claims of abuse. In cases of IPV, claims of abuse are often recanted. In such cases, police would usually leave without making an arrest.[18] If police did make an arrest, the assailant would be offered bail. If the accused were able to post bail, he or she would be out of jail in fewer than 3 days time.

Around the time of the Simpson murder trial, procedures began to shift from the way police departments traditionally handled domestic abuse situations. An arrest used to be made only in cases where a victim agreed to press charges, which meant following through with a prosecution until the end of a court trial. Use of the term "press charges" is now obsolete when referring to domestic abuse cases. If the prosecutor believes a victim's original account of an incident, charges are filed regardless of any later protest or wish to retract their story. Police officers now err on the side of caution when considering whether or not to arrest an assailant at the scene of the crime or take him or her into custody for questioning.[18]

In the Simpson case, evidence was used during trial for the purpose of demonstrating a pattern of abuse prior to the murders. Prosecutors exposed a history of domestic conflicts between Simpson and his ex-wife, Nicole Brown Simpson, citing at least 9 phone calls made by Nicole to the police asking for assistance with a domestic abuse incident. This revelation caused police agencies nationwide to take a good look at the way in which they handle domestic violence calls. Nine documented calls to their residence may have placed them in the informal category of "regulars" to police. Much like the boy who cried wolf, Nicole would state that she did not want to press charges when police responded to the home. Like many complainants in cases of IPV, Nicole Simpson may have wanted police assistance to stop the imminent threat and create a feeling of safety. From her perspective, arrest and prosecution may not have been necessary once that was accomplished. Unfortunately, once police identify a complainant as someone who will not follow through on criminal prosecution, they be less likely to put themselves at risk or to be as proactive as they might be with a first time caller.

During the time of the Simpson trial, police departments around the country experienced a surge in filed domestic abuse reports. In the city of Los Angeles alone, domestic violence calls went up by 80%.[19] News of Nicole Brown's murder and the preceding years of abuse she reported seemed to have empowered women to fight abuse.[19] Prior to this type of abuse making national news, women were reluctant to fight against IPV; many saw it as a losing battle. Even after Simpson was found not guilty at his criminal trial, the civil trial uncovered more details of domestic abuse. After learning that a famous athlete was the subject of numerous complaints and that the criminal justice system was taking it seriously, many women felt as if they, too, would be heard and taken seriously should they choose to fight against IPV.

The county's lawmakers responded swiftly by passing new legislation against domestic abuse and IPV. The City of New York passed a bill on domestic violence, which included new mandatory training for police officers to be completed prior to responding to IPV police calls.[19] The California State legislature lobbied for the passage of a bill that would require the confiscation of guns from those arrested for domestic abuse and for the creation of a state registry for those with restraining orders against them.[19] The state of Colorado immediately passed a law requiring police officers to take perpetrators into custody for the first violation of a restraining order and pushed to have officers arrest assailants at the scene of the crime.[19]

DETERRENCE AND IPV

Ideally, the remedy for IPV would be prevention. A report from the National Resource Center entitled "Advancing the Federal Research Agenda on Violence Against Women" specifies the need for variety and flexibility when dealing with the possibility of deterring IPV.[20] Successful deterrents vary from state to state, city to city, and precinct to precinct. Successful deterrents also depend heavily upon situational data. Factors such as perpetrators' characteristics, relationship with their partners, economic status, and criminal history, all play a vital role when determining effective strategies for deterring IPV. Terminated relationships should also be taken into consideration for prevention because victims are at the greatest risk when terminating a relationship.

Further complications for methods of deterrence are detailed in studies that found the most dangerous abusers are repeat offenders.[14] This data appears to demonstrate that arrests and other interventions are somewhat ineffective in deterring future abuse by known offenders. Repeat offenders are rarely threatened by the possibility of arrest and most abusers have a history of violence toward intimate partners, acquaintances, and strangers alike.

THE MINNEAPOLIS DOMESTIC VIOLENCE EXPERIMENT (MDVE)

In 1981-1982, police in the state of Minnesota conducted the Minneapolis Domestic Violence Experiment to evaluate the effectiveness of mandatory arrests and their correlation to the deterrence of domestic abuse. The inclusion criteria for the study specified that IPV incidents be included only when both the victim and the assailant were on the scene when law enforcement arrived. Once the inclusion criteria were met, each police officer was asked to do 1 of 3 things: (1) send the assailant away for a minimum of 8 hours by issuing a "no contact" or "protective" order; (2) offer both individuals advice and mediation through the utilization of social service programs; or (3) make an arrest.[21] Interviews of both victims and offenders were conducted during a 6-month follow-up to determine whether or not re-offending violence had occurred after 1 of the 3 aforementioned steps were taken.[22] Arrest was cited as the most effective police response for deterring future acts of IPV. Findings suggested that arrests reduced the re-offending rate against the same victim by half within the 6 months following the original offense.[23]

CRITICISM OF THE MDVE

Aforementioned sociologist Richard Davis criticized the MDVE in 2008. He questioned the results of the experiment and scrutinized the methodology used to collect data. He writes, "Some misinterpretations may be the fault of the MDVE co-authors, Lawrence W. Sherman and Richard A. Berk." They found "arrest was the most effective of 3 standard methods police use to reduce domestic violence" and discussed 3 standard methods used by police to reduce domestic violence. They described separating the abuser from the victim for 8 hours, offering counsel and advice through social workers, or making an arrest. Davis criticized the authors for demonstrating that arrest works best to reduce violence, and then described most of the cases called in to police as minor assaults. Though Davis agrees that the MDVE does demonstrate that arrest works for minor domestic violence, it does not work for serious battering behavior.[24] Davis cited this distinction as a troubling oversight in the study's data collection. He observed that after the results of the study were released, almost 90% of law enforcement agencies had encouraged or required that mandatory arrest policies be put in place and that by 2008, half of all agencies mandated arrest policy procedures.

Davis continued to describe other possibilities that could result in higher levels of deterrence outside of arrest. He writes "The National Institute of Justice (NIJ) and the Centers for Disease Control and Prevention (CDC) co-sponsored 5 programs, as suggested by the MDCE." One of these 5 programs was the Spouse Arrest Replication Program (SARP). Davis states that the authors did not associate significant reductions in repeated assault with the use of arrest, and they reported that the majority discontinued offending behavior without it. The SARP also suggested that violent offenders be identified and made the focus of the limited resources and personnel available to the criminal justice system.[24]

In concluding his article, Davis reflected on the findings of the study and states that they are not inherently erroneous in and of themselves. The problems, he said, were due to a few omissions in the data set. According to Davis, because the MDVE did not track the deterrence rate on the more violent instances of IPV, its findings prove unusable for a large portion of the problem areas regarding deterrence for domestic violence. As stated above, Davis suggested a more effective method for reducing violent crimes in the country by analyzing the risk factors associated with the most dangerous offenders and working to prevent the crimes before they even occur.[24]

As with any area of crime, many factors contribute to reducing the number of IPV conflicts in the US. Data from the MDVE suggests that mandatory on-scene arrests in any domestic violence dispute drastically reduce the percentage of recidivism. Richard Davis and other sociologists argue that a greater emphasis needs to be placed on identifying risk factors for the most violent offenders and stopping domestic crimes before they occur. Each state is at liberty to decide how best to deter IPV. The most effective methods for prevention involve all areas of a community working together to identify risk factors of IPV, to aid victims, and to punish domestic offenders.

HEIGHTENED AWARENESS TO AFFECT CHANGE

Recognition of IPV victims' rights has come a long way since the 'Rule of Thumb.' Change has been painfully slow at times, but certain events and movements have been catalyzed in the process. With the passage of the 19th Amendment to the United States Constitution, women were given the right to vote, and thereby attained a greater influence on their legal rights in the home. This, coupled with the civil rights movement in the 1950s and 1960s, laid the foundation for the feminist movement. As women rallied together through the feminist movement, groups specifically devoted to domestic violence came together, forming alliances such as the National Coalition Against Domestic Violence and the National Organization for Women (NOW). Battered women's shelters cropped up throughout the nation, providing protection and support for women affected by IPV.

Despite a new recognition of women's rights, instances of IPV continued to be swept under the rug by law enforcement agencies throughout the country during the 1970s and 1980s. Women decided to hold law enforcement responsible for their protection, and in 1976, battered women filed a class action law suit against the Oakland Police Department for failed intervention in Scott v. Hart.[25] A similar case was brought against the New York City Police Department in 1977.[26] The police departments in both cases settled and agreed to change policies. Almost 10 years later, Tracy Thurman filed and won her suit against a Connecticut police department for negligence and violation of her civil rights when police failed to protect her from her abusive husband.[13] The pressure created by these cases and others, as well as lobbying by women's rights groups and battered women's advocates, proved sufficient to give domestic violence a more prominent place in national politics.

Women began to campaign for legal reform and first found success in 1978 when the Civil Rights Commission recognized spousal abuse as a problem in the US.[27] The first major federal legislation focused on IPV was the Violence Against Women Act (VAWA), passed in 1994. In 1995, the Department of Justice formed the Office on Violence Against Women (OVW). The legislation addressing IPV has enjoyed revalidation and modification resulting in the Violence Against Women Act of 2000, reauthorized in 2005 and 2013.

It seems that the greatest social change has been effected by women's advocates taking legal action, whether legislative or judicial in nature. The publicity generated by this legal action makes the community aware not only of the specific cases or legislative action involved, but also heightens awareness of the problem of IPV in general; however, the presentation of IPV cases by prosecution in court is an ongoing challenge. In the recent landmark case Crawford v. Washington,[28] the US Supreme Court held that cross-examination is required to admit prior testimonial statements of witnesses who have since become unavailable. As is commonly the case with IPV, witnesses often change their mind, feel threatened or have other interpersonal challenges that make them unavailable for testimony in court. That makes it all the more difficult for prosecutors to present cases of IPV.

THE WAY FORWARD

As the nation has experienced a heightened awareness of IPV, the agencies and organizations involved in IPV response are primed and receptive to the concept of changes in policy and training, new methodology of education, and reinforcement of legislation. Law enforcement is at the forefront in responding to IPV and is most often the first place that victims turn for assistance. Legal cases were brought against unresponsive police officers during the early 1970s and 1980s. Additionally, the US Attorney General recommended that law enforcement establish written operational procedures for responding to IPV calls. As a result of these actions, most police departments in the US now have some form of a written policy in place outlining specific policies and procedures for officers responding to IPV calls.

In 2002, the appropriations for the Department of Justice included "$200 000 for the Attorney General to conduct a study and prepare a report…on the response of local law enforcement agencies to emergency calls involving domestic violence."[27] Another study, conducted in 2004, revealed that 77% of police departments have written operational procedures for responding to IPV calls.[27] The main factor in determining whether a department has a policy in place seems to be the size of the department, with larger departments receiving more IPV calls and being more likely to have an IPV policy in place.[27] Most existing policies clarify what relationships are considered to be domestic and what acts are considered to be domestic violence, and seem consistent in their scope; however, procedural issues vary, such as how to dispatch to scenes involving IPV, what questions to ask a caller and how to interact with the victim on the scene.[27]

While it is comforting that most police departments have written IPV policies, practical training is also necessary to ensure that officers have the tools to effectively execute the policies and appropriately respond to IPV calls. Townsend, Hunt, Kuck, and Baxter found that close to three quarters of law enforcement agencies require specialized IPV training for officers, with 63% requiring that the training occur during both in-service and recruit training.[27] However, local agencies have complete discretion over the length and content of the training. The type of training received can vary and the amount of time spent in training ranges from a few hours up to 1 week.[27] Grants from several federal agencies are available for IPV training, providing millions of dollars for law enforcement agency programs.[27]

In responding to IPV police calls, any training for officers is better than none; however, there is a need for more uniformity in both training and policies across the nation. Independent agencies, including the National Sheriff's Association and the National Institute of Crime Prevention, provide nationwide training programs, but these are neither required, nor is the content consistent between agencies. There needs to be more collaboration between state, local, and interstate agencies in order to ensure the best and most effective training and policies. A victim of IPV in rural Arkansas needs to be able to rely on local law enforcement to respond effectively, as does an IPV victim in downtown Los Angeles.

Although law enforcement is the primary and perhaps most important agency that responds to IPV, we must recognize that there are many different response organizations. Call centers and dispatchers that receive emergency calls, physicians and other medical workers that screen IPV victims as patients and provide medical care, and social workers that seek to rehabilitate IPV victims and their families are all important sources of assistance. Each of these agencies needs appropriate and uniform training.

CONCLUSION

IPV and domestic abuse continue to be problematic across cultures in the US. Historically, women have not had a strong legal voice and were forced to defend themselves against abusive husbands and partners. Over the last 50 years, legislation and court rulings have given more power to victims of abuse, but there still remains room for improvement.

Police departments in each state respond to instances of IPV differently, depending on their specific laws, policies, and procedures and the area's population base and specific criminal statistics. Federal laws apply to all states, but each state, city, and precinct interprets those laws to best fit the community it serves. Throughout the US, violent incidents have at times, though too often, occurred as a result of police officers not reacting to domestic abuse claims appropriately. As a result of such neglect, newly formed legislation has been put into place to provide further rights and protection for victims.

After the nationally publicized O. J. Simpson murder trial in 1995, many states changed domestic violence laws, as well as arrest policies and procedures for police officers responding to IPV conflicts. The increase in arrests has garnered some criticism by sociologists who claim arrests are not the only, nor are they the most effective means of deterring IPV. The United States is moving toward a more proactive stance in creating laws to increase protection for victims of IPV and domestic abuse, and to heighten awareness of these issues for the population at large.

REFERENCES

1. Saltzman LE, Fanslow JL, McMahon PM, Shelley GA. Intimate partner violence surveillance: uniform definitions and recommended data elements, version 1.0. Atlanta, GA: Centers for Disease Control and Prevention, National Center for Injury Prevention and Control; 2002.

2. Ross L. *The War Against Domestic Violence.* Boca Raton, FL: CRC Press; 2010.

3. Office of Women's Health, United States Department of Health and Human Services. Violence against women: stalking. Office of Women's Health Web site. http://www.womenshealth.gov/violence-against-women/types-of-violence/stalking.html. Accessed March 2012.

4. Meloy JR. *The Psychology of Stalking: Clinical and Forensic Perspectives.* New York, NY: Academic Press; 1998.

5. Lemon NKD. Domestic violence and stalking: a comment on the model anti-stalking code proposed by the national institute of justice. Minnesota Center Against Violence and Abuse. http://www.mincava.umn.edu/documents/bwjp/stalking/stalking.html. Accessed March 2012.

6. Rennison CM. *Intimate Partner Violence, 1993–2001.* Washington DC: US Department of Justice; 2003. NCJ 197838.

7. SafeNetwork: California's Domestic Violence Resource. Her story of domestic violence: a timeline of the battered women's movement. University of Virginia Web site. https://people.uvawise.edu/pww8y/Supplement/-ConceptsSup/Gender/HerstoryDomV.html. Accessed July 17, 2013.

8. Miller N. *Domestic Violence: A Review Of State Legislation Defining Police And Prosecution Duties And Powers.* Alexandria, VA: Institute for Law and Justice; 2004.

9. Roberts A, Roberts B. *Ending Intimate Abuse.* Oxford, UK: Oxford University Press; 2005.

10. Greer D. A transatlantic perspective on the compensation of crime victims in the United States. *J Crim Law Criminology.* 1994;85:333-401.

11. Violence Against Women Act, 42 USC § 13701-14040 (1994).

12. *United States v. Morrison,* 529 US 598 (2000).

13. *Thurman v. City of Torrington,* 595 F Supp 1521 (D Conn 1984).

14. Davis R. *Domestic Violence.* Boca Raton, FL: CRC Press; 2008.

15. *Macias v. IHDE,* 219 F3d 1018,1028 (9th Cir 2000).

16. DeJong C, Burgess-Proctor A, Elis L. Police officer perceptions of intimate partner violence: an analysis of observational data. *Violence Vict.* 2008;23(6):683-696.

17. Davis R. Exploring law enforcement's response to "intimate partner violence." Police One Web site. http://www.policeone.com/patrol-issues/articles/1788033-Exploring-law-enforcements-response-to-intimate-partner-violence/. Accessed March 2012.

18. Grimes DM. OJ Simpson and the evolution of domestic violence cases. Grimes and Warwick Web site. http://www.grimesandwarwick.com/DV_cases. Accessed May 20, 2013.

19. McCue M. *Domestic Violence: A Reference Handbook.* Santa Barbara, CA: ABC-CLIO, Inc; 2008.

20. Kruttschnitt C, McLaughlin B, Petrie C. Advancing the federal research agenda on violence against women. Washington, DC: National Academy Press; 2004.

21. Buzawa E, Buzawa C. *Domestic Violence: The Criminal Justice Report.* Thousand Oaks, CA: Sage Publications; 1990.

22. Gelles RJ. Constraints against family violence: how well do they work? *Am Behav Sci.* 2003;36(5):575–587.

23. Maxwell CD, Garner JH, Fagan JA. *The Effects of Arrest on Intimate Partner Violence: New Evidence From the Spouse Assault Replication Program.* Washington, DC: United States Department of Justice; 2001. NCJ 188199.

24. Davis R. The Minneapolis Domestic Violence Experiment. Police One Web site. http://www.policeone.com/police-products/training/articles/1690819-The-Minneapolis-Domestic-Violence-Experiment/. Accessed March 2012.

25. *Scott v. Hart*, No. C-76-2395 (ND Cal 1976).

26. *Bruno v. Codd*, 90 Misc. 2d 1047, 396 NYS2d 974 (Sup Ct 1977).

27. Townsend M, Hunt D, Kuck S, Baxter C. *Law Enforcement Response to Domestic Violence Calls for Service.* Washington, DC: United States Department of Justice; 2006.

28. *Crawford v. Washington*, 541 US 36 (2004).

Chapter 7

Intimate Partner Sexual Violence: Prosecution and Medical Issues

*Jennifer Gentile Long, JD
**Jenifer Markowitz, ND, RN, WHNP-BC, SANE-A, DF-IAFN

Key Points

1. Sexual assault is 1 of 5 main types of intimate partner violence (IPV). The majority of intimate partner sexual assaults occur within a physically abusive relationship.

2. Most victims of marital rape report multiple instances of rape. One third of women reporting martial rape have been raped more than 20 times.

3. Perpetrators may be involved in criminal activity and may coerce their victims into committing crimes themselves.

4. Due to their relationship with the perpetrator, victims of intimate partner sexual violence may have complex feelings about their assault. Their reaction to the abuse may seem illogical to a jury, and this is often a challenge to the successful prosecution of non-stranger sexual assault cases.

5. Counselors, psychiatrists, psychologists, victim advocates, social workers, and others who work with victims of sexual assault possess specialized knowledge of common victim behaviors and responses to trauma and can help lead to successful prosecutions.

Introduction

(T)he husband cannot be guilty of a rape committed by himself upon his lawful wife, for by their mutual matrimonial consent [and] contract the wife hath given up herself in this kind unto her husband, which she cannot retract . . . . (I)n marriage she hath given up her body to her husband.

— Sir Matthew Hale[1]

There was a time, not too long ago, when marital rape was not a crime. For example, it was not until 1995 that one statute reading, "a person commits a felony of the first degree when he engages in sexual intercourse with another person not his spouse: (1) by forcible compulsion. . ." was removed.[2] The decision, quoted above, was criticized when it was written in 1800. Nevertheless, it remained the law in many jurisdictions until it—and others like it—were overturned. According to the National Judicial Education Program (NJEP), "[b]y July 1993, marital rape was a crime, to some degree, in all

*Director, AEquitas: The Prosecutors' Resource on Violence Against Women
**Former Medical Advisor, AEquitas: The Prosecutors' Resource on Violence Against Women*

50 states. The Uniform Code of Military Justice eliminated the marital rape exception in 1995."[3-5] In many jurisdictions, however, the penalties and reporting requirements for intimate partner rapists are less severe than those imposed on stranger rapists.[6] The disparity in sentences reflects the common perception that intimate partner rapists are not as dangerous as stranger rapists, even though research demonstrates that abusers commonly use sexual abuse as a tactic to control and humiliate their victims.[7] In his article "Coercive Control," Evan Stark explains, "sexual violence…almost always occurs amid other forms of violence, intimidation and control."[7] In addition to weaker laws, society often minimizes intimate partner sexual assault and intimate partner rapists or blames the victim, which frequently leads to jury nullification in intimate partner sexual assaults. Black's Law Dictionary defines *jury nullification* as "a jury's knowing and deliberate rejection of evidence or refusal to apply the law either because the jury wants to send a message about some social issue that is larger than the case itself or because the result dictated by law is contrary to the jury's sense of justice, morality, or fairness."[8] These damaging attitudes range from the belief that women "give up their bodies to their husbands"[1] to a narrow definition of intimate partners that excludes many common perpetrators and victims, including same-sex couples or couples in which an abusive intimate partner also is sexually exploiting the victim. This category of perpetrator is discussed in further detail later in this chapter. These myths and attitudes also affect victims. For example, some victims of intimate partner sexual assault also may not know that the law prohibits their partners from raping them. Others blame themselves, minimize their assault, continue to love their rapists -- while hating and fearing the assaults, or are otherwise reluctant to reveal their sexually abusive partners. If these victims report their abuse, the reports are often delayed and filled with self-blame.

In order for allied professionals to more effectively respond to victims of intimate partner sexual assault, it is critical that they are able to: (1) recognize intimate partner sexual assault and its common dynamics; (2) understand its prevalence and seriousness; (3) identify its perpetrators and victims; (4) accept victim behaviors which may appear counterintuitive; (5) understand the typical progression of a case through the criminal justice system; and (6) prepare for the common legal issues surrounding a medical professional's testimony as a fact witness or expert. This section, therefore, briefly describes the dynamics, prevalence, perpetrators, and victims of intimate partner sexual assault. Next, it charts the progression of a criminal case from incident through disposition. Finally, it summarizes the legal issues relevant for medical and other allied professionals on the prosecution of intimate partner sexual violence.

THE SCOPE OF INTIMATE PARTNER SEXUAL VIOLENCE

DEFINITION AND DYNAMICS OF INTIMATE PARTNER VIOLENCE

The term *intimate partner violence (IPV)* "describes physical, sexual, or psychological harm [to an individual] by a current or former partner or spouse. This violence can occur among heterosexual or same-sex couples and does not require sexual intimacy."[9,10] Specifically, intimate partners are defined as "spouses or ex-spouses, boyfriends or girlfriends, and ex-boyfriends or ex-girlfriends."[9] IPV "occurs on a continuum, ranging from one hit . . . to chronic, severe battering."[9] Sexual assault is 1 of 5 main types of intimate partner violence, which also includes physical violence, threats of physical or sexual violence, psychological and emotional violence, and stalking.[11] Although some intimate partner perpetrators limit their violence to sexual assault, the majority of intimate partner sexual assaults occur within a physically abusive relationship.[12] For example, "marital rape is often more prevalent among women who also experience physical abuse within their intimate relationships."[12] Unfortunately, the crime has been overlooked by society for so long because marital rape is not considered "real rape."[12] Attitudes about marital rape reflect attitudes about all nonstranger rapes, which have been categorized by experts as "one of the most misunderstood forms of criminal violence. Many people do not believe that nonstranger rapes are 'real rapes'."[13]

All abusive relationships include some level of control or an attempt on an abuser's part to control his or her partner. It is important to remember that no single theory is applicable to all abusive relationships. There are, however, 3 well-known theories that may be used to understand common dynamics that may exist in particular abusive relationships. The first theory is power and control, exemplified by the Power and Control Wheel created by the Domestic Abuse Intervention Project in Duluth.[14] This wheel includes several spokes illustrating the various methods some abusers use to control their partners, including economic abuse, coercion and threats, intimidation, emotional abuse, isolation, minimization, denial and victim-blaming, using children, and using male privilege.[14] Abusive relationships vary in that they may involve a range of 1 to all of the spokes. Nevertheless, it is a useful tool for allied professionals to review in order to understand an abuser's ability to impact all facets of a victim's life. Another theory useful to understanding some abusive relationships is the transition that abusers move through, from abuse to contrition. This theory has been termed a *cycle of violence*, which was developed by Lenore Walker to describe 3 distinct phases in an abusive relationship: tension building, physical assault, and the honeymoon phase.[15] This cycle describes victims whose abusers are alternately contrite and violent. Further, as this theory has evolved, experts have recognized that not all abusers move through each phase of the cycle. A third theory describes abuser tactics as *coercive control.*[7] Stark uses this term to describe "an ongoing pattern of sexual mastery by which largely male abusive partners interweave repeated physical abuse with intimidation, sexual degradation, isolation, and control."[16] As stated above, although these theories are helpful in understanding intimate partner violence, not every relationship involves a cycle of violence or the dynamics featured in the Power and Control Wheel. Domestic Violence exists on a continuum,[14] and, therefore, most abusive relationships exist at some place or in many places along the continuum.

PREVALENCE OF INTIMATE PARTNER VIOLENCE

Intimate partner violence made up 70% of fatal violence among females in 2007, and females were murdered by intimate partners at twice the rate of men.[17] In a recent study, two-thirds of women who had been physically assaulted by an intimate partner had also been sexually abused by that partner.[18] Despite this statistic, the public still expects rapists to be weapon-wielding strangers who attack their victims in dark alleys. Researchers in Texas found that 68% of the abused women studied had been sexually assaulted and 80% reported repeated victimization.[18] Additionally, according to the Bureau of Justice Statistics, approximately 1640 women were murdered by an intimate partner in 2007.[17]

LETHALITY FACTORS: INDICATORS OF A
HEIGHTENED RISK OF DEATH FOR THE VICTIM

Once a court has determined that a crime is a domestic violence crime, it must then assess the risk of continuing or lethal violence.[3] This critical step must be taken in order to protect the victim from the accused both before and after any jail time is served. If the court determines that there is a high lethality risk in a particular case, normal batterer intervention programs may not provide enough protection for the victim; therefore, a judge must also consider "longer jail time for the offender, community custody programs, and/or 'no contact' provisions in orders for probation" when deciding the appropriate sentencing.[3] According to the research conducted by risk assessment expert Professor Jacquelyn Campbell,[6] in 1 multi-city study of attempted and completed domestic femicide cases, there was intimate partner sexual abuse in more than half;[6] however, because sexual violence that occurs in intimate relationships is frequently overlooked or unreported, a judge may never know about information that is crucial to appropriate sentencing.

The likelihood that an offender in a violent intimate relationship will murder his or her partner cannot be predicted with certainty; however, experts have identified several factors that, when present, contribute to an increased risk of lethality. One such factor is a history of forced or threatened sex acts.[19] According to Professor Campbell, a physically-abused woman also subjected to forced sex is over 7 times more likely than other abused women to be killed.[19] A study in Houston based on approximately 150 interviews with abused women seeking protective orders revealed that "the women who were being both physically and sexually abused reported more of the risk factors for femicide, such as strangulation and threats to children, than did those subjected to physical abuse only."[20] Such tragic consequences may be avoidable if evidence of sexual violence is made available to judges in the early stages of domestic violence cases.

Perpetrators of Intimate Partner Sexual Assault

Perpetrators occupy the lives and homes of their victims. The perpetrators' unparalleled access to their victims, results in repeated assaults. "Most victims of marital rape report being raped more than once, with at least one third of the women reporting being raped more than 20 times over the course of their relationship."[21] Perpetrators and victims also frequently share children. As a result, some perpetrators employ 2 powerful tools to control their victims: threatening harm to the victims' children or threatening to take away their children if the victim leaves the relationship or reports the abuse. Intimate partner perpetrators also possess an unmatched knowledge of their victims' weaknesses and vulnerabilities, including the victim's love for her abuser. This enables perpetrators to effectively use guilt, blame, threats, or intimidation to prevent their victims from seeking help or leaving the relationship.

Intimate partner offenders are often perceived as less dangerous; however, they are "more experienced; more invested; cross more boundaries; are safer from exposure; create more betrayal and family conflict; and are more psychologically/emotionally involved in offending."[22] Furthermore, intimate partner offenders commit multiple sexual assaults against their partners.[6] The rate of intimate partner sexual assault is also underestimated even though perpetrators of intimate partner sexual assault comprise 40% to 75% of sex offenders.[23] "In 7 out of every 10 assaults, the defendant is either the victim's intimate partner, other relative, friend, or acquaintance."[23] Significantly, offenders, who often commit lethal violence against their partners, do not admit to or recognize their behavior as sexual abuse. According to David Adams, men in one study who killed their intimate partners claimed to have never "been sexually violent or even coercive to the women they killed. The victims of abuse painted a very different picture. Nearly 3/4 of the women [who survived a near-murder] said their abusive partners had raped them."[6,24]

Intimate partner sexual assault perpetrators exist in every community. They may be, or at one time were, married to or dating their victims. They may be adults or adolescents. They may be heterosexual or lesbian, gay, bisexual, transgendered or queer/questioning (LGBTQ). They may be leaders or members of religious, cultural, law enforcement, or corporate communities.

In addition to abusing an intimate partner, the perpetrator also may be forcing the victim to engage in criminal activities. Allied professionals are frequently unaware of the dynamics of intimate partner violence in common criminal enterprises, such as pimping, trafficking, and gangs. As a result, a brief discussion of these perpetrators, and the closely linked criminal activity is included below.

Pimping and Trafficking

The following discussion regarding intimate partner violence in the context of pimping and trafficking is excerpted from a forthcoming monograph by Jennifer Long and Toolsi Meisner.[25]

Each year countless women and girls between the ages of 4 and 50,[26] are sexually exploited by family members, intimate partners, friends, and strangers. They are beaten, raped, and murdered by their exploiters, many of whom are also their intimate partners. Often undetected, overlooked, or ignored, the sexual exploitation of women and girls thrives in diverse urban, suburban, and rural jurisdictions across the country. The most common age of entry into the commercial sex industry in the United States is 12 years old.[27] As this statistic illustrates, entry is often coerced by relatives or family friends who force children into a life of exploitation. Notwithstanding the criminal justice system often ignores and even blames for their victimization the high percentages of prostituted women who experience violence at the hands of customers, pimps, intimate partners, family members, managers, police officers, and neighbors.[26]

While not always recognized as perpetrators of intimate partner violence,[28] significant others regularly force women and girls into prostitution and act as their pimps. In this capacity, women and girls are forced to have sex for money and then turn over that money to their intimate partner pimps. Interviews with prostituted women in one large metropolitan city found that an overwhelming majority suffered extensive physical and sexual violence and emotional trauma perpetrated by their significant others.[29] Furthermore, men who exploit women through prostitution frequently accept rape myths and justify the rape of these women.[30] For example, some clinicians do not know that victims may delay reporting—or choose not to report—their assault may not "forcefully" resist their attackers, may have a flat affect when reporting their assault, or, alternatively, may seem less distressed than a clinician would imagine.[31]

Women and girls may be forced to prostitute out of their own homes, the homes and businesses of their intimate partner pimps, or other locations.[32] Intimate partners also perpetrate violence against women engaging in sex for survival needs on the streets.[26] In one study, researchers found that intimate partners perpetrated up to 60% of the violence against women engaging in survival sex. It further found that women on the street identified intimate partners as being responsible for about one quarter of the violence they suffered.[26] In many instances, women who are addicted and/or in relationships with an addicted partner may trade sex for drugs or be forced to have sex with other men for money to support a partner's habit. Anecdotal information indicates that the exchange of sex for drugs is one of the most violent and degrading forms of sexual exploitation.[32]

Husbands and boyfriends who use wives and girlfriends in prostitution may also film the prostituted acts and make amateur pornography available to distributors or on the Internet. Amateur pornography sites, with titles like "Turning Wife into a Whore," "Forced White Wife: Watch as this Housewife is Raped and Humiliated," and "Wives that Whore from Home" are prevalent on the Internet. The pornography sometimes depicts intimate partners beating and raping the women they prostitute and justifies or incites other intimate partners' abuse against their own wives and girlfriends.[28] Furthermore, other pimps and exploiters may use this pornography as a training manual to groom young girls and women into prostitution.[28]

Gangs

An integral part of many gangs is an exploitive culture towards women and girls. This is demonstrated by terms used by gang members, use of violence against women in initiations and as punishment, and treatment of women as property. Less recognized, however, is the role of intimate partner sexual assault, perpetrated through abuse of girlfriends and partners by gang members, recruitment of girls and young women for the purpose of commercial sexual exploitation, and rape or assault of female gang members or non gang-affiliated girls and young women as part of gang initiation.

Women and girls in intimate relationships with gang members are frequently recruited into gangs by their desire for family. Many come from violent homes without any parental presence, and gang life offers them a "real" family. Some may also be lured into gangs by the power, money, and respect garnered by their intimate partners.

Intimate partner sexual assault in gang culture may be particularly brutal because of the violent culture that typifies gangs. In addition to violent rape, it can include branding, intimidation, and homicide. Furthermore, third-party sexual assaults directed by gang members against their intimate partners are also common. Status is an important part of gang dynamics. For example, young girls may be attracted to gang members because of their "status" as a "shot caller" or leader in the gang. If a gang member with higher status is upset with his girlfriend, one type of punishment is to "give" her to gang members with lesser status to be raped. In addition to rape, assault, intimidation, and homicide, intimate partners of gang members may also suffer reproductive coercion by being forced to have unprotected sex, have abortions, or carry unwanted pregnancies to term.[33]

VICTIMS OF INTIMATE PARTNER SEXUAL ASSAULT

A current or former relationship between the victim and the defendant can lead to additional complexities that often make the arrest, prosecution, and conviction of an intimate partner rapist even more difficult. Victims in a current or previous relationship with their perpetrators have a tend "to blame themselves, [and] there may also be complex feelings involved since they may love the offender but hate the offense."[34,35] Intimate partner sexual assault victims suffer psychologically because the assault is a betrayal of trust and intimacy.[34,35] Victims often "suffer long-lasting physical and psychological injuries as severe—or more severe—than stranger rape victims."[34,35]

Many victims may not recognize their rape as an assault. As previously mentioned, some are convinced that a spouse has the right to rape his wife. Some believe that the law protects their rapists. Others defer to their partners' insistence that spouses or other intimate partners who have previously given consent to a partner are unable to withdraw it. These beliefs, grounded in cultural bias, victim blaming, rape myth acceptance, and faulty expectations about victim behavior, create unique challenges to the successful prosecution of non-stranger sexual assault. For example, "[o]ne of the driving forces behind the widespread cultural invalidation has been the commonly held belief that marital rape is not 'real rape'.... Acquaintance rape is one of the most misunderstood forms of criminal violence. Many people believe that it is not 'real rape.'"[12]

An intimate partner victim's age, race, sexual orientation, or involvement in criminal activity may also impact the victim's reaction to - and willingness to disclose an assault or report the perpetrator. This may be due to many factors, such as distrust of police, misperceptions related to the victim or defendant's culture, or fear of exposing one's sexual orientation.

Victim Behavior

Despite the extent of research on domestic and sexual violence, many laypeople still believe stereotypes about sexual and physical abuse victim behavior.[36] For example, many people expect victims of physical abuse to accept responsibility, leave their batterers, and cooperate with police or prosecutors. They may also find victims who do not scream during their rape, "forcefully" resist their attackers, report immediately, remain vigilant following their attacks, and avoid their assailants to be acting in a "counterintuitive" manner. As one court notes, however, "[t]he lay notion of what behavior logically follows the experience of being raped may not be consistent with the actual behavior observed by social scientists studying rape victims."[37]

The reality is that intimate partner sexual assault victims often stay with their abusers, regularly minimize their abuse, recant, request the dismissal of charges against their batterers, or refuse to testify against or testify on behalf of their batterers.[38] They often do not scream or resist during a rape,[39] frequently delay reporting their rape, often do not remain hypervigilant, and may continue to have contact with their assailant. In fact, "[s]ometimes people reenact the traumatic moment with a fantasy of changing the outcome of the dangerous encounter. In their attempts to undo the traumatic moment, survivors may even put themselves at risk of further harm. . . . Reliving a trauma may offer an opportunity for mastery, but most survivors do not consciously seek or welcome the opportunity."[40] They may also "consent" to sexual activity with their assailant at some point following their assault.

Common victim behaviors are often counterintuitive to the public's expectations. Left without an explanation, a victim's behavior often becomes compelling evidence that the victim lacks credibility. Expert testimony on the general dynamics of intimate partner violence and common behaviors of intimate partner sexual assault victims may be necessary to explain certain behaviors. The introduction of this testimony is summarized later in this chapter. Allied professionals who understand that victims have individual responses to trauma are better able to provide victims with support and victim-centered care.

COORDINATED COMMUNITY RESPONSE TO INTIMATE PARTNER SEXUAL ASSAULT CASES

Sexual violence usually occurs in private, but like all crime, it impacts victims and entire communities.[41] Since many perpetrators of intimate partner sexual assault use sexual violence in the context of physically violent relationships, many victims face collateral consequences relevant to domestic assault. Prosecutors must, therefore, approach intimate partner sexual assaults in a multidisciplinary manner.[42] Unlike a victim of a random crime, an intimate partner sexual assault victim's involvement with the criminal justice system may put her at risk of losing her housing if her abuser is the primary household wage-earner; losing her employment if she repeatedly misses work in order to attend numerous court appearances that may accompany the criminal and civil hearings related to her abuse; losing custody of her children if a court feels she is unable to protect or provide for her children; losing financial support for herself and her children if her abuser loses his job once he is convicted or sent to prison; losing her immigration status if she is unable to qualify for a visa under VAWA provisions; and being prosecuted if her attempts to protect herself or her children are not recognized as self-defense. In addition, as discussed earlier, victims of intimate partner sexual assault may feel a deep sense of betrayal by their abusers and may engage in self-blame.

Many communities understand the need for collaboration among social systems and have formerly created Sexual Assault Response Teams (SART) to provide coordinated responses to sexual violence. These SARTs aim to provide victim-centered support and services to survivors. Hospital emergency departments and sexual assault nurse examiner

(SANE) programs can examine, document, and treat injuries; provide information about and prophylaxis for pregnancy and sexually transmitted infections; collect forensic evidence; provide mental health treatment and referrals; and offer discharge instructions. Victims' advocates may provide survivors with medical, legal, and court advocacy; provide crisis intervention; and offer counseling. The legal system can help address survivors' immediate safety concerns, inform them of their legal rights, and protect them and their community by holding offenders accountable in court.

In addition, prosecutors must identify and form relationships with community advocates and agencies to address the emotional distress caused by the violence and to resolve the collateral problems that intimate partner sexual assault victims face as a result of their abuse. By working with community advocates, prosecutors can help victims procure counseling, create a safety plan, obtain assistances with childcare, secure or maintain housing, and receive vocational training or assistance with a current employer (**Figure 7-1**).

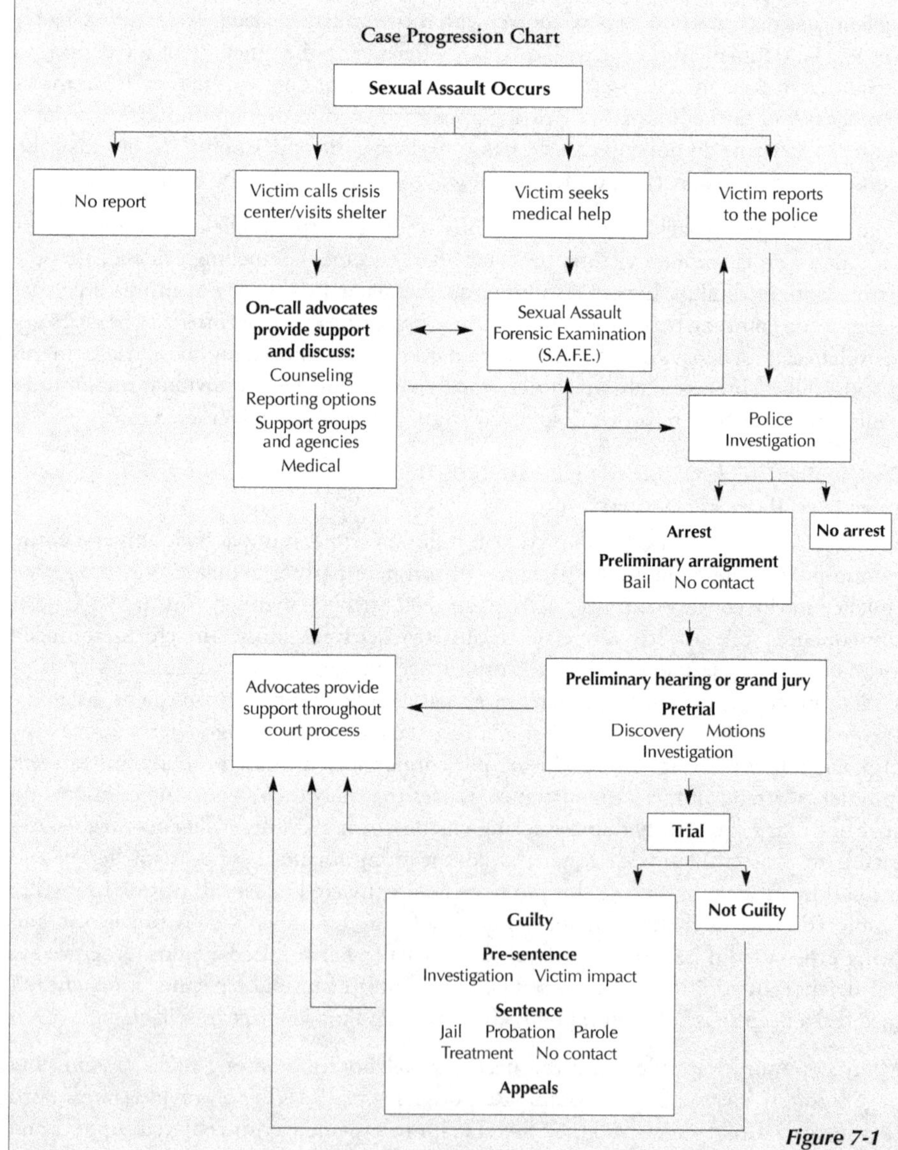

Figure 7-1. This chart represents victim reportage leading to legal intervention by way of and/or supported by assistance from community advocates. By maintaining advocate involvement throughout every step in the investigation, intervention, and prosecution, law enforcement and legal officials are better able to meaningfully support victims of sexual assault.

PROSECUTION OF INTIMATE PARTNER SEXUAL VIOLENCE: AN OVERVIEW OF COMMON LEGAL RULES AND ISSUES

Intimate partner sexual assaults pose significant challenges for prosecutors. Successful prosecutions require prosecutors to overcome cultural bias, victim blaming, and domestic and sexual violence myth acceptance. It is critical that prosecutors' approach to intimate partner sexual assault cases in coordination with allied professionals to detect all important evidence and to effectively support the victim. Some common issues, critical to understanding these cases are summarized below.

COMMON ELEMENTS OF RAPE AND SEXUAL ASSAULT OFFENSES

The definition and elements of rape and sexual assault offenses vary based on the jurisdiction in which it occurs (**Table 7-1**). Furthermore, intimate partner sexual assaults may include forcing a victim to engage in sexual intercourse,[2] engaging in sexual intercourse with a victim without her consent,[43] engaging in sexual intercourse with an unconscious or substantially impaired victim,[2] or having indecent contact with a victim through force or without her consent.[44]

Table 7-1. Definitions of Sexual Assault Terms[4,5]	
Rape	The definition of rape varies among jurisdictions. According to the definitions set forth by the National Institute of Justice, "Most statutes currently define rape as nonconsensual oral, anal, or vaginal penetration of the victim by body parts or objects using force, threats of bodily harm, or by taking advantage of a victim who is incapacitated or otherwise incapable of giving consent."[45]
Sexual Assault	The definition of sexual assault varies among jurisdictions. According to the National Institute of Justice, the term "[c]overs a wide range of unwanted behaviors - up to but not including penetration - that are attempted or completed against a victim's will or when a victim cannot consent because of age, disability or the influence of alcohol or drugs. Sexual assault may involve actual or threatened physical force, use of weapons, coercion, intimidation, or pressure and may include: intentional touching of the victim's genitals, anus, groin, or breasts; voyeurism; exposure to exhibitionism; undesired exposure to pornography; and public display of images that were taken in a private context or when the victim was unaware."[45]
Force, threat of force	Compulsion by use of physical, intellectual, moral, emotional, or psychological force, either express or implied. The term includes, but is not limited to, compulsion resulting in another person's death, whether the death occurred before, during, or after sex.[45]
Indecent Contact	Any touching of the sexual or other intimate parts of the person for the purpose of arousing or gratifying sexual desire, in either person.[46]

(continued)

<table>
<tr><td colspan="2">Table 7-1. Definitions of Sexual Assault Terms[4,5] (continued)</td></tr>
<tr><td>Consent</td><td>"Agreement, approval, or permission as to some act or purpose, especially given voluntarily by a legally competent person. Consent may be a defense to a crime if the victim has the capacity to consent and if the consent negates an element of the crime or thwarts the harm that the law seeks to prevent.[8] Consent can be express or implied. Implied consent may be inferred from one's conduct.</td></tr>
<tr><td>Penetration</td><td>The entry of the penis or some other part of the body or a foreign object into the vagina or other bodily orifice.[8]</td></tr>
<tr><td>Sexual Intercourse</td><td>In addition to its ordinary meaning includes intercourse, per os or per anus, with some penetration, however slight; emission is not required.[46]</td></tr>
<tr><td>Statute of Limitations</td><td>Enacted by the legislature and designed to prevent fraudulent and stale claims from arising after all evidence has been lost or after the facts have become obscure through the passage of time or the defective memory, death, or disappearances of witnesses. Once the statute has expired, the court lacks jurisdiction to try or punish a defendant. Criminal statutes of limitations apply to different crimes on the basis of their general classification as either felonies or misdemeanors. Generally, the time starts to run on the date the offense was committed, not from the time the crime was discovered or the accused was identified.[8]</td></tr>
</table>

In addition to specific sexual offenses set forth above, many forms of intimate partner sexual assault may be addressed through more general crimes, such as harassment, assault, intimidation, or extortion. For example, intimate partners frequently engage in conduct meant to degrade, humiliate, or embarrass the victim, such as showing naked pictures of the victim to friends or posting them online, surreptitiously video-recording sex acts and showing them to others or posting them online, biting or pinching breasts, removing victim's clothing or sexually grabbing/fondling in front of kids or others.

In a sexual assault criminal prosecution, defense attorneys routinely seek to admit evidence of a victim's other sexual activity in an effort to prove either that the victim consented or, that another perpetrator was the rapist; defense attorneys also may seek to introduce this evidence in an effort to prejudice the factfinder against the victim. Evidence of other sexual activity, even where relevant for medical treatment of a victim, may still be excluded at trial if it does not meet one of three requirements under the Federal Rule of Evidence 412, the Rape Shield Rule.[47]

Rape Shield

In a rape or sexual assault case, evidence that a victim engaged in other sexual behavior is generally inadmissible to prove the victim consented. If otherwise admissible under the rules of evidence, however, a party may introduce evidence of specific instances of sexual behavior by the alleged victim to prove that a person other than the accused was the source of semen, injury, or other evidence; evidence of specific instances of sexual behavior by the victim with respect to the accused offered by the accused to show consent or by the prosecution; or if the exclusion of the evidence would violate the defendant's constitutional rights.[47] The federal rules of evidence are not applicable to states; however, many states have adopted the rules, including Rape Shield, in their own state rules of evidence. Those without a law on point, have adopted the idea through case law. It is critical to check the laws of individual jurisdictions.

Other Crimes, Wrongs, or Acts

Evidence of other crimes, wrongs, or acts is not admissible to prove the character of a person to show action in conformity therewith. It may, however, be admissible for other purposes, such as proof of motive, opportunity, intent, preparation, plan, knowledge, identity, or absence of mistake or accident.[48]

— Evidence of Similar Crimes of Sexual Assault Committed by the Defendant: In a criminal case in which the defendant is accused of a sexual assault offense, evidence of the defendant's commission of another offense or offenses of sexual assault is admissible and may be considered for its bearing on any matter to which it is relevant.[49] The federal rules of evidence are not applicable to the states. Although many states have adopted these rules, they have not adopted 413. It is critical to check the laws of individual jurisdictions.

— Evidence of Defendant's Other Acts of Domestic Violence: In a criminal case in which the defendant is accused of a domestic violence offense, evidence of the defendant's commission of other domestic violence is admissible.[50] Please note, this is an extremely rare rule that currently exists only in Illinois, California, Colorado, and Minnesota.

NECESSITY OF CLINICAL OBJECTIVITY

Recent studies have found that approximately 40% to 65% of women physically assaulted by an intimate partner have also experienced co-occurring sexual abuse.[51-53] Clinicians must be prepared to provide comprehensive healthcare to victims of domestic violence that addresses the immediate medical-forensic needs and potential healthcare sequelae of acute and/or chronic sexual violence. This section will examine the needs of patients presenting after intimate partner sexual violence (IPSV), including identification, evaluation, and discharge and safety planning. The legal issues related to IPSV cases will also be reviewed, with special emphasis on the role of clinicians in educating judges and juries about the clinical presentation of IPSV during criminal proceedings.

IDENTIFYING SEXUAL VIOLENCE

Even when patients have disclosed intimate partner violence, sexual violence may still go undetected. Patients may have difficulty labeling forced sex by a partner as "rape." Patients may not necessarily recognize sexual assault can occur at the hands of an intimate partner. Therefore, specific and carefully worded screening questions are needed. They should be worded to be inclusive of different types of sexual violence, not just sexual assault; this includes a variety of activities, such as being forced to view pornographic material and reproductive coercion. (See **Table 7-2** for sample screening questions.)

Table 7-2. Sample Screening Questions

Have you ever been forced to have sex you didn't want to have?

Has your partner ever asked you to do things sexually that made you uncomfortable?

Have you ever been forced to participate in sexual practices you didn't want to do?

Has your partner ever interfered with your birth control?

There are many reasons to inquire about forced sex in intimate partner relationships, but the issue of paramount importance when discussing any type of intimate partner violence is discerning the potential level of dangerousness in the relationship.[19] Exploring sexual violence within the context of domestic violence may, then, occur at several points during the encounter: in initially identifying the immediate healthcare needs of the patient, and in discharge and safety planning, as a component of tools such as Campbell's Danger Assessment.[19]

ACUTE EPISODES OF SEXUAL ASSAULT

Patients who disclose acute sexual assault should be offered a medical-forensic exam. (See **Table 7-3** for an overview of examination components and evidence collection.) Clinicians should not assume that completion of the sexual assault evidence collection kit is unnecessary simply because the assailant is known. Time frames for kit completion vary among jurisdictions, with most falling between 72 and 120 hours. Patients refusing evidence collection should still be offered the examination, including sexually transmitted infection and pregnancy prophylaxis, as warranted per patient history and according to the patient's wishes.

Table 7-3. Sexual Assault Medical-Forensic Examination Components

EVALUATION OF PHYSICAL EVIDENCE, INCLUDING FOREIGN MATERIALS, FLUIDS, ETC., SHOULD BE COMPLETED PER PROTOCOL THROUGH THE EXAMINATION PROCESS.

General Physical Examination	Vital signs and physical appearance, including clothing
Demeanor	Behavior and orientation
Trauma Identification and Pain Assessment	Inquiry regarding any noted injury and levels of pain, preferably using a pain scale
Physiologic Changes	Noted alterations in function since the assault.
Anogenital Examination	External and perineal area for injury identification and physical evidence:

— Abdomen   — Clitorial hood and surrounding area

— Buttocks   — Periurethral tissue/urethral meatus

— Thighs   — Hymen

— Perineum   — Fossa navicularis

— Labia majora   — Posterior fourchette

— Labia minora

Anal examination

Rectal examination using anoscope, if appropriate

Oral examination looking for injury, such as frenal tears or palatal bruising following forced receptive oral copulation

(continued)

Table 7-3. Sexual Assault Medical-Forensic Examination Components *(continued)*

Documentation	— Narrative documentation of examination findings.
	— Diagramming of findings on body maps and traumagrams.
	— Photography, including genital photography, per jurisdictional policy
EVIDENCE COLLECTION	
Clothing Evidence	— Underwear or clothing worn next to genitalia for all patients
	— Other clothing as dictated by history and timing
Debris	— From patient's body
	— From under fingernails
Foreign Materials and Swabs from Body Surface	As noted on physical inspection and/or per patient history
Hair Combings	— Head hair
	— Pubic hair
Hair Reference Samples	— Head hair
	— Pubic hair*
Oral and Anogenital Swabs	— External genitalia: swab at least one dry and one moistened with a drop of sterile, distilled, or deionized water, according to jurisdiction policy.
	— Vaginal sample: swab vaginal vault, face of cervix.
	— Penile sample: moistened swabs along the shaft and glans.
	— Anal sample: moistened swabs perianally and swabs in anus, per patient history
	— Oral sample: swab along gum lines with history of forced receptive oral copulation.
	— Consider also: moistened swabs around the mouth and chin with history of forced receptive oral copulation
DNA Standard from Patient	— Bucchal swab
	— Draw blood with finger stick
	— Draw blood
	Toxicology samples, per history, patient presentation, or community protocol
	Note: Evidence collection should be completed according to jurisdictional polices and based on patient history.

** There is concern that the current scientific evidence does not support continued plucking of public hair or head hair given the limited hair analysis occurring in sexual assault cases, but this still may be protocol in some jurisdictions. Adapted from US Department of Justice, Office on Violence Against Women.[56]*

Anonymous Reports / "Jane Doe Rape Kit"

Anonymous or "Jane Doe" kits, the common names for the forensic evidence collected during a sexual assault examination of a victim who chooses not to report to law enforcement, enables a victim to have forensic evidence collected without revealing identifying information. Victims are given a code number or some other indicator they can use to identify themselves if they choose to report later, and they are not required to cooperate with law enforcement or criminal justice authorities. Many jurisdictions provide this voluntarily for victims who are not ready to report to law enforcement at the time of the examination.[54]

Forensic Compliance

The Violence Against Women and Department of Justice Reauthorization Act of 2005 (VAWA 2005), provides that states may not "require a victim of sexual assault to participate in the criminal justice system or cooperate with law enforcement in order to be provided with a forensic medical exam, reimbursed for charges incurred on account of such an exam, or both."[55] Under this provision, a state must ensure that victims have access to an exam free of charge or with full reimbursement, even if the victim chooses not to cooperate with police or participate in the criminal justice system. Prior to VAWA 2005, states were required to ensure access to such exams free of charge or with full reimbursement but could condition the exams on a victim's cooperation with law enforcement. (Additional information regarding forensic compliance and associated issues is available at http://www.evawintl.org/Forensic-Compliance.)

While conducting the medical-forensic examination, clinicians should consider some of the issues particularly important in caring for patients assaulted by an intimate partner.

Documentation of a Continuum of Injury

A patients presenting after IPSV may be seeking care following an acute episode of violence, but that episode is likely part of an ongoing pattern of violence in the patient's life. Clinicians should be careful to document all injury and, where possible, differentiate injuries resulting from the present episodes from previously inflicted injury. Past medical treatment and hospitalization from other episodes of violence may also be documented in patients' medical histories, and as potential support for discharge plans where appropriate.

Involvement of Children

Children are frequently present in the home during domestic violence incidents and may, in fact, be victims of co-occurring abuse. A recent study found that of more than 4500 children surveyed, 1 in 5 had witnessed some type of family violence in their lifetime and 10% had witnessed family violence in the previous year.[57] In their review of the research, Jouriles et al found that estimates of co-occurring child abuse ranged from 18% to 67%.[58] In working with patients, clinicians should inquire about child witnessing and abuse. Because many patients may be concerned that they will lose their children to either a child protection agency or the offending parent, clinicians must be aware of how screening occurs and, when necessary, how reports to child protection agencies are made. In a case where disclosure triggers mandatory reporting, clinicians may consider making a report with the patient present, in order to allow him or her to hear the details of the statement and potentially answer questions about the incident directly. Involving child protection professionals in regular multidisciplinary team meetings can facilitate communication in these types of situations and help clinicians navigate the child protection response in their own jurisdictions.

Safety and Discharge Planning

IPSV patients may require more extensive discharge planning than other types of sexual assault patients. Patients assaulted by an intimate partner have significantly different safety issues than patients assaulted by an acquaintance or a stranger. That is not to say IPSV patients are unique in their needs for safety planning. Clinicians should be aware, however, that preprinted discharge instructions frequently provided to sexual assault patients will be inadequate to address their highly individual situations and priorities. Clinicians should be prepared to involve other collaborating professionals, including victim advocates (from rape crisis, domestic violence, and general victim advocacy programs), agency social workers, and other experienced clinicians in order to effectively work with patients to craft their discharge and safety plans. Tools such as Campbell's Danger Assessment may be useful in working with patients to evaluate the degree of danger they face. An online training course for using the assessment tool is available at www.dangerassessment.org.

PAST AND CHRONIC SEXUAL VIOLENCE

Patients who do not fit the criteria for acute medical-forensic examination, or who choose not to partake in the evidence collection portion should still be offered comprehensive evaluation. Based on the history of the sexual violence, including recency and type of sexual violence, the following areas may be considered as part of the physical assessment and treatment:

— Head-to-toe physical assessment of the patient, looking for superficial, soft tissue, and underlying structural injury secondary to mechanisms of injury like strangulation, suffocation, and bite wounds

— Genital examination assessing for evidence of injury and infection

— Pregnancy screening and prophylaxis, if desired by the patient and within 120 hours of exposure

— Sexually transmitted infection screening and prophylaxis, depending on most recent exposure, including HIV, hepatitis, syphilis, gonorrhea, chlamydia, and trichomoniasis (Additional information regarding treatment guidelines for sexual assault post-exposure prophylaxis is available at http://www.cdc.gov/STD/treatment/default.htm for treatment guidelines, including sexual assault post-exposure prophylaxis.)

— Exploration of chronic health issues, including chronic pain complaints, and their association to and exacerbation by the sexual violence

— Screening and evaluation of mental health issues, including Post Traumatic Stress Disorder (PTSD) and suicidal ideation

HEALTHCARE SEQUELAE OF SEXUAL VIOLENCE

Patients who disclose sexual violence have the potential to develop a variety of physical and mental health sequelae. Understanding their associations will help clinicians identify and treat these issues. Furthermore, recognizing the interconnectedness of violence and health status can help decrease the likelihood of judgmental, inaccurate, and detrimental labels, such as "noncompliant" and "drug-seeking" from being assigned to patients. (See **Table 7-4** for an overview of violence-related healthcare sequelae.)

CLINICIAN COMPETENCY

Clinicians who care for patients presenting with complaints of domestic violence need to be careful not to separate sexual violence as a distinct and unrelated issue. Frequently, the 2 co-occur, and clinicians must be able to manage them simultaneously. For general,

<table>
<tr><td colspan="2">Table 7-4. Violence-Related Healthcare Sequelae[51,53,56-63]</td></tr>
<tr><td>CARDIOVASCULAR</td><td>HYPERTENSION</td></tr>
<tr><td>Gastrointestinal</td><td>— Digestive problems, such as diarrhea, spastic colon, constipation, nausea
— Loss of appetite, eating binges, self-induced vomiting</td></tr>
<tr><td>Genito Urinary</td><td>— Abdominal pain and cramping
— Pelvic pain
— Menstrual issues, dysmenorrhea
— Non-menstrual vaginal bleeding
— Bladder infection
— Painful urination
— Pain with intercourse or decreased sexual desire
— Gential irritation
— Rectal bleeding</td></tr>
<tr><td>Reproductive Health</td><td>— Unintended pregnancy
— Sexually transmitted infections</td></tr>
<tr><td>Musculo-skeletal</td><td>— Back and neck pain</td></tr>
<tr><td>Neurological</td><td>— Headaches or migraines
— Seizures or convulsions</td></tr>
<tr><td>Mental Health</td><td>— Depression or anxiety
— Post traumatic stress disorder
— Dissociative disorders
— Substance use or abuse
— Suicidality</td></tr>
<tr><td>Homicide</td><td>— Murder
— Murder-Suicide</td></tr>
</table>

primary, and acute care providers, this means being able to effectively screen and assess for intimate partner violence (IPV), as well as refer appropriately for sexual assault medical-forensic exams when appropriate. For specialists, such as sexual assault nurse examiners (SANEs), this involves individualizing the approach to sexual assault patients, with an understanding that the context of the assault should influence the course of treatment and discharge planning. Baseline education is needed for all clinicians caring for IPV patients, regardless of specialty, and several excellent examples of guidelines and core competencies are available.[64-66]

Admission of Hearsay Statements

Prosecutors frequently seek to introduce victim's statements to medical treatment providers in the prosecution of an intimate partner sexual assault. These statements may be admitted as prior inconsistent statements in the rare circumstance that an intimate partner sexual assault is prosecuted with a recanting or uncooperative victim.[67] They may also be admitted as prior, consistent statements in order to rehabilitate a victim after the defense has impeached her.[68] Under the medical hearsay exception, "[s]tatements made for the purpose of medical diagnosis or treatment in connection with treatment and describing medical history or past or present symptoms, pain, or sensations, or the inception or general character of the cause or external source thereof insofar as reasonably pertinent to diagnosis and treatment" are admissible.[69]

Impact of Crawford v. Washington and Its Progeny and Giles v. California

Crawford v. Washington and subsequent related court cases are only an issue when a victim is unavailable for cross-examination at trial, which does not frequently occur in sexual assault cases. Because of the difficulty in overcoming the consent defense, a prosecutor will rarely be able to successfully prosecute a sexual assault of a competent adult victim without the victim's cooperation. The term *competent adult* is used to represent those adult victims who are viewed by the legal system as able to understand and participate in criminal proceedings. It is important to refer to state laws for definitions or interpretations of what constitutes a competent adult in a given jurisdiction.

In the rare instance where the sexual assault of a competent adult is prosecuted without the victim's cooperation, SAFEs testimony may be objected to as "testimonial" under Crawford v Washington[70-72] and hearsay under the theory that the SAFE was acting as an arm of law enforcement. In Crawford, the Court held that testimonial statements of an unavailable witness could be admitted at trial only when the defendant has had a prior opportunity to cross-examine that witness. Although the Crawford holding offers examples of both testimonial and nontestimonial statements, it did not include a specific definition.

In Davis v. Washington,[73] the Court defined statements which are made to government agents for the primary purpose of receiving assistance in an ongoing emergency as nontestimonial. It defined statements made under circumstances that objectively indicate there is no ongoing emergency and the primary purpose of the interrogation is to establish or prove past events potentially relevant to a later criminal prosecution. The definition of emergency was further refined in Michigan v. Bryant.[74] Forensic nurses who perceive their primary role as law enforcement and conduct their practice with law enforcement goals, rather than medical goals, risk having their statements excluded as testimonial under Crawford and Davis. Forensic nurse examiners should be asked about, and must be able to articulate patient-centered, medically-focused practice philosophy.

When it is established that a victim's lack of cooperation is the result of a defendant's actions designed to cause the unavailability of a victim in order to prevent that victim from testifying in a current or future prosecution, the prosecution may introduce a witness' hearsay statements in a prosecution based on the doctrine of forfeiture by wrongdoing.[75] Forfeiture by wrongdoing is the legal rule under which prosecutors may introduce at trial a victim's or witness' testimonial statements. In order to establish forfeiture by wrongdoing, the prosecution must demonstrate that a victim's or witness' absence was caused by the defendant's wrongful act intended to prevent that victim or witness from testifying at a trial.[75]

If a victim is unavailable at trial, the prosecutor must determine whether the abuser caused her unavailability. If this is the case, prosecutors must prepare for a forfeiture hearing.[76] The prosecutor can introduce the history of abuse between the defendant and the victim; prior charges filed, even if they were withdrawn; testimony from prior cases; evidence from police, a prior prosecutor, family, or friends about the victim's fear of the defendant; evidence of the victim's fear of testifying in prior cases; and anything else that shows the defendant did something to prevent the victim from testifying. Establishing a coordinated community response can help a prosecutor uncover any threats or intimidation directed at a victim. Significantly, hearsay is permissible at a forfeiture hearing. If the prosecution successfully establishes forfeiture by wrongdoing, the defendant is precluded from objecting to the introduction of the victim's testimonial statements.

For healthcare providers, Crawford and its progeny do not change the priorities of the medical-forensic examination, which should continue to hold the health and well-being of patients to be of primary importance. The problem arises when clinicians are perceived to be investigators, rather than healthcare providers. Even in cases where a victim is cooperating in the prosecution of her perpetrator, statements made to the SAFE for the purpose of medical diagnosis and treatment may still be excluded as hearsay if it is established that the SAFE is acting as an arm of law enforcement rather than acting primarily as a medical treatment provider

USING EXPERTS IN AN INTIMATE PARTNER SEXUAL ASSAULT PROSECUTION

Medical experts may act as fact or expert witnesses. Qualified medical treatment providers and allied professionals may be called to testify as experts in an intimate partner sexual assault case to render medical opinions as well as to explain victim behavior. The following rules are relevant to the introduction of their testimony.

Federal Rule of Evidence 402: Establishing Relevance

Under the Federal Rules of Evidence, the admissibility of expert testimony is governed by liberal standards, and is first analyzed according to the general rules of relevance.[77] Federal Rule of Evidence 402 provides that "[a]ll relevant evidence is admissible" and "[e]vidence which is not relevant is not admissible."[78] Relevant evidence means evidence having a tendency to make the existence of any fact of consequence to the determination of the action more or less probable than it would be without the evidence.[79]

Federal Rule of Evidence 702: Proper Subject of Expert Testimony

Once relevance is established, prosecutors must show the subject of expert testimony satisfies the requirements of Federal Rule of Evidence 702. According to this evidence rule, if scientific, technical, or other specialized knowledge will assist the trier of fact to understand the evidence or to determine a fact in issue, a witness qualified as an expert by knowledge, skill, experience, training, or education, may testify thereto in the form of an opinion or otherwise, if (1) the testimony is based upon sufficient facts or data, (2) the testimony is the product of reliable principles and methods, and (3) the witness has applied the principles and methods reliably to the facts of the case.[80]

Qualifying the Expert

Under Federal Rule of Evidence 702, an expert must be qualified by "knowledge, skill, experience, training, or education."[80] Qualifications are defined broadly. Generally, an individual with reasonable pretense to specialized knowledge may be qualified as an expert based on his or her clinical experience, education, knowledge of relevant scholarly articles, authorships of articles, prior qualifications, or a combination of factors listed above.[80] "The trial court has discretion in determining the sufficiency of the expert's qualifications and its decision will be reviewed only for manifest error and injustice."[81] In addition, courts give much deference to their previous decisions and, therefore, experts who previously have been qualified to testify as an expert typically will be qualified again (eg, State v Townsend,[81] State v Ciskie,[82] State v Borelli[83]).

Expert Testimony to Explain Victim Behavior

The proper subjects of expert testimony are topics beyond the common knowledge of the average juror. Several decisions have adopted this very language when explaining the necessity of expert testimony to explain victim behavior; however, not all jurisdictions have found victim behavior that may be counterintuitive to victims to be beyond their understanding. One court concluded that expert testimony was not required to explain a victim's decision to stay with her abuser even when the defense argued that it was inconsistent with a real victim's behavior. The court concluded that the expert testimony was not required in the case because the "disputed element was adequately proved with lay testimony. Personal relationships, even abusive relationships, are within the realm of the jury's collective experience and common sense. The jurors [therefore] could evaluate the argument in light of human experience."[84]

In general, testimony by such an expert should be limited to background information about the dynamics of sexual violence, victim responses to sexual violence, and the impact of sexual violence on victims during and after being assaulted. The expert may testify to facts and opinions regarding specific types of victim responses and victim behaviors. For example, an expert might be asked: "In your experience, is it common for a victim of sexual assault to delay her report of the assault or to choose not to report the assault at all? What are some reasons for this?" The expert's response should focus on the behaviors that he or she has noted through his or her experience working with victims and should not be tied to a disorder or syndrome. The expert's opinion regarding the credibility of a witness is inadmissible.

Counselors, psychiatrists, psychologists, victim advocates, social workers, and others who work with sexual assault victims possess specialized knowledge about common victim behaviors and victim responses to trauma, and that expertise is beyond the experience and knowledge of the average juror.

CONCLUSION

Notwithstanding the prevalence of research, media, policy and legal attention to the topic of intimate partner violence, myths and misinformation about this crime persist and continue to impact the medical and prosecution response. To ensure victim safety and offender accountability, it is critical that allied professionals continuously seek information and resources regarding dynamics, appropriate healthcare responses, emerging issues, and current policies and laws.

ACKNOWLEDGMENTS

The authors of this Chapter would like to thank the following: staff of AEquitas: The Prosecutors' Resource on Violence Against Women: Toolsi Meisner, Attorney Advisor, for significant editing contributions; Christopher Mallios, Attorney Advisor, and Sarah Stanley, Legal Intern, for their assistance in creating the Case Progression Chart; and Bridget Kerlick, Legal Intern, for her assistance with Lethality Assessment research and in compiling the resources cited in this chapter.

REFERENCES

1.   Hale SM. *History of the Pleas of the Crown*. London, UK; 1736. Cited in: Commonwealth v. Chretian, 417 NE 2d 1203, 1207 (Mass 1981).

2.   18 Pa CS § 3121 (1994).

3.   National Judicial Education Program (NJEP). Intimate partner sexual abuse: adjudicating this hidden dimension of domestic violence cases. National Judicial Education Program Web site. http://www.njep-ipsacourse.org. Accessed June 28, 2010.

4.   Tracy CE, Fromson TL, Long JG, Whitman C. Rape and sexual assault in the legal system. http://sites.nationalacademies.org/dbasse/cnstat/currentprojects/dbasse_073316#.UKvuMI4QifR. Published Jun 5, 2012. Accessed September 10, 2013.

5. AEquitas. *Rape and Sexual Assault Analyses and Laws*. Washington, DC: AEquitas; 2014. AEquitas Web site. http://www.aequitasresource.org/Rape-and-Sexual-Assault-Analyses-and-Laws.pdf. Accessed September 10, 2013.

6. Schafran LH. Risk assessment and intimate partner sexual abuse: the hidden dimension of domestic violence. *Judicature*. 2010;93:161-163.

7. Stark E. *Coercive Control: The Entrapment of Women in Personal Life*. New York, NY: Oxford University Press; 2007.

8. Garner BA, ed. *Black's Law Dictionary*. 9th ed. Eagan, MN: West; 2009.

9. Centers for Disease Control and Prevention. Intimate partner violence: definitions. Centers for Disease Control and Prevention Web site. http://www.cdc.gov/Violence Prevention/intimatepartnerviolence/definitions.html. Accessed June 28, 2010.

10. Catalano S, Smith E, Snyder H, Rand M. *Female Victims of Violence*. Washington, DC: United States Department of Justice; 2009. Bureau of Justice Statistics Web site. http://bjs.ojp.usdoj.gov/content/pub/pdf/fvv.pdf. Accessed June 28, 2010.

11. Saltzman LE, Fanslow JL, McMahon PM, Shelley GA. *Intimate Partner Violence Surveillance: Uniform Definitions and Recommended Data Elements*. Atlanta, GA: Centers for Disease Control and Prevention, National Center for Injury Prevention and Control; 2002. Centers for Disease Control and Prevention Web site. http://www.cdc.gov/ncipc/pub-res/ipv_surveillance/intimate.htm. Accessed June 28, 2010.

12. Bennice JA, Resick PA. Marital rape: history, research, and practice. *Trauma Violence Abuse*. 2003;4(3):231-234.

13. Estrich S. *Real Rape*. Cambridge, MA: Harvard University Press; 1988.

14. Domestic Abuse Intervention Project. The power and control wheel. Domestic Abuse Intervention Programs Web site. http://www.theduluthmodel.org/pdf/PowerandControl.pdf. Accessed June 28, 2010.

15. Walker LE. *The Battered Woman Syndrome*. Fort Lauderdale, FL: Springer Publishing Company; 1984.

16. Stark E. Coercive control. *Fatality Rev Bul*. 2010:2-4.

17. Bureau of Justice Statistics, Office of Justice Programs. Intimate partner violence. http://bjs.ojp.usdoj.gov/index.cfm?ty=pbdetail&iid=4536. Accessed June 28, 2010.

18. Gaskin-Laniyan N, Taylor LR. Sexual assault in abusive relationships. *NIJ J*. 2007;256:12-14.

19. Campbell JC, Webster D, Koziol-McLain J, et al. Assessing risk factors for intimate partner homicide. *NIJ J*. 2003;250:14-19. National Criminal Justice Reference Service Web site. https://www.ncjrs.gov/pdffiles1/jr000250e.pdf. Accessed January 30, 2013.

20. McFarlane J, Malecha A, Watson K, et al. Intimate partner sexual assault against women: frequency, health consequences, and treatment outcomes. *Obstet Gynecol*. 2005;105(1):99-108.

21. Mahoney P. The wife rape fact sheet. Medical University of South Carolina Web site. http://www.musc.edu/vawprevention/research/wiferape.shtml. Accessed June 28, 2010.

22. Valliere VN. Understanding the non-stranger rapist. *Voice*. 2007;1(11):1-6.

23. Castalano SM. National Crime Victimization Survey: criminal victimization, 2004. http://www.bjs.gov/content/pub/pdf/cv04.pdf. Accessed September 10, 2013.

24. Adams D. *Why Do They Kill?: Men Who Murder Their Intimate Partners*. Nashville, TN: Vanderbilt University Press; 2007.

25. Long J, Meisner T, Kristiansson V, et al *Prosecutorial Response to Violence Against Sexually Exploited Women*. In press.

26. Raphael J, Shapiro DL. *Sisters Speak Out: The Lives and Needs of Prostituted Women in Chicago*. Chicago, IL: Center for Impact Research; 2002. Center for Impact Research Web site. www.impactresearch.org/documents/sistersspeakout.pdf. Accessed June 28, 2010.

27. Estes RJ, Weiner NA. *Commercial Sexual Exploitation of Children in the U.S., Canada, and Mexico*. Philadelphia, PA: University of Pennsynvania, School of Social Work, Center for the Study of Youth Policy; 2001. University of Pennsylvania School of Social Policy and Practice Web site. http://www.sp2.upenn.edu/restes/ CSEC_Files/Complete_CSEC_020220.pdf. Accessed June 28, 2010.

28. Hodgson C, Stark C. Sister oppressions: a comparison of wife battery and prostitution. In: Farley M, ed. *Prostitution, Trafficking and Traumatic Stress*. New York, NY: Haworth Press; 2003:17-32.

29. Sweet EM. *The Intersystem Assessment on Prostitution in Chicago*. Chicago, IL: Mayor's Office on Domestic Violence; 2006. City of Chicago Mayor's Office on Domestic Violence Web site. http://www.cfw.org/document.doc?id=168. Accessed June 28, 2010.

30. Durchslag R, Goswami S. *Deconstructing the Demand for Prostitution: Preliminary Insights From Interviews With Chicago Men Who Purchase Sex*. Chicago, IL: Chicago Alliance Against Sexual Exploitation; 2008. Chicago Alliance Against Sexual Exploitation Web site. http://www.slaverynomore.org/wp-content/uploads/2011/07/ Deconstructing-the-Demand-for-Prostitution.pdf. Accessed September 10, 2013.

31. Mallios C, Meisner T. Educating judges and juries in sexual assault cases: part I: using voir dire to eliminate jury bias. *Strategies*. July 2010;2:1-7. http://www. aequitasresource.org/EducatingJuriesInSexualAssaultCasesPart1.pdf. Accessed September 10, 2013.

32. Sponsler C. *Advocacy on Behalf of Women in Prostitution: A Handbook for Rural Advocates*. Duluth, MN: Praxis International; 2004. Praxis International Web site. http://www.praxisinternational.org/files/praxis/files/Women%20Used%20in%20 Prostitution/WomenUsedinProstitutioHandbook.pdf. Published 2007. Accessed January 30, 2013.

33. Harris L. When teen pregnancy is no accident. *The Nation*. May 24, 2010. http:// www.thenation.com/article/when-teen-pregnancy-no-accident. Accessed June 28, 2010.

34. Finkelhor D, Yllo K. *License to Rape: Sexual Abuse of Wives*. New York, NY: Free Press; 1985.

35. Russell DEH. *Rape in Marriage*. NewYork, NY: Macmillan Press; 1990.

36. Ben-David S, Schneider O. Rape Perceptions, Gender Role Attitudes, and Victim-Perpetrator Acquaintance. *Sex Roles*. 2005;53(5-6):385-399.

37. *People v Hampton*, 746 P.2d 947, 952 (Colo. 1987).

38. Buel SM. Fifty obstacles to leaving, a.k.a., why abuse victims stay. *Colorado Lawyer.* 1999;28(10):19-28.

39. Rennison CM. *Rape and Sexual Assault: Reporting to Police and Medical Attention, 1992-2000.* Washington, DC: United States Department of Justice; 2002. Bureau of Justice Statistics Web site. http://bjs.ojp.usdoj.gov/content/pub/pdf/rsarp00. pdf. Accessed June 28, 2010.

40. Herman J. *Trauma and Recovery.* New York, NY: Basic Books; 1992:38-42.

41. Mallios C, Markowitz J. Benefits of a coordinated community response to sexual violence. *Administrators' Corner.* 2010;March/April:7-9.

42. Kristiansson V, Long JG. Taking a process-oriented approach to domestic violence prosecutions. *Voice.* 2007;1(9):1-5.

43. 18 Pa CS § 3124.1.

44. 18 Pa CS § 3126.

45. National Institute of Justice. Rape and sexual violence. National Institute of Justice Web site. http://www.ojp.usdoj.gov/nij/topics/crime/rape-sexual-violence/ welcome.htm. Accessed June 28, 2010.

46. 18 Pa CS § 3101.

47. Fed R Evid 412.

48. Fed R Evid 404(b).

49. Fed R Evid 413.

50. Cal Evid Code §1109.

51. McFarlane J, Malecha A. *Sexual Assault Among Intimates: Frequency, Consequences, and Treatments.* Washington DC: United States Department of Justice; 2005. National Criminal Justice Reference Service Web site. http://www.ncjrs.gov/ pdffiles1/nij/grants/211678.pdf. Accessed June 28, 2010.

52. Cattaneo LB, DeLoveh HL, Zweig JM. Sexual A]assault within intimate partner violence: impact on helpseeking in a national sample. *J Prev Interv Community.* 2008;36(1-2):137-153.

53. Campbell JC, Soeken KL. Forced sex and intimate partner violence: effects on women's risk and women's health. *Violence Against Women.* 1999;5(9):1017-1035.

54. End Violence Against Women International. Forensic compliance: frequently asked questions. End Violence Against Women Internation Web site. http://www. evawintl.org/Forensic-Compliance/FAQs. Accessed August 8, 2013.

55. Violence Against Women Reauthorization Act of 2005, 42 USC 3402-15 (2005).

56. US Department of Justice, Office on Violence Against Women. *A National Protocol for Sexual Assault Medical Forensic Examinations: Adults/Adolescents.* 2nd ed. Washington, DC: United States Department of Justice, Office of Violence Against Women. Sexual Assault Forensic Examiner Technical Assistance Web site. http:// safeta.org/displaycommon.cfm?an=4. Accessed August 8, 2013.

57. Finkelhor D, Turner H, Ormrod R, et al. Violence, abuse, and crime exposure in a national sample of children and youth. *Pediatrics.* 2009;124(5):1411-1423.

58. Jouriles EN, McDonald R, Slep AM, et al. Child abuse in the context of domestic violence: prevalence, explanations, and practice implications. *Violence Vict.* 2008;23(2):221-235.

59. Temple JR, Weston R, Rodrigues BF, et al. Differing effects of partner and nonpartner sexual assault on women's mental health. *Violence Against Women.* 2007;13(3):285-297.

60. Campbell R, Lichty LF, Sturza M, et al. Gynecological health impact of sexual assault. *Res Nurs Health.* 2006;29:399-413.

61. Coker AL, Smith PH, Bethea L, et al. Physical health consequences of physical and psychological intimate partner violence. *Arch Fam Med.* 2000;9:451-457.

62. Campbell JC, Jones A, Dienemann J, et al. Intimate partner violence and physical health consequences. *Arch Internal Med.* 2002;162:1157-1163.

63. Pallitto CC, Garcia-Mareno C, Heise L, et al. Intimate partner violence, abortion, and unintended pregnancy: results from the WHO Multi-Country Study on women's health and domestic violence. *Int J Gynecol Obstet.* 2013;120(1):3-9.

64. Markowitz J, Pierce-Weeks J, Lewis-O'Connor A. *Intimate Partner Violence Education Guidelines.* Elkridge, MD: International Association of Forensic Nurses; 2012.

65. Ambuel B, Trent K, Lenahan P, et al. *Competencies Needed by Health Professionals for Addressing Exposure to Violence and Abuse in Patient Care.* Eden Prairie, MN: Academy on Violence and Abuse; 2011.

66. World Health Organization. *Responding to Intimate Partner Violence and Sexual Violence against Women: WHO Clinical and Policy Guidelines.* Geneva, Switzerland: World Health Organization, 2013. World Health Organization Web site. http://apps.who.int/iris/bitstream/10665/85240/1/9789241548595_eng.pdf?ua=1. Accessed August 8, 2013.

67. Fed R Evid 613(b).

68. Fed R Evid 801(d)(1).

69. Fed R Evid 803(4).

70. *Crawford v Washington,* 541 US §26 (2004).

71. AEquitas. *The Prosecutors' Resource on Crawford and its Progeny.* Washington, DC: AEquitas; 2012. AEquitas Web site. http://www.aequitasresource.org/The_Prosecutors_Resource_Crawford.pdf. Accessed September 10, 2013.

72. AEquitas. *The Prosecutors' Resource on Forfeiture by Wrongdoing.* Washington, DC: AEquitas; 2012. AEquitas Web site. http://www.aequitasresource.org/The_Prosecutors_Resource_Forfeiture_by_Wrongdoing.pdf. Accessed September 10, 2013.

73. *Davis v Washington,* 126 S Ct 2266 (2006).

74. *Michigan v Bryant,* 562 US 1143 (2011).

75. *Giles v California,* 128 S Ct 2678 (2008).

76. Tuerkheimer D. Forfeiture in the domestic violence realm. *Tex L Rev.* 2007;85:49-50.

77. Murphy S. Assisting the jury in understanding victimization: expert psychological testimony on battered woman syndrome and rape trauma syndrome. *Colum J L Soc Problems.* 1992;65:277-283.

78. Fed R Evid 402.

79. Fed R Evid 401.

80. Fed R Evid 702.

81. *State v Townsend*, 897 A2d 316, 328 (N J 2006).

82. *State v Ciskie*, 751 P2d 1165, 1169 (Wash 1988).

83. *State v Borelli*, 629 A2d 1105, 1112 (1993).

84. *State v Cooke*, 1997 Wash App LEXIS 1212 (1997).

Chapter 8

Winning in Court: Maximizing Protection through Prosecution

Aaron Holt, JD

Key Points

1. In 2000, a Massachusetts study of 350 IPV victims found that fewer than half wanted their cases to go to court; however, at the conclusion of the court process, however, 72% of victims felt satisfied with the final verdict. Surprisingly, the final disposition, whether jail, probation, or outright dismissal, did not directly relate to the victim's satisfaction with the court. Rather, the most important factor related to victim satisfaction was whether or not the court experience affected the personal safety of the victim.

2. The constitutional protections afforded to abusers when being questioned by law enforcement do not apply when being questioned by emergency room nurses, social workers, or professions unrelated to law enforcement. Thus, anything that frontline professionals learn from abusers may be used against them in court.

3. A 2000 National Institute of Justice study of 86 abused women who made 772 hospital visits found that one thrid of notes written by their doctors or nurses contained vital information that was also illegible.

4. A 1999 National Institute of Justice study found that 76% of victims wanted their abusers arrested after initial assaults, but that 45% of victims did not want their abusers subsequently prosecuted, and 14% of victims actively tried to stop prosecution.

5. Defenses in IPV cases fall into 4 categories: self-defense, provocation, diminished capacity, and actual innocence. Of these defenses, all but diminished capacity will directly oppose the victim's account of events.

6. Frontline professionals can help ensure a conviction via thorough documentation, including digital photographs and detailed written or computerized medical charting with exact quotes, documented histories of violence, and written statements from victims and third-party witnesses.

Introduction

Between 1976 and 2004, intimate partner homicide constituted 30% of all female murders in the United States.[1] Similar studies in Australia, Israel, and South Africa show that between 40% and 70% of all female homicide victims were murdered by their husbands or boyfriends.[2] The statistics are nothing new to those familiar with intimate partner violence (IPV). IPV is one of the oldest and often most culturally accepted crimes in our society, and it is this societal indifference that makes IPV cases difficult to prosecute.

The challenges associated with protecting victims from IPV crimes and preventing future occurrences are as varied as the victims themselves, including insufficient evidence, jury apathy, lack of cooperation by the victim, or simply no crime being reported. While there are various theories on the root causes of IPV, one goal remains constant: to protect victim from future acts of violence. One of the best and most effective means of accomplishing this goal is to effectively engage the legal system in providing protection for the victim and justice to the abuser. This goal can only be accomplished through the coordinated efforts of the criminal justice system and the front line professionals who work to end IPV. This chapter focuses on how frontline professionals can maximize the legal protections available to the victim through prosecution of the abuser.

Multidisciplinary Approach: A Frontline Defense

According to a survey of 14 000 police departments across the United States, 65% of departments have begun partnering with community-based victim advocacy groups.[1] Advocacy groups such as The National Center on Domestic and Sexual Violence assist the victim in meeting with local support providers, making social service referrals, counseling, and accompanying victims to court appearances.[2] This assistance helps victims cope with the psychological trauma often associated with victims reporting abuse. The partnership between local advocacy groups and police departments have been shown to improve overall police response, including number of arrests and successful prosecutions, as well as victim satisfaction.[3] However, the degree of participation and collaboration varies from department to department, and therefore the success of these partnerships also varies.[3] While the initial results of these collaborations are promising, progress toward eliminating IPV will only be made once the partnerships between advocacy groups and police departments are commonplace and victims are provided consistent assistance across all jurisdictions.

Prosecutorial Success

Rates

Prosecutorial success rates vary significantly across the country, due in large part to the varying approaches jurisdictions take toward prosecuting IPV. A 2009 U.S. Department of Justice study of 3750 IPV cases across 16 heavily populated counties found an average rate of conviction at 56%.[3] However, the rate of conviction from county to county varied from 17% to 89% at the outliers.[3] Another 2009 study by the National Institute of Justice analyzed 85 different studies of prosecutorial success rates of IPV cases across the country; they found an average conviction rate of 35%, with a high of 90% in Brooklyn, NY and a low of 8% in Milwaukee, WI.[4]

A significant contributing factor to this disparity among success rates is whether or not the prosecutors screen cases prior to filing criminal charges as opposed to the arresting officers filing charges directly. Allowing a prosecutor to screen cases prior to filing criminal charges gives the prosecutor discretion to decline charges based upon a lack of evidence. Screening cases also allows the prosecutor to direct further investigation and evidence gathering, if necessary, prior to charges being filed such as directing officers to take photographs or interview witnesses. Moreover, cases declined by the prosecuting attorney at the screening stage may always be refiled at a later time within the statute of limitations; additional time which can be profitably spent gathering additional evidence.

Of 16 counties surveyed in the 2009 Department of Justice study, only 9 counties allow prosecutors to screen their cases prior to filing charges.[3] In those 9 counties, the average rate of conviction was 72%, compared to 37% in counties that allowed officers to file cases directly.[3] Government resources and manpower are always finite. Allowing a prosecuting attorney to direct the investigation, evidence gathering, and the decision to file criminal charges allows prosecutors and police to focus on fewer cases with a greater likelihood of conviction, and protection for the victim.

What is a Successful Prosecution?

It is a inaccurate to view a prosecutorial "success" strictly in terms of whether or not an abuser is convicted. While conviction is the aim of every prosecutor who takes an IPV case to trial, the danger of recidivism or re-abuse in IPV cases is an ever-present and overriding concern. Success, as measured by the victim, is protection from further violence.

Legal Protection for Victims

Our legal system has a number of established protections specifically designed for IPV victims. These protections include protective orders, temporary protective orders, "no contact" orders, and no-trespassing affidavits. In addition, some states have adopted laws designed specifically for the protection of IPV victims. For example, the California Penal Code requires that an abuser convicted of IPV to serve a minimum of 3 years' probation, that protective orders must be issued to protect victims from further violence, and that defendants complete batterer re-education programs of no less than one year, and pay fines of up to $5000 to battered women's shelters.[5]

Punishment as Protection

The criminal justice system is designed to mete out punishment as deterrence according to the severity of a crime (**Table 8-1**), coupled with aggravating or mitigating factors, such as prior criminal history. Incarceration of abusers does provide some protection for victims in that it forces physical separation, albeit temporary. Generally speaking, perpetrators of the most severe crimes are given prison sentences, while perpetrators of lesser crimes are given jail sentences, and the remainder receives probation or some combination of jail and probation. A 2002 study of approximately 2000 IPV cases found that 82% of abusers received either a jail or prison sentence, while 17% received probation.[3]

Although temporary isolation from abusers does provide victims with temporary physical protection, the danger of recidivism is an ever-present threat to victims of IPV. The likelihood of recidivism will ultimately depend on the abuser, but some studies have shown a deterrent effect on abuser recidivism by invasive punishment.[6,7,8] A 2005 Ohio-based study of misdemeanor IPV cases found that with the application of invasive case dispositions, such as jail time, court-supervised electronic monitoring, and/or probation, 23% of abusers were re-arrested 1 year later, as compared with 66% of abusers who received non-invasive dispositions.[7]

Table 8-1. Severity of Punishment by Percentage, May 2002

Sentence Imposed	Percent of Abusers
Prison	7.4%
Jail	75.3%
Probation	17.3%

Adapted from: Smith EL, Farole DJ.[3]

While most agree an abuser's criminal history plays some role in the likelihood of recidivism, tit is unclear whether or not batterer intervention programs as a condition of probation have an effect on prevalence and incidence of recidivism.[9] In 1997, a New York study compared rates of recidivism among IPV abusers who received batterer intervention treatment and those who did not. Approximately 13% of abusers who did not receive treatment re-offended, while only 5% of those who received intervention treatment went on to re-offend.[10,11] In contrast, a 2003 National Institute of Justice study found that batterer intervention programs do not change the attitudes of abusers and have only a minor effect on behavior.[12] Although the content of batterer intervention programs varies, most involve either individual or group therapy. These therapeutic sessions may involve educational curricula, group psycho-therapy, or less structured discussions about relationships and anger-management skills.

BENEFITS OF SUCCESSFUL PROSECUTION

It is the role of IPV professionals to ensure the continued safety of victims. In 2000, a Massachusetts study of 350 IPV victims found that fewer than half wanted their case to go to court;[13] however, at the conclusion of the court process, 72% of victims felt satisfied with the final verdict.[13] Surprisingly, the final disposition, whether jail, probation or outright dismissal, did not directly relate to the victim's satisfaction.[13] The most important factor related to victim satisfaction was whether or not the court experience affected a victim's personal safety.[13] The study found that 88% of victims who felt a sense of increased personal safety also felt with the court process.[13] In other words, victim satisfaction and willingness to seek outside assistance in the future, correlates to the courts' providing a sense of safety.

TO REPORT OR NOT TO REPORT

Invoking the protections of the legal system through the court process is the first step to protecting victims of IPV. It is important to recognize that victims themselves need not start the process. Anyone who reasonably believes a crime has occurred or is about to occur may call the authorities, but reporting IPV is not easy. There is an inherent emotional and psychological element that leads some to question whether or not they should become involved. Nevertheless, if someone believes intimate partner violence is occurring, he or she has a moral, and often legal, obligation to report the abuse, even when a victim does not wish to file a report. Frequency of police response to a particular household or couple is often used as evidence in IPV trials; however, the police must first be called in order to create such a record.

RATES OF REPORTING FAMILY VIOLENCE

The number of violent crimes against family members is staggering. A study by the National Crime Victimization Survey found that from 1998 to 2002, a total of 3 534 150 non-fatal violent crimes against family members were reported to the police.[14] As **Table 8-2** shows, the percent of non-fatal violent crimes reported against family members varies depending on the crime.[14]

The same study by the National Crime Victimization Survey found that crimes against whites were less likely to be reported than crimes against other races. Violent crimes against white victims were reported 46% of the time, while violent crimes against non-white victims were reported 50% of the time.[14] Violent crimes committed by an intimate partner against white victims were reported at a rate of 50%, while violent crimes committed by an intimate partner against non-white victims were reported at a rate of 68%.[14]

Table 8-2. Percentage of Crimes Reported Against Family Members by Type between 1998 and 2002

Type of Offense	Percent Reported Against a Family Member
Rape	43.6%
Sexual Assault	26%
Robbery	70.6%
Aggravated Assault	63.3%
Simple Assault	57.5%
TOTAL	3 534 150

Adapted from Durose MR, Harlow C, Langan P, Motivans M, Rantala R, Smith E.[14]

Rates of Unreported IPV Cases

In 2005, the United States Department of Justice reported that nearly 34% of female IPV victims did not report abuse because they felt it was a private matter, 12% did not report abuse because they wanted to protect the offenders, and almost 9% thought the police would do nothing.[14] Regardless of whether or not victims wish to report incidents of IPV (**Table 8-3**), frontline professionals must consider that their wishes are not in the victims' best interest and may be life threatening.

Reporting Abuse

Multiple studies have shown that regardless of whether or not an arrest is made, police involvement in IPV cases has a strong deterrent effect.[15,16] The involvement of police and other authorities may alter existing power balance away from abusers.[16] This holds true whether or not a victim or a third party reports the abuse. One Department of Justice study found that 15% of all IPV cases were reported to police by third parties.[15,16]

MANDATORY REPORTING

Many states legally require health care providers to report suspected abuse to police. The purpose of mandatory reporting laws is to expose domestic abuse when medical professionals first observe it.

Table 8-3. Reasons for Not Reporting by Percent

Reason for Not Reporting	Percent
Private/personal matter	33.6%
Other reasons, including "I don't know"	24.1%
Protect the offender	12%
Not important to police	8.9%
Fear of reprisal	5.9%
Not important enough	5.4%
Reported to some other official	5.3%

Adapted from Durose MR, Harlow C, Langan P, Motivans M, Rantala R, Smith E.[14]

Several studies have examined the effects of mandatory reporting laws. One study involving over 1200 women across 12 emergency departments in California, a state with a mandatory reporting law, and Pennsylvania, a state without mandatory reporting law, found that 56% of abused women favored mandatory reporting, and 43% opposed such laws.[18] Of these abused women, nearly 8% did not want physicians to report the abuse and 36% preferred that physicians report only if they first obtained patient consent.[18] Another study of 577 victims found that 27% of victims would be more likely to seek medical care because of mandatory reporting laws, and 12% would be less likely to seek medical care due to mandatory reporting laws.[19]

It should also be noted that almost 71% of non-abused women support mandatory reporting, whereas only 29% oppose it.[20] Frontline healthcare providers and IPV professionals must be vigilant to spot and to report cases where intimate partner violence is suspected in order to take the first step in legally protecting IPV victims.

THE IMPORTANCE OF DOCUMENTATION

The importance of documentation in the prosecution of IPV cases cannot be overstated. Documentation may include photographs, emergency calls, police reports, medical records, and statements from neighbors or friends. Corroborative documentation bolsters the victims' credibility, which is usually a concern at trial. Too often, third parties believe their role ends when police arrive; however, once an arrest is made, law enforcement and the court system will independently evaluate a case to determine how best to proceed, and the ability of law enforcement and the courts to protect a victim largely depends on available evidence. If there is little evidence of prior abuse, a prosecutor's legal options may be limited when trying to keep an abuser in police custody and away from his or her victim. The following case study illustrates this point.

Case Study 8-1.

A husband has been abusing his wife for nearly 40 years. She is an immigrant who speaks very little English and, thus, depends on him socially and financially. One day, after an especially brutal attack, she decided to report the abuse to police; however, she had never before called the police or otherwise documented the abuse, except for infrequent visits to the hospital attributed to clumsiness. Because there was no prior documentation of abuse, the abuser could not be legally held in custody despite the fact that he had been beating his wife for nearly 4 decades. Had the prior abuse been documented, the abuser might have remained in custody up to the day of trial. Fortunately, a subsequent protective order and a "no-contact" order handed down by the judge were enough to protect the victim until a jury convicted her abuser.

CORROBORATION

IPV professionals who observe and document signs of abuse, may corroborate a victim's claim of abuse. An IPV professional's corroborating testimony may be highly damaging evidence to an abuser because the IPV professional, as an independent third party, has no reason to lie in court.

When an IPV professional realizes a victim is being abused, the professional should immediately document injuries—photographs are ideal, but if one is not available, then a detailed description of the injury will suffice. Documented records from medical professionals may prevent the abuser or his attorney from later changing that narrative at trial. If an abuser's testimony is inconsistent with an account reflected in medical records, his credibility will be hurt at trial.

Constitutional protections afforded to abusers when questioned by law enforcement do not apply when questioned by emergency room nurses, social workers, or professionals outside law enforcement. Thus, anything a medical professional learns from an abuser may be used against him in court. Of course, if law enforcement directs the medical professional to conduct this type of questioning, constitutional protections will apply. As **Table 8-4** illustrates, a statement from an abuser, regardless of how it was obtained, increases the likelihood of conviction more than any other factor.

Table 8-4. Likelihood of Conviction Based on Evidence Obtained	
EVIDENCE	NUMBER OF TIMES MORE LIKELY TO RESULT IN CONVICTION
Statement from the Defendant	2.04
Witness to the incident	1.73
Documented history of abuse	1.69
Physical evidence obtained	1.54
Adapted from Smith EL, Farole DJ.[3]	

A 2009 Department of Justice study of over 3300 incidents of abuse found that conviction was significantly more likely in cases where victims' accounts could be corroborated. In cases where physical evidence was obtained, abusers were 1.5 times more likely to be convicted.[3] Documented histories of abuse and third-party witnesses nearly doubled the likelihood of conviction.[3] Abusers' statements resulted in the highest likelihood of conviction.[3]

Corroborating victims' statements accomplishes a number of goals in the courtroom. First, it allows prosecutors and law enforcement to clearly track patterns of abuse and assists in protecting victims. For instance, a prosecutor's argument for any extraordinary legal protection is far more likely to succeed with a documented history of abuse. Second, corroboration supports victim credibility. It is common for victims of IPV to delay reporting their abuse. To the layperson serving on a jury, it seems unusual for someone to tolerate physical and/or emotional abuse for an extended period of time without reporting it. It is often difficult for jurors to understand, and thus believe, that abuse is occurring if there is no evidence other than the word of the victim. Because the state must prove its case beyond a shadow of a doubt, corroboration of the victim's account of events can often make a world of difference to the case and the victim.

Photographs: Seeing is Believing

Photographs may be the most significant evidence in an IPV case, and they are easy to obtain. Photography requires no expertise, and photographs may be admissible at trial regardless of whether or not the photographer testifies. As long as the photograph is a "fair and accurate" depiction of something relevant to the case, such as injuries to the victim or blood on the abuser, then the actual person who took the photograph does not need to testify or even be identified. Moreover, it is far easier and more powerful evidence to show a jury a photograph of facial bruising than it is to describe it verbally.

While any photograph is better than no photograph, the quality of an image may make a difference. A 2002 study in Queens, New York saw a spike in IPV-related convictions when police switched from Polaroid cameras to digital.[20] When the NYPD used the darker, grainy Polaroids, the conviction rate for IPV cases was 52%. but when the police switched to digital cameras, the conviction rate rose to 81%.

One study of 3750 IPV cases found that fewer than half of the victims were photographed during investigation.[3] Similar studies in Rhode Island, Ohio, and North Carolina found similarly poor results.[8,21,22] In Rhode Island, photos of victims' injuries were taken in only 17% of IPV cases.[21] The Ohio and North Carolina studies found that photos were taken in 15% and 14% of cases, respectively.[8,22] Given the evidential impact of photographs, and their essential role in explaining the cycle of abuse to juries, IPV professionals should take photographs of victims' injuries in all suspected IPV cases.

Other Documented Evidence

Other evidence commonly associated with IPV cases include medical records, 911 calls, and statements by victims and abusers. In 2009, emergency assistance calls were recovered in approximately 25% of all the IPV cases, and medical records were recovered in 3% (see **Table 8-5**).

Table 8-5. Types of Evidence Collected in IPV Cases

Type of Evidence Obtained	Percent of IPV Cases
Photos of the victim/defendant	46.5%
911 tape	25.9%
Statements from witness	45.9%
Statements from Defendant	10.2%
Medical records	3.4%
Forensic Evidence	3.3%
No evidence obtained	16.5%

Adapted from Smith EL, Farole DJ.[3]
NOTE: multiple types of evidence may be obtained per case

Statistics on 911 calls, forensic evidence, and medical records may be misleading because victims do not always call 911 or go to the hospital. Expecting medical records, forensic evidence. and 911 recordings in IPV cases is unrealistic given the reclusive nature of this type of crime and despite the fact that 90% of all IPV victims sustain some type of documentable injury.[3]

Recorded History of Abuse: Police Reports

Police reports offer one of the simplest and most effective means to establish a corroborative pattern of abuse for IPV prosecution. Police officers generally write reports after responding to domestic violence calls.[23] Any IPV professional encountering a police officer during investigation for IPV should ensure a report is filed, even when charges are not. A 2009 study by the United States Department of Justice found that 1 in 4 IPV victims had reported prior violence by their abusers to police.[3] The same study found that 46% of IPV cases involved defendants with prior histories of abuse toward the same victim and only 24% of their victims had reported the prior violence.[3] One unique aspect of calling the police regarding domestic violence is that a record of the call is generated automatically. Moreover, because studies have shown that abusers with documented histories of abuse are more likely to be convicted, police reports are especially important to successful prosecution and prevention of intimate partner violence.[3]

911 Calls

911 calls are often the most emotional exhibits in an IPV trial. The tone, infliction, and fear sometimes heard through these calls places the jury in the shoes of the victim like few other pieces of evidence. One of the hurdles prosecutors encounter when admitting 911 tapes is the anonymous caller. Although the desire not to get involved can play a role when concerned parties decide to call anonymously, it presents prosecutors with a real problem as to the admissibility of the evidence. Anonymous calls are potentially inadmissible because the defense is generally entitled to question any witness against the defendant.[24] Although a few exceptions exist which allow an anonymous 911 call to be admissible, those exceptions are outside the scope of this chapter. To better assist prosecution, a caller should as clearly as possible tell 911 operators his or her name and callback number and what he or she saw. Regardless of whether or not the 911 caller is a friend, a victim, or een a total stranger, the weight a 911 call carries in a courtroom cannot be overstated. Ensuring that these calls are given to law enforcement in an admissible form is of paramount importance.

Medical Records

A 2000 National Institute of Justice study of 86 abused women who made 772 visits to the hospital found that one third of notes written by their doctors or nurses contained vital information that was also illegible.[25] If a jury cannot read a doctor's diagnosis or a detailed description of a victim's injuries, then the value of the medical records in question is severely damaged. Frontline providers should be aware that every note and chart has the potential to be used as an exhibit at trial. Accuracy and legibility should be a primary concern for any medical professional.

Verbiage in medical records may present another problem in IPV cases. For example, consider these 2 sentences: "Patient was kicked in abdomen by husband." versus "The patient states that she was kicked in the abdomen by her husband." While both statements may have the same meaning medically, they are viewed differently by the legal system. The first statement is considered an evaluation by the doctor of the patient's injuries, whereas the second is a statement made by the victim herself. The difference may be subtle, but the legal effect is significant; therefore, medical professionals should document everything the patient or abuser says when speaking to an IPV victim about the injuries.

Table 8-6 includes some common wording mistakes, ideal wording suggestions, and the reasons why such wording may be helpful in an IPV trial.

RECANTATION

One of the most difficult challenges any prosecutor can face occurs when the victim recants and refuses to press charges. Recantation typically involves victim giving an alternate explanation of injuries differing from what was originally told to police or medical professionals. Examples include claiming to be the aggressor in a fight, minimizing injury, and claiming that injuries were the result of an accident. While the primary goal of prosecuting IPV case is to protect victims, recanting victims may frustrate this goal by refusing to answer basic questions, changing their account of events, or to appear in court. In such a case, prosecution must prove that an assault happened, and do so with a star witness acting against them.

There have been a number of high-profile cases involving IPV victims who recanted. Warren Moon, a hall of fame NFL quarterback, was arrested in 1996 for allegedly striking his wife and choking her to the point of unconsciousness.[26,27] On the stand, the victim took the blame for starting the fight. She told jurors that Moon was merely

Table 8-6. Significance of Wording in Medical Records

Poor Wording	Ideal Wording	Significance
3 cm laceration over eye	3cm laceration over left eye. Swelling/redness around both eyes. Patient states she walked into cabinet.	Swelling and redness around both eyes might indicate the injuries were caused by something other than a cabinet. Most people are right-handed, thus a blow from one's dominant hand will usually impact the left eye.
Bruises around throat	Five quarter-sized bruises around throat. Bruising consistent with a handprint. Patient refuses to say how she was injuried.	Even if a victim refuses to say how she received her injuries, her silence may be just as valuable at trial if she later testifies for the abuser.
Left eye swollen —patient walked into door frame	Left eye red and swollen. Patient states she walked into doorframe. Husband states he saw her walk into doorframe.	Locking an abuser into a story about a victims' injuries is invaluable. Once documented, he must stick to the story or explain why he lied to the doctor.

trying to restrain her.[27] The jury acquitted Moon in 27 minutes. In the case of Julio Lugo, a former baseball player for the Houston Astros, Lugo was arrested for assaulting his wife in 2003.[27] When the case went to trial, the victim said she had exaggerated her account of events and that Lugo had not intended to hurt her.[27] The jury acquitted Lugo. In order to win an IPV case with a recanting victim, the state must be able to rely on corroborating evidence of an assault. Without such evidence, recanting cases are very difficult.

RATES OF RECANTING AND VICTIM SATISFACTION

Advocacy and prosecution on behalf of IPV victims who does not wish to pursue charges ensure the long-term safety of the victim. A 1999 Massachusetts study found that nearly 47% of IPV victims did not want their case to go to court;[13] however, at the conclusion of court proceedings, 53% of victims felt their court experience gave them a "sense of control," 37% said it motivated them to end their abusive relationships and 39% said their court experience "made them safer."[14] Of the victims who did not want their cases to go to court, 72% felt satisfaction after the trial.[13]

A 1999 National Institute of Justice study of specialized prosecution programs across 4 states, including approximately 1 600 IPV cases, found that 76% of victims wanted their abusers arrested after initial assault, but 45% of victims did not want their abusers subsequently prosecuted.[13] Again we see the victim's desire to be protected in the high percentages who want their abuser arrested immediately after the assault. However, a significant number of victims do not wish to follow through in the court system by cooperating with the prosecution. Further frustrating matters, 14% of the victims studied actively tried to stop the prosecution.[13] However, these same victims were surveyed after trial, and the results were encouraging. 70% felt satisfied with police, 64% felt satisfied with prosecutors, and 67% were satisfied with their judges.[13] After trial, 85% of victims believed, in hindsight, that prosecution was helpful, and 79% said they would call the police if their abusers attacked in the future.[13] Victim testimonial statements were especially:

"I was mad at the time that they would not drop charges. Now, I am so happy they prosecuted. It was out of my hands. They had enough evidence to go through with it without my cooperation. I felt guilty I did this to him, but I am very grateful now."

"I called and wanted the prosecutor to make the charges more lenient. The prosecutor and the police said it was out of my hands. The case would be prosecuted. I wanted him (the defendant) to get counseling for alcohol and anger. In the long run, I am glad it was not up to me."[13]

RECANTATION AND ITS EFFECT ON CASES

Recantation is problematic for prosecutors. At the least, it gives the defense ammunition to use against the credibility of the victim. Logic and common sense dictate that two conflicting accounts given by the same person cannot both be true; therefore, the impact of recantation in a criminal case largely depends on the corroborating evidence available to the prosecutor.

A 2009 National Institute of Justice study found that prosecutors' handling of cases with uncooperative victims on days of trial may vary. The study found that if a victim failed to appear on the day of trial, prosecutors from Everett, Washington and Klamath Falls, Oregon tended to proceed without the victim in approximately two thirds of cases, and dismissed one third of cases.[13] Conversely, prosecutors in Omaha, Nebraska dismissed two thirds of IPV cases when the victim was not present on trial day.[13]

A prosecutor's willingness to take a recantation case to trial depends largely on the corroborating evidence available. If a victim's abuse can be chronicled through 911 tapes, photos, family members, nurses, IPV professionals, or any combination thereof, then a victim's recantation may not necessarily end his or her case.

RE-VICTIMIZATION

A constant concern for prosecutors and IPV professionals is to ensure that IPV victims are not re-victimized. Re-victimization may occur after a victim recants or otherwise refuses to cooperate and the state compels her to testify. When a recanting victim refuses to comply with a lawful subpoena, she may be forcibly brought to court by law enforcement. However, there is no such thing as a non-cooperative witness holding cell; therefore, victims are placed in the same holding cells with criminals present for a court. Such treatment is additionally traumatic for someone who has already been subject to physical and/or emotional abuse. Prosecutors and law enforcement must remember that the goal in prosecuting IPV cases is to protect victims and to see justice done. Re-victimization must be avoided if at all possible.

TRIAL

Trial may be an intimidating prospect for one unfamiliar with the court process. The court process, as it relates to IPV cases, can be broken down into 3 stages: (1) pre-trial, (2) trial, and (3) sentencing. IPV professionals, frontline providers, and victims may be required to appear at various stages for a number of reasons. This section will examine what to expect at each stage of trial, with regard to IPV cases.

PRE-TRIAL

A critical issue prior to trial is whether or not the abuser will be incarcerated until the court date. Multiple studies have shown that retaliation is a reality for IPV victims. One 4-site study across the United States found that between 32% and 39% of abusers re-assault their victims within 15 months of initial assault.[28] A 2005 Rhode Island study found that 38% of abusers were re-arrested for new domestic violence offenses within 2 years of their first IPV conviction.[29] A Bronx domestic violence court study placed recidivism rates at 48% during the same year as the initial assault.[30]

Some states have adopted laws to provide victims extra short-term protection. At least 2 states, Nevada and Tennessee, have adopted laws requiring a cooling-off period in which abusers must remain in jail for at least 12 hours after being arrested for IPV.[31,32] Whether or not an abuser is released prior to trial depends on whether a judge gives him an opportunity to post bail.

Bail

Bail involves giving the court something of value, usually money, as collateral to secure conditional freedom for the accused leading up to trial. Setting bail is one of the first steps in nearly every criminal case. By posting bail, a defendant puts up a specified amount of money as a promise he will abide by the court's rules and appear at each court setting for the duration of his case. Misconduct which might revoke bail typically includes failing to appear at a court setting, committing a new crime, or violating a court imposed condition of bail. Bail is set by a judge after weighing a number of factors, including the severity of the crime charged, the flight risk of the defendant, and the risk or further harm to the victim or the public.

In addition to setting the amount of bail, judges have discretion to set specific bail conditions. Such conditionsmay include random drug tests, regular meetings with a court officer, or any condition a judge deems necessary. For example, a common condition imposed in IPV cases prohibits further contact with victims for the duration of their cases. Violating a condition of bail may result in a defendant being placed in jail for the remainder of the court process, which could last from a few weeks to over a year.

A United States Department of Justice study published in 2005 showed that 51.4% of defendants charged with family assault were held in jail until the conclusion of their cases.[14] Only 40% were able to pay their bail.[14] The median bail set was $35 000 and the mean was $66 000.[15] Of the abusers who were able to make bail, 90% were released within one month of the assault, and 25% of those were released within 1 day of arrest.[14] Protection of the community, including the victim, is a primary concern for judges setting bail; therefore, most cases with documented abuse typically receive higher bail amounts, which decrease the chance that an abuser will be able to meet bail. Situations with thorough documentation of the history of abuse, photographs, and third-party testimony can be additionally effective in the pre-trial stage.

Protective Orders

A protective order is a legal order issued by a judge that prohibits an abuser from continuing to abuse a victim. A protective order may be issued at any time during the court process. An order may bar threatening or harassing communication, physical violence, or proximity to a victim, her home, or her place of work. A court may issue such an order even without pending criminal action.

A 1993 Boston study found that 68% of victims had left their abusers at least once, 15% had demanded their abusers leave their homes at least once, 78% had called the police at least once, 30% sought counseling, and 25% had called a hotline or gone to a shelter.[33] A 1997 National Institute of Justice multi-state study found that only 10% of victims obtained protective orders after a week of abuse, 14% experienced abuse for 1 to 2 years prior to obtaining protective orders, and nearly 25% of victims had endured abuse for more than 5 years before obtaining protective orders.[34]

Although some victims might not know about the legal protections available to them, many victims feel that any cooperation with law enforcement will bring retaliation from their abusers in the form of physical or emotional abuse. Whether or not protective orders deter further abuse is a question still up for debate. A 1999 protective order study in Texas found that 68% of victims were physically abusedan for 2 years prior to seeking a protective order.[35] The same study sampled abuse before and after a protective order and found that physical abuse dropped from 68% to 23% after the order was issued.[35] However, a 1996 Massachusetts study found that nearly 1/2 of abusers re-abused their victim within 2 years of a protective order being issued, and of those, only 34% were re-arrested for abuse.[36]

Research has been, however, consistent about the effect of protective orders on victims' state of mind. Eighty percent of victims felt safer knowing a protection order was in effect, and 95% of victims said they would seek protective orders again.[37] Regardless of whether or not protective orders deter abusers, they have a positive effect on the willingness of victims to cooperate with law enforcement. Moreover, protective orders give victims a sense of control and a feeling that the law is on their side and, therefore, shift the perceived power distribution in abusive relationships.

No-Contact Orders

No-contact orders differ from protective orders in that a no-contact order must be issued by a criminal court and there must be a pending criminal charge. Because a no-contact order is only good for as long as an abuser is on bail, the no-contact order ends with other bail conditions at the conclusion of a criminal case.

Some states have adopted mandatory no-contact orders in IPV cases. Rhode Island law provides that anyone charged with an IPV-related offense must appear before a magistrate for issuance of a no-contact order prior to release from jail.[37] Wisconsin law requires a no-contact order be issued prohibiting an abuser from having contact with his victim or her residence for 72 hours after arrest.[38]

A victim may obtain both a protective order and a no-contact order. The orders do not conflict with one another and call for varying punishments if violated. For example, a victim is assaulted by her husband. She files charges against her husband and obtains both a protective order and a no-contact order prohibiting her husband from coming within 100 feet of her residence. He then shows up at the victim's house asking her to reconcile and drop the charges. In this scenario, the husband is in violation of the no contact order and the protective order. He violated the no-contact order by initiating contact with his victim and by coming within 100 feet of her residence. Because the husband violated the no-contact order, the judge may keep him in custody until disposition of the assault case. The husband also violated the protective order by appearing at the victim's residence. Violation of the protective order is a new crime independent of any pending charge. Each of these orders operates independently, keep the abuser from the victim, and prevent re-abuse. IPV professionals should encourage victims to obtain as many layers of judicial protection as their jurisdiction allows.

AT TRIAL

The goal of this chapter is to prepare frontline providers and IPV professionals to more effectively assist and protect victims at trial. There are a number of occasions where frontline providers and IPV professionals may be used at trial to provide evidence through testimony. This section discusses how these professionals can maximize their effectiveness during trial.

Expert Testimony

Third parties may testify as expert witnesses in IPV trials. Expert testimony and qualification differ among jurisdictions, but the rules of evidence allow for a witness to be designated as an "expert" if his or her knowledge may assist a jury in understanding the evidence or in determining a fact at issue. Jurors are usually unfamiliar with the intricacies of IPV and, therefore, expert testimony. Any frontline professional with specialized or experiential knowledge of IPV may be deemed "expert" by a court and allowed to testify.[39,40]

Tips For Testifying

An IPV professional or third party may be called to testify at trial regarding their involvement in a specific case, or to share their specialized knowledge regarding IPV with the jury. When testifying in court, there are 3 things to keep in mind: appearance, reaction to questions, and credibility. As for appearance, the courtroom is not the place for high fashion or provocative dress. As a rule of thumb, one should dress professionally and conservatively.

Frontline professionals testifying as experts must keep in mind that they know more about the topic than the jurors and remember that an expert goes to court to help juries understand complicated subjects. In that capacity, expert witnesses should think of themselves as teachers rather than experts one might see on television who cannot use words with less than 3 syllables. Expert witnesses should speak confidently, share what they know, and try not to speak so forcefully as to seem arrogant.

At times, witnesses try to give their entire testimony between first and second introductory questions. This detracts from the effectiveness of their testimony and may make them appear nervous. A witness must remain calm and assertive while maintaining eye contact with the jury. Jurors are hesitant to believe witnesses who cannot look the jury in the eye while testifying.

Credibility is like glass: once broken it is difficult to repair. An expert witness should not embellish or elaborate beyond what he or she knows or remembers. It is always better to say, "I don't know" rather than embellish some minor detail. A good rule of thumb is to ask for a clarifying question when unsure of what is being asked. Guessing what a prosecutor or defense attorney is asking may cause inadvertent miscommunication and confusing testimony.

Cross Examination

In order to prepare for cross-examination, it is important to know what the defense at trial will be. Defenses in IPV cases fall into 4 categories: self-defense, provocation, diminished capacity, and actual innocence.[41] *Self-defense* is a theory of a case offered by the defense in order to show that an abuser's actions were merely defensive in nature. *Provocation defenses* are typically structured around an abuser's lack of intent.[41] For example, the abuser had no intent to harm the victim; the abuse happened in the heat of the moment. *Diminished capacity defenses* attempt to show an abuser was somehow less responsible for his or her actions. This defense typically blames the abuser's actions on alcohol, drugs, or a pre-existing psychological disorder.[41] The actual *innocence defense* attempts to establish a reasonable doubt in the minds of jurors as to whether a defendant truly perpetrated an act of violence.[41]

All of the above defenses, except for diminished capacity, directly attack the victim's account of the events. One 1999 study of IPV trials found that victims were directly attacked by the defense in 71% of murder cases and 37% of non-murder cases.[40] The most common defense attacks involve character assassination, or the introduction of negative evidence of a victim's past, such as mental health history; emotional problems; substance abuse; or a motive potentially affecting his or her testimony, such as child custody.[41] The motivation for character assassination by the defense is call into question a victim's character to the extent that her testimony may not be taken seriously.[41] This same study found that when the defense employed character assassination of a victim, the victim was commonly portrayed as mentally disturbed, "whoring" around, likely to cause trouble, spending too much time at bars, or "always drunk....skunkin' drunk."[41]

This type of defense tactic is strategically risky if there is corroborating evidence. If jurors may be convinced a victim's account by corroborative documentation, they may become resentful of attacks on the victim and may show their displeasure when sentencing the abuser.

Crawford v. Washington

In 2004, the United States Supreme Court issued one of the most significant decisions affecting IPV cases. *Crawford v. Washington* held that the 6th Amendment to the US Constitution required cross-examination of a witness when a testimonial hearsay statement of the witness was offered.[42-44] In other words, *Crawford* requires the in-court appearance of witness so that abuser has the opportunity to confront their accuser. This decision created a practical dilemma for prosecutors while simultaneously creating an additional incentive for abusers to keep their victims out of the courtroom.[45]

Crawford v. Washington offers abusers an additional incentive to reconcile with or to intimidate the victim in order to prevent his or her appearance in court. A survey of prosecutors from 3 mid-western states found that 65% of prosecutors felt that *Crawford* made IPV victims less safe and 76% indicated their office was more likely to dismiss charges when a victim recanted or refused to cooperate.[46]

However, there is an exception to the *Crawford* rule. The doctrine of forfeiture by wrongdoing allows prosecutors to use testimonial hearsay statements, barred under *Crawford*, if an abuser causes a witness to become unavailable.[47] If a defendant commits an act that leads to a witness' unavailability, he or she is deemed to have forfeited the right to confront the witness, and the defense may not profit from the defendant's wrongdoing. Thus, an abuser cannot threaten or coerce a witness to not testify, and then, when the witness does not appear, claim that he is still entitled to confront that witness.

In order for forfeiture by wrongdoing to apply, the state must show that an abuser intended to cause the unavailability of a witness.[47] A defendant's history of prior abuse, threats of abuse, or subsequent actions intended to dissuade a victim from resorting to outside help are seen as relevant as to whether the forfeiture doctrine should apply.[47] Again, documentation of the attack and the events thereafter may assist a prosecutor in protecting a victim by using this doctrine.

SENTENCING

Sentencing takes place after a jury returns a guilty verdict and the victim has an opportunity to tell the judge or jury how the crime impacted her life. All prior criminal history or bad acts of an abuser may be admitted, including testimony by former girlfriends, wives, or children who may have been abused by the defendant.

Again, documentation of prior assaults is invaluable because evidence of such acts may be admitted during sentencing and affect a defendant's ultimate sentence. Without such evidence, a prosecutor cannot show the habitual behavior of a defendant, who may, therefore, receive a lighter sentence.

Sentencing for IPV crimes is case-specific. While a felony aggravated assault will receive a much harsher punishment than a misdemeanor assault, the criminal history of the abuser and wishes of a victim can play a significant role. For example, a victim may not want a lengthy prison term for her abuser if she is financially dependent on him. Because the goal of most IPV prosecutions is to protect victims, monitored probation and batterers' intervention programs may be a more effective protection for the victim than actual jail time. Various studies of domestic violence courts across the country show that incarceration rates vary. Klamath Falls, Oregon incarcerates 76% of its IPV cases;[49] 71% are jailed in Cincinnati, Ohio;[22] 56% in Everett, Washington;[48] 52% in Omaha, Nebraska;[48] 30% in Milwaukee, Wisconsin;[49] 22% in Quincy, Massachusetts;[13] and 21% in San Diego, California.[48] Although this variance in rates of incarceration between different states is significant and worthy of further study, IPV cases should always be treated on a per case basis with severity of punishment depending on the circumstances of the victim, the nature of the abuser, and the severity of the crime itself.

CONCLUSION

Intimate partner violence permeates our society and may never be completely eradicated. Only a multi-disciplinary approach incorporating essential frontline professionals working with IPV victims will we see continued progress. Frontline professionals can help to ensure a conviction through documentation, including digital photographs, detailed and legible medical records, documented histories of violence, and written statements. By documenting and reporting abuse, with or without the victim's consent, frontline professionals protect victims and take a step towards bringing abusers to justice. By effectively documenting instances of abuse, IPV professionals and prosecutors can work together to more effectively prosecute perpetrators and protect victims.

REFERENCES

1. Klein AR. *Practical Implications of Current Domestic Violence Research: For Law Enforcement, Prosecutors and Judges.* Washington, DC: United States Department of Justice, Office of Justice Programs; 2009. National Criminal Justice Reference Service Web site. https://www.ncjrs.gov/pdffiles1/nij/225722.pdf. Accessed April 4, 2011.

2. Krug EG, Dahlberg LL, Mercy JA, Zwi AB, Lozano R, eds. *World Report on Violence and Health.* Geneva, Switzerland: World Health Organization; 2002. http://whqlib doc.who.int/publications/2002/9241545615_eng.pdf. Accessed April 23, 2011.

3. Smith EL, Farole DJ. *Profile of Intimate Partner Violence Cases in Large Urban Counties.* Washington, DC: United States Department of Justice; 2009. Bureau of Justice Statistics Web site. http://www.bjs.gov/content/pub/pdf/pipvcluc.pdf. Accessed April 4, 2011.

4. Garner J, Maxwell C. *Prosecution and Conviction Rates for Intimate Partner Violence.* Sherpherdstown, WV: Joint Centers for Justice Studies; 2008. Cited by: Klein A. *Practical Implications of Current Domestic Violence Research: For Law Enforcement, Prosecutors and Judges.* Washington, DC: United States Department of Justice, Office of Justice Programs; 2009. National Criminal Justice Reference Service Web site. https://www.ncjrs.gov/pdffiles1/nij/225722.pdf. Accessed April 4, 2011.

5. California Penal Code §1203.097.

6. Gross M, Cramer E, Forte J, Gordon J, Kunkel T, Moriarty L. The impact of sentencing options on recidivism among domestic violence offenders: a case study. *Am J Crim Justice.* 2000;24(2):301-312.

7. Ventura L, Davis G. Domestic violence: court case conviction and recidivism. *Violence Against Women.* 2005;11(2):255-277.

8. Friday PC, Lord VB, Exum ML, Hartman JL. *Evaluating the Impact of a Specialized Domestic Violence Police Unit.* Washington, DC: United States Department of Justice; 2006. National Criminal Justice Reference Service Web site. https://www.ncjrs.gov/pdffiles1/nij/grants/215916.pdf. Accessed April 4, 2011.

9. Thistlethwaite A, Wooldredge J, Gibbs D. Severity of dispositions and domestic violence recidivism. *Crime and Delinquency.* 1998;44(3):94-96.

10. Davis RC, Taylor BG. Does batterer treatment reduce violence? a synthesis of the literature. *Women and Criminal Justice.* 1999; 10(2):69-93.

11. Stith S, Rosen K, McCollum E, Thomsen C. Treating intimate partner violence within intact couple relationships: outcomes of multicouple versus individual couple therapy. *J Marital and Family Therapy.* 2004;30(3):305-318.

12. National Institute of Justice. *Do Batterer Intervention Programs Work? Two Studies.* Washington, DC: United States Department of Justice, Office of Justice Programs; 2003. National Criminal Justice Reference Service Web site. https://www.ncjrs.gov/pdffiles1/nij/200331.pdf. Accessed April 4, 2011.

13. Buzawa E, Hotaling GT, Klein A, Bynes J. *Response to Domestic Violence in a Pro-Active Court Setting.* Washington, DC: National Institute of Justice, United States Department of Justice; 1999. National Criminal Justice Reference Service Web site. https://www.ncjrs.gov/pdffiles1/nij/grants/181427.pdf. Accessed April 4, 2011.

14. Durose MR, Harlow CW, Langan PA, Motivans M, Rantala RR, Smith EL. *Family Violence Statistics: Including Statistics on Strangers and Acquaintances.* Washington, DC: United States Department of Justice, Office of Justice Programs; 2005. NCJ Publication No. 207846. National Criminal Justice Reference Service Web site. http://www.bjs.gov/content/pub/pdf/fvs.pdf. Accessed April 4, 2011.

15. Wordes M; National Council on Crime and Delinquency. *Creating a Structured Decision-Making Model for Police Intervention in Intimate Partner Violence.* NCJ Publication No. 182781. National Criminal Justice Reference Service Web site. https://www.ncjrs.gov/pdffiles1/nij/grants/182781.pdf. Accessed April 23, 2011.

16. Felson RB, Ackerman JM, Gallagher C. *Police Intervention and the Repeat of Domestic Assault.* NCJ Publication No. 210301. National Criminal Justice Reference Service Web site. https://www.ncjrs.gov/pdffiles1/nij/grants/210301.pdf. Accessed April 23, 2011.

17. Felson R, Pare P. *Reporting of Domestic Violence and Sexual Assault by Nonstrangers to the Police.* National Criminal Justice Reference Service Web site. https://www.ncjrs.gov/pdffiles1/nij/grants/210301.pdf. NCJ Publication No. 209039. National Criminal Justice Reference Service Web site. https://www.ncjrs.gov/pdffiles1/nij/grants/209039.pdf. Accessed April 23, 2011.

18. Rodriguez M, McLoughlin E, Nah G, Cambell J. Mandatory reporting of domestic violence injuries to the police: what do emergency departments think? *JAMA.* 2001;286:580–583.

19. Houry D, Feldhaus K, Thorson AC, et al. Mandatory reporting laws do not deter patients from seeking medical care. *Ann Emerg Med.* 1999;34:336–341.

20. Buckley C. In domestic abuse, digital photos can say more than victims. *New York Times*. May 7, 2007.

21. Klein A, Tobin T. Longitudinal study of arrested batterers, 1995-2005: career criminals. *Violence Against Women*. 2008;14(2):136-157.

22. Belknap J, Graham DLR, Hartman J, Lippen V, Allen G, Sutherland J. *Factors Related to Domestic Violence Court Dispositions in a Large Urban Area: The Role of Victim/Witness Reluctance and Other Variables*. Washington, DC: National Institute of Justice; 2000. NCJ Publication No.184112. National Criminal Justice Reference Service Web site. https://www.ncjrs.gov/pdffiles1/nij/grants/184112.pdf. Accessed April 23, 2011.

23. New York State Division of Criminal Justice Services, Office for the Prevention of Domestic Violence. *Family Protection and Domestic Violence Intervention Act of 1994: Evaluation of the Mandatory Arrest Provisions: Final Report to the Governor and Legislature, January 2001. New York, NY: New York State Division of Criminal Justice Services, Office for the Prevention of Domestic Violence;* 2001.

24. *Brown v. Keane*, 355 F3d 82, 94 (2dCir 2004).

25. Isaac NE, Enos P. *Medical Records as Legal Evidence of Domestic Violence*. Washington, DC: National Institute of Justice; 2000. NCJ Publication No. 184528. National Criminal Justice Reference Service Web site. https://www.ncjrs.gov/pdffiles1/nij/grants/184528.pdf. Accessed April 23, 2011.

26. Robinson LN. Professional athletes—held to a higher standard and above the law: a comment on high-profile criminal defendants and the need for states to establish high-profile courts. *I N Law J*. 1998;73(4):1313-1328.

27. Parameswaran L. Battered wives often recant or assume blame. Women's eNews Web site. http://www.womensenews.org/story/commentary/030730/battered-wives-often-recant-or-assume-blame. Published July 30, 2003. Accessed April 23, 2011.

28. Gondolf EW. *Characteristics of Batterers in a Multi-site Evaluation of Batterer Intervention Systems*. St. Paul, MN: Minnesota Center Against Violence and Abuse; 1996. MINCAVA electronic clearinghouse Web site. http://www.mincava.umn.edu/documents/gondolf/batchar.html. Accessed April 23, 2011.

29. Klein AR, Wilson D, Crowe AH, DeMichele M. *Evaluation of the Rhode Island Probation Specialized Domestic Violence Supervision Unit*. Washington, DC: National Institute of Justice; 2005. NCJ Publication No. 222912.National Criminal Justice Reference Service Web site. https://www.ncjrs.gov/pdffiles1/nij/grants/222912.pdf. Accessed April 23, 2011.

30. Rempel M, Labriola M, Davis R. Does judicial monitoring deter domestic violence recidivism? results of a quasi-experimental comparison in the Bronx. *Violence Against Women*. 2008;14(2):185-207.

31. Nev Rev Stat § 178.484(7).

32. Tenn Code Ann § 40-11-150(h)(1).

33. Ptacek J. *Battered Women in the Courtroom: The Power of Judicial Responses*. Boston, MA: UPNE; 1999.

34. Keilitz SL, Hannaford PL, Efkeman HS; National Center for State Courts. *Civil Protection Orders: The Benefits and Limitations for Victims of Domestic Violence.* Williamsburg, VA: National Center for State Courts; 1997. NCJ Publication No. 172223. National Criminal Justice Reference Service Web site. https://www.ncjrs.gov/pdffiles1/Digitization/172223NCJRS.pdf. Accessed April 23, 2011.

35. Carlson M, Harris S, Holden G. Protective orders and domestic violence: risk factors for re-abuse. *J Fam Violence.* 1999;14(2):205-226.

36. Klein A. Re-abuse in a population of court-restrained male batterers: why restraining orders don't work. In: Buzawa ES, Buzawa CG, eds. *Do Arrests and Restraining Orders Work?* Thousand Oaks, CA: Sage; 1996:192-213.

37. RI Gen Laws § 12-29-4.

38. Wis Stat § 968.075(5).

39. Zykorie L. Can a domestic violence advocate testify as an expert witness? follow the ABC's of expert testimony standards in Texas courts: assist the trier of fact, be relevant and reliable, credentials must be established. *T X J Women Law.* 2003;11(2):276-311.

40. Barnes CL. Admissibility of Expert Testimony Concerning Domestic Violence Syndromes to Assist Jury in Evaluating Victim's Testimony or Behavior, 57 ALR 5th 315 (2005).

41. Hartley CC, Ryan R. *Trial Strategies in Domestic Violence Felonies.* Washington, DC: National Institute of Justice, 2002. National Criminal Justice Reference Service Web site. https://www.ncjrs.gov/pdffiles1/nij/grants/194069.pdf. Accessed April 23, 2011.

42. *Crawford v Washington,* 541 US 36, 53-4 (2004).

43. US Constitution. Amendment VI.

44. Fed Rules of Evid 801(c).

45. King-Ries A. An argument for original intent: restoring Rule 801(d)(1)(A) to protect domestic violence victims in a post-Crawford world. *Pace Law Rev.* 2007;27(2):199-240.

46. Lininger T. Prosecuting batterers after Crawford. *V A Law Rev.* 2005;91(747):747-822.

47. *Giles v. California,* 128 S Ct 2678, 2684 (2008).

48. Smith BE, Davis R, Nickles LB, Davies HJ. *Evaluation of Efforts to Implement No-Drop Policies: Two Central Values in Conflict, Final Report.* Washington, DC: National Institute of Justice; 2001. NCJ Publication No 187772. https://www.ncjrs.gov/rr/vol2_3/15.html. Retrieved April 23, 2011.

49. Davis R, Smith B, Nickles L. The deterrent effect of prosecuting domestic violence misdemeanors. *Crime and Delinquency.* 1998;44(3):434-442.

Chapter 9

Intimate Partner Violence and Child Protection: The Journey to Collaborative Intervention Approaches

Casey Gwinn, JD
Gael Strack, JD

Key Points

1. Difficulties and tensions arise between the domestic violence movement and child protection services in cases where a child witnesses intimate partner violence (IPV). Often, these children are taken from their non-offending parent, who may be charged with failure to protect.

2. Years of tension came to a head in the 2001 *Nicholson v. Williams* case. The court ruled that child protective services could not presume guilt for neglect on the part of the non-offending partner, and encouraged cooperation between child abuse advocates and domestic violence advocates.

3. Strategies have been developed to help these groups collaborate, including cross-training child protection and domestic violence professionals, creating case teams involving both child abuse advocates and domestic violence advocates, and working with IPV victims to help them understand the impact of witnessing IPV on their children.

4. The National Family Justice Center Alliance seeks to identify and advocate against problematic practices in child protection groups, such as using the threat of removing children to force victims of IPV to perform certain actions, such as moving to a shelter or obtaining a protective order.

5. An integrated approach to this issue, involving multi-agency, multi-disciplinary centers as seen in the Family Justice Center model, is the best way forward to relieve the tensions between child protection and domestic abuse professionals.

A Survivor's Story

My name is Ming. I was born in China and came to the United States in 2005. I met my husband in 2006. He is a private investigator. I got pregnant about 6 months after we met. He did not hit me until I was pregnant. He always said it was my fault, and I believed him. I tried to do everything right, but he got mad at me all the time. He usually hit me with an open hand in the head or on the face, but sometimes he would grab my neck and choke me with his right hand. I called the police one time after he hit me, but when they came I was too scared to tell them what happened. I lied and just said we had an argument. He hit me again after they left and said they would never believe me anyway.

Right after our baby was born, he got really mad and choked me with his right hand. I tried to get away and then he threw me into the wall. The baby was screaming. The neighbors must have called the police, because about 2 hours later they knocked on our door. I told them everything was ok, but the baby was still screaming. The next day a social worker from Child Protective Services came to my house. She told me that I could not stay with my husband if he was hurting me. She did not tell me where to go or offer me many ideas about how to get away. My husband always told me that he would kill me if I left him. She warned me that if she had to come back that she might have to take my baby away.

When my little boy was 1 year old, my husband started hitting me really hard one night. He would not stop. Finally, I ran and called 911. He left as soon as I called. The police came, but they said they could not do anything because he was gone. The next day the CPS worker came to my house again and said that I had to come to her office with my son. We drove downtown, and she gave me a bunch of papers and told me that I had to go to a shelter and get a restraining order against my husband. Two days later, I went into the domestic violence shelter, and the day after that I got a restraining order against my husband.

About 2 weeks after I was at the shelter, I went outside one day and my husband was sitting in his car across the street. He motioned for me to come over. I was scared, but I did not want to make him mad. He told me to bring my son and go with him to lunch. I got in the car and went to lunch. After that, we took my son to the doctor because he had a bad cold. We got back about 2 hours later, and there was a police car in front of the shelter. They arrested my husband for violating the restraining order. The CPS worker was there too, and she told me she was taking my baby away with her. I wanted to die. An attorney that worked at the shelter asked if my boy could stay with me and everyone could have a meeting the next day, but she said "No." They took my son away, and now he lives in a foster home. I only see him twice a week. The CPS worker says if I divorce my husband I might be able to get my son back. But I have no money and no place to live.*

INTRODUCTION

Perhaps no issue is more complicated in the intimate partner violence intervention and prevention movement than the impact of such violence on children witnessing it. Ming's true story reminds us of how often the criminal, civil, and juvenile justice systems in this country continue to fail victims when child protection and domestic violence issues intersect. This chapter will provide an overview of the systemic challenges and tensions that any clinician, child protection worker, or other professional must understand, navigate, and address. It will provide practical guidance for professionals in promoting innovative initiatives in local communities and providing services, support, and advocacy to victims of intimate partner violence and their children. This chapter is not designed to focus on clinical practices for professionals in treating victims and their children but on the key steps and critical intervention processes that must be initiated to provide victims and their children with the support they need.

The co-occurrence of child abuse and intimate partner violence and the distinctly different intervention systems developed to address child abuse on the one hand and intimate partner violence on the other make those systems very difficult for victims to navigate. The child welfare movement and the domestic violence movements are 2 distinct social change movements with differing values, philosophies, and approaches and they have a long history of tension and conflict.

It is also clear that, in most communities, the juvenile, family, and criminal court systems are not integrated or coordinated. These separate systems have evolved with little coordination or integration, even though a majority of families dealing with violence and abuse must navigate them. In addressing the challenges of intimate partner violence and the child protection systems, key strategies and themes have emerged. The child welfare movement and intimate partner violence movements must build bridges and find common ground. Adult victims and their children need innovative, multi-disciplinary, and multi-agency approaches. Child protection agencies cannot handle domestic violence cases without advocates and allies with expertise in family violence. Domestic violence advocates need child protection professionals who will use the power of their position and the tools in their systems to help adult victims protect their children and themselves. Problematic practices in the child protection arena must yield to the analysis of abusive relationships from intimate partner violence researchers and professionals. Philosophical opposition to the child protection movement in the battered women's movement must ultimately yield to the profound needs of children exposed to violence, even as advocates seek to provide support and services to the adult victims.

The way forward is clear. Collaborative policies, multi-disciplinary teams, and co-located service delivery approaches can and do provide better support for victims of intimate partner violence and their children. Children are more likely to obtain the support and protection they need if their mothers or other non-violent adult care providers are safe, supported, and protected from an abusive partner. Offenders are more likely to be held accountable, and recurring violence is reduced by professionals working together to identify the evidence, support efforts to restrain offender from further acts of abuse, and prosecute the offender for provable criminal conduct.[1-5] The Family Justice Center model, coordinated community response approaches, and other collaborative models provide promising evidence for the future. Child welfare professionals and intimate partner violence professionals are slowly coming together and working together to provide the most effective and successful outcomes for victims of intimate partner violence and their children. Excellent examples include cross-training initiatives, multi-disciplinary team approaches, and co-located child advocacy centers and family justice centers where child welfare and domestic violence professionals work side by side.[6] One of the leading models of child protection and domestic violence professionals co-locating is found in Nampa, Idaho where the Nampa Family Justice Center and the Nampa Child Advocacy Center operate conjointly out of the same building.[7] This innovative approach and many others will be discussed later in this chapter.

THE NATURE OF THE PROBLEM

The starting point for any professional or clinician working with adult victims of intimate partner violence and their children is to understand the scope and breadth of the problem. Intimate partner violence is rarely the only abuse happening in homes with children present. Child abuse rarely happens without some amount of co-occurring verbal, emotional, physical, or even sexual abuse against another adult in the home. Nearly 20 years of research has provided solid evidence of co-occurrence, with studies identifying dual abuse dynamics in between 30% and 70% of all family violence–impacted homes.[8] One study revealed rates of co-occurrence for child abuse and intimate partner violence exposure in the range of 6% to 18% for community samples but nearly 40% for clinical samples.[9] Another study revealed child abuse and intimate partner violence overlapped in 30% to 60% of all identified cases.[10] In the earliest research, the percentages were lower, but they have increased with more aggressive research inquiries. One 1990 review of 200 substantiated child abuse reports in the Massachusetts Department of Social Services found that adult domestic violence was cited in 30% of the cases.[11] But in more recent studies, the number rose to 48%, which may reflect the training of caseworkers to specifically ask about possible adult abuse.[11] Case studies in Washington State found that 55% of physical and emotional abuse referrals involved domestic violence, and 47% of the emotional abuse–only referrals of children involved domestic violence.[12]

In medical settings, where the most injurious forms of child abuse and neglect are seen, a high incidence of domestic violence appears to coexist with child abuse. The seminal work of Stark and Flitcraft examined the hospital medical records of 116 children suspected of being abused or neglected and found that 45% of the mothers had medical histories that indicated or suggested abuse.[13] McKibben, De Vos, and Newberger[14] replicated the Stark and Flitcraft study at a Boston hospital and found that 59% of mothers of abused or neglected children had medical records that suggested they had been battered by their partners. Incidence of woman abuse was significantly greater than in a matched sample of mothers of non-abused and non-neglected children.[14] Other sources indicate that as many as 3 to 18 million children are exposed to intimate partner violence in some form each year in the United States even if they themselves are not being physically or sexually abused.[15,16] The US Department of Justice has reported that children were present in homes where intimate partner violence occurred in more than 1/3 (35.5%) of all documented cases.[17,18] In an additional 15.5% of cases, it was unknown if children were present.[17] Domestic violence is a significant risk factor for child verbal abuse, physical punishment, and physical abuse.[19-21]

While most studies focus on males as perpetrators of violence against both women and children, some research suggests that female victims of domestic violence are sometimes the perpetrators of child abuse. The results of a national survey of more than 6000 American families suggested that battered women were at least twice as likely to abuse their children physically, as opposed to women who were not abused.[22] A study of more than 400 battered women revealed that 28% of these women abused their children when living with violence, and 6% threatened to abuse their children. Moreover, 5% of the women used physical violence against their children when angry with an abusive partner.[23] Similarly, another study found that among a group of women who were violent toward their husbands, 24% also abused their children.[20] These rates are higher than child abuse rates for parents who were not violent toward each other.

In many households where intimate partner violence occurs, whether the perpetrator is the man or the woman, children are present and often witness both the physical and emotional pain and injuries suffered by the adult victims.[24] Other children may not witness the violence directly but are aware of violence in the home.[24]

While the effects of actual physical and sexual abuse on children have been studied more than the effect of children witnessing abuse, findings suggest that witnessing domestic violence similarly impacts child development.[25] Some of the earliest research found significant impacts on children exposed to violence. One researcher documented reactions of children at various ages who had been exposed to violence in their homes. The reactions of children from birth to 5 years ranged from sleep disturbances to bed wetting, separation anxiety, or failure to thrive. Children ages 6 to 12 exhibited eating disturbances, seductive or manipulative behavior, or fears of abandonment or loss of control, while adolescents tended to run away, become pregnant, experience suicidal or homicidal thoughts, or engage in drug or alcohol abuse.[26] Children from violent homes exhibit both more aggressive and delinquent behavior and more withdrawn, anxious behaviors in comparison to children from non-violent homes. Additionally, they perform significantly below their peers in such areas as school performance, organized sports, and social activities.[27] Most children, whether abused or exposed to abuse, exhibit some of these behaviors at times during their development. Child protective services practitioners and other professionals should be aware that if a child manifests several of these behaviors for an extended period of time, and they continue to increase in intensity, it is possible that the child may be witnessing intimate partner violence.

"When my father was arrested for abusing my mother, you ripped me away from the mother I wanted to protect and to be with and the siblings who I loved and wanted to protect. You moved us into foster homes outside of our own community, which ripped me away from every teacher who supported me and understood what was going on, from any friends who supported us and knew what was going on."

James Henderson, Battered Women's Justice Project, Report to the Attorney General's National Task Force on Children Exposed to Violence, 2012.

Whether children can be resilient to the effects of child abuse and exposure to intimate partner violence or develop resiliency is an issue of primary interest to both researchers and practitioners in the child welfare field.[28] Previous approaches that assume it is in the best interests of a child to always remove him or her from a non-abusing parent have been discredited, and today, well-trained professionals are much more focused on supporting the child, intervening with the abusing parent, and keeping the child in a strong, close relationship with the non-abusing parent.[29] But before looking at the practical, systemic, and personal advocacy efforts that every clinician should support, one must better understand the historical conflicts that still manifest themselves today between the domestic violence and child welfare movements.

HISTORY OF CHILD WELFARE AND DOMESTIC VIOLENCE MOVEMENTS

Practitioners or systems professionals dealing with intimate partner violence and children exposed to such violence need to understand the complex differences between the child welfare and intimate partner violence movements in order to effectively help victims navigate such systems. Uninformed observers often view the 2 movements as related, parallel, and closely connected. In reality, the 2 social change movements come from completely different origins, and those origins produced differences that continue to create conflict and tension today.[30]

CHILD WELFARE/CHILD PROTECTION

The origins of the modern child welfare movement date back to the late 1880s. The so-called 'Orphan Trains' were one of the earliest efforts in the United States to identify neglected and abused children and transport them to safe homes outside of the City of New York. The well-known case of Mary Ellen McCormack, a poor, neglected, and abused little girl in New York City, typifies the heart of the movement when wealthy, well-connected New York socialites supported the work of church-based volunteers seeking to protect Mary Ellen and remove her from an abusive home using animal cruelty laws as their vehicle. Modern juvenile dependency law was developed in the early 1960's, with the shift from a purely parens patriae approach and the state stepping into the role of an absent parent to a due process–based model that gives children independent constitutional and statutory rights, and continues to evolve.[31] Charles Wilson, the former Director of the National Child Advocacy Center in Huntsville, Alabama, and now the Director of the Chadwick Center for Children and Families, has identified the key elements in the foundations of the child welfare movement. He says, "The movement was born in paternalism, driven by caring community and business leaders, and focused entirely on the needs of children."[32] This orientation has often been characterized as a "rescue orientation."[33] This rescue orientation is strikingly different than the survivor-driven nature of the domestic violence movement.

As noted in the Mary Ellen McCormack case, the first efforts to create a legal framework around child welfare had no connection to violence against women or adults. Indeed, the first laws on child welfare were modeled after animal protection laws. The first organization to focus on abuse against children was the New York Society for the Prevention of Cruelty to Animals.[34] The origins of the child welfare movement are significant: born in paternalism, aligned with animal cruelty prevention efforts, oriented to "rescue" and "removal" of abuse victims, and driven by philanthropists and business leaders and not by survivors of the abuse. Remembering and understanding these early origins will help explain the tensions with the domestic violence and intimate partner violence movements.

The child welfare movement ultimately gave birth to the modern child protection system which began to evolve in the 1960s. The child protection movement grew out of medical recognition of the nature of abuse.[35] By the late 1970s, key medical profession leaders and researchers were focusing on the need for medical identification, treatment, and care for victims of physical and sexual abuse. The Child Advocacy Center model developed as medical professionals, social workers, therapists, and criminal justice professionals began to work collaboratively on the forensic issues surrounding the documentation of physical and sexual abuse of children. By the early 1980s, the Child Advocacy Center movement became core to the child protection movement. At the same time, child protection laws, policies, and procedures began to develop at the local government level across the United States. The origins of the child welfare movement were evident at every turn as the modern child protection movement developed: rescue orientation, paternalistic approaches, and no survivor-driven initiatives. As significant as any of these forces was the reality that during its developmental stages, the child welfare movement did not focus at all on the close relationship between child abuse and intimate partner violence.

DOMESTIC VIOLENCE/INTIMATE PARTNER VIOLENCE MOVEMENT

The modern domestic violence movement dates back to the mid-1900s. Its roots can be found in the women's suffrage movement and the efforts to outlaw alcohol during Prohibition.[36-39] The key foundational elements of the movement stand in juxtaposition to the origins of the child welfare movement. The domestic violence movement was feminist in orientation, a complete rejection of paternalism; connected to other efforts to empower and elevate women; and driven by female survivors of violence and abuse at the hands of violent men.[40]

In 1982, Susan Schecter did an excellent job of looking at the history of the domestic violence movement in the 1960s and 1970s.[41] But the history goes back much further than the development of the modern battered women's movement.[42] In 1868, the legal doctrine of "family privacy" was articulated by courts in North Carolina and across the country with the following statement: "However great are the evils of ill temper, quarrels, and even personal conflicts inflicting only temporary pain, they are not comparable with the evils which would result from raising the curtain and exposing to public curiosity and criticism the nursery and the bed chamber."[43]

Ellen Pence cited research looking back as early as 1640 for the genesis of the struggle against wife beating and the call for the government to play a role in providing protection for abused women.[44] Pence wrote:

The suffrage and progressive social reform movements of the late 19th century produced legislative changes, ending more than 200 years of regulating wife beating, and criminalized the practice regardless of the woman's behavior. By 1911, laws forbidding wife beating had been passed in every state. Because no infrastructure of local efforts existed to advocate for implementation of the new laws, they were noted in law books and shelved until 70 years later, when the next wave of feminism gained momentum and activists insisted on their enforcement.[45]

In the 1960s, the women's movement began to call on male-dominated institutions to pay attention to violence against women. Violence in intimate relationships was only one of many issues addressed by the women's movement, but it soon became a very identifiable movement in and of itself. The focus on culturally acceptable violence against women was new in the 1960s. Indeed, one of the first major legal decisions in America to address the new awareness of the issue was not published until 1964 when the North Carolina Supreme Court said it was better to "forgive and forget," but acknowledged the reality that some violence in the home had to be criminalized when it rose to such a level that serious injury or death occurred.[46,47]

In the 1970s, the battered women's movement began to grow out of the much larger women's movement and included the anti-rape movement. The battered women's movement was a loosely arranged group of survivors of family violence and feminist advocates who began to organize survivors into an identifiable group of activists. The movement grew slowly at first, but then more quickly as private shelters and privately-funded social service programs developed. Although it was made up primarily of women, small numbers of progressive men supported the movement even in the late 1970s and early 1980s. And though the movement was distinct from other powerful social change movements developing in America, it found common allies in the civil rights movement and later in the child abuse movement.

In the 1980s, feminist advocates began demanding legal protections for battered women. Del Martin's seminal book, *Battered Wives* published in 1980, became a clarion call for caring people across America to step forward and act to stop family violence.[48] Class action and individual lawsuits were filed by victims and survivors attempting to treat violence against women as a civil rights issue under state and federal law. One of the most famous lawsuits was litigated and became a published court decision in 1983 when Tracy Thurman successfully sued the City of Torrington, Connecticut, for violating her civil rights by failing to protect her from her violent and abusive husband, Buck Thurman.[49] As Joan Zorza points out, the effect of this one case was dramatic, not only because a federal jury awarded Tracy and her son $2.3 million, but it "was widely reported in popular press and in academic journals. It graphically confirmed the extreme financial penalty that could be imposed on police departments when they fail to perform their duties. In addition, it confirmed that in appropriate cases these massive liability awards would be upheld."[50]

Years later, the Tracy Thurman story became a movie and educated many about the terror and trauma of domestic violence. Many individual victims began using civil litigation to demand monetary compensation from law enforcement agencies that failed to protect them from their abusers. Mandatory arrest laws, restraining order laws, pro-prosecution policies, and a host of legal mandates came forward in legislatures across the country. Specialized police officers, advocates, and prosecutors sprang up in jurisdictions across the nation as the public began to realize the difficulty of dealing with domestic violence cases in the criminal justice system.

In 1984, then-Attorney General Edwin Meese created the first national task force on domestic violence issues, with the support of President Ronald Reagan. For the first time, the federal government looked at the broad nature of family violence issues. Still today, the Task Force Report is an excellent primer on the complex history of family violence issues in America. It also yielded a powerful set of recommendations that helped launch many initiatives in the mid-1980s.

As the newly established domestic violence intervention movement developed political power, more and more policy makers and elected officials began to advocate for resources, legislation, and policy changes related to violence in the home. Nationally and internationally, more and more attention was being given to the issue of domestic violence.

In the 1990s, the mainstream adoption of a feminist view of domestic violence (as a power and control behavior exercised through male privilege) continued. Specially trained police officers, prosecutors, and judges began advocating their views within the criminal justice system itself. In 1991, the National College of District Attorneys held its first-ever national conference on the prosecution of domestic violence. Judges, prosecutors, police officers, and advocates from across the country came together for the first time.

Prosecutors attending the first and subsequent conferences of the National College of District Attorneys learned how to prosecute cases even if the victim did not want to press charges. Evidence-based prosecution first advocated by law enforcement agencies in Minnesota and later adopted in major cities was endorsed by the National College of District Attorneys as the best approach to victim safety and abuser accountability. Simply put, evidence-based prosecution was the strategy to prosecute a batterer even if the victim refused to press charges or testify. Jurisdictions such as San Diego, California; Quincy, Massachusetts; and Baltimore, Maryland led the way in training prosecutors in newly developed prosecution techniques. For the first time anywhere in America, the responsibility for law enforcement intervention in family violence cases was removed from the shoulders of victims and placed squarely on the criminal justice system itself. Advocates, police officers, prosecutors, and judges began working together cooperatively to develop coordinated approaches to deal with the long-neglected crime of domestic violence. While controversy swirled around so-called mandatory arrest laws and no-drop prosecution policies, more and more jurisdictions began treating domestic violence as seriously as any other major crime.

Though the issue remains somewhat controversial in some jurisdictions, the thesis of aggressive prosecution with or without victim participation is simple. If we don't ask victims of other serious crimes if they want to press charges, why should we ask intimate partner violence victims? If someone robs a bank, no one asks the bank teller if she wants to press charges. Why? Because bank robbery has been defined as a serious crime in this country, and bank robbers get held accountable whether or not the teller in the bank wants to testify, or prosecute. Slowly, jurisdictions began applying the same principle to both misdemeanor and felony domestic violence cases.

As the process of change continued, judges from across the country began joining in the criminal justice focus on domestic violence. In 1992, the first-ever National Judges Conference on Domestic Violence was funded by the State Justice Institute and organized by the National Council of Juvenile and Family Court Judges. The Chief Justice of each state Supreme Court named a delegation to attend the conference and work on statewide plans to train judges, educate court personnel, and revise court policies and procedures to better protect the rights of domestic violence victims. The conference, held in San Francisco, California, became a catalyst for organizing efforts in court systems across the nation and inspired many of the specialized domestic violence courts that have subsequently developed.

Without question, the 1990s saw an ongoing expansion of laws related to domestic violence, child custody issues, child support issues, and other related legal issues that impact families torn apart by violence. Policy-based legislation was only one part of the national legislative focus. The first major federal funding for domestic violence initiatives in American history finally occurred in 1994. The Violence Against Women Act (VAWA) was a landmark piece of legislation. Passed by Congress and signed by President Bill Clinton, VAWA created federal criminal offenses related to domestic violence,[51-53] mandated legal protections for battered women,[54-56] and authorized funding for shelters, tribal communities, law enforcement agencies, prosecutors, and a variety of intervention initiatives in every state.

VAWA was a far-reaching, historic, bipartisan step forward in the effort to address domestic violence issues in the United States. Within a similar time frame, laws were passed and funding was being made available in Canada, Australia, and many other countries in the Western world. Notably, the Violence Against Women Act was structured to remain completely separate from funding streams and federal laws related to Child Advocacy Centers and child protection. Feminist advocates did not want funding for violence against women to be aligned with the child welfare movement and the child welfare movement did not want their funding jeopardized or threatened by the funding needs of the domestic violence movement.

THE O. J. SIMPSON CASE

In June 1994, the O. J. Simpson case focused America, and much of the Western world, on domestic violence issues as never before. International, national, and local media were captivated by the terror and tragedy of domestic violence. As the case developed and later went to trial, it was covered worldwide. Simpson's acquittal in the criminal case, though stunning to many, did nothing to dampen the public fervor to seek justice for victims of family violence.

Media saturation of the O. J. Simpson case caused widespread public awareness. In 1996, Newsweek reported that 96% of Americans deemed domestic violence to be a major social problem in need of attention. More laws were passed, more specialized services were created, and more funding was allocated as public interest skyrocketed. The chilling 911 tapes and other evidence of prior violence by O. J. Simpson that preceded Nicole Brown Simpson's murder caused many to question whether the Los Angeles intervention system had failed to protect her when she was in obvious danger. ABC, NBC, CBS, CNN, Court TV, and other networks produced hundreds of stories on issues surrounding family violence. Print media devoted thousands of column inches to telling the stories of domestic violence victims, abusers, and system responses to such violence in jurisdictions across the country.

During the 1990s, America focused on domestic violence issues as never before. Task forces formed in local communities and at the state and federal level; arrest and prosecution became standard procedure in family violence incidents; counseling and support groups for victims proliferated; batterer intervention programs multiplied across the country; more specialized resources were devoted to family violence than at any time in our history; and some of the first major public awareness campaigns were launched at the local, state, and national level.

Notably, little of the history of the modern domestic violence movement includes a focus on the co-occurrence of child abuse and domestic violence. The community-based domestic violence organizations and shelter professionals were keenly aware of child abuse and providing services to children, but there was little interaction or connection between the burgeoning child protection movement and the domestic violence movement. While the history of these 2 movements is complex, it is critical to understanding the challenges experienced in the last 15 years by child protection and intimate partner violence professionals and the challenges clinicians and professionals still face in helping victims understand the systems they must navigate. The 2 movements developed separately, often still operate separately, and do not naturally align themselves with consistent intervention approaches.

NICHOLSON V. WILLIAMS

In 2001, the tensions between the child welfare movement and the domestic violence movement that had been building for years played out in a federal court room in New York City. The case of Nicholson v. Williams (sometimes referred to as Nicholson v. Scoppetta) is an ideal case study in the tensions between the domestic violence and child protection movements, and it provides an outline for the issues addressed in this chapter.[57] It also provides the research which clinicians need to address the intersection of intimate partner violence and children exposed to such violence.

Attorneys focused on protecting battered women filed suit against the New York City's Administration for Child Services (ACS) in 2001 for a blanket policy that removed children from homes where domestic violence was occurred and routinely resulted in mothers being prosecuted for failure to protect their children. The ACS placed primary responsibility on the mother for not escaping the violence and assumed major negative impacts on the children exposed to the violence without any examination or evidence. In the case's early hearings, ACS workers testified that by removing children from abusive environments, even without a court order, they could then force mothers to participate in any services they required before getting their children back. The lawsuit started out with 3 different plaintiffs, in 3 different cases, but the cases were eventually consolidated into 1 class action suit. After a 24 day trial, the judge granted a preliminary injunction in favor of the plaintiffs and against ACS. The trial judge ruled that:

— Removing a child exposed to violence, without additional evidence of long-term mental impairment, was a violation of the child's rights and the mother's rights.

— Child protection professionals must assist mothers with access to shelter and protection orders.

— Child protection professionals must receive training in domestic violence and the research regarding children exposed to domestic violence.

— A monitoring process to ensure ACS compliance with the court's findings was necessary.

— Findings must be made in each case as to whether a domestic violence victim/mother has exercised a minimum degree of care in the effort to protect her children before deciding if she is liable for any form of neglect.

— Any court determining whether a domestic violence victim has exercised a minimum degree of care must consider the risks attendant to leaving (the violent abuser), the risks attendant to staying, the risks attendant to seeking assistance through government channels, the risks attendant to criminal prosecution of the batterer, the risks attendant to relocating, the severity and frequency of the violence, and the resources available to the adult victim.[58]

The judge's findings were challenged by ACS The case was removed from federal court, and went to the New York State Court of Appeals. The Court of Appeals affirmed the trial court's rulings and found that a "blanket presumption" of neglect against a domestic violence victim when a child is exposed to violence was improper and that removal of the child may do more harm than good.[58] The court also called for efforts by child protection authorities to seek a protection orders against abusers and offer more services to mothers and children before pursuing removal of children from their mother.[58] The court expressed a strong preference for a court order before removal of the children from their mother and an even stronger preference for removing abusers instead of blaming their victims.[58]

The Nicholson case still stands as one of the most important court cases in the last 30 years in the ongoing issues between child protection systems and domestic violence movement advocates. Though many other states have not followed the exact findings in the Nicholson case, the overall tenets of the case and the research that was presented to the court has helped shape the future of collaborative approaches to domestic violence now evolving all over the country. Major challenges still remain in the policies, protocols, and procedures that guide professionals in these 2 distinct worlds including the approach of child advocacy centers in America.

The National Child Advocacy Center certification standards are promulgated through the National Children's Alliance to guide the process for the creation and operation of Child Advocacy Centers throughout the United States.[59] The standards provide an excellent framework for professionals seeking to work in multi-disciplinary teams to address incidences of child physical and sexual abuse and neglect.

While the standards are well-regarded and strongly supported by child protection professionals across the country, a careful analysis of the standards points again to the disconnection between the child welfare and domestic violence movements. A recent analysis of the standards identified the use of the term "domestic violence" only once in 88 pages.[60] There is not a single reference to intimate partner violence.[60] Indeed, the only reference to domestic violence in the standards is not a discussion of the impact of violence and abuse on the adult care provider but a lone reference to the psychological impacts of witnessing violence on children.[35] Even the language in child protection is not humanizing or friendly to the adult victim of domestic violence.[35] The standards and most local and state regulations on child protection refer euphemistically to domestic violence victims as "the non-offending parent."[35] Such an approach acknowledges neither the humanity nor frailty of a parent experiencing violence and abuse, while also witnessing violence against and abuse of their children.

While the National Family Justice Center Alliance continues to advocate for changes in these standards, it is important to understand the tendency of the child protection movement to focus only on children and the impacts of abuse and witnessing violence on children instead of focusing on the critical nature of their relationship with their mother.[61]

ADDRESSING THE CHALLENGES

Practitioners and clinicians providing advocacy, support, and case management services to victims of domestic violence and their children must be aware of and be prepared to address the challenges faced by victims and their children in accessing criminal and civil justice system services. The key to all intervention strategies is collaboration and joint approach addressing both child abuse and domestic violence issues. To properly address issues in communities, systems, and individual cases, clinicians and professionals should focus on awareness, understanding, responses and strategies, and general community collaborative efforts.

AWARENESS

The first challenge to every professional working with families exposed to child abuse or intimate partner violence is awareness of research. Many child victims of physical abuse and neglect witness intimate partner violence in their homes. Many adult victims of domestic violence have children who may be experiencing physical abuse, sexual abuse, or neglect at the hands of adult caretakers. Research has confirmed that adult victims of domestic violence may emotionally, verbally, or physically abuse their children as well (see **Table 9-1**). A basic understanding of the prevalence of co-occurrence should motivate professionals to probe and inquire about other potential forms of abuse.

UNDERSTANDING

The second challenge is to fully understand the dynamics and impact of intimate partner violence. Children in violent homes face 4 major risks: observing traumatic or violent events; being abused themselves, being neglected, and intervening in witness violence. Though they may care deeply for their children, adult victims of domestic violence often find it difficult to protect their children from violence and abuse that they themselves experience. Appreciating the complexity of these dynamics will make concerned professionals much more effective in advocating for and empowering adult

Table 9-1. Research Into Domestic Violence Victims' Efforts to Protect Their Children

Battered parents make decisions for their children in the context of their lives, considering all the risk factors, and not just domestic violence. For example, a battered mother might decide her child witnesses her boyfriend's controlling behavior, he will be OK, even though he witnesses her boyfriend's controlling behavior, as long as she can put food on the table and a roof over his head, and keep him in his current school, which means she will need to stay with her abusive partner.[62]

Victims of domestic violence worry about the safety of their children, but research on the protective strategies they use is relatively sparse. In one small study of 17 battered women with children, 65% described removing their children from scenes of violence by moving away from them or putting them in their bedrooms.[63] In the same study, almost half spoke of reassuring their children and emphasizing to them that the fighting was not their fault. Some mothers try to teach their children to make nonviolent choices in their own relationships.[63,64]

victims of domestic violence to protect their children and work with intervention systems critical to creating accountability for abusers. A clinician trained in child welfare should work with an intimate partner violence professional or advocate in order to effectively support adult victims of domestic violence, and a clinician specialized in domestic violence may need to reach out to a child welfare professional after identifying trauma in children.

Dr. Jeff Edelson and others have argued that witnessing violence should be viewed as a potential risk factor rather than conclusive evidence of child maltreatment. Most of the research confirms that children witnessing violence and suffering physical abuse suffer confirms children witnessing violence alone, who in turn suffer a more traumatic impact than children who witness no violence at all.[65] In most of the research, children witnessing violence and experiencing violence are referred to as "abused witnesses." Children simply witnessing violence are referred to as "non-abused witnesses." Some researchers have found significant differences between non-abused child witnesses and abused child witnesses.[66] In comparison to non-abused witnesses, abused witnesses are more likely to exhibit more aggressive behaviors. Abused witnesses perceive the quality of father-child relationships as more negative and are more likely to live in families with a greater frequency and severity of intimate partner violence and less relationship satisfaction (**Table 9-2**).

As noted earlier, some victims of domestic violence are so fearful of the abusive partner's focusing their anger on the children that the adult victim (usually the mother) over-disciplines them in an effort to control the children's behavior and protect them from what they perceive as greater abuse from the abusive partner. Given the consequences of witnessing domestic violence for children, many professionals in the field are grappling with whether or not exposure to domestic violence is itself a form of child maltreatment.[67] Research in this area initially focused on documenting the co-occurrence of domestic violence and child maltreatment. Subsequently, the focus of research shifted to the effects on children witnessing domestic violence. Recently, some researchers have drawn the conclusion that exposure to domestic violence is in fact a form of child abuse. Edelson and others advise caution in interpreting findings regarding the impact of witnessing domestic violence because each child will experience domestic violence in unique ways depending on a variety of factors, including the child's gender, age, and relationship with adults in the home.[68] In addition, many studies of child witnesses have drawn primarily from children residing in shelters, thereby contributing more extreme

Table 9-2. Key Principles for Child Protection Advocates

— The best way to protect a child who has been exposed to domestic violence is to keep his or her non-offending parent safe and ensure that the non-offending parent is able to engage in a safe, secure, and nurturing relationship with the child.

— Respecting a child's developmental needs requires keeping safety paramount and ensuring that a child maintains a continuous relationship with his/her offending parent.

— A non-offending parent should not be held responsible for the behavior of an offending parent.

— It is essential to recognize the protective behaviors that abused parents engage in while remaining in the home.

findings than may actually exist; therefore, findings may be more dramatic than is usual in the general public. Many children may, in fact, demonstrate resilience to violence by coping in a number of constructive ways.[69] Thus witnessing abuse does not, in every case, rise to the level of psychological abuse. Many battered women do attend to the psychological needs of their children. Clinicians and child protection professionals should view witnessing violence as a potential risk factor rather than conclusive evidence of child maltreatment.

RESPONSES AND STRATEGIES

In recent years, specific responses and strategies in addressing child protection and intimate partner violence intersections have been identified and recommended for clinicians, practitioners, and child protection worker. A number of these recommended responses should be central to the response of child protection professionals and others working with victims of domestic violence and their children.

Focus on the Perpetrator

Most researchers and professionals have identified the overall need for greater focus on the predominately male perpetrators of intimate partner violence and co-occurring child abuse. As noted, criminal prosecution of the offender does reduce recidivism or alter a perpetrator's strategies with his partner and children. Juvenile and dependency courts can and should issue protection orders against male perpetrators more often instead of focusing primary intervention efforts on victims and their actions in response to violence and abuse. Greater coordination between juvenile courts; family courts; dependency courts, where most child protection cases are heard; and the criminal courts, where most domestic violence offenders are prosecuted, produces more accountability for perpetrators of violence and abuse, as opposed to focusing on the limited authority of the civil courts to address perpetrators of violence.

While batterer intervention program effectiveness is debated by many researchers, there is strong evidence that increased monitoring of, consequences for, and attention to offenders does alter their behavior and often mitigates their violence. Longer programs tend to be more effective than shorter programs in altering behavior, and specialized courts, specialized probation, and parole monitoring seem to be more effective with offenders than general court dockets and supervision. An evaluation of the court review process for men referred to batterer's counseling from the Domestic Violence Court in Pittsburgh.

The evaluation found that court review dramatically increases compliance with batterer counseling and that court review and batterer's counseling together lower recidivism.[70]

Research has also found that aggressive misdemeanor prosecution of domestic violence offenders reduces repeat violence and increases victim safety.[71] As noted earlier, the Nicholson court rulings, based on research, focused on the importance of courts issuing orders against perpetrators and seeking to hold them accountable for their behavior and found that to be more effective than blaming victims or attempting to prosecute them for neglect or failure to protect.[72]

Cross-Train Child Protection and Domestic Violence Professionals

Many of the earliest initiatives to improve outcomes for adult victims and children exposed to violence found that conducting regular cross-trainings between domestic violence professionals and child welfare professionals produced more effective and coordinated intervention approaches. From 1991 to 1993, the first cross-training efforts in San Diego built a foundation for communication, coordination, and understanding between child welfare and domestic violence professionals.

Similar initiatives were promoted by the federal government and by local communities across the country. Between 1994 and 1996, 26 federal Domestic Violence/Child Protective Services Collaboration grants were awarded to support the development of training, intervention protocols, and screening tools that could be applied when domestic violence is encountered during investigation by Child Protective Services. A number of other federal agencies, including the Office of Justice Programs and the Centers for Disease Control and Prevention, began administering grant programs focused on the relationship between domestic violence and child abuse. A number of those early cross-training efforts produced long-term systemic change. Michigan's family preservation program, Families First, began a dialogue with the Governor's Domestic Violence Prevention and Treatment Board in 1993. After learning about each other and establishing common goals, Families First staff requested a domestic violence in-service training seminar for family preservation workers. This led to co-sponsorship, with the Family Violence Prevention Fund (now Futures Without Violence), of a national curriculum on domestic violence for family preservation workers. In 1995, Michigan became the first state to institutionalize mandatory training, provided jointly by Families First trainers and domestic violence advocates, for all family preservation managers, supervisors, and workers. This cooperation led to the first family preservation effort within domestic violence programs when family preservation teams were placed in battered women's shelters. Since 1995, the collaboration has expanded to include Child Protective Services (CPS), with mandatory training on domestic violence for all CPS supervisors and workers, and CPS policy on how to handle child abuse and neglect cases of domestic violence. Portions of this curriculum are highlighted later in this chapter but the beginning of the systems change happened through cross-training. But such cross-training between intimate partner violence and child protection professionals should be regularly occurring in every community in the United States.

The National Curriculum for Child Protective Services developed by Futures Without Violence includes excellent guidance for conducting such trainings and provides guidance for individual practitioners. The first focus area, which can benefit all practitioners includes the basic facts about the risk domestic violence perpetrators pose to children, as outlined in **Table 9-3**.[73]

Child protection professionals and others working in the child welfare movement can gain valuable information about individual domestic violence perpetrators by collaborating

Table 9-3. Domestic Violence Perpetrators Pose the Following Risk to Children

— Domestic violence perpetrators may physically abuse children.

— Domestic violence perpetrators may sexually abuse children.

— Domestic violence perpetrators may endanger children through neglect. The domestic violence perpetrator may focus so much attention on controlling and abusing his adult partner that he ignores and neglects their children.

— Domestic violence perpetrators may also prevent adult victims from caring for their children, resulting in neglect.

— Domestic violence perpetrators may harm children by coercing them into abusing their mothers or other adult caretakers.

— Domestic violence perpetrators may endanger children emotionally and physically by creating environments in which children witness assaults against their mothers.

— Domestic violence perpetrators may endanger children by undermining the ability of CPS and other community agencies to intervene and protect children.

with domestic violence advocates, law enforcement officers, and prosecutors handling domestic violence cases.

The authors have also spent time observing batterer intervention programs; meeting with convicted domestic violence offenders; and reviewing police reports, 911 tapes, and other evidence in cases to gain an understanding of perpetrators. In addition, hosting focus groups with survivors of family violence outside of the adversarial courtroom setting or system intervention process also provides valuable insight and training for child protection professionals in understanding how offenders think and operate.

All child protection professionals and other clinicians should also be familiar with the Futures Without Violence curriculum's summary information on symptoms in children who witness domestic violence against their mothers (see **Table 9-4**).[73]

Engage Child Abuse and Domestic Violence Advocates in Case Teams

Many of the early cross-training efforts also resulted in cross-assignment of child welfare and domestic violence advocates. Carter and Schechter[74] identified a 4-step approach that enables child protective services and domestic violence programs to collaborate for the safety of the entire family; the 4 steps are screening, investigating, assessing, and intervening. Intake/assessment procedures incorporate questions about both child abuse and domestic violence, and interventions are crafted for the family unit, not just the child or just the woman. Around this approach, the 2 workers from different service perspectives can organize their separate but related activities. Some of the earliest team approaches evolved in communities like Jacksonville, Florida, where Hubbard House, a local domestic violence program, partnered an advocate with each CPS worker on cases with children and domestic violence; Cedar Rapids, Iowa, where YWCA domestic violence advocates attended CPS case consultation meetings and accompanied CPS workers on home visits; communities across Oregon, where CPS hired part-time domestic violence advocates to attend weekly case staffing meetings; and throughout the State of Massachusetts, where the Massachusetts Department of Social Services (DSS) hired its first domestic violence advocate to provide education and consultation to CPS staff in 1990 and eventually created a statewide domestic

Table 9-4. Possible Symptoms in Children Who Witness Their Mothers' Abuse

— Sleeplessness, fears of going to sleep, nightmares, dreams of danger

— Headaches, stomach aches

— Anxiety about being hurt or killed, hyper-vigilance about danger

— Fighting with others, hurting others or animals

— Temper tantrums

— Withdrawal from other people and activities

— Listlessness, depression, little energy for life

— Feelings of loneliness and isolation

— Substance abuse

— Suicide attempts or engaging in dangerous behavior

— Fears of going to school or of separating from mother, truancy

— Stealing

— Frozen watchfulness or excessive fear

— Acting perfect, overachieving, behaving like small adults

— Worrying, difficulties in concentrating and paying attention

— Bed-wetting or regression to earlier developmental stages

— Eating problems

— Medical problems like asthma, arthritis, ulcers

— Denial of any problem or dissociation

— Identification with the aggressor

violence unit with domestic violence specialists placed in local DSS offices. This team approach has now been codified into state law in places such as Massachusetts, New Hampshire, and Kentucky, and has been implemented by protocol in many communities across the country.

Engage in Safety Planning with Children and with Adult Victims

Professionals should engage in individual safety planning efforts with adult victims and their children. Risk assessment with victims is critical in evaluating how much danger victims are in based on the actions and mental state of their perpetrator. But once risk assessment is completed, safety planning must be conducted on a regular basis. Conducting a risk assessment with the victim, such as the Danger Assessment Tool developed by Dr. Jacquelyn Campbell, will help the victim understand the need for not only developing a personalized Safety Plan for herself but also for her children.[75] Safety planning for adults has many components and is usually customized based on the victim's unique situation, her level of danger and available support system, the danger to her children or others, and her plan of action. Safety plans have been developed to assist victims when preparing to leave; during an explosive incident; identifying the things to take with them; safety in the home; safety on the job and in public; safety for her children, safety after leaving the relationship; and safety with technology.[76]

Professionals working with abused victims and children can also assist children in developing safety plans for their own plans based on their age, level of danger, comfort level, and family dynamics. Safety planning for children helps to empower children, helps them to overcome feelings of helplessness or fear, and ultimately enhances their safety. Safety planning with children should include:

— Use of a code word, such as the child's pet's name or another safe word or sentence, and an explanation of what to do if the code word is used

— Identification of a safe place to go if someone is getting hurt

— Description of how the child can get to that safe place

— Instructions for the child on when and how to call 911[77]

The American Bar Association Commission on Domestic Violence has developed a model safety plan for children to assist professionals working with children.[78] Professionals can help victims stay safer by customizing safety plans for victims and their children as well as linking victims to specialized intimate partner violence services or advocates.

Work with the Domestic Violence Victim to Help Her Understand the Impact on Children

Many child protection professionals fail to constructively help victims of intimate partner violence understand the impacts of witnessing the abuse on their children. The research is clear that victims of domestic violence are most likely to leave their abusers and cooperate with intervention professionals when they realize the impacts of the abuse on their children. Blaming the victim for what the children are experiencing does not tend to motivate constructive action. Victims already blame themselves for their partners' violence and placing blame on the victim for the actions of the perpetrator often drives the victim away from the intervention process. The Domestic Violence: National Curriculum for Child Protection Services includes excellent questions (see **Table 9-5**) to ask the adult victim and, in the process of this dialogue, help the victim to see the impacts of her partner's abuse on their children.

The most critical component in helping the victim to initially understand the impact of domestic violence on her children is for the clinician or professional to engage in a dialogue with the victim about the impacts of the violence on the children. It is important that this be a dialogue that seeks to help the victim "self-discover" the impacts of the violence on the children. The questions in **Table 9-5** are recommended by the authors for such an assessment interview.

Professionals should always view such an assessment interview with a mother whose children are exposed to domestic violence as a dialogue and partnership.

Utilize Evidence-Based Therapeutic Practices With the Victim and Children

The most promising therapeutic practices in co-occurring cases of child abuse and domestic violence now include child-parent psychotherapy therapy and parent-child interactive therapy. Child-parent interactive therapy and other forms of individual and group counseling clearly help children process the trauma of witnessing violence and abuse. **Table 9-6**, below, describes the approach and the initial results.[79]

Other therapeutic practices have been identified as an evidence-based practice in working effectively with children exposed to domestic violence and their parents including parent-child interaction therapy (see **Table 9-7**).

9-5. Interview Questions for Assessing the Impact of Domestic Violence on Children

1. Injuries or health impact to children?

What kind of health issues does your child have? Injuries? Bruises, broken bones, black eyes, burns, pain, unconsciousness due to hitting or choking? Injuries from weapons?

2. Psychological and emotional impact?

Have there been any emotional changes? Withdrawal, depression, increased irritability, anxiety, nightmares? Are you aware of any suicidal thoughts or acts by the child?

3. Behavioral Problems?

Have your children had behavioral problems in family, school, and peer relationships? Have your children used physical force or threats of physical force against you or others? Are your children dealing with anger in ways that disturb you? Problems in eating, sleeping, running away, alcohol or drug abuse, cutting themselves, harming animals, destroying toys?

4. Social Problems?

Have your children suffered social disruption due to the domestic violence: moves, changing schools, isolation from friends, loss of family members, etc.? Are their social relationship problems with family, peers, other adults?

5. How does the domestic violence impact your parenting of the children?

Is the domestic violence interfering with your ability to take care of the child, to consider the child's best interest, to keep the child safe? Do you feel supported by in parenting your child?

6. How does domestic violence impact the parenting of the domestic violence perpetrator?

Is the perpetrator able to take care of the child, to consider the child's best interests, to keep the child safe? Does the perpetrator support your parenting? Does the perpetrator undermine you? Does the perpetrator use the children to control you? Does the perpetrator use physical force against the children?

Table 9-6. Child-Parent Psychotherapy Helps Children Exposed to Domestic Violence

Pioneered at San Francisco General Hospital, psychiatrist Alicia Lieberman and psychologist Patricia Van Horn instituted an effective approach to ameliorating the effects of trauma on young children resulting from exposure to domestic violence.

The model begins with assessment meetings focused on the child's individual functioning and quality of the relationship with the caregiver, who is also a participant. After the assessment, joint parent-child psychotherapy is provided for a year and can be provided in the home if it is safe and the parent elects to have it there. The treatment is offered in multiple languages and focuses on strengthening the parent-child relationship and assisting the parent in understanding the child's experience so that she more effectively protects the child.

Randomized controlled trials of this approach have demonstrated effectiveness and durability of parent-child psychotherapy in remediating the effects of trauma resulting from preschool age children's exposure to domestic violence and setting (or re-setting) young children on their appropriate developmental trajectories.

Table 9-7. Parent-Child Interaction Therapy*

Parent-child interaction therapy (PCIT) is an empirically-supported treatment for conduct-disordered young children that places emphasis on improving the quality of the parent-child relationship and changing parent-child interaction patterns. In PCIT, parents are taught specific skills to establish a nurturing and secure relationship with their child while increasing their child's pro-social behavior and decreasing negative behavior. This treatment focuses on two basic interactions: child-directed interaction (CDI) is similar to play therapy in that parents engage their child in a play situation with the goal of strengthening the parent-child relationship; parent directed interaction (PDI) resembles clinical behavior therapy in that parents learn to use specific behavior management techniques as they play with their child.

**For a summary of PCIT and information about the future research directions of PCIT see research by Zisser and Eyberg from 2010.[80]*

Identify and Advocate Against Problematic Practices in Child Protection

The National Family Justice Center Alliance has identified a number of problematic practices in child protection that continue to be utilized in some states and certain communities. Clinicians and other professionals working with victims of domestic violence should be aware of these practices and advocate against them on a systems and individual case basis. First, child protection agencies sometimes order domestic violence victims to obtain a restraining order against their partner under threat of having their children removed. This practice is problematic on a variety of levels. The victim cannot obtain an order unless she is in imminent danger of bodily harm. Seeking an order and not obtaining it may empower the offender and create further danger for the victim. Protection orders, if granted, tend to create more danger for victims because separation heightens risk for the adult victim of abuse.[81] Risk assessment and safety planning procedures should be in place if any protection order is going to be put in place. As noted earlier, however, compelling a victim to obtain a protection order may be much less effective than child protection services actually seeking the order against the offender. The better practice is to develop a team of professionals to work collaboratively with the adult victim and develop a cooperative approach with the adult victim in order to protect the children.

The second problematic practice identified by the Alliance is any effort by child protection services that seeks to compel a victim to enter a domestic violence shelter in order to separate her from the abuser. No adult victim of domestic violence should be forced into a shelter against her will. First, she will become more likely to disclose her location to her abuser thereby endangering other shelter residents. Second, scarce shelter beds should be available to victims in immediate danger of serious injuries or death. If CPS attempts to coerce a victim into shelter against her will, the victim is likely to leave the shelter sooner or not participate in programs as fully and may be more likely to disclose the location of the shelter to her abuser.

The third problematic practice identified by the Alliance is more broadly described as any case or service plan developed by child protection professionals that does not include participation from domestic violence advocates, prosecutors, and civil legal service providers working to protect adult victims and prosecute abusers. It is difficult for victims to navigate the various criminal, civil, and social systems. In Ming's case, described at the beginning of the chapter, she had a juvenile dependency case pending in juvenile court, a domestic violence case pending in criminal court, and a protection order pending in family court. She was also in a shelter receiving counseling and support services. While she had an advocate working with her at the shelter, none of these systems or professionals were working together or sharing information. There was no one to help Ming navigate through the various systems; coordinate information sharing; or alert professionals to key information that might have enhanced victim safety, child protection, or offender accountability in all the cases.

The overarching problematic practice in co-occurring child abuse and domestic violence cases is simply the failure of all professionals to coordinate their work with victims and their children. Across the United States, legal services for victims of domestic violence and their children are fragmented, inaccessible, and often ineffective. The complex coordination necessary to address family court, criminal court, and juvenile court cases is further confounded by the failure of the civil legal services approach to integrate needed social services, child advocacy services, and health-related assistance.

Beyond these problematic practices, is the daunting reality of trauma, fear, lack of transportation, unavailability of safe housing, and failure of intervention and prevention systems to coordinate their activities with the pressing legal issues of victims that leaves many victims disempowered and lost in a maze of systems they do not understand and cannot navigate. As a result, victims of domestic violence face adverse court rulings daily across America related to protective orders, child support, child custody, divorce, immigration status, wrongful termination, landlord-tenant matters, and bankruptcy.

As noted throughout this chapter, intimate partner violence must be addressed in all child protection cases and child abuse issues must be evaluated in all intimate partner violence cases. The short-term results and long-term outcomes all appear to improve with multi-agency, multi-disciplinary approaches.

GENERAL COMMUNITY AND SYSTEMS COLLABORATIVE EFFORTS

In recent years, collaborative models have evolved in a variety of communities and systems with demonstrated success in providing better coordination and cooperation among child welfare and domestic violence professionals when working on cases involving child protection and intimate partner violence issues. In the early 1980s, as noted earlier, Child Advocacy Centers began developing multi-disciplinary approaches for the investigation, documentation, prosecution, and treatment of child physical and sexual abuse cases. The research has validated the effectiveness of these multi-agency, multi-disciplinary centers in producing better cases, services, and community responses for child abuse cases. Many communities do not yet have a certified Child Advocacy Center, but the efficacy and success of such a model is well established.[82]

In the 1990s, the Edna McConnell Clark Foundation and others demonstrated that collaborations between child abuse and domestic violence advocates and members of the community can make families safer. One of the first funded projects, known as the Community Partnership for Protecting Children, enlisted the entire community to respond to domestic violence and child abuse by adopting and funding prevention and intervention efforts that used the resources of neighbors, friends, churches, and other non-traditional supports for families.[74,83] More recently, many communities have developed multi-agency, co-located service models, which bring together child welfare and domestic violence professionals under one roof. The federal Greenbook Initiative found that co-location of professionals enhanced services for victims and their children, facilitated cross-training and information sharing, and produced better outcomes in cases intimate partner violence and children witnessing such violence.[84]

In 2002, the first Family Justice Center was created in San Diego, California where child welfare professionals and domestic violence professionals came together under one roof to provide services for victims of domestic violence and sexual assault and their children.[6] The San Diego Family Justice Center brought together professionals from more than 25 agencies for the first time – working together day to day to address domestic violence, sexual assault, stalking, elder abuse, and child abuse cases. Working in close partnership with the Chadwick Center for Children and Families in San Diego, then San Diego City Attorney Casey Gwinn and Police Chief David Bejarano included a focus on children exposed to domestic violence as a key service area within the center.

President George W. Bush endorsed the Family Justice Center model in 2003 with the creation of the President's Family Justice Center Initiative to fund 15 additional centers in diverse communities across the United States. In 2005, Congress added Family Justice Centers to Title I of the Violence Against Women Act and provided a funding stream for the creation of more such centers. Most recently, communities such as Nampa, Idaho have developed Family Justice Centers and Child Advocacy Centers under the same roof with the goal of coordinating services for children and adult victims in a more effective and timely manner.

The early outcomes in Family Justice Centers point toward better long-term outcomes for adult victims and expedited services for children when all the services are co-located. The US Department of Justice has hailed Family Justice Centers as a "best practice" in the field of family violence intervention and prevention:

The documented and published outcomes have included: reduced homicides; increased victim safety; increased autonomy and empowerment for victims; reduced fear and anxiety for victims and their children; reduced recantation and minimization by victims when wrapped in services and support; increased efficiency in collaborative services to victims among service providers; increased prosecution of offenders; and dramatically increased community support for services to victims and their children through the family justice center model.[85]

All communities and all allied professionals working with victims of intimate partner violence and their children should take seriously their responsibility to advocate for and participate in partnerships, cross-trainings, collaborative service delivery approaches, and co-located service models that seek to produce more effective and efficient intervention, treatment, and long-term healing services for victims and their children. Child protection professionals and others should also recognize that closer collaboration produces more accountability for perpetrators of abuse against adult partners and children. The Family Justice Center model, multi-disciplinary teams, and multi-agency approaches all produce better results than individual agencies, courts, or professionals seeking to handle child protection matters without the support of allied professionals.

Ming's Story: When Intervention is Done Well

Our dream for the future is a different ending for Ming and other abused women and children. We dream of a day when child protection professionals and domestic violence professionals will work together whenever a mother and her children are both being abused. Victims like Ming need a comprehensive, multi-agency team of legal professionals to provide criminal and civil legal services and comprehensive social and medical services. These services should include risk assessment, safety planning, access to public benefits, assistance with short- and long-term housing, representation in all civil legal matters, including child custody, child support, dissolution, contempt hearings, immigration-related legal services, housing/tenancy issues, credit restoration and protection, and restitution matters.

If Ming's case were handled properly, CPS would refer her to a local Family Justice Center or community-based domestic violence program for advocacy and support services immediately. No other CPS action would be taken until a multi-disciplinary team could be put together to meet with each other and Ming. In a Family Justice Center community, a general client intake process would occur. A clinical assessment, risk assessment, and safety plan would be completed for Ming. One of the services at the Center would be the FJC Legal Network or some other agency providing civil legal services. The Family Justice Center would continue to provide social services to Ming to ensure her needs were met related to counseling, social services, safety planning, transportation, and medical issues. If the FJC Legal Network enrolled her, however, her legal needs would then be addressed in a coordinated fashion. Assuming Ming was eligible, wanted to participate, and signed the necessary waivers for information sharing, the legal network coordinator would then convene a case conference with all the players involved, including the FJC staff to make sure everyone's efforts on Ming's behalf were coordinated. Ming's legal needs, in coordination with her social and medical service needs, would be coordinated through a joint team consisting of one case manager for social services and one case manager for legal services. The FJC team would operate in a model that includes case conferencing with all team professionals, coordination of related social services for Ming and her children, court accompaniment, case management services, short-term and long-term housing support, medical services, and technology-based assistance, including cell phones for all clients with real-time communication between the client and her legal team regarding court dates, appointments, and case conferencing.

Thousands of women like Ming need child protection and domestic violence professionals to cross-train each other, work together, develop team approaches, share information, and develop approaches to work with victims instead of 'acting on victims' or attempting to control and order victims to take certain actions. We long for a day when Ming will not lose custody of her children, will not be blamed for her abuser's violence, and her abuser will be held accountable for his abuse in criminal, family, and juvenile court.

CONCLUSION

Intimate partner violence and child protection professionals have begun the long journey of cross-learning, collaboration, and coordinated responses to the common co-occurrence of child abuse and domestic violence. All professionals have realized the significance of children exposed to domestic violence even if they are not physically or sexually abused. Children exposed to such violence may be seriously affected and the effect of witnessing the violence and also experiencing physical abuse may produce greater negative effects than one factor alone. The child welfare and domestic violence movements are different social change movements with often conflicting philosophical underpinnings. Understanding these differences and seeking common ground can help mitigate the conflicts and tensions that still exist between the systems and the well-meaning professionals that work in both fields. Collaborative responses and team approaches can produce powerful results and, ultimately, systemic changes. Co-located service models such as Child Advocacy Centers, Family Justice Centers, and other forms of multi-agency, multi-disciplinary teams often produce better results for victims and their children and more accountability for perpetrators of violence and abuse.

Individual relationships and collaborative agency relationships help to produce more informed and effective case plans and intervention strategies. Excellent model protocols now exist to help guide child protection professionals in working with adult victims of domestic violence and trained domestic violence advocates and professionals even while maintaining their primary focus on the best interest of the child. Indeed, a great deal of research now points to the reality that one cannot protect children if one does not protect their mothers. Protecting adult victims of domestic violence clearly requires a diverse and well-trained team.

There is growing evidence that reform in service delivery in the intersection between child protection and intimate partner violence can happen if domestic violence professionals and child protection professionals work closely with law enforcement officers, prosecutors, civil legal service providers, and court systems to come together, stay together, and learn together (**Table 9-8**). Hundreds of thousands of women like Ming need a comprehensive approach to civil, criminal, and juvenile justice system intervention in family violence cases. Every professional has a role to play in bringing together such a team when working with individual victims.

Table 9-8. Select Websites for Further Information on the Intersection Between Child Protection and Intimate Partner Violence

Administration for Children and Families (ACF)

http://www.acf.hhs.gov/programs/opa/facts/domsvio.htm

This online fact sheet describes ACF-funded activities that reflect the Department of Health and Human Services' current focus on domestic violence, child maltreatment, and child welfare issues.

Futures Without Violence

http://www.futureswithoutviolence.org/

Futures Without Violence, formerly the Family Violence Prevention Fund, is a national non-profit organization that focuses on domestic violence education, prevention, and public policy reform. The Fund co-sponsored the development of 2 national domestic violence and child welfare training curricula, "Domestic Violence: A National Curriculum for Family Preservation Practitioners," and "Domestic Violence: A National Curriculum for Children's Protective Services." This site includes fact sheets on the effects of domestic violence on children and other resources.

MINCAVA

http://www.mincava.umn.edu

The Minnesota Center Against Violence and Abuse (MINCAVA) operates this electronic clearinghouse, which provides scholarly papers on battered women and their children, a searchable database on the link between child maltreatment and woman battering, bibliographies, and links to additional resources.

National Family Justice Center Alliance (Resource Library)

http://www.familyjusticecenter.com

The Alliance provides a free online resource library with a host of resources on collaborative service delivery models that bring together child welfare and domestic violence professionals including Child Advocacy Centers, Family Justice Centers, and other types of multi-disciplinary teams.

Office on Violence Against Women (OVW)

http://www.ovw.usdoj.gov/domviolence.htm

This US Department of Justice site provides summaries of the grant programs authorized by the Violence Against Women Act (VAWA) that foster collaboration among domestic violence programs and child protection service agencies and provide services to battered women and their children. Full text Federal legislation and regulations regarding domestic violence and child victimization, including VAWA, and links to a number of related resources, including the Violence Against Women Grants.

References

1. Smith BE, Davis RC. *An Evaluation of Efforts to Implement No Drop Policies: Two Central Values Conflict.* NCJ 199719. https://www.ncjrs.gov/pdffiles1/nij/199719.pdf. Accessed August 19, 2011.

2. Gwinn C, Strack G. *Hope for Hurting Families: Creating Family Justice Centers Across America.* Volcano, CA: Volcano Press; 2006:100-101.

3. Spears L. *Building Bridges Between Domestic Violence Organizations and Child Protective Services.* Harrisburg, PA: Natinal Center on Domestic Violence; 2000. National Online Resource Center on Violence Against Women Web site. http://www.vawnet.org/Assoc_Files_VAWnet/BCS7_cps.pdf. Accessed July 6, 2013.

4. Listenbee R, Torre J, Boyle G, et al. *Report of the Attorney General's Task Force on Children Exposed to Violence.* Washington, DC: United States Department of Justice; 2012. Department of Justice Web site. http://www.justice.gov/defendingchildhood/cev-rpt-full.pdf. Accessed July 8, 2013.

5. Durose MR, Harlow CW, Langan PA, Motivans M, Rantala RR, Smith EL. *Family Violence Statistics: Including Statistics on Strangers and Acquaintances.* Washington, DC: United States Department of Justice; 2005. NCJ 207846. Bureau of Justice Statistics Web site. http://www.bjs.gov/content/pub/pdf/fvs.pdf. Accessed August 19, 2011.

6. Gwinn C, Strack G. *Dream Big: A Simple, Complicated Idea to Stop Family Violence.* Tucson, AZ: Wheatmark Press; 2010.

7. Nampa Family Justice Center Web site. http://www.nampafamilyjusticecenter.org. Accessed Aug 6, 2013.

8. United States Department of Health and Human Services, Administration on Children, Youth and Families. *Child Maltreatment, 2007.* Washington, DC: United States Department of Health and Human Services, Administration on Children, Youth and Families; 2009. Cited by: Sousa C, Herrenkohl TI, Moylan CA, et al. Longitudinal studies on the effects of child abuse and children's exposure to domestic violence, parent-child attachments, and anti-social behaviors in adolescence. *J Interpers Violence.* 2011;26(1):111-136.

9. Appel AE, Holden GW. The co-occurrence of spouse and physical child abuse: a review and appraisal. *J Fam Psychol.* 1998;12:578-599. Cited by: Sousa C, Herrenkohl TI, Moylan CA, et al. Longitudinal studies on the effects of child abuse and children's exposure to domestic violence, parent-child attachments, and anti-social behaviors in adolescence. *J Interpers Violence.* 2011;26(1):111-136.

10. Edleson JL. The overlap between child maltreatment and woman battering. *Violence Against Women.* 1999;5:134-152.

11. Dykstra CH, Alsop RJ. *Domestic Violence and Child Abuse.* Englewood, CO: American Humane Association; 1996.

12. English D. Co-occurrence: child abuse and domestic violence. Paper presented at: 6th Forum on Federally Funded Research on Child Abuse and Neglect; March 25, 1998; Washington, DC.

13. Stark E, Flitcraft AH. Women and children at risk: a feminist perspective on child abuse. *Int J of Health Services.* 1988;18(1):97-118.

14. McKibben L, De Vos E, Newberger EH. Victimization of mothers of abused children: a controlled study. *Pediatrics.* 1989;84:531-535.

15. Tajima EA, Herrenkohl TI, Moylan CA, Derr AS. Moderating the effects of childhood exposure to intimate partner violence: the roles of parenting characteristics and adolescent peer support. *J Res Adolesc.* 2011;21(2):376-394.

16. McDonald R, Jouriles E, Ramisetty-Mikler S, Caetano R, Green CE. Estimating the number of American children living in partner-violent families. *J Fam Psychol.* 2006;20(1):137-142.

17. US Department of Justice. Intimate partner violence in the U.S., victim characteristics. Bureau of Justice Statistics Web site. http://www.bjs.gov/content/intimate/victims.cfm. Accessed August 19, 2011.

18. Finkelhor D, Turner H, Ormrod R, Hamby S. Violence, abuse, and crime exposure in a national sample of children and youth. *Pediatrics.* 2009;124(5):1-14.

19. Kerker BD, Horwitz SM, Leventhal JM, Plichta S, Leaf PJ. Domestic violence in the home; pediatric and parental reports. *Arch Pediatr Adolesc Med.* May 2000;154(5):457-462.

20. Ross SM. Risk of physical abuse to children of spouse-abusing parents. *Child Abuse Neglect.* 1996;20:589-598.

21. Finkelhor D, Turner H, Ormrod R, Hamby S, Kracke K. *Children's Exposure to Violence: A Comprehensive Survey.* Washington DC: United States Department of Justice; 2009. National Criminal Justice Reference Service Web site. https://www. ncjrs.gov/pdffiles1/ojjdp/227744.pdf. Accessed August 6, 2013.

22. Straus MA, Gelles RJ. *Physical Violence in American Families: Risk Factors and Adaptations to Violence in 8 145 Families.* New Brunswick, NJ: Transaction Publishers; 1990.

23. Walker LE. *The Battered Woman Syndrome.* New York, NY: Springer Publishing Company, Inc.: 1984.

24. Fantuzzo J, Boruch R, Beriama A, Atkins M, Marcus S. Domestic violence and children: prevalence and risk in five major US cities. *J Am Acad Child and Adolesc Psychiatry.* 1997;36(4):425-435.

25. Curie C. Animal cruelty by children exposed to domestic violence. *Child Abuse Negl.* 2006;30:427.

26. Sinclair D. *Understanding Wife Assault: A Training Manual For Counselors and Advocates.* Toronto, ON: Ontario Government Bookstore, Publications Services Section; 1985.

27. Kolbo JR. Risk and resilience among children exposed to family violence. *Violence Vict.* 1996;11:113-128.

28. Herrenkohl TI, Sousa C, Tajima EA, Herrenkohl RC, Moylan CA. Intersection of child abuse and children's exposure to domestic violence. *Trauma Violence Abuse.* 2008;9:84-89.

29. Pecora P, Whittaker J, Maluccio A, et al. *The Child Welfare Challenge; Policy, Practice, and Research.* Piscataway, NJ: Transaction Publishers; 2010.

30. Beeman SK, Hagermeister AK, Edleson JL. Child protection and battered women's services: from conflict to collaboration. *Child Maltreat.* 1999;4(2):116-126.

31. Wu CN. Introduction to Dependency Law, Chapter 1. In: Continuing Education of the Bar – California. *California Juvenile Dependency Practice 2010.* Oakland, CA: Continuing Education of the Bar – California; 2010; See also http://www. courts.ca.gov/documents/JournalVol5.pdf (Accessed July 6, 2013).

32. Wilson C. Presentation at: 8th Annual International Family Justice Center Conference; April 23, 2008; San Diego, CA. Recording available upon request to the Family Justice Center Alliance at info@nfjca.org.

33. Schene P. Past, present, and future roles of Child Protective Services. *Future Child.* 1998;8(1):23-38. http://futureofchildren.org/futureofchildren/publications/ docs/08_01_01.pdf. Accessed August 23, 2011.

34. Mason PT Jr. Child abuse and neglect part I: historical overview, legal matrix, and social perspectives. *North Carolina Law Rev.* 1971;50:293.

35. Jaffe P, Crooks C, Poisson S. Common misconceptions in addressing domestic violence in child custody disputes. *Juvenile and Family Court J.* 2003; 61.

36. Krout JA. *The Origins of Prohibition.* New York, NY: Knopf; 1925.

37. Asbury H. *The Great Illusion: An Informal History of Prohibition.* New York: Doubleday, 1950.

38. Gusfield JR. *Symbolic Crusade: Status Politics and the American Temperance Movement.* Urbana, IL: University of Illinois Press, 1963

39. Sack EJ. Battered women and the state: the struggle for the future of domestic violence policy. *Wis Law Rev.* 2004;35:1658.

40. Miccio G. House divided: mandatory arrest, domestic violence, and the conservatization of the battered women's movement. *Houston Law Rev.* 2005;42(237):248.

41. Schecter S. *Women and Male Violence: The Visions and Struggles of the Battered Women's Movement.* Cambridge, MA: South End Press; 1982.

42. Pleck E. *Domestic Tyranny: The Making of Social Policy Against Family Violence From Colonial Times to the Present.* Champaign, IL: University of Illinois Press; 1987:3-13.

43. *State v. Rhodes*, 51 NC 453 (1886).

44. Pence E, Shepard M. *Coordinating Community Responses to Domestic Violence: Lessons From Duluth and Beyond.* Thousand Oaks, CA: Sage Publications; 1999:2-6.

45. Dobashand RE, Dobash RP. *Women, Violence, and Social Change.* New York, NY: Routledge Kegan Paul; 1992. Cited by: Pence E, Shepard M. *Coordinating Community Responses to Domestic Violence: Lessons from Duluth and Beyond.* Thousand Oaks, CA: Sage Publications; 1999:6.

46. *State v. Oliver*, 70 NC 44 (1874).

47. *State v. Rhodes*, 61 NC 453, 459 (Phil. Law 1868).

48. Martin D. *Battered Wives.* Volcano, CA: Volcano Press; 1976.

49. *Thurman v. City of Torrington*, 595 F. Supp. 1521 (DC Conn. 1984).

50. Zorza J. The criminal law of misdemeanor domestic violence, 1970-1990. *J Crim Law Criminol.* 1992-1993;83:46-72.

51. Interstate Stalking, 18 USC, Section 2261A.

52. Interstate Travel to Commit Domestic Violence, 18 USC, Section 2261.

53. Interstate Violation of a Protection Order, 18 USC, Section 2262.

54. Full Faith and Credit, 18 USC, Section 2265, 2266.

55. Full Faith and Credit for Child Support Orders Act 28 USC, Section 1738B.

56. Civil Rights, 42 USC, Section 13981, 2000.

57. *Nicholson v. Williams*, 203 F. Supp. 2d 153,199 (EDNY 2002)

58. *Nicholson v. Scoppetta*, 820 NE2d 840, 844–55 (NY 2004).

59. National Children's Alliance. Standards for accredited members. National Children's Alliance Web site. http://www.nationalchildrensalliance.org/index.php?s=76. Accessed May 21, 2013.

60. National Family Justice Center Alliance Web site. www.familyjusticecenter.org. Accessed May 21, 2013.

61. Davies J. *Advocacy Beyond Leaving: Helping Battered Women in Contact With Current or Former Partners.* San Francisco, CA: Family Violence Prevention Fund; 2009. http://www.futureswithoutviolence.org/userfiles/file/Children_and_Families/Advocates%20Guide(1).pdf. Accessed July 7, 2013.

62. Haight WL, Shim WS, Linn LM, Swinford L. Mothers' strategies for protecting children from batterers; the perspectives of battered women involved in child protective services. *Child Welfare.* 2007;86(4):41-62.

63. Holt S, Buckley H, Whelan S. The impact of exposure to domestic violence on children and young people: a review of the literature. *Child Abuse Negl.* 2008;32:797-810.

64. Edleson JL. Problems associated with children's witnessing domestic violence. VAWnet. www.vaw.umn.edu. Published 1997. Accessed August 4, 2011.

65. O'Keefe M. Predictors of child abuse in martially violent families. *J Interpers Violence.* 1995;10:3-25.

66. In Re Heather A., 52 Cal. App. 4th 183 (1996).

67. In harm's way: Domestic violence and child maltreatment. Adoption.com Web site. http://library.adoption.com/articles/in-harms-way-domestic-violence-and-child-maltreatment.html. Accessed August 12, 2011.

68. Peled E. *The Experience of Living with Violence for Preadolescent Witnesses of Woman Abuse* [PhD dissertation]. Minneapolis, MN: University of Minnesota; 1993.

69. Gondolf EW. The impact of mandatory court review on batterer program compliance: an evaluation of the Pittsburgh Municipal Courts and Domestic Abuse Counseling Center (DACC). MINCAVA Electronic Clearinghouse Web site. www.mincava.umn.edu. Published 1998. Accessed August 4, 2011.

70. Smith BE, Davis RC. An evaluation of efforts to implement no-drop policies: two central values conflict. NCJ 199719. https://www.ncjrs.gov/pdffiles1/nij/199719.pdf. Published 2004. Accessed August 19, 2011.

71. Aron LY, Olson, KK. *Efforts By Child Welfare Agencies To Address Domestic Violence: The Experiences Of Five Communities.* Washington, DC: United States Department of Justice; 1997.

72. Domestic violence: national curriculum for child protection services excerpts. Sociology Center Web site. http://thesociologycenter.com/GeneralBibliography/EndAbuseOrg.pdf. Accessed August 19, 2011.

73. Carter J, Schechter S. *Child Abuse and Domestic Violence: Creating Community Partnerships for Safe Families.* San Francisco: Family Violence Prevention Fund; 1997.

74. Campbell J, Webster D, Glass N. The danger assessment: validation of a lethality risk assessment instrument for intimate partner femicide. *J Interpers Violence.* 2009;24:4653-4674.

75. Davies J, Lyon EJ, Monti-Catania D. *Safety Planning with Battered Women: Complex Lives/Difficult Choices*. Thousand Oaks, CA: SAGE publications; 1998.

76. Domestic violence and child safety planning. New york State Office for the Prevention of Domestic Violence Web site. http://www.opdv.state.ny.us/professionals/childwelfare/dvchild_safetyplan.html. Accessed August 20, 2011.

77. Safety tips for you and your family. American Bar Association Web site. http://apps.americanbar.org/abanet/common/print/printview.cfm?Ref=http://apps.americanbar.org/tips/publicservice/safetipseng.html. Accessed August 21, 2011.

78. Rosewater A, Moore K. Addressing domestic violence, child safety and well-being: collaborative strategies for California families, 2010: recommendations from the California Leadership Group on Domestic Violence and Child Well-being. California Partnership to End Domestic Violence Web site. http://www.cpedv.org/Calendar%20Documents/DV%20Report. Published 2010. Accessed August 21, 2011.

79. Zisser A, Eyberg SM. Treating oppositional behavior in children using parent-child interaction therapy. In: Kazdin AE, Weisz Jr, eds. *Evidence-Based Psychotherapies for Children and Adolescents*. 2nd ed. New York, NY: Guilford; 2010:179-193.

80. Campbell JC, Webster D, Koziol-McLain J, et al. Assessing risk factors for intimate partner homicide. *Nat Inst Justice J*. 2003;250:14-19.

81. Cross T, Jones L, Walsh W, et al. Evaluating children's advocacy centers' response to child sexual abuse. Washington, DC: United States Department of Justice; 2009. National Criminal Justice Reference Service Web site. https://www.ncjrs.gov/pdffiles1/ojjdp/218530.pdf. Accessed August 24, 2011.

82. Carter J. Addressing domestic violence: the vision of the community partnerships. *Safekeeping*. 1998;3(1):1-5.

83. The Greenbook National Evaluation Team. *The Greenbook Initiative Final Evaluation Report*. Fairfax, VA: Greenbook National Evaluation Team; 2008. Office of the Assistant Secretary for Planning and Evaluation Web site. http://aspe.hhs.gov/hsp/08/sr/greenbook/report.pdf. Accessed August 24, 2011.

84. The President's Family Justice Center Initiative best practices. United States Department of Justice Web site. http://www.justice.gov/archive/ovw/docs/family_justice_center_overview_12_07.pdf.Accessed August 19, 2011.

Chapter 10

SAFETY PLANNING

Kathy Bell, MS, RN

KEY POINTS

1. Safety planning is intended to reassure and instill confidence in victims of intimate partner violence (IPV), not to frighten or discourage. Whether or not IPV victims decide to stay with their abusive partners, safety planning should provide enough information to keep them safe.

2. Safety planning can be done by anyone, but someone knowledgeable about domestic violence and safety issues will be best equipped to assist a victim in creating a safety plan. The role of health care professionals in particular can be of vital importance.

3. A danger or risk assessment is a good way to begin the process of safety planning as it establishes the level of risk the victim is in.

4. A health care professional should not be shy in asking about IPV. A good knowledge of local community services for victims of IPV can help a clinician give the best possible advice to patients.

5. It is important to take other factors, such as children or pets, into account when developing a safety plan. It is important to be aware of advances in technology that may make it easier for perpetrators to find out where their victims are.

6. Most important for many victims is that they feel supported and safe when talking to a health care provider about safety planning and IPV.

INTRODUCTION

Case Study 10-1-a.

Heidi is a 22-year-old female who is 28 weeks pregnant. She states that she and A. were walking to a friend's house when they argued, and he began to punch and kick her numerous times, including in the stomach. He pulled out a gun and began holding it to her back as they walked. Then he shoved her into a puddle and began to choke her. His anger escalated and he began to "pistol whip" her on the right side of her face. He dragged her back to his home where he pulled her clothes off and raped her. Upon examination, it is found that both of her eyes are swollen with the left one almost completely shut. The very outer edge of the sclera is deep blood red. Inspection of her mouth reveals distinct lacerations and abrasions to the inside lower lip. Both arms have abrasions and contusions. She has tenderness on the left side of her lower abdomen. Fetal heart tones are present. She has contusions along the outside edge and back of both legs.

A person in a violent relationship without a safety plan is in an extremely vulnerable position. Imagine what this person might be feeling immediately after such a violent attack. What are her most immediate needs? Health care providers do an excellent job of treating injuries and putting plans in place for follow-up care of injuries, but what about safety plans? How might clinicians prevent another episode of violence? What if health care providers could lessen the injuries associated with the next episode of violence? What if they could prevent a child from witnessing violence between their parents and the associated consequences of that? Or prevent a child from being injured in a violent event?

Case Study 10-1-b.

Heidi also stated that she has been in this relationship for over 8 months and that the frequency of the abuse has become more frequent. Heidi stated that A. has made threats to not only kill himself but to kill her and her family. She lives with her mother and 2-year-old son. A. is not the father of the 2 year old. He has made the comment to Heidi that he is not afraid to use the gun and he will bury her deep. A. is unemployed and abuses alcohol and drugs, such as crack cocaine and marijuana. The police are looking for A. but have not yet found him. Heidi also has a history of self-injury. She has a danger assessment score of 30 and rated each re-assault question at a 9, both indicating extreme danger and high risk for re-assault.

(How the danger assessment score and re-assault questions scores are derived will be discussed later in the chapter)

How would the plan of care change based on this additional information? Working with people who have experienced violence offers a tremendous opportunity to make a difference in their lives and the lives of their children. One goal of safety planning is to promote optimal change, and this may or may not involve leaving the partner. In order to do this, one has to understand that change is a process, not an event. Optimal change may be very different from one person to another. Safety is the main focus. One also needs to know that change may come at a great expense, not only in the relationship with their partner, but also with family and friends.

The intent of a safety plan is not to convince someone to leave their partner, but rather for them to be safe in whatever decision they have made at that moment regarding staying or leaving. People assisting a patient with safety planning need to understand that they are not dealing with a simple task but rather helping a complex person who may have children, injuries from physical abuse, grief over the loss of a relationship, emotional trauma, guilt, sadness, and shame.[1]

These plans are not put into place to scare or frighten but to calm and give confidence that the victim will know what to do in the future. There is no "one size fits all" in safety planning. Each person's plan needs to be unique to their circumstances and ability to abide by the plan. Once a safety plan is developed, it needs to be reviewed regularly so the person maintains a familiarity with it and changes it as the situation changes.

Safety in a battering environment must be based on the self-protective capability of the victim.[2] The development of a safety plan and knowledge of important matters to be considered when discussing a plan for the individual's future well-being is important at every health care encounter, not just when they come in for abuse-related complaints.

WHAT IS SAFETY?

Hermann[2] states that recovery from a traumatic event occurs in 3 stages, with the first stage being safety. The meaning of *safety* may be very different from one person to another. For one person it might mean not getting hit and belittled on a daily basis, for another it might be sleeping soundly at night, and for yet another it might involve no more intrusive thoughts about harming oneself.

In her classic work, *Trauma and Recovery*, Hermann defines personal safety and environmental safety as they pertain to individuals that have experienced a traumatic event.[2] Helping a person obtain personal safety includes not only discussing locations safe from the abuser but a safe atmosphere within which the victim can regain control, begin to heal, and move on with his or her life. Hermann suggests a patient will be far less frightened by being prepared for symptoms of hyperarousal, intrusion, and numbing. She recommends that information on adaptive coping strategies be discussed. Self-medicating with drugs or alcohol, risk-taking behaviors, and seclusion are common in trauma survivors. These actions have helped the individual get through the trauma, but they are unhealthy, and assistance in finding more positive coping methods may promote better health and safety. Maintaining a non-judgmental approach is likely to be key in keeping survivors engaged as they work through these issues.

Post-traumatic stress disorder (PTSD) can develop in anyone who experiences trauma. Johnson states that recent research suggests that PTSD symptoms in intimate partner violence (IPV) victims are associated with increased risk of re-abuse.[3] Not everyone who experiences a traumatic event will experience PTSD, and not everyone with PTSD directly experienced one specific traumatic event. Symptoms of PTSD are typically classified into 3 categories. Re-experiencing symptoms may manifest when certain words, objects, or situations occur that remind a patient of the traumatic event. Avoidance symptoms cause a patient to change their personal routine. Hyperarousal symptoms are usually constant rather than triggered by something else and include things like feeling on edge, being easily startled, and having difficulty with sleeping.[4] It is not unusual for people who have experienced a traumatic event to have some of these symptoms. These symptoms may last for a few weeks, but when they last for more than that and when they become an ongoing problem, they need to be addressed by a professional. A patient will be well served during the safety planning process by discussions on self-care of their body, such as sleep, healthy diet, and exercise. A clinician should explore options with them for what to do when intrusive thoughts about the event creep into their awareness, what to do if nightmares occur, or what to do if some reminder of the event sets off physical symptoms such as pounding heartbeat or rapid breathing. Warnings about self-destructive behavior are important to address. Some of the harmful behaviors could be diverted by identifying healthy social support systems as another component of safety planning. Family, friends, or self-help support groups may be included in the list of options. Hermann recommends that a careful review of the important relationships take place, assessing each as a potential source of protection, emotional support, or practical help as well as a potential source of danger.

How a person is coping with a situation can impact the safety planning process. Coping is an ongoing dynamic process.[5] Nurius, Macy, Nwabuzar, and Holt explains that understanding a person's perception of vulnerability, as it relates to his or her partner, impacts how he or she will cope with a situation. Vulnerability may be expressed as feeling trapped, loss of power and control, or physical and psychological danger.[5] In general, the higher the severity of violence resulting in injury, the more involved in safety planning a person likely will be.[5] Many studies show who women that have experienced violence are more apt to seek services for chronic health issues, such as chronic pain, gynecological and reproductive problems, sleep disorders, and gastrointestinal disorders, than women who have not experienced violence. Assessment of an individual's unique circumstances, such as degree of violence, feelings of vulnerability and depression, and socialization, can all help guide the development of a safety plan.

WHAT IS A SAFETY PLAN?

Davies[6] describes *safety planning* as an individualized plan to reduce the risks women and their children face. A description given by Campbell[17] is that safety planning is an opportunity for an abused person to gain information in order to strategize her responses. Warrant officers would not go into what is known to be an unsafe environment without first strategizing their approach and responses. A cardiovascular surgeon cannot perform a potentially lethal procedure without knowing their resources. The knowledge and plans that the warrant officer and the cardiovascular surgeon use do not occur to them out of the blue one day. They spent time learning about the situation, looking at the experience of others, trying out different approaches, and reaching out to others to be able to develop the best plan to be safe. Victims of violence should have the same opportunities to develop tactics to stay safe. Assisting a person with putting a safety plan in place can ease some of the difficulties they are experiencing.

Many individuals do not seek help for the violence they are experiencing. A safety plan may be nothing more than planting a seed through assessing and inquiring about IPV in such a manner that shows that the clinician is safe and willing to discuss very difficult topics.

Developing a safety plan can be approached similarly to the strategic planning process that organizations use constantly to help guide them.[8] What is this person's vision? What do they have in the way of strengths, such as employment, family support, or spirituality? Weaknesses could include chemical or alcohol dependence, fear, and limited financial resources. What are the barriers? Examples of this often include embarrassment, wants the partner to change, or wants the relationship to be like it seemed in the beginning.

Another question to ask is what resources the victim has working for her. There are hard resources, such as transportation, education, skill, childcare, and finances, and soft resources, such as things as awareness of the community IPV services.

Effective Communication

Communication is key in safety planning discussions; however, even at its best, sometimes clear communication only causes confusion. Of the various communication models that exist, Betts[9] favors the Tubbs Communication Model because it involves just 2 people and crosses a variety of communication settings. Safety planning frequently involves just 2 people, with one person as the sender/receiver and the other as the receiver/sender. Messages are typically sent either verbally or nonverbally. Some are sent intentionally and others unintentionally. Betts provided the descriptions for each of these types of communication, as defined by Tubbs and Moss in *Human Communication: Principles and Contexts.*[10]

— *Verbal:* any type of spoken communication that uses one or more words

— *Intentional verbal:* conscious attempts we make to communicate with others through speech

— *Unintentional verbal:* the things people say without meaning to

— *Nonverbal:* all of the messages people transmit without words or over and above the words people use

— *Intentional nonverbal messages:* the nonverbal messages people want to transmit

— *Unintentional nonverbal messages:* the nonverbal aspects of human behavior transmitted without control

Development of some level of trust is a key component to effective communication about safety planning. Trust between nurses and patients are explored many times in the nursing literature. It is clear that trust has a major influence on patients' acceptance of care and treatment from health care professionals.[11] Trust in something, whether it be in oneself, the people around oneself, in the surrounding world, or in some phenomena or power, can empower a victim with the necessary strength needed to accomplish change.[12] A patient that feels accepted and noticed will be more likely to participate in developing a trusting relationship with the person performing the safety planning.

Gladwell, in his book *Blink*, gives example after example of how a situation or person is sized up in the blink of an eye.[13] That quick judgment may be right, or it may be wrong depending on factors such as stress, emotions, other interests, and attitudes. Given that there are many variables in the equation of developing a trusting relationship, how can a health care provider talk about safety planning with an individual who is experiencing a violent time in her life?

In face-to-face communication, individuals almost exclusively rely on the senses of hearing, sight, and touch.[10] Hearing is different than listening and is critical because it is the first element of the listening process.[10] Betts[9] states that the International Listening Association defines listening as "the process of receiving, constructing meaning from, and responding to spoken and/or nonverbal messages." Although controversial, Mehrabian stated in her book, *Silent Messages*,[14] that communication can be broken down into 3 elements. These elements are nonverbal, tone, and words. Some research indicates that tone of voice is more important than posture, and both of these are more important than the words that are used.[9]

In order for communication about safety to be useful, the conversation should be done where the victim is comfortable and safe. A private, calm, quiet area, free of noise and bright lights is ideal. Distractions should be minimized. If children are present, a safe place nearby, preferably where the mother can still see them, will allow the victim to better focus on the conversation.

WHO DOES SAFETY PLANNING?

Safety planning can be done by anyone, but someone knowledgeable in the dynamics of domestic violence and safety issues will be best equipped to assist a victim in developing a workable plan. Safety planning is often provided by victim advocacy agencies, and they are well-trained for this; however, many individuals do not access the advocacy system, and it is imperative that health care professionals acquire the knowledge and make the time to assist patients with safety planning. Ideally, health care would involve the local advocacy centers in safety planning, but much work remains to be done to accomplish that in every community.

THE ROLE OF HEALTH CARE PROFESSIONALS

Health care providers have a tremendous opportunity to make a difference in the lives of women and children affected by intimate partner violence. Most do not realize how important their role may be in saving lives affected by IPV. According to the femicide study, only 4% of the women killed accessed advocacy systems for services in the year prior to their killing;[15] however, 56% had been seen in the health care system for something during the previous year.[15]

Health care providers can be judgmental, hurried, and unaware of resources, all of which can make it virtually impossible for individuals experiencing abuse to access information in a health care setting. It is imperative that the system and the safety planning process not re-victimize the patient.

Some of these patients come in scared, wishing the professional could read their minds. They are often waiting for the health care provider to ask the one question that opens the door so they can tell what really happened to them or make the one statement that conveys concern and lets them know it is safe to talk to them. Others come in hoping that you do not ask or discover they are a victim of violence. They may have concerns about the stigma of violence in their relationships. All this combined makes effective communication about abuse difficult. Chang[16] provided empirical support about asking about IPV. She concluded that victims of violence want to be asked in an unaccompanied, safe, confidential setting. They want a nonjudgmental, kind, relaxed, and open manner from the professional.[16] Common sense hints that time and good listening skills will elicit disclosure and discussion.

Health care providers often do not understand the victim's reluctance to leave her abuser. In a 2003 project , Hendy et al[17] descibed fear of loneliness, childcare needs, financial problems, social embarrassment, poor social support, fear of harm, and hope that things will change as some of the factors a victim has to address before making the decision to stay or leave. Sometimes the change that a person would have to make, given these hurdles, is more than they can bear. Not only do victims have these internal fears and problems, but their abusers are often manipulating them. Daniel Sheridan's HARASS instrument[18] describes many partner behaviors that can cause varying degrees of distress and affect a victim's decision about leaving or staying. Whether she leaves or stays can result in the same outcomes. She could be killed in either case; her children could be harmed; her credibilty could be damaged; she could lose her job, friends, or family; and there could be an emotional impact. The goal of safety planning is to maximize her well-being in whatever she decides. Health care providers need to understand that the changes a victim has to make in order to be in a safer environment, emotional state, or relationship is often a slow process with many ups and downs.[19] The focus of the conversations should be on the woman. She cannot change the perpetrator's behavior, but she can take steps that will reduce risk and exposure to the perpetrators behavior and actions.

The Change Model described by Chang et al states that most people move through predictable stages as they start to change behavior. During the *precontemplation stage*, they may not recognize or feel a need to change. The *contemplation phase* is when the individual realizes that change is needed. The *preparation stage* is when plans are made to actually change. This stage is followed by *maintenance*, when efforts are made to reinforce and sustain the desired behavior. According to Chang these stages are not necessarily linear and patients may move backwards into a previous stage. They may cycle through the stages multiple times before achieving sustained change.[19] It is important for the health care provider to be aware of the change process in order to have some understanding where the patient is on the Change Model, so that the activites taken will have a better chance of surviving. Actions such as listening for readiness for change, providing information to raise awareness, identifying support persons, and engaging in activities that support self-efficacy and promote empowerment can be employed by health care providers.[8] Readiness for change can be discerned to some extent in discussing challenges and barriers. Health care providers should make sure they have access to resources and information to help victims of IPV, as this can be an important component of readiness for change. These resources can give patients valuable options and support for any changes they make.

HOW ARE SAFETY PLANS FORMED?

Assessment of risk and danger that the person is currently experiencing gives a starting point for development of the safety plan. There are a lot of different danger and risk assessments that can be done in domestic violence cases. One of the most important assessments is how the individual perceives her circumstances. Danger and risk assessment is a fairly young concept so it is still developing. Although criteria varies from one author to another, some of the most common risks for harm from homicide in the domestic violence context include:[20]

— Abuser's access to firearms

— Use of weapons in prior abusive incidents

— Threats with weapons

— Drug and alcohol abuse

— Forced sex

— Possessiveness/extreme jealousy/extreme dominance

— Threats of suicide

There are risks for clinicians in performing risk assessments too. What happens if a clinician over-predicts the danger? If done consistently, the risk assessment tools could lose effectiveness. A misleading result could scare someone senseless without good cause. But what happens if a clinician under-predicts the danger? Someone could be killed. Knowledge and experience in working with the assessments is necessary to limit each of these extremes. By doing a thorough job with risk assessment and safety planning, clinicians can assist in saving lives.

DANGER ASSESSMENT

It can be difficult to predict human behavior. How do we know when a particular situation will become lethal? It has been suggested that a validated risk assessment performed by a skilled clinician combined with a woman's self-perception of her danger will give some guidance.[20] The Danger Assessment developed by Dr. Jacquelyn Campbell was specifically designed for the health care setting. The Danger Assessment is designed to assess a victim's awareness of safety planning and service provision for those experiencing IPV. It is a 20-question assessment that can be administered by a health care professional or an IPV advocate and is scored between -3 and 37. It assesses for increased, severe, or extreme danger; incorporates a calendar; and is performed in conjunction with an interview of the victim. The Danger Assessment gives the victims a sense of validation that what they are experiencing is really happening, and it is dangerous. This is where assessment and associated safety planning provides the tremendous opportunity to make a difference in the lives of those suffering from IPV and in the lives of their children.

A victim's perception of re-assault is also a good predictor and, when combined with danger assessment, provides better information for safety planning.[20] Re-assault can be assessed by asking the patient to answer 2 questions, using a scale of 1-10 (see **Table 10-1**).

Table 10-1. Re-Assault Assessment
— What is the likelihood your partner will physically abuse you in the next year?
— What is the likelihood your partner will seriously hurt you in the next year?

STARTING THE CONVERSATION

Opening statements could include something similar to "I'd like to talk to you about ways of keeping you and your children safe."[21] Safety planning in varying degrees can be used in every encounter with patients. Victims of interpersonal violence are often open to change immediately after a crisis or episode of violence.[22] If the opportunity is missed or delayed, many victims will employ defense mechanisms such as minimization of the event, denial, or ambivalence.[23]

IDENTIFYING RESOURCES

Abused women use all kinds of methods to be safe, such as placating their abusers, seeking services from formal and informal institutions, and resisting or fighting back.[8] A health care provider should ask patients what methods they are using now. If a provider listened carefully while gathering information, he or she may already have some of this information. In order to be most effective, a patient needs to be an active participant. What are the threats that she perceives? A safety plan needs to be a plan that will work for a specific patient, not a generic plan. Another good question to ask is what current protective actions are being used. That question can then be followed up with discussing how these protective actions can be strengthened.

Case Study 10-2.

Samantha left her abusive relationship 3 weeks ago. Her husband spent a few days in jail after beating and strangling her to near unconsciousness. While he was in jail Samantha moved to another apartment. In an effort to keep her husband from knowing where she now lives, she put a variety of plans in place, including:

— Direct discussions with close family and friends not to disclose to anyone where she now lives, because of the danger she is in

— Closing accounts and opening others on utilities rather than just transferring the account

— Changing how her children were transported to school

— Registering for a confidential address program (an example of this can be viewed at the Oklahoma Confidentiality Address Program web site[24])

— Using a third party to exchange her children on the dates her husband is to have them

She attended a Family Safety Center for a follow-up. In a review of her current safety plan, the discussion moved to the above changes she has made in her routine. She has also changed:

— Where she shops for groceries

— Where she banks

— The park where her children play

— The time of the church service she regularly attends.

During this conversation it was discovered that on the fourth of each month, she goes to the pharmacy and picks up a refill prescription for one of her children. Based on this review of the plan, she then changed the pharmacy location and eliminated one more possible way for the abuser to find her.

IDENTIFYING READINESS FOR CHANGE

A woman's perception of her abilities to increase safety will affect her willingness to attempt those behaviors.[25] Does she want to live with the abuser, live separately from the abuser, or is she planning to leave? Safety planning will be approached differently in each of these situations. If she is planning to leave she should not have any contact with the abuser about it. Some women feel that they owe the abuser and should tell him face-to-face. Leaving is an especially dangerous period. A note or phone call later will suffice.

It became apparent in a study by Cluss et al[25] that a woman who are living with abuser soften take actions that decrease their exposure to the abuse but are not aimed at leaving. In this study, women hid money or set up their own bank accounts associated with working from their home. This provided them with a sense of safety because it gave them some options while they were still living with the abuser. It is well known that many women attempt to leave relationships many times before they succeed. This becomes very frustrating to family, friends, co-workers, and health care professionals. How this is framed can eliminate some of the frustration. Instead of blaming and stigmatizing the individual because she goes back to her abuser, it is important to remember that we get better at something by practicing it, sometimes over and over and over again. A victims in a violent relationship needs to be coached and supported through safety planning rather than chastised for the predicament she is in at the moment.

Basic Safety Behaviors

General basic safety behaviors often include things like:

— Hiding money

— Hiding an extra set of house and car keys

— Establishing a code word for danger with family and friends. This word is an alert that help is needed. The receiver knows to leave and get help. It is especially important that kids know how to respond to these code words. Children often want to help but are liable to get hurt if they come to the rescue. They must be taught that getting outside help is best. Safety words are useful in a range of situations and should be established in all families as a safety measure.

— Asking a neighbor to call police if violence begins

— Removing weapons

— Hiding a bag with extra clothing

They need to have available:

— Social security numbers (her own, her abuser's, and those of any children)

— Rent and utility receipts

— Birth certificates (her own and the children's)

— Driver's License (her own and the children's)

— Bank account numbers

— Insurance policies and numbers

— Marriage license

— Valuable jewelry

— Important phone numbers

— Copy of protection order (if applicable)

The National Center for Victims of Crime has developed safety plan guidelines that outline considerations in different stages and scenarios within a relationship. These have been included at the end of the chapter with their permission.

Be Prepared

This girl scout and boy scout motto will serve healthcare providers well. A person tends to shy away from doing things they are not familiar with or do not know how to do. One way to be prepared for the needs of patients when safety planning is to know what resources there are in one's community for victims of intimate partner violence and have information on those resources readily available. A sample listing of some of these resources can be found at the end of this chapter. Contact with social services or local advocacy centers may show they already have a similar document prepared that they would be willing to share.

SPECIAL CONSIDERATIONS

CHILDREN

Millions of children are exposed to IPV each year.[26] In a single day in 2008, 16 458 children were living in a domestic violence shelter or transitional housing facility, and another 6 430 children sought services at a non-residential program.[27]

What the mother thinks her child is aware of is sometimes very different than what the child actually knows.[21] Most often the child knows a lot more about what is going on around them than the mother realizes.[28] Exposure to violence against a mother is included on the list of adverse childhood experiences that can have an effect on a person decades later.[29] A child exposed to abuse at an early stage in life may lead to re-victimization, perpetration of a cycle of violence as well as a wide array of diseases, social problems, and untimely deaths.[29] Differences in children's responses to violence have been attributed to protective factors that include well-developed interpersonal skills, intelligence, special talents, social support, and supportive nurturing adults.[26]

In many cases, the best way to protect a child is to protect the mother.[28] Including information specific to their children is part of safety planning for women with children. For some mothers, discussions about their children's safety are very scary and they fear that Child Protective Services will be contacted and their children will be taken away. Feder et al[30] stated that studies have shown that proximity to the caregiver is an important modulator of a child's sense of safety when facing trauma.

An individual's genetic make-up and particular history of environmental stressors determine the degree of adaptability of neurochemical stress response systems.[30] Genetics research into resiliency is an area of focused study that is getting a lot of attention at this time. Much is being learned about how hormonal, neurotransmitter function and neuropeptides affect stress. An individual's gene interaction with the environment and how that shapes the neural circuitry and neurochemical function that end up being expressed in behaviors is another area being studied.[30] Until more understanding of these factors is established and applied in the day-to-day care of children, safety planning is one way to promote protective factors that will enhance resiliency.

Children can be assessed for development of the appropriate type and amount that they can tolerate and retain. Depending on their stage of development, discussions with children about safety could include questions such as:

— What would you do if you came home from school and your front door was already open or unlocked?

— What is a safe way for you to answer the phone when your parent is not home or is not available?

— What is a safe way for you to get out of your home in an emergency?

— What would you do if a stranger or someone you do not know tries to talk to you?

— Tell me about an unsafe situation.

— What would you do for help in this situation?

— What is a safe place?

— Who can you talk to when you feel worried or scared?

— In an emergency, who can you call for help?

— If you call 911, what do you tell them?

— Do you have a code word with your parent?

— How do you know when violence is about to happen?

— The last time there was a fight or your mom got hurt, what did you do?

— If this happens again, what can you do to be safe?

— If you need to hide, where are some safe places?

There are some important messages that a child needs to hear in regards to safety planning.

— Do not get in the middle of a fight.

— It is not your fault.

— Know how to call 911.

— Talk to someone safe when you are feeling unsafe.

— Go to a safe place if home is not safe. (The route to this location should be discussed with the clinician. For example, many communities designate the fire station as a safe place; however, if the child has to cross a busy street to get to it, it is not a safe option.)

— It is not unusual or bad for you to have feelings of love toward your abusive parent.

Case Study 10-3.

Juanita is a 35-year-old woman who came to the Family Justice Center after having been struck in the face by her husband. They have been married 14 years and the violence has been occurring since the beginning of the relationship. Recently he has strangled her twice and that has never happened in the past. Juanita is also concerned about some of the behaviors she is seeing in her 13-year-old son. He is becoming aggressive toward his father and overly protective of her. She came in today for medical treatment, and she has some questions. She does not want to involve the police and does not authorize the release of medical records. She tells the nurse that she is planning on leaving the relationship but cannot do it yet because it is not safe for her as long as her husband is around. She already has been working on a plan that she intends to put into place when her husband goes to visit relatives in another state. That event is set to happen 6 weeks from now. Her plan is to go to another state where she has made arrangements to initially live with an old high school girlfriend that he doesn't know of. Her 13-year-old son will be going with her, and he does not yet know of the plan. She is going to file a complaint with the police the day that he leaves the state, and at that time, authorize the release of information contained in her medical record as well as the photographs, all of which were memorialized the day she went to the Family Justice Center.

The Older Patient

Case Study 10-4.

June B, a 76-year old woman, reports that last night, her 28-year-old granddaughter pushed into her house, knocking her to the floor. She went to the kitchen where she knew that her grandmother kept her medications. They had just been refilled, but because they had been stolen before ,June had put them in a different location in the house. When her granddaughter could not find them she grabbed June and shook her, leaving bruises on her arms. The earlier fall left abrasions on June's legs. June told her granddaughter where the medications were, and she left with them. June is frail and has a poor gait. She has a standing prescription for Lortab 15/500 due to degenerative hip issues. She also takes Celexa and Wellbutrin for depression and Temazepam for sleep. A similar event has happened 5 times prior to this. June has obtained EPOs in the past but has never continued with them past the emergency period.

Abuse of the elderly is often domestic abuse [21] but also occurs in the context of other familial relationships. The elderly patient may not report abuse for fear of losing some of their autonomy. For this reason and many others, such as fear of retaliation, fear of loneliness, and fear of embarrassment, the elderly may recant the initial histories.

When working with older victims, it is important to ascertain if they know how to use a cellphone and if they are comfortable using one. It cannot be assumed that they are or are not familiar with today's technology. It is necessary to ask, and sometimes, it may be necessary to help them learn the new technology. Paying close attention to any disabilities that they might have that may impede communication is important. Making sure that they can hear and see, that they are not too cold, and that they are able to communicate will help facilitate a conversation about safety planning.

Pets

Some people will not leave their pets at any cost. In many homes where animal abuse occurs, research indicates that child maltreatment or domestic violence may also be present.[31] When a victim is worried about pets in an abusive home, the pets can be incorporated into the safety plan by taking the following actions:

— Develop an emergency plan for sheltering the pets.

— Establish ownership of the pets (obtain an animal license, proof of vaccinations or veterinary receipts in victim's name to help prove they own the pets).

— Collect vaccination and medical records, collar and identification, medication, bowls, bedding, etc.

— Ask for assistance from law enforcement or animal care and control officers to reclaim the pets if left behind.

Stalking and Technology

The National Center for Victims of Crime have a Stalking Resource Center with a plethora of information related to the issues of stalking. There one will find publications, videos and educational materials to use in your work with victims in which stalking is a part of the crime. An extensive Safety Plan can be accessed at the National Center for Victims of Crime web site.[32] Some of the suggestions within that plan include:

— Journal events of abuse.

— Keep emails, text messages, etc. that detail the abuse.

— Identify witnesses.

— Make trusted family and friends aware.

— If being followed, do not go to an isolated location. Go to a public place, preferably a law enforcement agency or specific location designated as a safe place. Call 911.

Technology is such an integral part of everyday life that most individuals may not be thinking about how this technology can make them vulnerable as they move about in their day-to-day activities. Cell phones now have GPS components that can be used to track individuals, putting them into a vulnerable, potentially dangerous situation. However, this same technology can be applied to enhance safety and privacy. When safety planning discussions are held, use of phones and computers should be included. There is a myriad of resources available that discuss the issues surrounding technology and intimate partner violence. Some basic concepts to be communicated during the safety planning process include:

— Cordless, wireless, and mobile phones do not provide the same level of confidentiality as a corded phone.

— There are a variety of phone services available that can be accessed to provide some level of confidentiality and privacy.

— Email is not confidential. Passwords and login names the abuser could not guess are recommended.

— Use a "safe" computer.[33]

Some resources on stalking and technology are included here:

National Network to End Domestic Violence.
http://nnedv.org/resources/safetynetdocs/93-technology-safety-planning-with-survivors.html

National Center for Victims of Crime
Stalking Resource Center
http://www.ncvc.org/src/main.aspx?dbID=DB_Safety_Plan_GuideLines333

Minnesota Center on Violence and Abuse
http://www.mincava.umn.edu/documents/commissioned/stalkingandtech/stalkingandtech.html

National Sexual Violence Resource Center
http://www.nsvrc.org/projects/internet-safety-online-resource-collection

POSITIVE MESSAGES

No matter what the unique variables are for each person a health care provider assists with safety planning, and there are some common, clear messages that can and need to be conveyed. Often, the victim needs to hear phrases such as "I'm sorry this happened to you." and "You are always welcome here, no matter what your situation is." However, if a clinician is honestly scared for the victim and her children, he or she should make that known to the patient. Health care providers should advise their patients to trust their instincts.

Many individuals that have experienced violence have been put into the situation of questioning their own instincts due to the offender telling them how worthless, crazy, and stupid they are. Other individuals have been raised from the time of their childhood not to make waves, not to cause a commotion, or not to embarrass themselves or others. They have learned not to listen to those subtle inner thoughts and instincts that are tell them something is wrong, or they need to be more aware, or that they need to react. Any one of these situations can put a person in a compromised position. Learning to trust one's decisions and instincts again is an activity well worth the time and effort.

Safety planning may involve nothing more than planting a seed that there is hope and that there are resources available to anyone experiencing violence in their lives. Just asking about IPV and opening the door to the possibility gives a person knowledge that this is a safe and open place to discuss violence if it is happening or if it ever happens in the future. An individual may not feel comfortable enough at that first encounter to disclose abuse, but the seed has been planted.

There is no one recipe for safety planning. Every individual is different, their resources are different, and their needs are different. By taking the time to individualize their strategies for safety, workable plans can be developed.

It is important to never give up on patients in violent relationships. They may suddenly develop the courage to disclose or ask for help. Patients will be better served if health care professionals have a plan for developing a safety plan and are prepared to deal with the situation when it arises.

Case Study 10-5.

Marcy is a 28-year-old who came to the emergency department with the complaint of abdominal pain. All through the visit her husband hovered around her. Having noticed the husband's behavior, when they were separated the nurse took the opportunity to ask Marcy about domestic abuse. Marcy denied it. Shortly afterwards the husband was again at her side. The medical treatment options for the abdominal complaints were addressed. The subject of abuse never came up again. The nurse provided Marcy with discharge instructions and had her sign the form. Much to the nurse's amazement, instead of signing her name, Marcy had written "Help Me."

APPENDIX 10-1

Appendix 10-1. Domestic Violence Safety Plan Guidelines

One of the most important things you can do when developing your safety plan is to talk to a victim advocate who can help you fully consider safety issues, understand your legal rights, and identify community resources (eg, shelters, sources of financial assistance, or food banks). You can locate a victim advocate through a local domestic violence agency, which provides services at no charge to victims. The National Crime Victim Helpline (1-800-FYI-CALL) can also help you prepare a safety plan and find victim assistance within your own community. The following safety suggestions have been compiled from safety plans distributed by state domestic violence coalitions from around the country. Following these suggestions is not a guarantee of safety, but could help improve your safety situation.

PERSONAL SAFETY WITH AN ABUSER

— Identify your partner's use and level of force so that you can assess danger to you and your children before it occurs.

— Try to avoid an abusive situation by leaving.

— Identify safe areas of the house where there are no weapons and where there are always ways to escape. If arguments occur, try to move to those areas.

— Don not run to where the children are as your partner may hurt them as well.

— If violence is unavoidable, make yourself a small target: dive into a corner and curl up into a ball with your face protected and your arms around either side of your head, fingers entwined.

— If possible, have a phone accessible at all times and know the numbers to call for help. Know where the nearest pay phone is located. Know your local battered women's shelter phone number. Don't be afraid to call the police.

— Let trusted friends and neighbors know of your situation, and develop a plan and visual signal for when you need help.

— Teach your children how to get help. Instruct them not to get involved in the violence between you and your partner. Plan a code word to signal that they should get help or leave the house.

— Tell your children that violence is never right, even when someone they love is being violent. Tell them that neither you nor they are at fault or cause the violence, and that when anyone is being violent, it is important to keep safe.

(continued)

Appendix 10-1. Domestic Violence Safety Plan Guidelines *(continued)*

— Practice how to get out safely. Practice with your children.

— Plan for what you will do if your children tell your partner of your plan or if your partner otherwise finds out about your plan.

— Keep weapons like guns and knives locked up and as inaccessible as possible.

— Make a habit of backing the car into the driveway and keeping it fueled. Keep the driver's door unlocked and the other doors locked for a quick escape.

— Try not to wear scarves or long jewelry that could be used to strangle you.

— Create several plausible reasons for leaving the house at different times of the day or night.

— Call a domestic violence hotline periodically to assess your options and get a supportive, understanding ear.

Getting Ready To Leave

— Keep any evidence of physical abuse, such as photographs of bruises and torn clothing.

— Know where you can go to get help; tell someone what is happening to you.

— If you are injured, go to a doctor or an emergency room and report what happened to you. Ask that they document your injuries.

— Plan with your children and identify a safe place for them, such as a room with a lock or a friend's house where they can go for help. Reassure them that their job is to stay safe, not to protect you.

— Contact your local battered women's shelter and find out about laws and other resources available to you before you have to use them during a crisis.

— Keep a journal of all violent incidents, noting dates, events, and threats made.

— Acquire job skills as you can, such as learning to type or taking courses at a community college.

— Try to set money aside or ask friends or relatives to hold money for you.

— Store some belongings with a friend or relative. Leave clothing, medications, your social security card, a credit card (if possible), citizenship documents, children's school and medical records, children's toys, insurance information, copies of birth certificates, money, and other valued personal possessions with them.

The Day You Leave

— Leave when it is least expected, for example, during times of agreement and calm.

— Create a false trail. Call motels, real estate agencies, and schools in a town at least 6 hours away from where you plan to relocate. Ask questions that require a call back to your house in order to leave those phone numbers on record.

(continued)

Appendix 10-1. Domestic Violence Safety Plan Guidelines *(continued)*

GENERAL GUIDELINES FOR LEAVING AN ABUSIVE RELATIONSHIP

— Make a plan for how you will escape and where you will go.

— Plan for a quick escape.

— Put aside emergency cash as you can.

— Hide an extra set of car keys.

— Take with you important phone numbers (of friends, relatives, doctors, schools, etc.) as well as other important items, including:

  — Driver's license

  — Regularly needed medication

  — List of credit cards (account number and date of expiration) held by self or jointly, or the credit cards themselves if you have access to them

  — Pay stubs

  — Checkbooks and information about bank accounts and other assets.

IF TIME IS AVAILABLE, ALSO TAKE:

— Citizenship documents, such as your passport, or greencard

— Titles, deeds, and other property information, and tax returns

— Medical records

— Children's school records and immunization records

— Insurance information

— Copy of marriage license, birth certificates, will, and other legal documents

— Verification of social security numbers

— Welfare identification

— Valued pictures, jewelry, or personal possessions.

AFTER LEAVING THE ABUSIVE RELATIONSHIP

If you are getting a restraining order and the offender is leaving:

— Change your locks and phone number.

— Change your work hours and route taken to work.

— Change the route you take to transport children to school.

— Keep a certified copy of your restraining order with you at all times.

— Inform friends, neighbors, and employers that you have a restraining order in effect.

(continued)

Appendix 10-1. **Domestic Violence Safety Plan Guidelines** *(continued)*

— Give copies of the restraining order to employers, neighbors, and schools along with a picture of the offender.

— If available in your community, register with VINE Protective Order ™ (https://www. vineprotect.com) to be notified immediately when the order is served, when hearings will be held, and when any amendments to the order are filed. Ask your victim advocate or sheriff's office about this service.

— Call law enforcement to enforce the order.

— Carry a charged mobile phone preprogrammed to 911.

IF YOU LEAVE

— Consider renting a post office box for your mail.

— Be aware that addresses are listed on restraining orders and police reports.

— Be careful to whom you give your new address and phone number.

— Change your work hours if possible.

— Alert school authorities about the situation.

— Consider changing your children's schools.

— Reschedule any appointments that the offender is aware of when you leave.

— Use different stores and frequent different social spots.

— Alert neighbors and request that they call the police if they feel you may be in danger.

— Talk to trusted people about the violence.

— Replace wooden doors with steel or metal doors.

— Install security systems if possible.

— Install a lighting system that turns on when a person is coming close to the house.

— Tell people you work with about the situation and have your calls screened by one receptionist if possible.

— Tell people who take care of your children which individuals are allowed to pick up your children. Explain the situation to them and provide them with a copy of the restraining order.

Courtesy of the National Center for Victims of Crime.

APPENDIX 10-2

Appendix 10-2. IPV Community Resources

1. **Domestic Violence Shelter**

   Contact number:____

   After hour contact: ____

   How are patients transported to the shelter?:_________________

   Do they accept children?: __________________________________

   What arrangements are available for male victims?: ___________

2. **Child protective Services**

   Local contact number: _____________________________________

   State hotline number:______________________________________

   Shelter information: ______________________________________

3. **Adult Protective Services**

   Local contact number: _____________________________________

   State hotline number: _____________________________________

   Is there shelter available?: ________________________________

4. **Health Services**

   Medical Free or Sliding Scale

   Medical care clinic: _______________________________________

   Contact: ____

   Number: ____

   Hours of operation: ______________________________________

   Financial arrangement:_____________________________________

   Medical care clinic: _______________________________________

   Contact:____

   Number: ____

   Hours of operation: ______________________________________

   Financial arrangement:_____________________________________

   Medical care clinic: _______________________________________

   Contact number: ____

   Hours of operation: ______________________________________

   Financial arrangement:_____________________________________

   Pharmacy

   Pharmacy: ____

   Contact number:____

(continued)

<table>
<tr><td>Appendix 10-2. IPV Community Resources (continued)</td></tr>
</table>

Hours of operation: _______________________________________

Financial arrangement: ____________________________________

Pharmacy: ____

Contact number: ____

Hours of operation: _______________________________________

Financial arrangement: ____________________________________

5. **Law Enforcement (most common agencies in your community)**

Agency 1 name: ____

Dispatch number: ____

DV investigator: ____

Contact number: ____

Agency 2 name: ____

Dispatch number: ____

DV investigator: ____

Contact number: ____

Agency 3 name: ____

Dispatch number: ____

DV investigator: ____

Contact number: ____

6. **Counseling**

Agency: ____

Contact name: ____

Contact number: ____

Agency: ____

Contact name: ____

Contact number: ____

7. **Protective Order**

Where do they file?: ______________________________________

What do they need to bring to file?: ________________________

8. **Animal Shelter**

Contact number: ____

9. **Food Assistance**

Contact number: ____

Contact number: ____

10. **Child Care Assistance**

Contact number: ____

Appendix 10-3

1. It appears you are in danger now. I'd like to talk with you about your safety.

   a. Is there anything else you would like to tell me?

   b. DVIS/Call Rape has a shelter. Would you like to go to the shelter?   Yes   No

2. DVIS offers free counseling for you and your children. Walk-in crisis counseling is available without an appointment M-F 8:30am-5pm at 4300 S Harvard. The 24-hour crisis line is available 7 days a week at 918-7HELPME. (918-743-5763)

3. What are the plans for the night?

   a. Where will you be staying?

   b. Do you have a safe place to go/be right now?

   c. Who can you call for support?

   d. If you are going to stay in your home:

      i. Has it been secured?

      ii. Have you thought about the quickest way to get out of the house in an emergency?

      iii. Call 911 immediately if the person who harmed you returns.

4. If you have to leave your house quickly, is there a safe place you could go?

   a. Friend/Relative/Neighbor?

   b. Can you talk to that person and let them know that in case of an emergency you are considering going there?

5. Can you pack a bag and put it where you could get to it quickly if you need to leave because of your safety?

   a. Include important documents, medicine, money, etc.

   b. Leave it by the door, in the trunk of a car, or with a neighbor, friend or relative.

6. Are you planning to return to work in the next 48 hours?

   a. Can you let your supervisor, security staff, or co-workers know that you might be in danger?

   b. Walk with someone to and from parking lot/have someone screen calls/move office.

7. Did you know that you can apply for a protective order?

   a. Protective order paperwork can be done at the Family Safety Center, Monday-Friday at 9am, at 3010 S. Harvard.

   b. Advocates are there to provide additional safety planning and provide resources for you whether you want a protective order or not.

   c. If you receive a protective order, keep a copy on your person at all times and give copies to your supervisor at work, your children's school, and your landlord.

8. Is it okay if we get a safe telephone number to call and follow-up with you?

Adapted from Domestic Violence Intervention Services. 48-hour Safety Plan. Tulsa, OK.

REFERENCES

1. Lindhorst T, Nurius P, Macy RJ. Contextualized assessment with battered women: strategic safety planning to cope with multiple harms. *J Soc Work Educ.* 2007;41(2):331-352.

2. Herman JL. *Trauma and Recovery.* New York, NY: Harper Collins Publishers; 1992.

3. Johnson DM, Zlotnick C, Perez S. Cognitive behavioral treatment of PTSD in residents of battered women's shelters: results of a randomized clinical trial. *J Consult Clin Psychol.* 2011;79(4):542-551.

4. National Institute of Mental Health. Post-traumatic stress disorder. National Institute of Mental Health Web site. http://www.nimh.nih.gov/health/publications/post-traumatic-stress-disorder-ptsd/nimh_ptsd_booklet.pdf. Accessed January 11, 2012.

5. Nurius PS, Macy RJ, Nwabuzar I, Holt VL. Intimate partner survivors' help-seeking and protection efforts: a person-oriented analysis. *J Interpers Violence.* 2011;26(3):539-566.

6. Davies J. *Safety Planning.* Hartford, CT: Greater Hartford Legal Assistance; 1997. http://www.vawnet.org/Assoc_Files_VAWnet/SafetyPlanning.pdf. Accessed May 16, 2011.

7. Campbell JC. Safety Planning based on lethality assessment for partners of batterers in intervention programs. *J Aggression Maltreat Trauma.* 2001;5(2):129-143.

8. Lindhorst T, Nurius P, Macy RJ. Contextualized assessment with battered women: strategic safety planning to cope with multiple harms. *J Soc Work Educ.* 2007;41(2):331-352.

9. Betts K. Lost in translation: importance of effective communication in online education. *Online J Distance Learning Adm.* 2009;7(2). http://www.westga.edu/~distance/ojdla/summer122/betts122.html. Accessed May 24, 2011.

10. Tubbs SL, Moss S. *Human Communication: Principles and Contexts.* 10th ed. Boston, MA: McGraw-Hill Companies; 2006.

11. Belcher M. Graduate nurses' experiences of developing trust in the nurse-patient relationship. *Contemp Nurse.* 2009;31(2):142-152.

12. Erickson I, Nilsson K. Preconditions needed for establishing a trusting relationship during health counseling - an interview study. *J Clin Nurs.* 2008;17(17):2352-2359.

13. Gladwell M. *Blink.* New York, NY: Little, Brown and Company; 2005.

14. Mehrabian A. *Silent Messages.* Belmont, CA: Wadsworth; 1971.

15. Campbell JC, Sharps P, Sachs C, Yam M. Medical lethality assessment and safety planning in domestic violence cases. *Clin Fam Pract.* 2003;5(1):101-111.

16. Chang JC, Cluss PA, Ranieri L, et al. Health care interventions for intimate partner violence: what women want. *Womens Health Issues.* 2005;15:21-30.

17. Hendy HM, Eggen D, Gustitus C, McLeod KC, Ng P. Decision to leave scale: perceived reasons to stay in or leave violent relationships. *Psychol Women Q.* 2003;27(2):162-173.

18. Thompson MP, Basile KC, Hertz MF, Sitterle D. *Measuring Intimate Partner Violence Victimization and Perpetration: A Compendium of Assessment Scales.* Atlanta, GA: Centers for Disease Control and Prevention; 2006. Centers for Disease Control and Prevention Web site. http://www.cdc.gov/ncipc/pub-res/IPV_Compendium.pdf. Accessed May 21, 2013.

19. Chang JC. Understanding behavior change for women experiencing intimate partner violence: mapping the ups and downs using the stages of change. *Patient Educ Couns.* 2006;62(3):330-339.

20. Campbell JC, ed. *Assessing Dangerousness.* New York, NY: Springer Publishing Company LLC; 2007.

21. Campbell JC. Helping women understand their risk in situations of intimate partner violence. *J Interpers Violence.* 2004;19(12):1464-1477.

22. McFarlane J, Malecha A, Gist J, et al. Increasing the safety-promoting behaviors of abused women. *Am J Nurs.* 2004;104(3):40-50.

23. Waldrop AE, Resick PA. Coping among adult female victims of domestic violence. *J Fam Violence.* 2004;19(5):291-302.

24. Oklahoma Office of the Attorney General. Oklahoma Address Confidentiality Program (ACP). Oklahoma Office of the Attorney General Web site. http://www.oag.state.ok.us/oagweb.nsf/v-acp.html. Accessed May 24, 2011.

25. Cluss PA, Chang JC, Hawker L, et al. The process of change for victims of intimate partner violence: support for a psychosocial readiness model. *Womens Health Issues.* 2008;16:262-274.

26. Ewen BM. Failure to protect laws: protecting children or punishing mothers. *J Forensic Nurs.* 2007;3(2):84-86.

27. Futures Without Violence. The facts on domestic, dating and sexual violence. Futures Without Violence Web site. http://www.futureswithoutviolence.org/userfiles/file/Children_and_Families/DomesticViolence.pdf. Accessed May 16, 2011.

28. Humphreys J, Campbell JC. *Family Violence and Nursing Practice.* Philadelphia, PA: Lippincott, Williams and Wilkins; 2004.

29. Anda RF, Felitti VJ, Nordenberg D, et al. Insights into intimate partner violence from the adverse childhood experiences (ACE) study. In: Salber P, Taliaferro E , eds. *The Physician's Guide to Intimate Partner Violence and Abuse: A Reference for All Health Care Professionals.* Volcano, CA: Volcano Press; 2006.

30. Feder A, Nestler EJ, Charney DS. Psychobiology and molecular genetics of resilience. *Nat Rev Neurosci.* 2009;10(4):46-457.

31. DeGue S, DiLillo D. Is animal cruelty a "Red Flag" for family violence?: investigating co-occurring violence toward children, partners and pets. *J Interpers Violence.* 2009;24(6):1036-1056.

32. National Center for Victims of Crime. Stalking safety planning. National Center for Victims of Crime Web site. http://www.victimsofcrime.org/our-programs/stalking-resource-center/help-for-victims/stalking-safety-planning. Accessed May 24, 2011.

33. Some safety considerations around using technology. National Online Resource Center on Violence Against Women. http://www.vawnet.org/print-document.php?doc_id=430&find_type=web_sum_GC . Published 2011. Accessed March 14, 2011.

Chapter 11

AN OVERVIEW OF BEST AND PROMISING PRACTICES TO PREVENT INTIMATE PARTNER VIOLENCE

Linda Chamberlain, PhD, MPH

KEY POINTS

1. Routine assessment combined with anticipatory guidance on healthy relationships can lead to more informed choices and prevent intimate partner violence (IPV).

2. Home visitation interventions have demonstrated promising results for reducing the risk of IPV.

3. Premarital prevention programs have reported positive outcomes, including an improvement in couples' conflict development skills and higher relationship satisfaction.

4. Programs focusing on dating violence prevention among young people, particularly in schools, have been shown to be successful in raising awareness of the prevalence and warning signs of unhealthy relationships and preventing dating violence.

5. Community-based prevention projects have grown increasingly popular. These aim to reduce IPV by changing social norms tolerant of violence and promoting social responsibility for IPV.

6. The Centers for Disease Control and Prevention (CDC) has taken a leadership role in promoting primary prevention of IPV and sexual violence throughout the US.

INTRODUCTION

Prevention strategies can be classified into 3 levels of prevention, primary, secondary, and tertiary, based on what time the intervention is implemented relative to when the problem occurs.[1] These 3 levels of prevention create a continuum of opportunities to prevent violence from ever occurring, to intervene early, and to minimize the after-effects of intimate partner violence (IPV). Primary prevention strategies are implemented before violence occurs to remove the cause or prevent the occurrence of known risk factors. Further along the continuum there are opportunities for secondary prevention strategies to identify a problem before it becomes evident and intervene as soon as possible to prevent the problem from occurring or progressing.[2] Tertiary prevention occurs at the opposite end of the continuum, after the problem has occurred, to minimize the consequences and restore health and safety. Comprehensive prevention initiatives use multiple strategies along the prevention continuum.

The purpose of this chapter is to describe the best and most promising practices for preventing IPV with emphasis on primary prevention. There is no universally accepted definition of "best practices." A best practice is usually supported by rigorous evaluation, has demonstrated success, and can be replicated. There is limited data on best practices for primary prevention of IPV, however. A promising practice may have inconclusive evidence of success or evidence of partial success and little or no evidence demonstrating successful replication. While addressing risk factors such as alcohol and drug abuse that also has the potential to prevent IPV, prevention strategies designed to address other risk behaviors that are associated with IPV are beyond the scope of this chapter.

This chapter begins with a discussion of how clinical responses, as basic as assessing patients for IPV and providing information on referrals and healthy relationships, can be preventive. Early detection of IPV can lead to more accurate diagnoses, interventions to reduce the effects of victimization on patients and their children, prevent revictimization, and interrupt the intergenerational cycle of violence. The next section examines the potential of home visitation programs, an increasingly popular primary prevention strategy for child maltreatment and IPV. This is followed by a brief discussion on premarital programs as a prevention strategy for IPV. The most rigorously evaluated primary prevention strategy that has been proven to be effective for IPV is school-based programs addressing teen dating violence. Several evidence-based curricula and innovative programs are described. There is increasing emphasis on developing broader community responses to change social norms that support interpersonal violence and to promote prosocial behaviors to prevent IPV and sexual violence. Bystander approaches and programs to engage men and boys have shown promise and are included in this chapter. The chapter closes with information about large-scale public health initiatives to prevent IPV.

ASSESSMENT AS A HEALTH PROMOTION TOOL

Studies have demonstrated that assessing patients for IPV and offering referral information are associated with increased safety behaviors,[3] reduced physical violence,[4,5] fewer depressive symptoms,[6] and less psychological abuse.[7] The prevention potential of screening for IPV extends beyond preventing revictimization. Assessment can be a health promotion tool to reduce the disease burden associated with IPV and educate clients about healthy relationships before the violence occurs. While assessment is an example of secondary prevention, anticipatory guidance about healthy, nonviolent relationships provides an opportunity for primary prevention in the clinical setting.

IPV, a hidden risk factor for many common women's health problems including depression,[8] gastrointestinal problems,[9] chronic pain,[10] and gynecological problems,[11] accounts for 7.9% of the overall disease burden for women, ages 18-44.[12] Research has shown that women exposed to ongoing IPV report increased physical symptoms over time.[13] Health care providers can use routine assessment as an opportunity to educate patients about the connection between victimization and many common health problems and unhealthy coping behaviors. Nicolaidis and Touhouliotis[14] have applied the chronic care model to IPV. A key strategy in this model is to increase patients' self-awareness so that they can employ self-support tools to manage comorbid conditions and develop safety plans. The ultimate goal, from a prevention standpoint, is to minimize the long-term health effects and prevent revictimization.

The role of assessment in preventing the long-term consequences of IPV extends beyond the adult victim. In a 2-arm, clinical trial, there was a significant reduction in behavioral problems among children exposed to IPV when their mothers were either screened and offered wallet-size referral cards or screened and offered referral cards along with nurse case management sessions.[15] Educating caregivers about how exposure to IPV impacts children and providing referrals to parenting classes, children's support groups, and other trauma-informed services can help to minimize the acute and long-term effects of childhood exposure to IPV. Because growing up in a home with IPV is associated with an increased risk of perpetrating IPV or being a victim of IPV as an adult for both men and women,[16,17] addressing childhood exposure to IPV has the potential to stop the transmission of IPV to the next generation.

Moving further along the continuum towards primary prevention, routine assessment and anticipatory guidance create opportunities to talk with all patients about healthy relationships and the health effects of victimization. Starting early by talking with adolescents as they are forming values about relationships and beginning to date can plant the seeds for prevention. Hearing this information from health care providers will help to elevate the importance of IPV as a health concern. In a randomized controlled trial with female patients (ages 16-29 years) seen at family planning clinics, when assessment was combined with anticipatory guidance using a business-size-card intervention resource, patients who received the intervention were more likely to report ending a relationship because it was unhealthy or because they felt unsafe regardless of IPV status.[18] Raising awareness and increasing individuals' knowledge about IPV provides the foundation to support boarder environmental and system-level changes to change social norms about violence. In summary, clinicians have a wide range of options to promote prevention as an integral part of routine assessment as shown in **Table 11-1**.

Table 11-1. Strategies to Integrate Prevention into Assessment for IPV
— Educate and offer patients information about the impact of IPV on health.
— Educate patients about the effects of IPV on children and provide referrals.
— Use the chronic care model as a framework to empower patients to take an active role in managing the health effects of abuse and increasing personal safety.
— Integrate anticipatory guidance on healthy relationships into routine assessment with adolescent and adult female patients.

SUPPORTING FAMILIES: HOME VISITATION

Home visitation services have been used to address a wide range of public health issues, including adverse pregnancy outcomes, poor parenting skills, child maltreatment, and IPV. Home visits can reduce the isolation that victims experience while providing social support, a protective factor that can reduce the long-term physical and mental health effects associated with IPV victimization.[19] Home visitation programs usually employ nurses or paraprofessionals to provide support services in a client's home setting. These programs vary significantly in terms of goals, philosophical orientation, the type of service providers involved, eligibility requirements, how clients are enrolled, and the range and intensity of services offered. Home visitation services are typically provided through public health departments, hospitals, or social service agencies and are frequently targeted to pregnant women and new families. In addition to providing social support to clients and their children, home visitation services usually offer referrals to community resources and may include education on parenting, child development, and/or healthy relationships. Evaluation studies of home visitation programs have provided important insights into the need for routine assessment and intervention for IPV and the potential of home visitation as a prevention strategy.

THE NURSE-FAMILY PARTNERSHIP

The Nurse-Family Partnership (NFP) model, developed by Dr. David Olds, is a perinatal home visitation program that has been rigorously evaluated. Home visitation services were offered to first-time–pregnant, low-income women who were visited by registered nurses during their pregnancy and through the child's second birthday. A randomized trial of the NFP model was conducted in Elmira, New York with a large sample of predominantly Caucasian mothers. Findings indicated that the NFP was effective in reducing several risk factors for child maltreatment and improving children's health status. In the Elmira trial, nurse-visited children had fewer state-verified reports of child abuse and neglect, fewer visits to the emergency room, and fewer physician visits for injuries and ingestions compared to children in the control group.[20] Other findings included that nurse-visited families had more informal social support and used more community services. Nurse-visited teen mothers used less punishment with their infants and provided safer, more developmentally-appropriate home environments.[21] These findings are highly relevant to IPV prevention due to the very high prevalence of IPV among home-visited families and the strong correlation between IPV and child maltreatment, and because several of the malleable risk factors for child maltreatment are also risk factors for IPV.

The promising results of the NFP model in Elmira, New York led to replication trials in Memphis, Tennessee and Denver, Colorado. The follow-up of the Elmira trial was also extended to 15 years. One of the challenges in comparing results between these trials is that while the core home visitation services offered were basically the same in all 3 trials, the study populations, comparison services, and outcome measures differed. The Memphis trial served predominantly black families, while the replication in Denver was with a large sample of Hispanic families. Results from the Denver study provided evidence that home visitation can prevent future IPV. Two years after the program had ended, nurse-visited women who were living with partners reported significantly less IPV compared to women who had not received home visits.[22] It is important to note that routine assessment and intervention for IPV were not in place during the intervention which makes this finding particularly poignant. While a statistically significant reduction in IPV was not found in the other 2 trials, the 3 trials were different as noted above. In the Memphis trial, nurse-visited mothers reported fewer incidents of IPV compared to mothers who were not home visited, but the difference was not statistically significant in a follow-up study measuring outcomes 7 years after the intervention ended.[23]

In the long-term follow-up of the Elmira trial, the program effects of NFP on preventing state-verified reports of child abuse and neglect increased between the children's fourth and 15th birthdays.[24] However, the effectiveness of the NFP intervention on reducing child maltreatment was attenuated in the presence of moderate to high levels of IPV.[25] A 5 year project to develop and evaluate a NFP intervention to reduce IPV during pregnancy and the first 2 years postpartum has recently been completed, but results are still forthcoming.[26] Research is currently underway to identify strategies to strengthen the NFP's response to IPV. The model has been replicated in hundreds of locations across the nation through a combination of funding sources including Temporary Assistance for Needy Families, Medicaid, Maternal and Child Health Block Grants, and child abuse and crime prevention dollars.[27] Based on findings from the 3 NFP trials, it is estimated that this model saves $18 054 per family. It is anticipated that the cost effectiveness of this model will be even greater with an integrated response to IPV.

HAWAII HEALTHY START

Hawaii Healthy Start is an early childhood home visitation program designed to promote child health and prevent child maltreatment by enhancing family functioning and reducing malleable risk factors, such as IPV. Paraprofessional home visitors offer direct services that includes teaching clients about child development, modeling positive parenting and problem solving strategies, and linking clients to other community services such as mental health services and IPV shelters and advocacy programs. Home visits begin within 1 week of an infant's birth and are offered for at least 3 years. Services are offered to women who have infants at high risk for maltreatment based on an extensive assessment at the time of birth.

A randomized, controlled trial was conducted with English-speaking mothers who were not currently involved with child protective services and had newborn infants at risk for child maltreatment.[28] The racial/ethnic composition of the intervention group was 34% Native Hawaiian or Pacific Islander, 28% Asian or Filipino, 10% white, and 28% no primary ethnicity or other; the control group was comparable in race and ethnicity. Approximately two-thirds of intervention and control mothers had graduated from high school. In this study, the average rates of IPV victimization and perpetration as well as the rates of specific types of IPV (physical, verbal, sexual, and injuries) were measured over 3-year intervals (during program implementation and at long-term follow-up when the child was 7 to 9 years old).

During the first year, families in the intervention group received an average of 13.6 home visits. Ninety percent of the families participated in home visits when their child was 3 months old; at 6 months of age, 70% participated; at 11 months, 49% participated; and by 36 months of age, one-fourth of families in the intervention group were still receiving home visits. During the first 3 years of the child's life, intervention mothers reported significantly lower rates of IPV victimization and perpetration. Analyses for specific types of IPV indicated a significant reduction in maternal IPV perpetration and a reduction in maternal victimization for physical assault but not for sexual violence, verbal abuse, or injuries. The rates of maternal IPV victimization and perpetration also decreased over long-term follow-up, but the differences between intervention and control mothers were not statistically significant. The authors noted that these findings contrast with an earlier evaluation of Hawaii Healthy Start during the implementation phase that did not show reductions in IPV.[29] In that study, IPV was measured as a dichotomous outcome (present/absent), which may have compromised the study's power to detect a difference. In the more recent analyses, Bair-Merritt et al measured IPV as a count variable and compared specific rates which avoids the problem of selecting an arbitrary "cut point" of the number of IPV acts as being present or not present.[28]

This is the first randomized, controlled study of a home visitation intervention to report reduced rates of female-perpetrated IPV. Two important considerations in interpreting these findings are that program content on IPV was minimal at the time of the study and that few families participated in the expected number of visits. Nevertheless, this study illustrates the potential for preventing IPV in high-risk households.

HEALTHY FAMILIES ALASKA

The complexities of measuring the impact of home visitation services on IPV and understanding how IPV influences the impact of home visitation services is evident in the evaluation of Healthy Families Alaska. A paraprofessional home visitation program designed to prevent child maltreatment by promoting healthy family functioning and supportive parenting, Healthy Families Alaska offers weekly visits during the first 6-9 months of an infant's life to parents who scored 25 or higher on the Kempe Family Stress Checklist.[30] A randomized, controlled trial was conducted with an ethnically diverse population of 325 families (23% Alaska Native, 54% Caucasian, 10% multiracial, and 13% other). Approximately one-third of mothers (32% of intervention mothers and 34% of mothers in the control group) disclosed some form of IPV which was defined as either partner having engaged in 3 or more incidents of violence toward the other partner in the past year. Follow-up data collected when children where 2 years old revealed that there was no program impact on child maltreatment or parental risk factors including IPV. The program did demonstrate marginal effects on the quality of home environment, reductions in maternal high parenting stress, and improved maternal sensitivity to infant cues.

Duggan et al[31] conducted additional analyses with the same randomized, controlled trial data to examine maternal depression and attachment insecurity as moderators of the impacts of Healthy Families Alaska home visitation services. At baseline, 28% of all mothers met criteria for depression. Scores for attachment anxiety and discomfort with trust/dependence varied considerably. The baseline prevalence of depression, attachment anxiety, and discomfort with trust/dependence were higher among mothers who disclosed IPV. Findings indicated that program impacts were moderated by both maternal depression and attachment insecurity for several outcomes, including IPV. Among depressed mothers with relatively low discomfort with trust/dependence, home visiting was associated with a significant decrease in IPV. These results highlight the importance of considering the impact of other co-occurring factors such as depression in program evaluations.

HOME VISITATION INITIATIVES DESIGNED TO ADDRESS IPV

Home visitation programs have been developed for families experiencing IPV and have been shown to be effective in preventing future incidents of physical violence against mothers and reducing adverse outcomes for children exposed to IPV. An important difference between the home visitation programs to address IPV and the previously reviewed home visitation programs is the level of prevention. Since all of the women and children being served by these programs have already experienced IPV, the programs in this section are examples of tertiary prevention, or intervening after the violence has occurred to minimize the after-effects on mothers and their children. The home visitation programs reviewed in the previous section are primary prevention strategies that focus on preventing child maltreatment and other maternal and child health outcomes from ever occurring while reducing malleable risk factors. Since some of those risk factors, such as IPV, may already be occurring with at risk-families, there is also an element of secondary prevention when assessment and early intervention are implemented. As we learn more about the prevention potential of home visitation for IPV, it is likely that we will see programs that address all levels of the prevention continuum by targeting families at risk for IPV and offering services to prevent IPV from ever occurring.

Sullivan and Bybee[32] conducted the first randomized trial of a home visitation program designed to address the needs of women who had experienced abuse. Women were recruited immediately upon exit from domestic violence shelters and randomly assigned to an intervention or control group. The age range of women in the study population was 17 to 61 years old; the mean age was 29 years. Forty-five percent of the women were African American; 42 percent were Caucasian; 7 percent were Latino; and the remaining women were Native American, Arab American, or of mixed heritage. Women in the intervention group were visited by trained advocates in their homes over a 10-week period. The advocates provided social support while helping clients with safety plans and accessing community services, including housing, employment, legal assistance, transportation, education, child care, services for children, and health care.

Home-visited women reported less physical violence, increased quality of life, higher social support, fewer depressive symptoms, and less difficulty obtaining community resources compared to women in the control group. Across 2 years of post-intervention follow-up, more than twice as many women receiving advocacy home visits experienced no violence compared with women who were not home-visited. The intervention was effective in preventing revictimization by the original abuser as well as preventing IPV by any new partners partners; however, the program's effect on the risk of abuse by a new or former partner did not continue when follow-up was extended to 3 years post-intervention.[33] The program's positive effect on women's quality of life and level of social support did persist 3 years after the program ended. Women who reported that they had people in their networks who provided practical help and/or were available to talk about personal matters at the 2-year follow-up were at less risk for abuse at 3 years post-intervention. These findings reiterate the importance of social support as a protective factor.

Lessons learned from the NFP model were combined with an evidence-based, empowerment intervention for pregnant women experiencing IPV to develop the Domestic Violence Enhanced Home Visitation Intervention Project (DOVE). Using a town and gown partnership approach, university-based researchers partnered with county prenatal home visitation programs to provide home visits to pregnant women who have experienced IPV in the past 2 years. The goal of the intervention is to prevent abuse around the time of pregnancy. Public health nurses visit clients in their homes 3 times during their pregnancies and 3 times postpartum. The intervention includes a brochure that is used interactively with clients to discuss their experiences and options. Qualitative research during the implementation phase of DOVE has provided strategic information on barriers to identifying and addressing IPV within the context of home visits.[34] These barriers include home visitors' challenges of dealing with their own emotions particularly stress and frustration when working with victimized clients, comfort levels for initiating conversations with clients about violence, and safety concerns when working in homes where IPV may escalate at any time. A randomized, controlled trial was recently completed with sites in Baltimore, Maryland; rural areas of Missouri; and Kansas City, Missouri to evaluate the efficacy of public health nurse home visits on reducing IPV and children's exposure to IPV and a publication of the promising results is in progress.

Home visitation services have been shown to prevent adverse outcomes in children exposed to IPV. Project SUPPORT provided home visits to abused women who had recently stayed at a domestic violence shelter and had at least 1 child exhibiting oppositional defiant disorder or conduct disorder. Mothers and their children received 1-hour weekly visits from a therapist for up to 8 months after leaving the shelter. Offering social support was the primary goal of the intervention; therapists assisted mothers with problem-solving skills, child management, and nurturing skills that were designed to reduce their children's behavioral problems. In a randomized, controlled trial, 15% of the children in the intervention group had clinical levels of conduct problems compared to 53% of children in the control group at 2 years post-treatment.[35] Home-visited mothers were less likely to return to their abusive partners compared to mothers in the control group. Home-visited mothers were also less likely to use aggressive child management strategies, a finding that is similar to the improvement in parenting skills that were reported for nurse-visited women during the NFP trials. A summary of home visitation programs that have demonstrated an impact on IPV and/or are designed to address IPV is provided in **Table 11-2**.

Premarital Prevention Programs

Premarital prevention programs are typically knowledge- and skill-based training that are offered to nondistressed couples. Since premarital prevention programs are designed to maintain relationship satisfaction over time and prevent divorce, these interventions

Table 11-2. Home Visitation Programs with IPV Outcomes

PROGRAM	FOCUS	TYPE OF HOME VISITOR	STUDY POPULATION	IPV OUTCOMES
Nurse-Family Partnership;[22] **Denver, Colorado**	Improve pregnancy outcomes, promote children's health and development, and strengthen families' economic self-sufficiency	Nurses and paraprofessionals	Predominantly Hispanic sample of first-time–pregnant women who were recruited from antepartum clinics serving low-income families	Nurse-visited women who lived with a partner during the 2 year period before the interview reported less IPV from partners during the past 6 months.
Hawaii Healthy Start[28]	Prevent child maltreatment and promote child health by improving family functioning and reducing malleable risk factors	Paraprofessionals	Ethnically diverse sample of English-speaking women who had recently given birth, were not involved with child protective services, and infants at high risk for maltreatment	Home-visited women reported lower rates of IPV perpetration and victimization during the first 3 years of their children's lives.
Healthy Families Alaska[31]	Prevent child maltreatment by promoting healthy family functioning and supportive parenting	Nurses and paraprofessionals	Sample of English-speaking women (54% white and 23% Alaska Native) identified as high-risk during pregnancy or post partum	IPV in the past year decreased among home-visited, depressed mothers with low-to-moderate attachment insecurity at follow-up when the child was age 2.
Community-based Advocacy Michigan[32]	Provide social support, increase access to community resources, and prevent revictimization by an abusive partner	Advocates	Women who had experienced IPV and spent at least one night in a domestic violence shelter	Home-visited women reported less IPV over a 2 year period; reduction in violence not sustained at 3-year follow-up.
DOVE; Baltimore, Maryland[34]	Empowerment model to prevent abuse around the time of pregnancy	Nurses	Pregnant women who have experienced IPV in the past 2 years	Randomized, controlled trial in progress
Project SUPPORT;[35] **Houston-Galveston area, Texas**	Provide mothers and children with social and instrumental supports; teach mothers child management and nurturing skills	Therapists	Mothers leaving domestic violence shelters with at least one child exhibiting oppositional defiant disorder or conduct disorder	At 20-month follow-up, children had reductions in conduct problems and mothers had fewer psychiatric symptoms and used less inconsistent and harsh parenting.

are oriented towards the future of the relationship versus working on current problems. Physical aggression by a marital partner is a significant predictor of divorce.[36] In a review study by Stahmann and Salts,[37] the authors found relative consistency in the topics addressed in premarital programs. These topics included communication, conflict resolution, roles in marriage, commitment, financial management, sexuality, parenting expectations, and partners' families of origin. In a meta-analytic review by Carroll and Doherty,[38] the mean effect size for premarital prevention programs was .80, or stated differently, the average participant receiving this type of intervention experiences a 30% improvement in outcome measures. Of the 13 experimental studies where control groups were used, only 1 study failed to find that the experimental group had improved interpersonal skills. Outcome effectiveness was similar for the 10 nonexperimental studies that were reviewed; couples reported an improvement in skills including conflict resolution skills and higher relationship satisfaction. The authors concluded that premarital prevention programs produced significant immediate and short-term gains in interpersonal skills and relationship quality when compared to couples who did not participate in these programs.

Although premarital prevention programs address skills, such as conflict resolution and conflict management, that are very relevant to IPV, published evaluation studies of these programs have not systematically reported findings on violence perpetrated in relationships, with one exception. The Premarital Relationship Enrichment Program (PREP) is the most long-term follow-up study of a premarital program to date. Couples participating in PREP reported fewer instances of physical violence compared to control couples over a 5 year period.[39] Offered to couples that are planning to marry, the conceptual framework for PREP is based on behavioral marital therapy with emphasis on building skills for effective communication, problem-solving, and conflict management.

The intervention was offered to 85 couples of which 33 couples (39%) completed the program, 43 (50%) declined to participate, and 9 (11%) partially completed the program. Fifty couples who were not offered PREP served as controls and couples who declined to participate served as a second control group to examine differences in couples who chose not to participate. The average age of male study participants was 24 years old and females, on average, were 23 years old. No information on ethnicity or race was included in the study. Intervention couples attended a total of 5 sessions, approximately 3 hours each, in small groups of 3 to 5 couples and also worked with a trained consultant throughout the program. Consultants were undergraduate or graduate psychology students who received 20 hours of training and worked under supervision. IPV was measured by couples' self-report at 1.5, 3, 4, and 5 years post-intervention.

Eight intervention couples were not included in the outcome analyses because they received a different form of the program. Across follow-ups from year 3 through year 5 following the intervention, the mean frequency of physical violence per year was lower for the 25 intervention couples compared to control couples. There was, however, no significant difference in the frequency of physical violence among intervention couples compared to couples who declined to participate in the intervention. Other significant findings included greater use of communication skills, greater positive affect, more problem-solving skills, and more support and validation among intervention couples at the 4-year follow-up. While a lower prevalence of physical violence persisted among intervention couples at 5 years post-intervention, most of the other study effects diminished between the 4- and 5-year follow-up periods. The authors recommended that booster sessions be offered on an annual basis as part of marital prevention programs. A significant limitation in this study was potential selection bias due to the significant proportion of couples who declined to participate in the intervention.

Halford et al[40] conducted a randomized, controlled trial of a modified version of PREP. Noting that self-regulation strategies have been well documented as being instrumental in the long-term maintenance of adaptive relationship behaviors, the authors expanded the standard PREP content to include self-regulation skills (Self-PREP). Two key predictors of relationship satisfaction and stability were selected for defining high–risk couples: female partners whose parents were divorced or male partners whose parents were reported to have been physically aggressive towards each other. Eighty-three couples who were involved in committed relationships and planned to marry within 11 months were recruited through media outreach. Mean ages were 31.8 years for men and 28.9 years for women; 49 percent of couples were living together. Information on the ethnic background of participants was not included in the publication. Couples were stratified into high- or low-risk groups for relationship distress. The high- and low-risk intervention groups participated in Self-PREP while the control condition consisted of guided reading and group discussion that was reflective of a standard relationship program without training in relationship or self-regulation skills. Physical aggression was only measured before the intervention was implemented. As anticipated, self-reported physical aggression was higher for men and women in high-risk couples compared to low-risk couples. At 1 year follow-up, high-risk couples who received Self-PREP exhibited significantly fewer negative nonverbal behaviors than control couples. Across 4 years of follow-up, high-risk couples had higher relationship satisfaction compared to controls. An unexpected finding was that relationship satisfaction was higher in control couples compared to low-risk couples by the end of the study.

More research is needed to examine the positive and negative effects of skill-based relationship education for couples with varying levels of risk for relationship problems.

Given the popularity of premarital prevention programs, this intervention can provide another pathway for promoting healthy relationships and nonviolence. Routine, periodic assessment for IPV should be integrated into these programs and measured as an outcome in evaluation studies. Any adult who discloses victimization or perpetration should be referred to appropriate intervention services. As we learn more about predictors for IPV, these programs may be able to screen for risk factors and offer more intensive intervention and follow-up for participants who are at high-risk for IPV perpetration and victimization. Using a vulnerability-stress-adaptation framework, Langer et al[41] identified personality traits that were predictive of physical aggression in relationships. Husbands' aggressiveness and impulsivity predicted physical aggression against their wives while wives who were more physically aggressive towards their husbands had more impulsive personalities and were married to husbands with aggressive personalities. Information on IPV including the health effects on adult victims and their children should be woven throughout the program content to help couples recognize how abuse affects every aspect of a relationship.

HEALTHY RELATIONSHIP CURRICULA AND PROGRAMS FOR YOUTH

Adolescence is a developmental window of opportunity to promote healthy relationship skills as teens begin dating and developing attitudes and beliefs about intimate relationships. In a longitudinal study with adolescent African American females, lack of understanding about healthy relationships was predictive of dating violence victimization.[42] Increased awareness of the high rates of dating violence, the correlation between dating violence and other adolescent risk behaviors, and dating violence as a predictive factor for IPV in adulthood has led to a proliferation of dating violence prevention programs. Only a few of these programs have been rigorously evaluated. Whitaker et al[42] conducted a systematic evidence review of interventions for the primary prevention of IPV that were published from 1990 to 2003. All but 1 of the 11 programs that met inclusion criteria for the review were delivered in the school setting and were offered universally to all students. There were only 2 interventions that were longer than 5 hours in duration. While more than half of the studies used experimental designs, the quality of the studies was poor overall due to high attrition rates, poor measurement, and short follow-up periods. Two exceptions were the Youth Relationship Project and the Safe Dates Program, which were evaluated with randomized designs and demonstrated significant program effects on dating violence over extended follow-up periods with acceptable attrition rates. The discussion below begins with a community-based dating violence prevention initiative, the Youth Relationship Project, targeted to at-risk youth. This is followed by an overview of Safe Dates, a universal primary prevention program, and several other school-based programs that have published evaluation results since the systematic review by Whitaker et al.[43]

Youth Relationships Project

The Youth Relationships Project (YRP) is the only curriculum-centered prevention program implemented outside of the classroom that has demonstrated a significant intervention effect on dating violence perpetration.[44] YRP was designed for youth who are at higher risk of dating violence due to childhood exposure to family violence. The project was evaluated in a randomized, controlled trial in Canada with adolescents (92 boys and 99 girls), 14 to 16 years old, who had a history of child maltreatment and/or witnessing IPV. Youth were referred to the YRP from active caseloads of child protection service agencies and received financial incentives to participate in the intervention. Study participants were typically from low-income homes and 60% were living outside of the home. Eighty-five percent of the youth were white, 8% were First Nations, 3% were of Asian descent, and 4% were black Canadians.

Social workers and other community professionals delivered the 18-session curriculum combined with other community-based activities. The curriculum uses group discussion and interactive exercises to address power and control in relationships, sexism, media and sexism, and gender-based violence. The control group continued to receive existing care, usually bimonthly visits from social workers and other basic care. Over the 16-month follow-up period, intervention youth perpetrated less physical violence in relationships compared to the control group. There were no significant differences in the perpetration of emotional abuse or threatening behaviors between the intervention and control groups. An incidental finding was that youths who received the intervention reported fewer symptoms of emotional distress compared to youths in the control group.

Safe Dates

The Safe Dates Program is a school-based intervention to prevent and reduce adolescent dating violence. Safe Dates consists of a 10-session curriculum that is taught by teachers, a poster contest, and a theater production performed by peers.[45] Some of the topics addressed in the curriculum are defining healthy relationships, recognizing patterns of abusive behaviors, improving communication skills, dealing with anger, and how to help a friend who is being abused (see **Figure 11-1**). Each 45-minute session includes interactive exercises such as a dating bingo game, role plays, peer panels, and a feelings diary. The play script, "There's No Excuse for Dating Violence," was developed by high school drama students. A fact sheet and sample letter for parents are provided. Safe Dates has been recognized as a model program by the National Registry for Effective Programs.

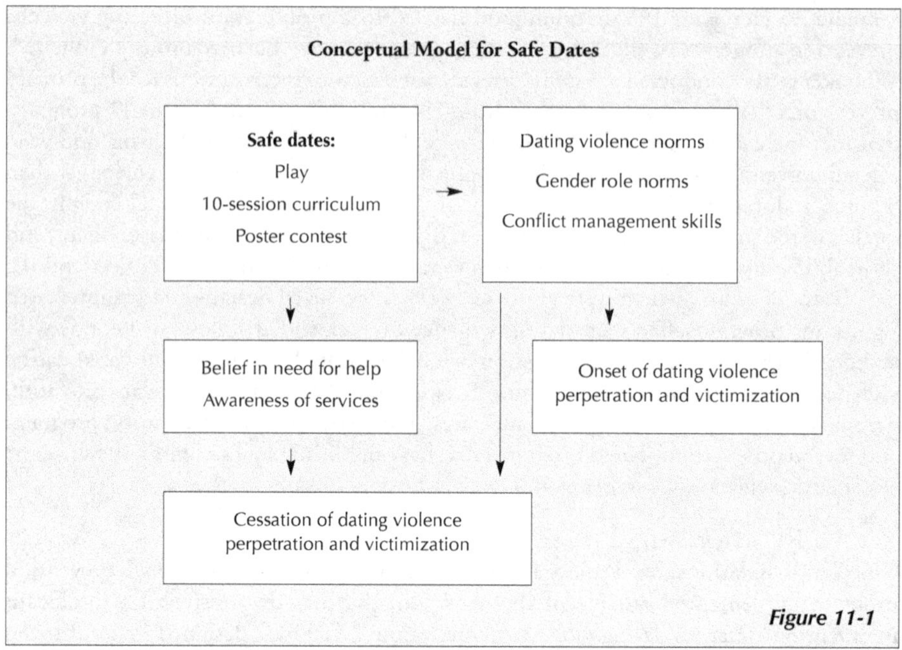

A randomized, controlled trail was conducted with a large sample of middle and high schools in rural North Carolina. Nearly three-fourths of the students were white and approximately one-fifth was African American. Across a period spanning 4-years post-intervention with several waves of data collection, adolescents who received Safe Dates in the eighth or ninth grade reported less perpetration of psychological, moderate physical, and sexual dating violence compared to adolescents who did not receive Safe Dates.[46] Students also reported significantly less moderate physical dating violence victimization, but only marginal effects were found for sexual victimization. Compared to controls, adolescents who received the intervention reported 56% to 92% less dating violence victimization and perpetration at the 4-year follow-up. There was no difference in program effects for boys and girls.[47] The program was equally effective for adolescents who had no history of perpetrating dating violence at baseline and those who had disclosed a positive history of perpetrating dating violence prior to the intervention. Program effects were mediated by changes in dating violence norms, gender role norms, and adolescents' awareness of community services. These findings stress the importance of reaching youth early while attitudes and beliefs about relationships are being developed.

FOURTH R

The Fourth R is a school-based, comprehensive program to promote healthy relationships and prevent risk behaviors that are linked with dating violence.[48] A key premise of the Fourth R is that relationship skills can and should be taught just like reading, writing, and arithmetic. As shown in **Figure 11-2**, the program employs a combination of strategies to inform students, help them to clarify values, and provide opportunities to develop and practice decision-making and other skills that are essential to building healthy relationships and preventing sexual risk-taking behaviors and substance abuse. The Fourth R uses a gender-specific approach that recognizes the issue of gender inequity in violent relationships. While, the program was designed to be delivered to same-sex groups with opportunities for students to come together for group discussions, it is also used in coed classrooms. Messages are crafted to fit with adolescents' realities and experiences while recognizing that these are different for boys and girls.

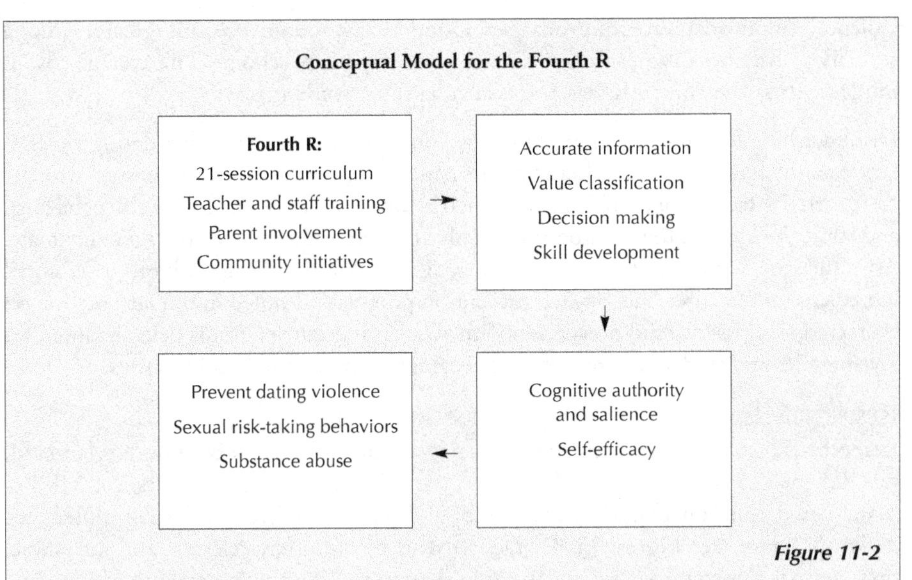

Figure 11-2.
Conceptual Model for the Fourth R.

The core strategy is a 21-session, skill-based curriculum. The ninth grade curriculum has 3 units: personal safety and injury prevention, healthy growth and sexuality, and substance use and abuse. The first unit focuses on developing skills for effective relationships with emphasis on communication, negotiations, and problem solving. This unit includes content on same-sex relationships, cyber-bullying, and media violence.

The curriculum has been adapted for seventh and eighth graders. Another version of the curriculum, "The Aboriginal Perspective" has been developed for indigenous Canadian populations. All versions of the Fourth R are designed to meet educational requirements so that the lessons can be embedded into existing coursework.

In addition to the classroom curriculum, there are additional strategies to actively involve schools, communities, and parents. School interventions include training for staff and teachers and the formation of student-led Youth-Safe-Schools Committees. These student committees forge links with community partners by arranging guest speakers, organizing field trips, arranging agency open houses, and developing media campaigns. In addition to a parents' orientation about the program, parents also receive information about adolescent development and parenting strategies. The content of 4 consecutive parent newsletters is coordinated with the unit of the curriculum that is being covered in the classroom.

The Fourth R was evaluated in ninth grader health classes at 20 public schools in southwestern Ontario, Canada.[48] Using a cluster randomized trial design, students were followed from the ninth grade through the 11th grade (2.5 years from baseline). The study population was predominantly Caucasian. More than one-half of the students' parents had college diplomas or university degrees, and more than three-fourths of the students came from homes where both parents were employed. By the end of the 11th grade, students in the control school were nearly 2 1/2 times (adjusted odds ratio = 2.42) more likely to report using physical violence in a dating relationship compared to students at the intervention schools. The intervention effect varied significantly by gender. Boys in intervention schools were significantly less likely to perpetrate dating violence than boys in control schools (2.7% vs. 7.1%); girls in the intervention and control schools reported similar rates (11.9% and 11.0% respectively). There were no significant differences between control and intervention groups for physical peer violence. Additional subgroup analyses found that condom use was greater among sexually active boys in intervention schools than in control schools. The average cost of implementing the Fourth R was $16 (Canadian) per student.

Distinguishing features and strengths of the Fourth R compared to other dating violence curricula include its comprehensive prevention approach which addresses strongly correlated risk factors for dating violence, such as substance abuse and sexual risk behaviors, and strategies beyond the classroom to involve parents and influence the school climate. As is the case with Safe Dates, the Fourth R is a skill-based curriculum, an essential ingredient for effective school-based prevention programs as noted in the next section on characteristics of successful prevention with youth. The curriculum is being adapted for lower grades and students from different geographic and cultural backgrounds.

RESPECT ME

Respect ME, an arts-based dating violence prevention initiative in Baltimore, Maryland, was designed to reach younger students in the middle school grades. Respect ME has 3 arts-based components: a theatre group, a visual arts project, and a computer web design program (see **Figure 11-3**). Designed to be culturally relevant and adaptable, these activities encourage students to explore healthy and unhealthy relationships while considering the influences of culture, race, gender, and ethnic stereotyping. The arts-based strategies are augmented with discussion advocacy groups and a 4-session curriculum that engages students through role plays. Teachers and school staff also receive training. Using a quasi-experimental pre- and post-test comparison group design, an evaluation of Respect ME was conducted in 4 urban middle schools with predominantly African American seventh graders.[49] All of the students at the intervention schools received the curriculum component while approximately half of the students participated in at least 1 of the 3 arts-based components or discussion advocacy groups. Of the arts-based components, the theatre project (38%) had the highest participation rate while the website project had the lowest participation rate (2%).

The curriculum was offered in the fall semester and follow-up was conducted during the spring semester. Perpetration for physical, emotional, and lifetime dating violence was significantly lower in the intervention group compared to the comparison group. There was

Figure 11-3.
Conceptual Model for Respect ME.

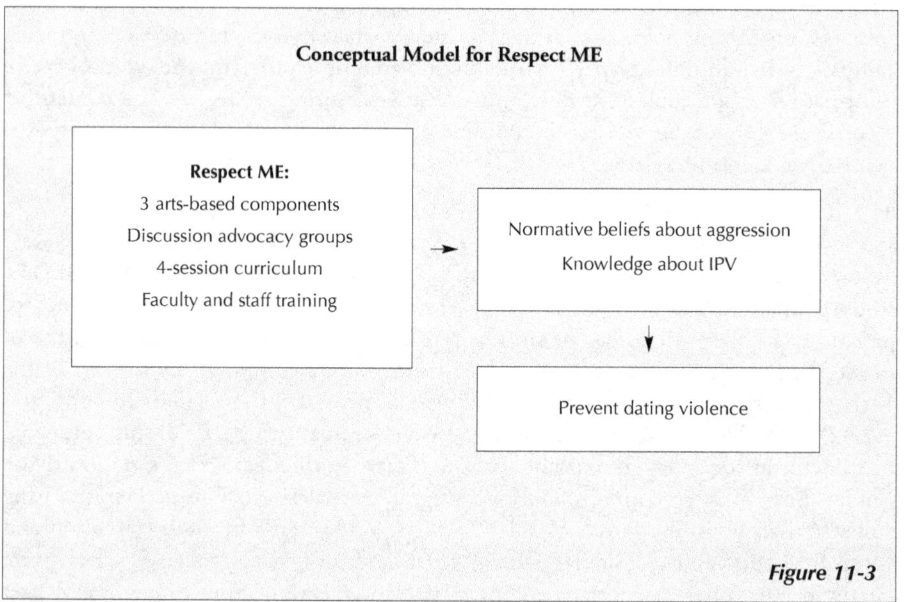

a 60% increase in past-year dating violence among the comparison group from the fall to spring semesters compared to a slight reduction in past-year dating violence in the intervention schools during this period (41% to 35%). Intervention students demonstrated a significant increase in knowledge about dating violence; however, their attitudes about dating violence did not differ significantly from students in comparison schools. The intervention effect did not vary by students' gender. A significant challenge and limitation to this study was obtaining parental consent which resulted in an overall response rate of 31%.

ENDING VIOLENCE

Ending Violence: A Curriculum for Educating Teens about Domestic Violence and the Law focuses on the legal aspects of dating violence.[50] As shown in the conceptual model for Ending Violence (see **Figure 11-4**), this brief curriculum consists of 3 sessions that can be incorporated into existing health curricula. Designed to be taught by attorneys, a primary objective of the intervention is to increase young people's comfort level when speaking with attorneys while at the same time being informed about legal services and the role of the legal system in protecting victims and punishing perpetrators. The curriculum provides an overview of dating and domestic violence with content on legal options in the criminal and civil justice systems. Students participate in a mock hearing role play which walks them through the process of obtaining a restraining order.

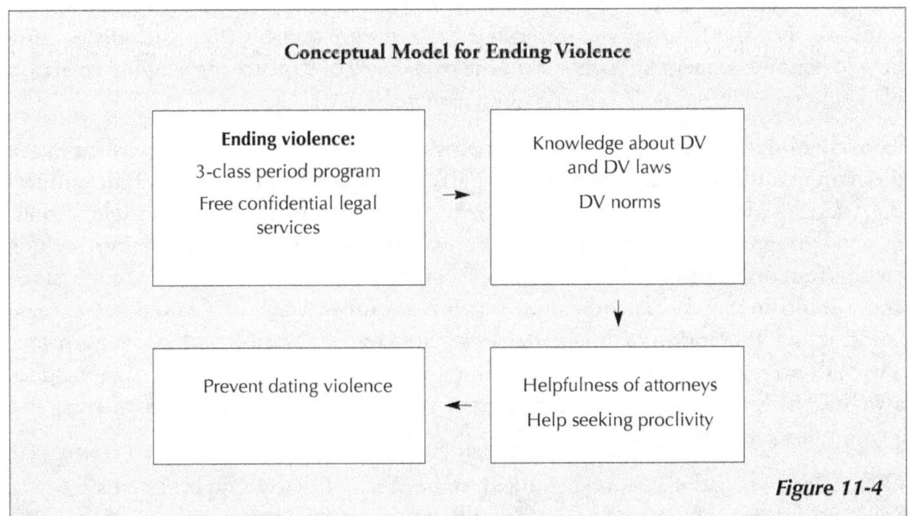

Figure 11-4.
Conceptual Model for Ending Violence.

A randomized, controlled trial was conducted with ninth grade students at 10 public schools in Los Angeles, California. The students were predominantly Latino (92%);,75% were US-born, and 11% had lived outside of the US for at least 10 years. The program was implemented by bilingual, bicultural attorneys and included free legal services to youth. Immediately following the intervention, students who received the curriculum showed improved knowledge, less acceptance of female-on-male aggression, and increased likelihood of seeking help from professionals, particularly police and lawyers. There were no significant differences in recent abusive or fearful dating experiences or violence victimization or perpetration. Acceptance of male-on-female violence in response to provocation also did not differ between intervention and control classrooms; however, intervention effects on improvements in knowledge and the perceived helpfulness of talking with an attorney about dating violence persisted at 6-month follow-up. The short duration of this intervention and its focused approach to legal aspects of dating violence may be limiting factors in changing attitudes and actual behaviors compared to the longer, skill-based curricula previously described.

EXPECT RESPECT

Expect Respect, a 3-prong school-based dating violence initiative developed in Austin, Texas, uses an ecological approach combining primary and secondary prevention strategies to address a broader continuum of abuse that includes dating violence, bullying, and sexual harassment.[51] At the secondary level of prevention, Expect Respect support groups are offered to youth who have been exposed to IPV, have experienced sexual abuse, and/ or have already been involved in an abusive dating relationship. Students are referred by school staff and self-referred through posters and flyers. A 24-session curriculum supports the group sessions which are gender-specific and designed to be held outside of the classroom setting. The skill-based curriculum includes content on expressing feelings, assertive communication, recognizing the warning signs of dating violence, resolving conflicts, handling anger, and setting healthy boundaries. The Expect Respect program provides training for school administrators, counselors, teachers, parents, and other professionals on how to respond to and prevent dating violence and harassment.

Primary prevention strategies consist of a service learning component on youth leadership and a school-wide awareness campaign. The SafeTeens youth leadership training is designed to be integrated into school or community activities. The 8-session curriculum addresses bullying, sexual harassment, and dating violence. The content focuses on developing skills to reduce the risk of victimization and knowing how to help someone else who is being victimized. Leadership development skills include learning how to conduct student assessments on the prevalence of violence, developing an action plan, and creating Public Service Announcements (PSAs).

The school-wide awareness campaign employs 3 key strategies that are described in the program manual: assessing the school climate, developing a school policy, and conducting a school-wide awareness campaign. Sample school climate survey and school policies on dating violence are provided. School-wide awareness campaign activities include faculty/staff orientation, parent seminars, facilitator training for teacher and counselors, and a multi-modal media campaign utilizing resources from the Centers for Disease Control and Prevention's Choose Respect Campaign on dating violence prevention. The wide array of resources developed through the Choose Respect Campaign includes a website in English and Spanish, posters, TV and PSAs, cinema advertisements, and a community action kit.

Quantitative evaluation results are limited to the Expect Respect support groups.[52] A pre- and post-test design was used to evaluate the impact of the support groups with a small sample of middle school and high school students from ethnically diverse backgrounds (50% Hispanic or Latino, 23% African American, 10% multiracial, and 14% Caucasian). A total of 26 support groups (13 boy groups and 13 girl groups) participated in the evaluation study. Students in the intervention group reported a significant increase in healthy/positive conflict resolution; a positive change in relational security, defined as students feeling less worried about being rejected or betrayed and less likely to engage in controlling behaviors; and a decrease in sexual violence victimization. Girls reported a positive increase in identifying abusive behavior which was identified as a mediator for decreased perpetration of dating violence. These findings are consistent with the findings from a qualitative empowerment evaluation that was conducted with the same study population described above.[51] Group participants reported an increase in healthy relationship skills, new knowledge, increased awareness of their own and their peers' abusive behaviors, and changes in relationship norms. A more rigorous evaluation design with comparison groups, larger sample sizes, and long-term follow-up will provide much needed data to measure the effectiveness of this comprehensive prevention approach.

LESSONS FROM THE FIELD OF YOUTH PREVENTION SCIENCE

There is a substantial body of empirical evidence on effective strategies for preventing adolescent risk behaviors. The National Institute of Health (NIH) State-of-Science Conference on Preventing Violence and Related Health-Risking Social Behaviors in Adolescents employed systematic literature reviews, presentations, and deliberations by a panel of experts to identify the key characteristics of successful prevention with youth.[52] Several key characteristics of effective prevention programs to prevent adolescent risk behaviors were identified that can be used as a checklist to evaluate whether a prevention strategy addresses these lessons learned (see **Table 11-3**). The dating violence curricula described in this chapter have incorporated many of these key characteristics, such as being derived from sound theoretical rationale, being developmentally appropriate, focusing on skills including social competency, and having capacity for delivery with fidelity.

Table 11-3. Key Characteristics of Effective Prevention Strategies with Youth

— Derived from sound theoretical rationale

— Multimodal and multicontextual

— Address strong risk factors

— Involve long-term treatments

— Developmentally appropriate

— Follow a cognitive behavioral strategy

— Focus on improving social competency and other skill development strategies

— Capacity for delivery with fidelity

— Not delivered in coercive settings

The NIH recommendations are consistent with findings from other systematic evidence reviews and meta-analyses of effective prevention programs with youth.[53-58] The design, implementation, and evaluation of adolescent dating violence prevention initiatives should be considered within the context of what we have learned about successful prevention initiatives for other adolescent risk behaviors. Multimodal and multicontextual prevention strategies have the advantage of combining different levels of prevention; for example, if a universal primary prevention strategy designed to prevent dating violence is offered to all high school students in a study population, there would be a significant proportion of students who have already experienced dating violence. There will also be a substantial number of students who witnessed IPV and/or experienced child maltreatment, which are risk factors for dating violence and adult IPV.[59-61] A comprehensive approach that combines strategies along the prevention continuum to meet the needs of both unexposed and exposed youth in different settings, while also addressing strong risk factors will increase the reach of the program and the probability of success. Expect Respect, as described above, is an example of a multi-level prevention initiative that combines primary and secondary strategies.

COMMUNITY-BASED PREVENTION

There is growing interest in broader community prevention initiatives that are aimed at changing social norms tolerant of violence and that offer skill-based training to prepare everyone for a positive role in prevention. Empowering bystanders, media campaigns, and social diffusion are examples of community engagement strategies that promote social responsibility for preventing relationship violence. The Centers for Disease Control and Prevention (CDC) recommends using a public health approach to prevent violence against women through community-based prevention programs that give everyone an active role in prevention.[61] The public health approach, which integrates a variety of strategies to address complex problems with different segments of the population, has the potential to address multiple levels of prevention.

BYSTANDER EDUCATION

The bystander approach has been implemented with men and women on college campuses across the United States to address sexual violence and IPV.[63-66] Bystanders learn skills that prepare them to speak out against social norms that tolerate violence, to interrupt situations that are likely to lead to violence, to safely intervene during violent incidents, and to support survivors.[67] Banyard and colleagues conducted an experimental study to evaluate the effectiveness of a peer-facilitated bystander education program to prevent sexual violence on a college campus.[64] The authors had previously developed a tool to measure outcomes related to bystander attitudes, decision making, and behaviors that was used in this study.[68] Male and female undergraduate students were randomly assigned to a 1-session program, a 3-session program, or a control group. A booster session was offered to participants in the treatment groups approximately 2 months after the interventions. The study population was predominantly Caucasian. The training session(s) employed interactive learning exercises with role plays to promote skill development and the opportunity to practice intervention and personal safety skills. Participants in the treatment groups developed a personal bystander plan and signed a bystander pledge.

Results indicated that up to 2 months after participating in the 1- or 3-session programs, there were significant differences in participants' pre-test and post-test scores for greater efficacy, knowledge, willingness to help, appreciation of the "pros" of helping, and lower rape myth acceptance compared to the control group scores. Participants who received the longer, 3-session intervention had greater increases in knowledge, more positive bystander attitudes, and lower rape myth acceptance than participants in the 1-session group which suggests a dose-response relationship between the number of sessions and the study outcomes. The treatment groups also had significantly higher increases in self-reported bystander behaviors compared to the control group. Analyses to examine the differential effect of the program by gender indicated that while women scored higher on many of the outcomes, the program was effective for both men and women. An exploratory analysis with much smaller sample sizes at 4- and 11-month follow-ups suggested that many of the program effects for efficacy, knowledge, and attitudes persisted over time.

Overall, these study findings are consistent with an earlier exploratory formative evaluation of the same bystander intervention with a small sample of undergraduate university students by Moynihan et al.[65] The study population, composed of 14 women and 12 men, was predominantly Caucasian (23 white and 3 multiracial or biracial). Nearly one-half (46.2%) of the students were freshmen, 30.8 percent were sophomores, and the remaining 23 percent were juniors or seniors. Based on a comparison of pre-test and post-test scores, participants demonstrated greater disagreement with statements favorable to date rape, greater knowledge about sexual violence, and greater knowledge about behaviors shown to be predictive of intervening in situations of sexual violence. Study participants also had higher scores on the Bystander Efficacy Scale which measures beliefs that sexual violence can be prevented and that bystanders have a role in prevention.

Media campaigns are a well-established strategy in community-wide prevention initiatives that have the potential to reach a broad spectrum of the population.[69,70] Potter et al[70] used a post-test–only design with a convenience sample of predominantly Caucasian college students (87% white) to evaluate the efficacy of a poster campaign to promote prosocial bystander behaviors for sexual violence against women on campus. Nearly two-thirds (62%) of the study population was female. Twenty-seven percent were first-year students and 28% lived off campus. Students who saw the posters reported greater awareness of the problem and greater willingness to get involved in reducing violence against women compared to students who did not see the posters. The 4-poster series used empowering language and featured a triptych of friends reaching out and supporting friends who have experienced sexual violence. While this exploratory study has major limitations due to the lack of an experimental design, it provides preliminary data on a prevention strategy that is frequently used and rarely evaluated.

The Mentors in Violence Prevention (MVP) is a leadership development program and curriculum that is based on an empowered bystander approach to prevent interpersonal violence.[71] Developed at the Center for Study of Sport in Society at Northeastern University, the program originally trained male college student–athletes to mentor high school student–athletes on issues related to violence against women. The MVP program has been an innovator in working with men as allies to prevent violence against women. The program has been expanded to include female high school leaders. The sessions are facilitated by mixed gender, multi-racial trainers.

The curriculum is usually delivered in 6 or 7 sessions. Student leaders and athletes learn about the effects of abuse and how to be proactive bystanders. Resources include the MVP Playbook, which provides interactive exercises and case scenarios that are designed for male-only and female-only groups. A quasi-experimental evaluation was conducted with 211 high school students using a pre-test–post-test design with a nonequivalent comparison group.[72] There were substantial differences in the ethnic background of students in the intervention and comparison groups (61% Caucasian and 44% Caucasian, respectively). At the end of the program, pre-test and post-test scores indicated a strong program effect for males and females. Due to small sample sizes, gender differences could not be statistically evaluated. Students in the intervention group had greater knowledge and awareness about gender-based violence, less acceptance of negative attitudes about gender violence, and improved self-efficacy and confidence about their personal ability to prevent and/or intervene in situations involving male violence against women. Student satisfaction with the program was measured with qualitative survey questions. The majority of MVP participants said that they would recommend the program to a friend and had spoken with at least one other person about the program.

Green Dot Kentucky is a state-wide, multifaceted violence prevention initiative developed at the University of Kentucky.[73] This innovative program combines the bystander approach with adaptations of social diffusion theory to change how communities think about and respond to violence against women. Using a theory-driven approach, Green Dot Kentucky uses the bystander research to provide examples of targeted behavior to safely intervene and prevent violence. The bystander approach describes what needs to happen while social diffusion theory explains who needs to take action to influence behavior change.

According to social diffusion theory, behavior change in a population can be initiated and diffused through the influence of popular opinion leaders (POLs) who endorse and recommend innovative behaviors. Numerous community-level trials using POLs have demonstrated the effectiveness of this approach in HIV prevention.[74] In a randomized, community-level field design study, cities where popular homosexual men endorsed and spread risk reduction behaviors among their peers had significantly lower rates of sexual risk behaviors compared to control cities.[75] The study population of 1116 men in 8 cities was 90% white with a mean age of 31.1 years. Twenty-eight percent had completed college and 40% had attended but not graduated from college.

By adapting social diffusion theory to violence prevention, Green Dot Kentucky has applied a targeted recruitment strategy to develop a critical mass of POLs who endorse and demonstrate behaviors that are proactively and visibly intolerant of violence against women and children. POLs receive skills-building training called SEEDS (Students Educating and Empowering to Develop Safety) to learn how to prevent IPV and safely intervene when they are in the role of bystander. By using detailed perpetrator information to inform bystander responses, Green Dot broadens the role of the bystander beyond helping victims to identifying potential high-risk perpetrator behaviors that can lead to early intervention. Using a train-the-trainer model to provide statewide coverage, certified Green Dot trainers offer training to communities, businesses, and other organizations. The media campaign component of the initiative includes flyers, posters, and an informational Web site where users view statistics about IPV, learn about effective prevention strategies, obtain a bystander pledge, and share their stories or "green dots" on a map of Kentucky that visually tracks the initiative's progress. A pilot study with a random sample of 7945 college undergraduates indicated that students who received bystander training reported more active bystander behaviors than non-exposed students.[76] Trained students also had significantly lower rape myth acceptance scores compared to students who did not participate in Green Dot training. A 5-year, randomized, controlled trial is currently underway to evaluate the effectiveness of Green Dot with high school students, according to its principal investigator, Dr. Ann Coker. The Green Dot approach is being replicated in communities across the United States.

PROGRAMS TO ENGAGE MEN AND BOYS

Research with men and boys from many different cultures has shown that gender role socialization and inequitable gender norms influence health including sexual risk behaviors and IPV.[77-79] There is a growing number of programs with boys and men that use a gender perspective. These programs address a wide range of health-related issues including sexual and reproductive health, maternal and child health, fatherhood, and gender-based violence. Batterers intervention programs use a gender perspective to help men examine how rigid gender roles and specific norms related to masculinity compromise their relationships and contribute to violence against women.

The World Health Organization (WHO) conducted an international systematic evidence review of programs to engage men and boys in changing gender-based inequities in health, including violence against women.[78] A total of 58 evaluation studies of interventions with men and boys from different countries and cultures were analyzed. Programs were categorized as gender-neutral, gender- sensitive, and/or gender-transformative. Gender transformative was defined as programs that "seek to transform gender roles and promote more gender-equitable relationships between men and women." Programs that were assessed as gender-transformative had a higher rate of effectiveness compared to programs that were assessed as gender-neutral or gender-sensitive. Gender-transformative programs rated as effective in the WHO report included Soul City in South Africa, Violence against Women: A Disaster We Can Prevent in Nicaragua, and the Safe Dates Program. While more rigorous, long-term evaluation studies that include cost data are needed, the report concluded that there is compelling evidence that well-designed programs with men and boys lead to changes in behavior and attitudes.

Coaching Boys into Men, a US-based program, was rated as a gender sensitive, promising practice in the WHO report.[78] Developed through a joint partnership between Futures Without Violence and the Advertising Council, Coaching Boys into Men uses community engagement and mobilization to engage men as fathers, coaches, teachers, uncles, and mentors to teach boys that violence against women is wrong. The program centers around a public service advertising campaign using television, radio, posters, and other print media to encourage men to talk with boys about gender roles and healthy relationships. An evaluation was conducted of a national campaign that piloted a series of Public Service Announcements (PSAs) that were rolled out in several waves.

Over a 4-year study period, awareness of the campaign increased fourfold.[80] Results from random digit dial telephone surveys indicated that 41% of men reported talking to boys at the sixth wave of tracking, nearly 4 years after the campaign began, compared to 29% of men before the first PSA was released. This rate had plummeted to 33%, 7 months later. This reduction was attributed to a significant decrease in donated media coverage and demonstrates the importance of maintaining a high level of exposure and monitoring impact throughout a media campaign. Respondents who saw the "The Wrong Way Around" PSA were significantly more likely to have spoken to a boy about violence against women, spoken to other adults about preventing IPV, and gone to a Web site or called a phone number for more information than respondents who did not see the PSA. "The Wrong Way Around" PSA combines humor with a heavy dose of reality to encourage men to start talking with boys early; an uncle, a coach, and a postman are approached by young boys expressing confusion over mixed messages about violence against women and asking for help with shaping their attitudes.

While demographic information about the study population was not provided, differences in outcomes by different characteristics, including age, ethnicity, and income level, were reported. African American men (54%) were more likely say that they had spoken to a boy about violence against women and girls compared to white (32%) and Hispanic (38%) men. Higher income level ($25-$50K vs. <$25K) and younger age (35-54 years old vs. age 55+) were also associated with an increased likelihood of talking to boys about violence against women. African American and Hispanic men were more likely to say that they talked to other adults about preventing IPV and obtained information about preventing IPV by going to a Web site or called a phone number. Overall, these findings suggest that a gender approach to engage men and boys should be part of a broader prevention strategy for IPV and that media campaigns should be included in the evaluation plan for any prevention initiative.

A new tool, the "Coaching Boys into Men Playbook," has been developed to engage coaches and young athletes in violence prevention. The playbook provides step-by-step strategies for coaches, ranging from a pre-season motivational speech to post-season activities, to discuss dating violence and sexual assault with students. The CDC has funded a cluster-randomized trial of the "Coaching Boys into Men Playbook" across 16 high schools in California. Data is collected before and immediately after the sports season, as well as one year later. In addition to measures of changes in coaches' attitudes and behaviors, key study outcomes include male athlete knowledge about what constitutes disrespectful and abusive behaviors, gender-equitable attitudes, and bystander behaviors (greater likelihood to intervene when witnessing disrespectful and harmful behaviors).

PUBLIC HEALTH RESPONSE

The CDC has taken a leadership role in promoting primary prevention of IPV and sexual violence. The CDC uses a 4-level ecological model as a framework to prevent violence.[62]

The ecological model supports a comprehensive public health approach by addressing risk factors at 4 levels: individual, relationship, community, and societal. The ecological model, presented in the World Report on Violence and Health,[81] accommodates the inclusion of risk and protective factors across multiple domains that influence IPV.[26] Two large-scale CDC initiatives that support using the ecological model to prevent IPV and sexual violence are described below.

Domestic Violence Prevention and Leadership Through Alliances (DELTA) is a CDC-sponsored project to promote primary prevention at the state-level through leadership development, capacity building, and partnerships.[82] Domestic violence coalitions in 14 states received funding to develop and implement primary prevention activities that can be integrated into Coordinated Community Responses (CCRs) or other community-based collaborations. CCRs coordinate efforts between the criminal justice system and social service agencies in violence against women cases through improved communication, implementation of protocols, and community education. The mission of DELTA is to expand the scope of the CCRs' collaborative work to include strategies that prevent violence against women from ever occurring. The CCRs receive prevention-focused technical assistance, training, and funding from the domestic violence coalitions. The evaluation plan includes a cross-site evaluation of DELTA to measure program effectiveness in developing, integrating, and sustaining primary prevention activities within the CCR model and an environmental scan of CCR prevention activities in participating states.

Another CDC public health initiative to end violence against women is the Rape Prevention Education (RPE) program.[82] Authorized under the Violence Against Women Act (VAWA), this program provides funding to all 50 states, the District of Columbia, and US territories. The core activities of this program, which are legislatively mandated, include educational seminars, hotlines, informational materials, training for professionals, student/campus education and training, and date rape drug education. The overarching goal of RPE is to translate science into practice and build capacity for prevention activities. To achieve this goal, states participate in videoconferencing and annual meetings to facilitate cross-program exchanges and share lessons learned. While DELTA and RPE are separate initiatives, growing recognition of the tremendous overlap between IPV and sexual violence has led to more collaboration between the programs.

CONCLUSION

IPV is not inevitable. The evidence base on preventing IPV has grown substantially over the past 2 decades. Lessons learned from the extensive body of research on effective prevention with youth parallel what we are learning about preventing relationship violence among adolescents and adults. IPV is a complex social problem with predictable long-term health effects for victims and their children. There is a continuum of opportunities for health care providers to engage in prevention that begins with assessment and counseling patients on healthy relationships and extends to being a well-informed advocate for community-level prevention.

There are significant gaps in the research on IPV prevention that need to be addressed, including the need for more rigorous research designs with control groups; more long-term follow-up for outcome variables and untoward effects; cost-effectiveness studies to demonstrate the potential cost savings of prevention; and comprehensive evaluation plans that address all aspects of a prevention initiative, including media campaigns and community outreach. Evaluation studies need to be replicated in a variety of settings with ethnically diverse study populations. While acknowledging existing limitations, there are several common characteristics of the best and promising practices for preventing IPV that were reviewed in this chapter. Prevention strategies for IPV should be comprehensive and multifaceted to address individual, relationship, community, and societal risk factors. Strategies must extend beyond education and skill-building programs to promote broader changes in systems, policies, and social norms. Green Dot Kentucky combines the bystander approach and social infusion theory to educate individuals and change behaviors. The statewide public education campaign is using several forms of media to change social norms.

To address the high levels of victimization in any population, prevention activities for IPV should combine different levels or layers of prevention that are appropriately timed to meet people where they are at in their life experiences. Using an ecological approach, Expect Respect embeds support group for teens that have been exposed to violence into its broader primary prevention focus to educate youth on healthy relationships during this developmental window of opportunity. IPV prevention strategies should include gender transformative approaches to engage men and boys and provide proactive, positive roles in preventing violence against women. The Fourth R, the Safe Dates Program, Mentors in Violence Prevention, and Coaching Boys into Men demonstrate how the gender approach can be incorporated into different types of prevention strategies.

IPV prevention strategies need to be dynamic and adaptable to meet the sociocultural needs of diverse communities. A persistent challenge in implementing any prevention program is the fidelity of implementation, or staying true to the original design of the program; however, program designers and implementers need to be flexible and willing to adapt programs to be culturally sensitive and relevant to the populations being served. While the Fourth R curriculum has been adapted for Aboriginal youth, the designers and trainers recognize that additional adaptations are necessary to accommodate regional and cultural differences between Aboriginal communities.

The common characteristics of effective prevention strategies for IPV are consistent with characteristics of effective prevention programs identified in a review of reviews by Nation and colleagues.[83] By applying a systematic public health approach that applies the most current knowledge on best and promising practices, professionals in the field have the potential to prevent the predictable health consequences of victimization, prevent future violence, and interrupt the intergenerational transmission of IPV.

REFERENCES

1. Chamberlain LA. A prevention primer for domestic violence: terminology, tools, and the public health approach. VAWnet: The National Online Resource Center on Violence Against Women Web site. http://www.vawnet.org/summary.php?doc_id=1313&find_type=web_sum_AR. Accessed February 22, 2011.

2. Chrisler JC, Ferguson S. Violence against women as a public health issue. *Ann NY Aca Sci.* 2006:1087:235-249.

3. McFarlane J, Parker B, Soeken K, Silva C, Reel S. Safety behaviors of abused women after an intervention during pregnancy. *J Obstet Gynecol Neonatal Nurs.* 1998;27(1):64-69.

4. McFarlane J, Soeken K, Wiist W. An evaluation of interventions to decrease intimate partner violence to pregnancy women. *Public Health Nurs.* 2000;17(6):443-451.

5. McFarlane J, Groff JY, O'Brien JA, Watson K. Secondary prevention of intimate partner violence: a randomized, controlled trial. *Nurs Res.* 2006;55(1):52-61.

6. Tiwari A, Tak Fong DY, Yuen KH, et al. Effect of an advocacy intervention on mental health in Chinese women survivors of intimate partner violence. *JAMA*. 2010;304(5):536-543.

7. Tiwari A, Leung WC, Leung TW, Humphreys J, Parker B, Ho PC. A randomized, controlled trial of empowerment training for Chinese abused pregnant women in Hong Kong. *BJOG*. 2005;112(9):1249-1256.

8. Caetano R, Cunradi C. Intimate partner violence and depression among whites, blacks, and Hispanics. *Ann Epidemiol*. 2003;13(10):661-665.

9. Lesserman J, Drossman DA. Relationship of abuse history to functional gastrointestinal disorders and symptoms. *Trauma Violence Abuse*. 2007;8(3):331-343.

10. Wuest J, Merritt-Gray M, Ford-Gilboe M, Lent B, Varcoe C, Campbell JC. Chronic pain in women survivors of intimate partner violence. *J Pain*. 2008:9(11):1049-1057.

11. Mark H, Bitzker K, Rauchfuss M. Gynaecological symptoms associated with physical and sexual violence. *J Psychosom Obstet Gynacol*. 2008;29(30):164-172.

12. Vos T, Astbury J, Piers LS, et al. Measuring the impact of intimate partner violence on the health of women in Victoria, Australia. *Bull World Health Organ*. 2006;84(9):739-744.

13. Gerber MR, Wittenberg E, Ganz ML, Williams CM, McCloskey L. Intimate partner violence exposure and change in women's physical symptoms over time. *J Gen Intern Med*. 2008;23(1):64-69.

14. Nicolaidis C, Touhouliotis V. Addressing intimate partner violence in primary care: lessons from chronic illness management. *Violence Vict*. 2006;21(1):101-115.

15. McFarlane J, Groff JY, O'Brien JA, Watson K. Behaviors of children following a randomized, controlled treatment program for their abused mothers. *Issues Compr Pediatr Nurs*. 2005;28(4):195-211.

16. Ehrensaft MK, Cohen P, Brown J, Smailes E, Chen H, Johnson JG. Intergenerational transmission of partner violence: a 20-year prospective study. *J Consult Clin Psychol*. 2003;71(4):741-753.

17. McKinney CM, Caetano R, Ramisetty-Mikler S, Nelson S. Childhood family violence and perpetration and victimization of intimate partner violence: findings from a national population-based study of couples. *Ann Epidemiol*. 2009:19(1):25-32.

18. Miller E, Decker MR, McCauley HL, Tancredi DJ, Levenson RR, Waldman J, Schoenwald P, Silverman JG. A family planning clinic partner violence intervention to reduce risk associated with reproductive coercion. *Contraception*. 2011:83(3):274-280.

19. Coker AL, Smith PH, Thompson MP, McKeown RE, Bethea L, Davis KE. Social support protects against the negative effects of partner violence on mental health. *J Womens Health Gend Based Med*. 2002;11(5):465-476.

20. Olds DL. Prenatal and infancy home visiting by nurses: from randomized trials to community replication. *Prev Sci*. 2002;3(3):153-172.

21. Olds DL, Henderson CR, Kitzman H. Does prenatal and infancy nurse home visitation have enduring effects on qualities of parental caregiving and child health at 25 to 50 months of life? *Pediatrics*. 1994;93(1):89-98.

22. Olds DL, Robinson J, Pettitt L, et al. Effects of home visits by paraprofessionals and by nurses: age 4 follow-up results of a randomized trial. *Pediatrics*. 2004;114(6):1560-1568.

23. Olds DL, Kitzman H, Hanks C, et al. Effects of nurse home visiting on maternal and child functioning: age-9 follow-up of a randomized, controlled trial. *Pediatrics*. 2007;110(4):e832-e845.

24. Olds DL, Eckenrode J, Henderson CR , et al. Long-term effects of home visitation on maternal life course and child abuse and neglect: fifteen-year follow-up of a randomized trial. *JAMA*. 1997;278(8):637-643.

25. Eckenrode J, Ganzel B, Henderson CR, et al. Preventing child abuse and neglect with a program of nurse home visitation: the limiting effects of domestic violence. *JAMA*. 2000;184(11):1385-1391.

26. World Health Organization. *Preventing Intimate Partner And Sexual Violence Against Women: Taking Action And Generating Evidence.* Geneva, Switzerland: WHO; 2010.

27. Donelan-McCall N, Eckenrode J, Olds DL. Home visiting for the prevention of child maltreatment: lessons learned during the past 20 years. *Pediatr Clin North Am*. 2009;56(2):389-403.

28. Bair-Merritt MH, Jennings JM, Chen R, Burrell L, McFarlane E, Fuddy L, Duggan AK. Reducing maternal intimate partner violence after the birth of a child: a randomized, controlled trial of the Hawaii Healthy Start home visitation program. *Arch Pediatr Adolesc Med*. 2010;164(1):16-23.

29. Duggan A, Fuddy L, Burrell L, et al. Randomized trial of a statewide home visiting program to prevent child abuse: impact in reducing parental risk factors. *Child Abuse Negl*. 2004;28(6):623-643.

30. Duggan AK, Caldera D, Rodriguez K, Burrell L, Rohde C, Crowne SS. Impact of a statewide home visiting program to prevent child abuse. *Child Abuse Negl*. 2007;31(8):801-827.

31. Duggan AK, Berlin LJ, Cassidy J, Burrell L, Darius Tandon S. Examining maternal depression and attachment insecurity as moderators of the impacts of home visiting for at-risk mothers and infants. *J Consult Clin Pyschol*. 2009;77(4):788-799.

32. Sullivan CM, Bybee DI. Reducing violence using community-based advocacy for women with abusive partners. *J Consult Clin Psychol.*1999:67(1):43-53.

33. Bybee D, Sullivan CM. Predicting re-victimization of battered women 3 years after exiting a shelter program. *Am J Community Psychol.* 2005;36(1-2):85-96.

34. Eddy T, Kilburn E, Chang C, Bullock L, Sharps P. Facilitators and barriers for implementing home visit interventions to address intimate partner violence: town and gown partnerships. *Nurs Clin N Am*. 2008;43(3):419-435.

35. McDonald R, Jouriles EN, Skopp NA. Reducing conduct problems among children brought to women's shelters: intervention effects 24 months following termination of services. *J Fam Psychol*. 2006;20(1):117-136.

36. Rogge RD, Bradbury TN. Til violence do us part: the differing roles of communication and aggression in predicting adverse marital outcomes. *J Consult Clin Psychol.* 1999;67(3):340-351.

37. Stahman RF, Salts DJ. Educating for marriage and intimate relationships. In: Arcus ME, Schvanevedlt JD, Moss JJ, eds. *The Handbook for Family Life Education.* Vol 2. Newbury, CA: Sage Publications; 1993:33-61.

38. Carroll JS, Doherty WJ. Evaluating the effectiveness of premarital prevention programs: a meta-analytic review of outcome research. *Fam Relat.* 2003;52(2): 105-118.

39. Markman HJ, Renick MJ, Floyd FJ, Stanley SM, Clements M. Preventing marital distress through communication and conflict management training: a 4- and 5-year follow-up. *J Consult Clin Psychol.* 1993;61(1):70-77.

40. Halford WJ, Sanders MR, Behrens BC. Can skills prevent relationship problems in at-risk couples? four-year effects of a behavioral relationship program. *J Consult Psychol.* 2001;15(4):750-768.

41. Langer A, Lawrence E, Barry RA. Using a vulnerability-stress-adaptation framework to predict physical aggression trajectories in newlywed marriage. *J Consult Clin Psychol.* 2008:76(5):756-768.

42. Raiford JL, Wingood GM, DiClemente RJ. Prevalence, incidence, and predictors of dating violence: a longitudinal study of African American female adolescents. *J Women's Health.* 2007;16(6):822-832.

43. Whitaker DJ, Morrison S, Lindquist C, et al. A critical review of interventions for the primary prevention of perpetration of partner violence. *Aggress Violent Behavior.* 2006;11(2):151-166.

44. Wolfe DA, Wekerle C, Scott K, Straatman A, Grasley C, Reitzel-Jaffe D. Dating violence prevention with at-risk youth: a controlled outcome evaluation. *J Consult Clin Psychol.* 2003;71(2):279-291.

45. Foshee VA, Bauman KE, Arriaga XB, Helms RW, Kock GG, Linder GF. An evaluation of Safe Dates, an adolescent dating violence prevention program. *Am J Public Health.* 1998;88(1):45-50.

46. Foshee VA, Bauman KE, Ennett ST, Linder F, Benefield T, Suchindran C. Assessing the long-term effects of the Safe Date Program and a booster in preventing and reducing adolescent dating violence prevention and perpetration. *Am J Public Health.* 2004;94(4):619-624.

47. Foshee VA, Bauman KE, Ennett ST, Suchinran C, Benefield T, Fletcher Linder G. Assessing the effects of dating violence prevention program "Safe Dates" using random coefficient regression modeling. *Prev Sci.* 2005;6(3):245-258.

48. Wolfe DA, Crooks C, Jaffe P, et al. A school-based program to prevent adolescent dating violence: a clustered randomized trial. *Arch Pediatr Adolesc Med.* 2009;163(8):692-699.

49. Campbell J, Soeken K, Kub J, et al. *Evaluation Of "Respect Me": An Arts-Based Dating Violence Prevention Program For Urban Middle School Adolescents.* Unpublished manuscript.

50. Jaycox LH, McCaffrey D, Eiseman B, et al. Impact of a school-based dating violence prevention program among Latino teens: randomized, controlled effectiveness trial. *J Adolesc Health.* 2006;39(5):694-704.

51. Ball B, Kerig PK, Rosenbluth B. "Like a family but better because you can actually trust each other:" the Expect Respect Dating Violence Prevention Program for at-risk youth. *Health Promot Pract.* 2009;10(1):45S-58S.

52. Ball B. *Preliminary Evaluation results for Expect Respect Support Groups: brief report.* Austin, TX: SafePlace; March, 2008.

53. Johnson RL. The National Institutes of Health (NIH) state-of-the-science conference on preventing violence and related health-risking social behaviors in adolescents—a commentary. *J Abnorm Child Psychol.* 2006;34(4):471-474.

54. Elliott DS. *Prevention Programs That Work For Youth: Violence Prevention.* Boulder, CO: Center for the Study of Violence, Institute of Behavioral Science, University of Colorado; 1998.

55. Mihalic SF, Fagan A, Irwin K, Ballad D, Elliott D. *Blueprints for Violence Prevention.* Washington, DC: US Department of Justice, Office of Justice Programs, Office of Juvenile and Delinquency Prevention; 2004.

56. United States Public Health Service and Office of the Surgeon General. *Youth violence: a report of the Surgeon General.* Washington, DC: United States Department of Health and Social Services; 2000.

57. Tobler NS, Roona MR, Ochshom P, Marshall DG, Streke AV, Stackpole KM. School-based adolescent drug prevention programs: 1998 meta-analysis. *J Prim Prev.* 2000;20:275-336.

58. Tobler NS. Lessons learned. *J Prim Prev.* 2000;20:261-274.

59. Reitzel-Jaffe D, Wolfe DA. Predictors of relationship abuse among young men. *J Interpers Violence.* 2001;16(2):99-115.

60. Kingsfogel KM, Grych JH. Interparental conflict and adolescent dating relationships: integrating cognitive, emotional, and peer influences. *J Family Psychol.* 2004;18(3):505-515.

61. McCloskey LA, Lichter EL. The contribution of marital violence to adolescent aggression across different relationships. *J Interpers Violence.* 2003;18(4):390-411.

62. Centers for Disease Control and Prevention. *Sexual violence prevention: beginning the dialogue.* Atlanta, GA: Centers for Disease Control and Prevention; 2004.

63. DeKeseredy WS, Schwartz MD, Alvi S. The role of profeminist men in dealing with women on the Canadian college campus. *Violence Against Women.* 2000;6(9):918-935.

64. Banyard VL, Moynihan MM, Plante EG. Sexual violence prevention through bystander education: an experimental evaluation. *J Community Psychol.* 2007;35(4):463-481.

65. Moynihan MM, Banyard VL, Plante EG. Preventing dating violence—a university example of community approaches. In: Kendall-Tackett KA, Giacomoni SM, ed. *Intimate Partner Violence.* Kingston, NJ: Civic Research Institute; 2007:17-1 to 17-15.

66. Potter SJ, Moynihan MM, Stapleton JG, Banyard VL. Empowering bystanders to prevent campus violence against women: a preliminary evaluation of a poster campaign. *Violence Against Women.* 2009;15(106):106-121.

67. Banyard VL, Plante EG, Moynihan MM. Bystander education: bringing a broader community perspective to sexual violence prevention. *J Community Psychol.* 2004;32(1):61-79.

68. Baynard VL, Plante EG, Moynihan MM. *Rape Prevention Through Bystander Education: Final Report To NIJ For Grant 2002-WG-BX-009.* Durham, NH: University of New Hampshire; 2005.

69. Cavill N, Bauman A. Changing the way people think about health-enhancing physical activity: do mass media campaigns have a role? *J Sport Sci.* 2004;22(8):771-790.

70. Potter SJ, Stapleton JG, Moynihan MM. Designing, implementing, and evaluating a media campaign illustrating the bystander role. *J Prev Interv Community.* 2008;36(1-2):39-55.

71. Katz J. *Mentors in Violence Prevention (MVP) Trainer's Guide.* Boston, MA: Northeastern University Center for the Study of Sport in Society; 1994.

72. Ward KJ. *2000-2001 Mentors in Violence Prevention Evaluation Report.* Boston, MA: Northeastern University; 2001.

73. Green Dot Kentucky Web site. http://www.kdva.org/greendot. Accessed November 20, 2009.

74. Kelly JA. Popular opinion leaders and HIV prevention peer education: resolving discrepant findings, and implications for the development of effective community programmes. *AIDS Care.* 2004;16(2):139-150.

75. Kelly JA, Murphy DA, Sikkema KJ, et al. Randomized, controlled, community-level HIV-prevention intervention for sexual-risk behavior among homosexual men in US cities. *Lancet.* 1997;350:1500-1504.

76. Coker AL, Cook-Craig PG, Williams CM, et al. Evaluation of Green Dot: An active bystander intervention to reduce sexual violence on college campuses. *Violence Against Women.* 2011;17(6):777-796.

77. Barker G. *What About Boys: A Literature Review On The Health And Development Of Adolescent Boys.* Geneva, Switzerland: World Health Organization; 2000. World Health Organization Web site. http://whqlibdoc.who.int/hq/2000/WHO_FCH_CAH_00.7.pdf. Accessed November 19, 2009.

78. World Health Organization. *Engaging Men And boys In Changing Gender-Based Inequity In Health: Evidence From Programme Interventions.* Geneva, Switzerland: World Health Organization; 2007.

79. Marston C, King E. Factors that shape young people's sexual behaviour: a systematic review. *Lancet.* 2006;368(9547):1581-1586.

80. Family Violence Prevention Fund. *Add Council Domestic Violence Prevention Tracking Survey.* San Francisco, CA: Family Violence Prevention Fund; 2005.

81. Dahlber LL, Krug EG. Violence-a global public health problem. In: Krug EG et al, eds. *World report on violence and health.* Geneva, Switzerland: World Health Organization; 2002:3-21.

82. Graffunder CM, Noonan RK, Cox P, Wheaton J. Through a public health lens. Preventing violence against women: an update from the U.S. Centers for Disease Control and Prevention. *J Womens Health.* 2004;13(1):5-16.

83. Nation M, Crusto C, Wandersman A, et al. What works in prevention: principles of effective prevention programs. *Am Psychol.* 2003;58(6-7):449-256.

The World Health Organization, United Nations, and Red Cross: Approaches to Intimate Partner Violence

Kimberly Adams Tufts, DNP, WHNP-BC, FAAN

Key Points

1. Intimate partner violence (IPV) highlights the relationship context of the violence. IPV is violence perpetrated by a current or ex-spouse, or a current or ex-boyfriend or girlfriend.

2. IPV extends beyond the scope of the violent act and can impact physical, psychological, and behavioral well-being.

3. The scope and complexity of IPV requires the multi-sectorial approach provided by international organizations such as the World Health Organization (WHO), United Nations (UN), and Red Cross.

4. The WHO's approach to addressing IPV has been to increase awareness of the impact of IPV, generate scientific evidence about IPV, and develop strategies to prevent IPV.

5. The UN has used various UN agencies and offices to mount a truly creative effort that stresses policy changes, mobilization of various constituencies, and partnering with others, including law enforcement, health officials, school officials, and industry. The UN has generally approached the global issue of IPV as a social, political, and health problem that needs local intervention.

6. The Red Cross asserts that protecting the health and welfare of women via humanitarian efforts is integral to the general welfare of communities. From the Red Cross viewpoint, the prevention of sexual violence during armed conflicts has the potential to prevent IPV.

Introduction

Intimate partner violence (IPV) is a deliberate physical and/or psychological emotional injury[1] visited by one person on another. IPV remains a pervasive public health concern, which has proven to be difficult both to prevent and treat.[2] The term IPV highlights the relationship context of the violence, as IPV is violence perpetrated by a current or ex-spouse, or a current or ex-boyfriend or girlfriend.[3] The impact of IPV extends beyond the scope of the violent act and can impact physical, psychological, and behavioral well-being.[4-6] IPV has been linked to a myriad of social and economic ills including the incidence and prevalence of HIV/AIDS,[7,8] other health problems,[4,9,10] poor childhood adjustment,[6] and loss of days of productivity.[4]

IPV is a global problem. The World Health Organization (WHO) asserts that IPV "occurs in all countries, irrespective of social, economic, religious or cultural group."[11] Although both men and women may be victims of as well as perpetrators of IPV, women most often bear the brunt of IPV.[12] IPV is estimated to affect 1 in 3 women globally.[13] The United States Department of Justice (DOJ) declares that women are 4 times more likely to report incidents of abuse when compared to men.[12] IPV is the leading cause of injury for women ages 15-44.[9] Approximately 65% of victims murdered by intimate partners are women.[14] Homicide that occurs during battering is a leading cause of death for pregnant women.[15] Violence against pregnant women impacts maternal mortality rates in a range of countries including Bangladesh, India, and the United States.[16] Frequently, IPV is the result of gender inequity and gender disparities that result in relationship power differentials.[17,18]

In 2002, the Centers for Disease Control and Prevention (CDC) published a set of standard definitions for types of IPV. This was an attempt to promote consistency of IPV surveillance and to provide a broad sense of the types of IPV. Saltzman, Fanslow, McMahon, and Shelley[19] published comprehensive definitions of IPV (see **Table 12-1**).

Table 12-1. Forms of Intimate Partner Violence[19]

Physical Violence	Sexual Violence	Threat of Physical or Sexual Violence	Psychological/ Emotional Abuse
Physical violence is the intentional use of physical force with the potential for causing death, disability, injury, or harm. Physical violence also includes eliciting others to execute any of these acts. This type of violence includes but is not limited to: — Scratching — Shaking — Pushing — Poking — Shoving — Hair — Throwing pulling — Grabbing — Slapping — Biting — Punching — Choking — Burning — Use of a weapon (gun, knife, or other object) — Use of restraints or one's body, size, or strength against another person	Sexual violence manifests 3 ways: — Use of physical force to compel a person to engage in a sexual act against his or her will. — An attempted or completed sex act involving a person who is unable to understand the nature or condition of the act, or decline participation, (eg, because of illness, disability, or the influence of alcohol or other drugs, or due to intimidation or pressure). —Any sexual behavior perceived as abusive by victim.	Threats include the use of words, gestures, or weapons to communicate the intent to cause death, disability, injury, or physical harm. Also includes the use of words, gestures, or weapons to communicate the intent to compel a person to engage in sex acts or abusive sexual contact when the person is either unwilling or unable to consent.	Psychological and emotional violence may take the form of acts, threats of acts, or coercive tactics. These acts are considered emotionally abusive and traumatic if they are perceived as such by the victim.

A review of Saltzman and colleagues' definitions,[19] underscores that IPV consists of a variety of behaviors and can significantly impact victims and their families.

Consequently, IPV is a complex issue requiring a multi-sectorial approach.[20] Hence, the prevention of IPV has been addressed from a global perspective by leading organizations such as the World Health Organization, United Nations, and the International Red Cross/Red Crescent. Although, all of these organizations have introduced campaigns and created standards for IPV prevention and treatment,[21-23] during the past decade the WHO has been at the forefront of efforts targeted at decreasing the incidence and prevalence of IPV.[4,13,24]

WHO Global Campaign for Violence Prevention

The WHO defines IPV as "any behavior within an intimate relationship that causes physical, psychological or sexual harm to those in the relationship."[25] The WHO's approach to addressing IPV has been to increase awareness of the impact of IPV, generate evidence about IPV, and develop strategies to prevent IPV.

Increasing Awareness and Generating Evidence of IPV

In 2002, the WHO released a landmark report on the worldwide scope of violence; the forms of violence, whom it affects, and the potential for prevention. IPV was one of the most common forms of violence encountered during the WHO assessment.[13] Population-based surveys conducted in 48 countries revealed a lifetime battering rate that ranged from 10% to 69%.[13] In 2005, the WHO presented the results of another WHO study. The study was conducted in 10 countries (N=19 568) across Europe, Asia, and South America.[26] A reported association between a partner's controlling behavior and physical and/or sexual violence was found across all study sites. In addition, there was a positive association between current or previous IPV and negative effects on physical, sexual, and mental health. The WHO reported a strong association between ever experiencing IPV and of an array of self-reported health problems, including memory loss, challenges with activities of daily living, and pain.[27] As a result of the findings from this descriptive study, the WHO concluded that there was a need for further research exploration of several issues: (1) potential determinants, or predisposing and protective factors for IPV; (2) an in-depth analysis of the relationship between violence and health outcomes; (3) risk profiles for perpetrators; and (4) exploration and development of standardized definitions for emotional abuse.

The WHO also released recommendations that address the strengthening of national response and commitment, promote primary prevention, involve the education sector, enlist the assistance of the health sector, and underscore the need for research collaboration. Their recommendations are listed below[26(pp91-97)]:

1. Promote gender equality and women's human rights, and compliance with international agreements.

2. Establish, implement, and monitor multi-sectorial action plans to address violence against women.

3. Enlist social, political, religious, and other leaders in speaking out against violence against women.

4. Enhance capacity for data collection to monitor violence against women and the attitudes and beliefs that perpetuate it.

5. Develop, implement, and evaluate programs aimed at primary prevention of intimate-partner violence and sexual violence.

6. Prioritize the prevention of child sexual abuse.

7. Integrate responses to violence against women into existing programs such as for the prevention of HIV and AIDS and for the promotion of adolescent health.

8. Make physical environments safer for women.

9. Make schools safe for girls.

10. Develop a comprehensive health sector response to the various impacts of violence against women.

11. Use the potential of reproductive health services as entry points for identifying women in abusive relationships and for delivering referral and support services.

12. Support research on the causes, consequences, and costs of violence against women and on effective prevention measures.

These recommendations set the stage for the WHO's IPV-related activities over the course of the next 7 to 8 years. Thus, over the next several years, the WHO released a number of publications, aimed at increasing international awareness of IPV and its resultant societal ills (see **Table 12-2**). These publications highlighted less than optimal family function, poor health outcomes, and IPV's impact on the economy,[4,11,26] and presented exemplars of potentially effective interventions.[24,28,29]

Table 12-2. Chronology of WHO Intimate Partner Violence Publications *(continued)*

TITLE OF PUBLICATION	YEAR PUBLISHED	FOCUS OF PUBLICATION
World Report on Violence and Health http://www.who.int/violence_injury_ prevention/violence/world_report/en/	2002	Detailed results of a 48 country assessment of the incidence and prevalence of IPV
Guidelines for Medico-Legal Care for Victims of Sexual Violence http://whqlibdoc.who.int/ publications/2004/924154628X.pdf	2003	Standards for the provision of both health care and forensic services to victims of sexual violence
WHO Multi-Country Study on Women's Health and Domestic Violence Against Women: Initial Results on Prevalence, Health Outcomes, and Women's Responses http://www.who.int/gender/violence/ who_multicountry_study/en/index.html	2005	Preliminary results of 10 country study of prevalence of IPV, impact of IPV on health outcomes, and factors that put women at risk for IPV
Primary Prevention of Intimate-Partner Violence and Sexual Violence: Background Paper for WHO Expert Meeting May 2–3, 2007 http://www.who.int/violence_injury_ prevention/publications/violence/IPV-SV.pdf	2007	Underscores strategies for reducing new instances of IPV and identifies protective factors for intimate-partner violence, and/or sexual violence, and action to address those factors

(continued)

Table 12-2. Chronology of WHO Intimate Partner Violence Publications *(continued)*

TITLE OF PUBLICATION	YEAR PUBLISHED	FOCUS OF PUBLICATION
Intimate Partner Violence and Women's Physical and Mental Health in the WHO Multi-Country Study on Women's Health and Domestic Violence: An Observational Study Lancet. 2008;371(9619):1165-1172.	2008	Summarizes the results of a 10-country study that focused on IPV's impact of women's mental and physical health status
Violence Prevention the Evidence: Promoting Gender Equality http://whqlibdoc.who.int/publications /2009/9789241597883_eng.pdf	2009	Examines the relationship between gender roles and violence; highlights a 3- pronged approach for violence prevention
Violence Prevention the Evidence: Changing Cultural and Social Norms that Support Violence http://www.who.int/violence_injury_ prevention/violence/norms.pdf	2009	Highlights interventions that challenge cultural and social norms that support violence
Preventing Intimate Partner and Sexual Violence Against Women: Taking Action and Generating Evidence http://whqlibdoc.who.int/ publications/2010/9789241564007_eng.pdf	2010	Provide evidenced-based information for policy makers and planners to facilitate the development of data-driven and evidence-based programs for preventing IPV and sexual violence against women

DEVELOPING PREVENTION STRATEGIES

In the third milestone report, the WHO Secretary General declared that the WHO's role must change from that of "advocacy, normative guidance and the planting of programme seeds in many countries…to scaled-up country level implementation, accompanied by a concerted effort to measure the effectiveness of interventions using the outcomes that really matter – rates of violence-related deaths, non-fatal injuries and other violence-related health conditions."[4] Hence, the WHO released a 2010 report entitled "Preventing Intimate Partner and Sexual Violence Against Women: Taking Action and Generating Evidence." This groundbreaking report classifies the evidence related to IPV prevention and intervention. The WHO taxonomy for evidence-based classification is listed below:

1. Effective: strategies which include 1 or more programs demonstrated to be effective as supported by multiple well-designed studies focused on the prevention of and/or the experience of intimate partner violence;

2. Emerging evidence of effectiveness: strategies which include 1 or more programs for which evidence of effectiveness is emerging due to the implementation of a rigorous intervention study that focused on prevention of and /or the experience of intimate partner violence. Emerging evidence can also refer to studies that show positive changes in knowledge, attitudes and beliefs;

3. Effectiveness unclear: strategies which include 1 or more programs of unclear effectiveness due to insufficient or mixed evidence;

4. Emerging evidence of ineffectiveness: strategies which include 1 or more programs for which evidence of ineffectiveness is emerging as regards to the prevention of intimate partner violence and/or changes in knowledge, attitudes and beliefs;

5. Ineffective: these strategies include 1 or more programs shown to be ineffective when analyzed by trialed in multiple well-designed studies related to intimate partner violence;

6. Probably harmful: there is at least 1 well-designed study that found an increase in perpetration and/or experiencing of intimate partner and/or sexual violence or negative changes in knowledge, attitudes and beliefs.[24])

In addition to interventions being evidence-based, the WHO asserts that IPV prevention strategies must take a 3-pronged comprehensive approach; including school-based interventions, community-based approaches, and media programming.[28]

School-Based Interventions

School-based interventions must be directed at adolescents and young adults in order to impact attitudes and beliefs before they are deeply engrained. The WHO suggests that such interventions speak to gender norms, dating violence, and sexual abuse.[28] When discussing the state of the evidence, the WHO declares that only a select few school-based programs that focus on the prevention of violence within dating relationships can be classified as effective. In *Violence Prevention the Evidence: Promoting Gender Equality To Prevent Violence Against Women*,[28] the WHO highlights several effective school-based programs (see **Table 12-3**) that may be used as exemplars for those considering implementing IPV prevention programming for adolescents and young adults. The WHO stresses that the state of the science is such that most evaluations of these programs are taking place in the United States (US) and other high-income countries, yet there is a need to conduct rigorous evaluations in developing countries. Evidence-based programs must be adapted for use in developing countries with the caveat that well designed evaluation procedures must be integrated into all prevention programming,[24] including community-based programming.

Community-Based Interventions

Support of community-based programming is essential to the WHO approach to addressing IPV, due to the WHO perspective that IPV is often a result of gender inequities and cultural norms regarding male and female societal roles.[26] The WHO brings attention to community-based programming as a normative guidance strategy.

Community-based programs that provide economic resources to women have often been supported by the WHO, including microfinance schemes. South Africa's Intervention with Microfinance for AIDS and Gender Equity (IMAGE) is an example of such a program. This program targets male and female rural populations, combining financial services with information on HIV prevention, cultural norms for gender roles, and IPV prevention.[33] IMAGE aims to positively increase women's influence in their households and to teach them conflict resolution skills. IMAGE has been formally evaluated via a randomized controlled trial; women who participated in IMAGE reported fewer incidents of physical violence and controlling behaviors. Other community-based programs that have been highlighted by the WHO include Uganda's Raising Voices and Centre for Domestic Violence Prevention initiatives and Nicaragua's Mi Familia.[24,34] The focus of these community-based interventions is to facilitate a change in social norms and values. Media interventions can also be used to impact community-based social norms and values.

Table 12-3. School-based IPV Prevention Programs: Highlighted by WHO

Program	Program Description	Age of Participants	Gender of Participants	Country of Implementation	Evidence
Safe Dates	10-session curriculum, educational theatre, and support for affected teens	13-15	Male and female	USA	Randomized controlled trial; participants reported less physical and psychological violence against a significant other 1 month after participation and 4 years later.[29]
Youth Relationships Project	Educational sessions highlighting the difference between healthy and abusive relationships, conflict resolution, and communication skills and social action activities	14-16	Male and female	Canada	Randomized controlled; concluded that intervention had a positive effect, ie, a reduction of incidents of physical and emotional abuse and symptoms of emotional distress during the 16-month follow-up period.
The Men's Program	College-based rape prevention program targeted at increasing empathy for rape survivors; changing attitudes and behavioral intent related to committing rape or sexual assault	19-21	Male	USA	Two years later, 79% of participants report an attitudinal or behavioral change.[30]
Safe Dates	10-session curriculum, educational theatre, and support for affected teens	13-14	Male and female	South Africa	Evaluation in progress
The Fourth R: Skills for Youth Relationships	21-session, peer-based curriculum; focused on developing positives strategies for conflict resolution	14-15	Male and female	Canada	Decreased rates of dating related physical violence reported by male participants[32]

Media Interventions

The WHO has tracked and highlighted IPV-related media interventions that are designed to alter social norms, provide information, change attitudes, and alter behaviors.[28] Media interventions encompass TV, newsprint, radio, magazines, and the internet. The WHO states that the most effective media interventions are those that initially assess the behaviors of the intended audience and collaborates with audience members during the development of the intervention.[4] One such example is *Series #4*, a TV and radio series from South Africa. *Series #4* was developed by Soul City Institute for Health and Development Communication; it highlights IPV issues and is accompanied by information brochures that are distributed throughout the country.[35] A formal evaluation of the program concluded that changes in attitudes about IPV were associated with exposure to the Soul City series; ie, there was a 10% increase in respondents who disagreed that IPV was a private affair.[36]

Some media interventions specifically target men; Violence against Women–It's Against All the Rules is an example of this type of program. Based in Australia, this media intervention featured anti-IPV messages delivered by sports figures. These athletes stressed that violence is not masculine and that violence against women is never tolerable.[37] However, the WHO declares that most media interventions as well as school-based and community-based interventions have not been rigorously evaluated. Hence, no intervention should be replicated without an integration of evaluations procedures into program implementation.

The WHO puts forth that the magnitude of IPV must be accurately measured and that standardized definitions must be consistently used by institutions to report cases of IPV and used as operational definitions during the implementation of research; therefore, standardized definitions for IPV and accurate measurers of IPV must be incorporated into any program evaluation. Hence, the WHO has generated operational definitions to be used in surveillance, monitoring, and when conducting research studies (see **Table 12-4**).[26]

The WHO has also stressed that intervention with and prevention of IPV must also specifically address cultural and social norms. Interestingly, the WHO has stated that, although men may be victims of IPV and women may be perpetrators of relationship violence, IPV against men most often happens in countries with more equalized gender relationships.[4] Thus, given that most societies still support power differentials between men and women as cultural and social norms, women continue to experience higher rates of IPV victimization. For that reason, WHO has brought to light many of the cultural and social norms that create environments that put women at risk for violence.[29] Examples include beliefs that: a) violence is an acceptable way to resolve conflict with one's partner (eg, in South Africa); b) a woman is responsible for the success of a marriage (eg, in Israel); c) a man is socially superior to a women (eg, in Nigeria, India, and Ghana); d) a man has a right to discipline a woman (eg, in China); and e) a woman's sexual behavior can affect a man's honor (eg, in Jordan).[29] The WHO proclaims that effective interventions against IPV must address entrenched beliefs and social norms that support gender inequities as well as engage all sectors of society to rectify the resultant inequality that place women at risk for IPV.[28]

The WHO has brought attention to several initiatives that have focused on changing cultural and social norms. In the 2009 publication on changing cultural and social norms that support violence, it features a US-based organization, Men of Strength Clubs. This organization has implemented the Men Can Stop Rape program. This program aims to teach male youth that men can prevent violence against women. The program emphasizes alternative views of male masculinity and stresses that youth can

Table 12-4. WHO Operational definitions for Measuring IPV: Physical and Sexual Violence, Emotional Abuse, and Controlling Behaviors

PHYSICAL VIOLENCE	SEXUAL VIOLENCE	EMOTIONAL ABUSE	CONTROLLING BEHAVIORS
Moderate			
Slapped or had something thrown at her that could hurt her Pushed, or shoved, or had hair pulled	Physically forced to have sexual intercourse when she did not want to Had sexual intercourse when she did not want to because she was afraid of what partner might do	Insulted or made to feel bad about herself Belittled or humiliated in front of other people	Kept her from seeing friends Restricted contact with her family of birth
Severe			
Hit with fist or something else that could hurt Kicked, dragged, or beaten up Choked or burnt on purpose Partner threatened to use or actually used a gun, knife, or other weapon against her	Forced to do something sexual that she found degrading or humiliating	Partner did things to scare or intimidate her on purpose, eg, by the way he looked at her, yelling, or smashing things Partner threatened to hurt someone she cared about	Partner insisted on knowing where she was at all times Partner ignored her and treated her indifferently Partner got angry if she spoke with another man Partner often suspicious that she was unfaithful Partner expected her to ask permission before seeking health care for herself

build relationships with women that are built on gender equity.[38] The WHO also brought attention to a Centers for Disease Control and Prevention initiative, called Choose Respect. This national initiative targets young adolescents (ages 11-14) with the purpose of motivating them to challenge harmful ideas about dating violence and giving them strategies for developing healthy dating relationships.[39] The WHO 2009 publication[29] also featured an Australian television and radio campaign intended for perpetrators and potential perpetrators of IPV. Called Freedom From Fear, the campaign featured messages that stressed the impact that IPV has on children and called on perpetrators to be accountable for their behavior, encouraging them to access a telephone helpline if needed.[40] Although the WHO states that the Freedom From Fear campaign was formally evaluated, the WHO continues to emphasize that most programs are not evaluated and that formalized mechanisms for conducting research on IPV interventions and prevention strategies must be widely implemented.

SEXUAL VIOLENCE RESEARCH INITIATIVE

The WHO's leadership regarding the necessity of conducting rigorous evaluations of IPV interventions and prevention strategies has led to the establishment of the Sexual

Violence Research Initiative *(http://www.svri.org)*. The Sexual Violence Research Initiative (SVRI) aims to address the lack of research on sexual violence, to generate empirical data that will bring the attention of media and policy makers to this specific component of IPV, moving IPV, including sexual violence, out of the arena of the private sphere to status as a high priority public health problem.[41] This is especially important because knowledge of what constitutes effective provision of health services for victims of sexual violence is limited, particularly in developing lands. The SVRI is housed in South Africa. The SVRI also engages in capacity-building activities that increase the research skills of workshop participants. The SVRI Web site highlights a successful research workshop that was facilitated by the SVRI, wherein 19 participants from around the globe learned about various research methods including the use of qualitative methods to explore women's responses to IPV and using court records for research purposes, among others. Recent SVRI-sponsored research studies include a review of effective service models, an appraisal of sexual violence legislation, and a state of affairs analysis of medico-legal services in selected developing countries.[29] The WHO states that knowledge gleaned from the SVRI will be used to inform policy-making. Yet, according to the WHO, research regarding IPV has to move beyond just SVRI efforts to generate evidence about effective prevention and intervention strategies for sexual violence. Research must address all aspects of IPV including health related issues, protective factors, factors that place women at risk for IPV, the impact of IPV on the economic welfare of communities, and the long term impact of IPV on children and families. Only when there exists a well-established, data-driven, and evidence-based repository of resources for high income, middle income, and low income countries will health professionals, communities, and policy-makers be able to effectively address IPV from a global perspective.

The WHO has taken on a primary leadership role regarding IPV and has worked to bring a global perspective to the issue of IPV. The WHO consistently highlights the best examples of IPV intervention and prevention, from programs that have focused on violence prevention from a particular perspective, such as human rights or criminal justice reform, to those which focus on a specific sector or level of administration (ie, at the local, national, regional, or international level). Notably, the WHO has reported both on programs that were directly dependent on WHO support and on programs that were more or less independent of WHO assistance.[4] In summary, the WHO's pervasive and targeted global focus on the prevention of IPV, as well as on the care and treatment of victims of IPV, has resulted in other international organizations taking up the mantle against IPV, including the United Nations.

UNITED NATIONS: UNiTE TO END VIOLENCE

In 2008, the United Nations Secretary General, launched the UNiTE to End Violence against Women campaign. The United Nations (UN) campaign calls on parties from all sectors of society, including private industry, civil society, governments, women organizations, and young people to come together to address violence, particularly violence against women. Like the WHO, the UN asserts that IPV is a global problem impacting the lives of women cross-continentally. The UN Web site features statistics on IPV from Africa, Asia, Australia, Europe, and the Americas.[23] The UN declares that early marriage is a form of sexual violence exposing young girls to health problems such as uro-gynecological fistulas, poor sexual functioning, and the risk of HIV infection. The United Nations concludes that the economic viability of these girls and their families is adversely impacted due to decreased school attendance. The UN Web site draws attention to the fact that in many lands honor killings are used to punish women for real and imagined moral violations. The United Nations Population Fund (UNFPA) concludes that each year approximately 5 000 women die due to honor killings. The UN states that IPV clearly impacts the lives of women across the globe, hampering their potential for a better quality of life. Hence, the UN proposes that the following goals be realized globally by 2015[42]:

1. Adopt and enforce national laws to address and punish all forms of violence against women and girls.

2. Adopt and implement multi-sectorial national action plans.

3. Strengthen data collection on the prevalence of violence against women and girls.

4. Increase public awareness and social mobilization.

5. Address sexual violence in conflict.

The UN published a benchmarking document, entitled, "Unite to End Violence Against Women, Framework for Action: Programme of United Nations Activities and Expected Outcomes, 2008-2015."[43] This document sets forth the UN's key objectives in combating violence against women (ie, raise awareness, reduce prevalence, create supportive environments, etc.), a broad framework for action, and measurable outcomes for the campaign.

The UN has substantially invested in their campaign against IPV as evidenced by charging multiple UN offices and agencies to work together to collaborate on the UN's approach to preventing IPV. Those charged to work together to achieve these goals include the Office of the High Commissioner for Human Rights, the Inter-Agency Network on Women and Gender Equality, the United Nations Children's Fund (UNICEF), and UNFPA, among others.[44] The Secretary General of the UN has taken a leadership role related to ending violence against women. In 2010, Ban Ki-moon, the Secretary General, continued to call for action from diverse sectors of the community. In an UN-sponsored speech marking the occasion of the International Day for the Elimination of Violence Against Women, he stressed that corporations must also take a stand against IPV and to actively come to the table bringing funds and other resources. Under the leadership of the Ban Ki-moon, the UN set up the UN Trust Fund in Support of Actions to Eliminate Violence against Women and established an annual goal of $100 million to support projects. The fund is currently funded at just $20 million dollars, yet there are some 26 projects underway in 33 countries and territories.[45]

Broadly speaking, the UN's approach to addressing IPV is three-fold: a) influencing laws and policies; b) mobilizing various constituencies to take a stand regarding IPV; and c) partnering with others to develop and implement strategies.[46]

INFLUENCING LAWS AND POLICIES

As regards influencing laws and policies, the UN has taken a multilateral approach; for example in the area of family law, the UN Development Fund for Women (UNFEM) has supported the passage of several laws against domestic and sexual violence as well as rape in several countries, including Zimbabwe, Vietnam, and Columbia. Recognizing the role of sexual violence in the Rwandan genocide, the UN Development program provided substantial support to female parliamentarians who then drafted legislation criminalizing gender-based violence.[46] The UN has carried out research for the purposes of shaping policy by conducting surveys on violence against women and using the results to influence policy decisions. Accordingly, the UN used research conducted in Jamaica to provide data for that country's national anti-violence action plan. The UN partnered with community partners and local governments to create the global "Virtual Knowledge Centre to End Violence against Women and Girls," for the purpose of helping advocates influence policy. The information available from the Centre can be accessed in over 50 languages and contains more than 700 tools to help those interested in shaping law and policy, including a detailed guide on how to develop legislation.[47]

MOBILIZING AGENCIES AND COMMUNITIES AGAINST IPV

In addition to directly working to influence laws and policies, the UN aims to mobilize others to take a stand against violence. In Asia and the Pacific Rim, the UN organized a multi-agency initiative (UNDP, UNFPA, and UNIFEM) called Partners for Prevention: Working with Boys and Men to Prevent Gender-based Violence. This project is a public awareness campaign that focuses on mobilizing boys and men to do more to prevent violence, reaching them through campaigns that are presented in their local languages.[46] The UN has also utilized art forms to mobilize others around the issue of IPV. Recently the UN produced *Congo /Women: Portraits of War,* a photographic exhibit. The purpose of the exhibit was to raise awareness about violence against women. Although the use of violence as a tool of war is not explicitly IPV, often women who are raped or sexually assaulted during war become victims of IPV, due to the resultant social ostracism from family members and significant others. This exhibit was shown throughout the United States. Currently, the photographic exhibit, along with people's reactions to seeing it, can be accessed online at *http://www.unfpa.org/congowomen/.*

Creating community-based dialogue has also been used by UN agencies to mobilize specific populations around IPV. For example, the UNDP assisted Cambodian village facilitators with the organization of community conversations that focused on the social and legal ramifications of IPV. Approximately 2500 Cambodian villagers participated in these discussions.[46] In addition, UNICEF partnered with the South Africa Development Fund to sponsor the One Man Can campaign.[46] This campaign was produced by Sonke Gender Justice with the purpose of increasing awareness about the scope and consequences of IPV and to provide resources to men who want to take action against IPV. In addition to locally-based mobilization efforts, such as the Cambodian Village Project and One Man Can, the UN makes use of strategies with broader spheres of influence, such as the internet, to bring increased awareness to the issues of IPV. One such example is Say No—Unite to End Violence Against Women (www.saynotoviolence.org), a social mobilization Web site. This Web site uses social networking (ie, Facebook) to showcase IPV advocacy efforts. In addition, in 2009, the UN released a "global one stop shopping" database for those who are seeking information about issues related to IPV (http://sgdatabase.unwomen.org/home. action). This database contains extensive resources for victims and their families, model legislation and awareness raising strategies for policy-makers and advocates, statistics on the scope of the problem, and a summary of the criminal justice response.

PARTNERING WITH LOCAL COMMUNITIES

The UN also approaches the prevention and treatment of IPV by partnering with other advocacy groups, including law enforcement, health care workers, and school officials. The UN sees the engagement of local law enforcement as an essential factor in protecting women from IPV and as an effective strategy for successful intervention when IPV does occurs. In concert with this point of view, UNIFEM supported education about violence against women for Nigerian policemen.[46] The UN has also provided assistance and training to health care workers in several countries. Examples include sensitivity training for workers in Russia, Lebanon, Nepal, and Ecuador, among others.[46] The UN has capitalized on school officials' opportunity to intervene with children and to affect their attitudes about IPV early on. Thus, UNICEF has garnered the assistance of football coaches by providing materials about IPV and asking football coaches to discuss the consequences of violence against girls and women with their players.[45] Recently, the UN capitalized on the global window of opportunity that the 2010 World Cup in South Africa provided. The UN used the occasion to put the topic of violence on center stage, generating the worldwide release of the *Breakaway* videogame. This videogame uses football as a platform to speak to violence against women, asking "will you follow the popular path or breakaway?" *(http://www.breakawaygame.com/).*

Taking the perspective that IPV can and will take place in all settings, the UN has continued to be creative about who to partner with and in what settings, including during times of armed conflict and natural disasters with populations who are experiencing displacement. Hence, in Liberia the UN refugee agency (UNHCR) partnered with local offices to develop a community health center. Sexual and gender-based violence training was a component of the core training provided to community health workers. UNFPA stressed the importance of addressing violence against women among the survivors of 2010 floods in Pakistan, stating that women and girls are often more vulnerable to violence during times of crisis. UNFPA provided financial and technical support to those providing health care to victims of violence.[48]

In summary, the UN has undertaken a multilateral approach to intervening with IPV. The UN has used various UN agencies and offices to mount a truly creative effort that stresses policy changes; mobilization of various constituencies; and partnering with others, including law enforcement, health officials, school officials, and industry. The UN has generally approached the global issue of IPV as a social, political, and health problem that needs local intervention. This is in contrast to the International Red Cross; the Red Cross primarily takes a humanitarian perspective to addressing violence against women.

INTERNATIONAL RED CROSS/RED CRESCENT: A HUMANITARIAN APPROACH

The International Red Cross/Red Crescent (Red Cross) has taken a rather broad approach to addressing violence against women. They take a humanitarian perspective on violence prevention as well as institute-specific programs aimed at preventing and intervening with IPV.

The Red Cross also approaches the issue of violence against women through a humanitarian lens, specifically making statements about their commitment to addressing violence against women that occurs during times of war or armed conflict, vowing to protect women and girls since they are particularly vulnerable to assaults and sexual violence in conflict situations.[49] The Red Cross uses a rights-based approach that is framed by International Humanitarian Law (IHL), advocating for nations to ensure a woman's right to be free from violence and coercive acts. In 1999, the ICRC committed to addressing the special needs of women and girls, specifically with a focus on sexual violence.[22] The Red Cross supports UN Security Council Resolution 1325 on women, peace, and security.[50,51] This resolution calls on all parties to undertake concerted efforts to protect women and girls from all forms of violence, including sexual violence, during times of conflict. The Red Cross asserts that protecting the health and welfare of women via humanitarian efforts is integral to the general welfare of communities. Women often play an essential part in rebuilding communities once a conflict has been resolved.[52] The Red Cross acknowledges that a woman's role in rebuilding her community may be stunted due to the social ostracism and IPV that often follows sexual violence that occurred during an armed conflict. The following broad strategies are used by the Red Cross to address violence against women and girls: a) promoting adherence to IHL by all nation states; b) stressing the importance of nation states engaging in prevention of sexual violence in times of conflict rather than waiting to react to incidences of sexual violence; and c) using the humanitarian platform as a mechanism for raising awareness about IPV, including sexual violence.

Thus, from the Red Cross viewpoint, the prevention of sexual violence during armed conflicts has the potential to prevent IPV. However, Horn[53] conducted a focus group study that focused on the nature and consequences of IPV with 157 male and female refugees residing in a refugee camp in north-west Kenya and she reported that from the perspective of the refugees, only the most serious or intransigent case of IPV received the attention of the UN or its implementing agencies during times of armed conflict or displacement. Refugees reported that there was hierarchy of responses to reported IPV cases. These reports were triaged, and only the most severe cases reach the UN High Commission for Refugees; hence, they perceived the UN to be ineffective. Horn concluded that, although large-scale community-based responses such as those proposed by the Red Cross might often be useful, the findings from her study suggested that they do not necessarily result in protection of women. This may suggest that the Red Cross should consider expanding programs such as the Canadian RespectED to multiple nations, in addition to its multi-national humanitarian efforts.

RESPECTED

For the last 30 years, the Canadian Red Cross has provided violence prevention programming under the umbrella of RespectED. RespectED shines a light on violence prevention, focusing on preventing child maltreatment, family violence, emotional abuse, and dating violence. Two programs are structured around the prevention of intimate partner violence, It's Not Your Fault and What's Love Got To Do With It. It's Not Your Fault is designed for youths aged 12 and above; it uses case studies, video games, and interactive discussions to teach about emotional, physical, and sexual abuse.[54] What's Love Got To Do With It is aimed at students in secondary school ages 14 and older. This program uses group work to explore adolescents' general experiences with violence as well as issues of intimate partner violence.[55] This type of programming is specifically aimed at educating potential perpetrators and victims of IPV about the consequences of violence and how to prevent it.

CONCLUSION

IPV is a pattern of coercive behavior in which an individual establishes and maintains power and control over someone with whom he or she has a current or previous relationship.[55] IPV affects all people who are touched by it, including children who witness it.[56,57] IPV results in short-term and long-term health consequences for those affected by it.[58-60] IPV may also impact the economic welfare of victims, including lost days of productivity.[61] Hence, IPV is a global public health problem that requires a multi-faceted approach.

The WHO, United Nations, and Red Cross have each taken such an approach, assuming a leadership role, and setting the pace for national, regional, and local communities regarding the development of IPV prevention and intervention strategies. The WHO has taken a very comprehensive public health approach to intervening with IPV.[62] They have conducted studies that defined and measured the scope of the problem, identified risk and protection factors for IPV, conducted evaluations of IPV intervention, and disseminated information about effective strategies for preventing and intervening with IPV. The WHO has provided technical and monetary support to parties on 6 of 7 continents, stressing that a three-fold approach of using school-based, community-based, and media interventions must be undertaken. The WHO has also emphasized that rigorous evaluations of interventions and programming must be conducted as part of any planned implementation before these strategies should be replicated. The United Nations' approach has underscored that one size does not fit all, that local approaches to solutions are best. In this vein, the United Nations has used the resources of multiple United Nations agencies and affiliates to support on the ground approaches to intervening, partnering with local law enforcement, health care professionals, community leaders, and school officials. For the Red Cross, IPV is primarily seen via a humanitarian lens, takes the form of sexual violence, and often occurs in the midst of or as a result of larger conflicts such as wars and ethnic cleansings. A review of all 3 approaches emphasizes that all are relevant to successfully preventing IPV and to effectively intervening when it does occur. Thus, all who desire to intervene with this difficult issue may well benefit from reviewing the various approaches of these global organizations.

REFERENCES

1. Association of State and Territorial Health Officials. Injury prevention fact sheet – intimate partner violence. 2006. http://www.astho.org/pubs/IPVfactsheet.pdf Accessed April 25, 2011

2. Anderson JE, Abraham M, Bruessow DM, et al. Cross-cultural perspectives on intimate partner violence. J *Am Acad Physician Assistants*. April 2008;21(4)36-44.

3. Centers for Disease Control and Prevention. Intimate partner violence: definitions. Centers for Disease Control and Prevention Web site. http://www.cdc.gov/ViolencePrevention/intimatepartnerviolence/definitions.html. Published September 20, 2010. Accessed November 1, 2010.

4. Harvey A, Garcia-Moreno C, Butchart A. Primary prevention of intimate partner violence and sexual violence: background paper for WHO expert meeting May 2-3, 2007. http://www.who.int/violence_injury_prevention/publications/violence/IPV-SV.pdf. Published May 2007. Accessed December 16, 2010

5. Campbell R, Greeson MR, Bybee D, Raja S. The co-occurrence of childhood sexual abuse, adult sexual assault, intimate partner violence, and sexual harassment: a mediational model of posttraumatic stress disorder and physical health outcomes. *J Consult Clin Psychol*. 2008;76(2):194–207.

6. Graham-Bermann SA, Perkins S. Effects of early exposure and lifetime exposure to intimate partner violence (IPV) on child adjustment. *Violence Vict*. 2010;25(4):427-439.

7. Silverman JG, Decker MR, Saggurti N, Balaiah D, Raj A. Intimate partner violence and HIV infection among married Indian women. *JAMA*. 2008;300(6):703-710.

8. Tufts KA, Clements PT, Wessell J. When intimate partner violence against women and HIV collide: challenges for healthcare assessment and intervention. *J Forensic Nurs*. 2010;6(2):66-73

9. Centers for Disease Control and Prevention. Violence and reproductive health. Centers for Disease Control and Prevention Web site. http://www.cdc.gov/reproductivehealth/violence/index.htm. Published February 25, 2009. Accessed November 10, 2010.

10. Lafta RK. Intimate-partner violence and women's health. *Lancet*. 2008;371(9619): 1140-1422.

11. World Health Organization (WHO). Global campaign for violence prevention. World Health Organization Web site. http://www.who.int/violence injury prevention/violence/global campaign/en. Accessed May 22, 2013.

12. Catalano S, Smith E, Snyder H, Rand M. Female victims of violence: Bureau of Justice statistics selected findings. Bureau of Justice Statistics Web site. http://bjs.gov/content/pub/pdf/fvv.pdf. Published October 23, 2009. Accessed May 22, 2013.

13. Krug EG, Dahlberg LL, Mercy JA, Zwi AB, Lozazno R, eds. *World Report on Violence and Health.* Geneva, Switzerland: World Health Organization; 2002. http://www.who.int/violence_injury_prevention/violence/world_report/en/.

14. Fox J, Zawitz M. Homicide trends in the United States. Bureau of Justice Statistics Web site. http://www.bjs.gov/content/pub/pdf/htius.pdf . Published July 1, 2007. Accessed May 22, 2013.

15. Chang J, Berg JB, Saltzman LE, Herndon J. Homicide: a leading cause of injury deaths among pregnant and postpartum women in the United States, 1991–1999. *Am J Public Health.* 2005;95(3):471–477.

16. Garcia-Moreno C, Heise L, Jansen HA, Ellsberg M, Watts C. Public health: violence against women. *Science.* 2005; 310(5752):1282–1283.

17. Germain A. With women worldwide: a compact to end HIV/AIDS. Presented at the meeting of Physician for Human Rights; February 2008; Washington, DC.

18. Nagae M, Dancy BL. Japanese women's perceptions of intimate partner violence (IPV). *J Interpers Violence.* 2010;25(4):753-766.

19. Saltzman LE, Fanslow JL, McMahon PM, Shelley GA; Centers for Disease Control and Prevention. Intimate partner violence surveillance: uniform definitions and recommended data elements, version 1.0. Centers for Disease Control and Prevention Web site. http://www.cdc.gov/ncipc/pub-res/ipv_surveillance/Intimate%20 Partner%20Violence.pdf. Published 2002. Accessed May 22, 2013.

20. International Committee of the Red Cross. Women and war: the ICRC's response. International Committee of the Red Cross Web site. http://www.icrc.org/eng/ resources/documents/misc/women-icrc-response-020307.htm. Published February 3, 2007. Accessed May 22, 2013.

21. Lindsey-Curtet C, Holst-Roness FT, Anderson L. *Addressing the needs of women in armed conflict: An ICRC guidance document.* Geneva, Switzerland: International Committee of the Red Cross; 2007.

22. United Nations. United Nations secretary general's campaign to end violence against women, the situation. United Nations Web site. http://www.un.org/en/women/ endviolence/situation.shtml. Published 2010. Accessed November 11, 2010.

23. World Health Organization, London School of Hygiene and Tropical Medicine. *Preventing Intimate Partner and Sexual Violence Against Women: Taking Action and Generating Evidence.* Geneva: World Health Organization; 2010.

24. Heise L, Garcia-Moreno C. Intimate partner violence. In: Krug et al, eds. *World Report on Violence and Health.* Geneva: World Health Organization; 2002:87-122.

25. Garcia-Moreno C, Jansen HA, Ellsberg M, Heise L, Watts C. *WHO Multi-Country Study on Women's Health and Domestic Violence Against Women: Initial Results on Prevalence, Health Outcomes and Women's Responses.* Geneva: World Health Organization; 2005. World Health Organization Web site. http://www.who.int/ gender/violence/who_multicountry_study/en/. Accessed October 16, 2010.

26. Ellsberg M, Jansen HA, Heise L, Watts CH, Garcia-Moreno C; WHO Multi-country Study on Women's Health and Domestic Violence against Women Study Team. Intimate partner violence and women's physical and mental health in the WHO Multi-Country Study on women's health and domestic violence: an observational study. *Lancet.* 2008;371(9619):1165-1172.

27. World Health Organization. Violence prevention the evidence: Promoting gender equality to prevent violence against women. World Health Organization Web site. http://whqlibdoc.who.int/publications/2009/9789241597883_eng.pdf. Published 2009. Accessed November 08, 2010

28. World Health Organization. Violence prevention the evidence: changing cultural and social norms that support violence. World Health Organization Web site. http://www.who.int/violence_injury_prevention/violence/norms.pdf. Published 2009. Accessed December 17, 2010.

29. Foshee VA, Bauman KE, Ennett ST, Linder GF, Benefield T, Suchindran C. Assessing the long-term effects of the Safe Dates program and a booster in preventing and reducing adolescent dating violence victimization and perpetration. *Am J Public Health.* 2004; 94(4):619-624.

30. Foubert JD, Godin EE, Tatum JL. In their own words: sophomore college men describe attitude and behavior changes resulting from a rape prevention program 2 years after their participation. *J Interpers Violence.* 2010;25(12):2237-2257.

31. Wolfe DA, Crooks C, Jaffe P, et al. A school-based program to prevent adolescent dating violence: a cluster randomized trial. *Arch Pediatr Adolesc Med.* 2009;163(8):692–699.

32. Kim JC, Watts CH, Hargreaves JR, Ndhlovu LX, Phetla G, Morison LA, Busza J, Porter JDH, Pronyk P. Understanding the impact of a microfinance-based intervention on women's empowerment and the reduction of intimate partner violence in South Africa. *Am J Public Health.* 2007;97(10):1794–1802.

33. Schopper D, Lormand J-D, Waxweiler R. *Developing Policies to Prevent Injuries: Guidelines for Policy-Makers and Planners.* Geneva: World Health Organization; 2006.

34. Soul City Institute. *Soul City Series 4.* http://soulcity.org.za/projects/soul-city-series/soul-city-series-4/soul-city-series-4-1. Updated 2010. Accessed December 16, 2010.

35. Usdin S, Scheepers E, Goldstein S, Japhet G. Achieving social change on gender-based violence: a report on the impact evaluation on Soul City's fourth series. *Soc Sci Med.* 2005;61(11):2434–2445.

36. Flood M. Engaging Men: strategies and dilemmas in violence prevention education among men. *Women Against Violence.* 2002;13:25–32.

37. Men Can Stop Rape Web site. http://www.mencanstoprape.org. Updated 2010. Accessed December 20, 2010.

38. Centers for Disease Control and Prevention. Choose respect. http://www.cdc.gov/women/az/violence.htm. Updated 2010. Accessed December 20, 2010.

39. Freedom from Fear Web site. www.freedomfromfear.wa.gov.au. Published 2010. Updated April, 2013. Accessed December 20, 2010.

40. Activities of the SVRI: promoting research. Sexual Violence Research Initiative Web Site. http://www.svri.org/activities.htm#promoting. Accessed November 12, 2010.

41. United Nations. UNiTE goals. United Nations Web site. http://www.un.org/en/women/endviolence/goals.shtml. Published 2010. Accessed November 12, 2010.

42. United Nations. *UNiTE to End Violence Against Women, Framework for Action: Programme of United Nations Activities and Expected Outcomes, 2008-2015.* New York, NY: United Nations Department of Public Information; 2009.

43. United Nations. UNiTE we are. United Nations Web site. http://www.un.org/en/women/endviolence/who.shtml. Published 2010. Accessed November 12, 2010.

44. United Nations. UN calls on corporate sector to help eliminate violence against women. United Nations Web site. http://www.un.org/apps/news/story.asp?NewsID=36844. Accessed November 23, 2010.

45. United Nations UNiTE What we do. United Nations Web site. http://www.un.org/en/women/endviolence/what.shtml. Published 2010. Accessed November 18, 2010.

46. Virtual Knowledge Centre to End Violence against Women and Girls Web site. http://www.endvawnow.org/. Accesses November 18, 2010.

47. Pakistan: UN addresses gender-based violence against flood victims. United Nations Web site. http://www.un.org/apps/news/story.asp?NewsID=36881&Cr=pakistan&Cr1. Accessed November 27, 2010.

48. International Committee of the Red Cross. Advancement of women: ICRC statement to the United Nations, 2010. International Committee of the Red Cross Web site. http://www.ikrk.org/eng/resources/documents/statement/united-nations-women-statement-2010-10-14.htm. Published October 14, 2010. Accessed November 30, 2010.

49. International Committee of the Red Cross. Wartime violence against women: States must do more to end it. International Committee of the Red Cross Web site. http://www.ikrk.org/eng/resources/documents/statement/women-statement-2010-10-31.htm. Published November 2, 2010. Accessed December 1, 2010.

50. United Nations Security Council. Resolution 1325 (2000). United Nations Web site. http://www.un.org/events/res_1325e.pdf. Published October 31, 2000. Accessed November 30, 2010.

51. International Committee of the Red Cross. Women protected under international humanitarianlaw. International Committee of the Red Cross Web site. http://www.ikrk.org/eng/war-and-law/protected-persons/women/overview-women-protected.htm. Published October 29, 2010. Accessed December 1, 2010.

52. Horn R. Responses to intimate partner violence in Kakuma refugee camp: refugee interactions with agency systems. *Soc Sci Med.* 2010;70(1):160-168.

53. Ungar M, Tutty LM, McConnell S, Barter K, Fairholm J. What Canadian youth tell us about disclosing abuse. *Child Abuse Negl.* 2009;33(10):699-708.

54. McColgan MD, Dempsey S, Davis M, Giardino AP. Overview of the problem. In: Giardino AP, Giardino ER, eds. *Intimate Partner Violence: A Resource for Professionals Working with Children and Families.* St. Louis, MO: STM Learning, Inc; 2010:1-29.

55. Kearney JA. Women and children exposed to domestic violence: Themes in maternal interviews about their children's psychiatric diagnoses. *Issues Ment Health Nurs.* 2010;31(2):74-81.

56. Taft A, Broom DH, Legge D. General practitioner management of intimate partner abuse and the whole family: qualitative study. *BMJ.* 2004;328(7440):618-621.

57. Emenike E, Lawoko S, Dalal K. Intimate partner violence and reproductive health of women in Kenya. *Int Nurs Rev.* 2008;55(1):97-102.

58. Rose L, Bhandari S, Soken K, Marcantonio K, Bullock L, Sharps P. Impact of intimate partner violence on pregnant women's mental health: mental distress and mental strength. *Issues Ment Health Nurs.* 2010;31(2):102-111.

59. Sarkar NN. The impact of intimate partner violence on women's reproductive health and pregnancy outcome. *J Obstet Gynaecol.* 2008;28(3):266-271.

60. Centers for Disease Control and Prevention. Costs of Intimate partner violence against women in the United States. Centers for Disease Control and Prevention Web site. http://www.cdc.gov/ncipc/pub-res/ipv_cost/IPVBook-Final-Feb18.pdf. Published March 2003. Accessed December 27, 2010

61. Teti M, Chilton M, Giardino AP. Looking ahead: the public health approach to intimate partner violence prevention. In: Giardino AP, Giardino ER, eds. *Intimate Partner Violence: A Resource for Professionals Working with Children and Families.* St. Louis, MO: STM Learning, Inc; 2010:327-353.

Chapter 13

IPV AND SEXUAL ASSAULT: A GLOBAL PERSPECTIVE

Nancy Cabelus, DNP, MSN, AFN-BC

KEY POINTS

1. Intimate partner violence is a global problem. In most countries, between 30% and 60% of women report physical and/or sexual violence over the course of their lifetimes.

2. Incidences of sexual abuse often go unreported. In the US, up to 54% of sexual assaults are not reported to law enforcement. In Bangladesh, 66% of women reported their abuse for the first time in the study interview.

3. Cultural assumptions about domestic violence vary from country to country, and these assumptions have an impact on the prevalence of IPV and on the level of reporting. Other practices, such as widow cleansing, female genital mutilation, and honor killing, are also embedded in the local culture.

4. Victims of sexual assault face severe health consequences. Women who have their first sexual experience before the age of 15, many of whom are sexually abused, are 3 times more likely to become HIV-infected than men.

5. Forensic nurses who educate themselves on other cultures will be able to provide culturally sensitive care to their patients.

INTRODUCTION

Since the 1980s, violence against women has shifted from being a private issue to being recognized as a public issue.[1] A 2008 report of the United Nations Trust Fund to End Violence Against Women declared that, "Intimate partner violence is a global emergency, but it is happening behind closed doors." The report further stated that while political commitment to end violence against women has never been higher, gender-based violence occurs in every country regardless of age, race, or ethnicity.[2]

Nearly 50% of all sexual assaults worldwide target girls aged 15 or younger.[3] Such acts of sexual violence not only have a hand in the oppression of women's rights, they also strike at the status of global health. United States Secretary of State Hillary Clinton stated, "We cannot stop the epidemic of HIV unless we also address the epidemic of violence against women."[4] Despite international policies and donor initiatives currently underway to combat sexual and gender-based violence, especially in developing countries, more awareness of the violence is needed, and a global force is necessary to stop it. This chapter provides a glance beyond the borders of the United States to discuss in a broad context the types of sexual assault and intimate partner violence, primarily against women, that are occurring regularly around the world; to identify the health implications of these forms of violence; and to raise awareness of international policy efforts being made to prevent these violent acts from happening.

GLOBAL PREVALENCE

Prevalence of sexual assault and intimate partner violence is well documented in the media and in international research literature. The World Health Organization's (WHO) Multi-Country Study on Women's Health and Domestic Violence Against Women collected data from over 24 000 women living in 15 sites in 10 countries featuring diverse cultural settings: Bangladesh, Brazil, Ethiopia, Japan, Namibia, Peru, Samoa, Serbia and Montenegro, Thailand, and the United Republic of Tanzania.[5] The study verified that the home is not a safe haven for women and revealed that women are more at risk of experiencing violence in intimate relationships than anywhere else.[5] Investigation found that:

— Physical and/or sexual violence committed by an intimate partner and reported over a lifetime, ranged from 15% in Japan city to 71% in Ethiopia province. This wide variation speaks volumes to the different cultural underpinnings within countries.

— In most countries the prevalence of IPV ranged from 30% to 60%. In more than ½ of the sites, over 30% of women who reported that their first sexual encounter occurred before age 15 said that their first sexual experience was forced.

— Women who experienced violence were also significantly more likely to report their general health status as being poor or very poor compared to women who had never experienced violence.

— Women who experienced IPV were significantly more likely to have contemplated suicide than women who had not experienced IPV.

— Women were often kept isolated by their batterers from potential sources of help.

— A significant number of women surveyed had told someone about the violence; however, 20% of the respondents in Brazil and 66% of women surveyed in Bangladesh reported the violence for the first time during the study interview.

The findings of the WHO study speak volumes about the global prevalence of violence against women. Alarmingly, researchers found that the attitude of most women interviewed is that violence against women by an intimate partner is normal behavior. Respondents found it difficult to answer questions effectively when intimate partner violence was the normal way of life in their culture. Compensating for this difficulty could mean that violence across all cultures is probably happening more regularly than respondents disclosed. A woman interviewed in Bangladesh reported, "My husband slaps me, has sex with me against my will, and I have to conform. Before being interviewed I didn't really think about this. I thought this is only natural. This is the way a husband behaves."

"Woman-battering or domestic violence exists within the greater societal context because it is rooted in the historical oppression of women."[6] Some discriminative forms of gender violence may even begin before birth. Son preference is common in many parts of the world where prenatal tests are sometimes used to detect the sex of the fetus. Female fetuses in these cultures may be aborted before birth.[3] Even when these girls are born, female babies unwanted by families in male-dominated societies are often killed by their own mothers.[7,8]

If survivors accept sexual assault and intimate partner violence as normalized behavior, it may be because they are often uneducated with regard to human rights. Some are not aware that their human rights have been violated or that human rights exist. This lack of awareness could be an underlying reason for victims' failure to report acts of violence. Worldwide, large numbers of abused women suffer in silence without ever telling a family member or making a report to the police. In the US, 54% of sexual assaults are not reported to law enforcement according to the Rape, Abuse & Incest National Network.[9] In Canada 28%, in the United Kingdom 38%, and in Bangladesh 68% of battered victims have kept their abuse a secret.[3] With the under-reporting of abuse, research statistics on the exact numbers of acts of sexual assault and intimate partner violence are unknown.

FORMS OF VIOLENCE

Acts of violence against women take many forms, sometimes public but most often private and always with disregard for human rights. Some forms of intimate partner and sexual violence are specific to a culture or region of the world and may be unfamiliar to clinicians who work within the United States. Yet patients, whether US citizens or visitors from another country, may perceive the health care system as an entry point for seeking assistance or safety. It is important for clinicians to take note of these practices to better prepare themselves and to understand health implications associated with these crimes.

INTIMATE PARTNER VIOLENCE

There are forms of violence other than battering or rape that oppress women's rights and that can affect mental health and well-being. Restriction of personal and social freedoms by "holding women in their place" is a violation of human rights whether done in public or in a private space.[3] Restraints on female freedom and the countries where such restrictions are enforced include: requiring a husband's permission to work or to open a bank account (Democratic Republic of the Congo), restricting women from obtaining a driver's license without male authorization (Qatar), isolating women within their homes (India, Afghanistan, Iraq), and barring women from leaving their houses without their husbands' consent (Yemen). Disobedience by the wife or violating the house rules could result in torture, injury, or death.

Boy and Kulczycki state that Middle Eastern women have been conditioned to believe that beatings are not only justified but are their fault.[9] The top 3 reasons for domestic violence as identified by researchers in the Middle East are "dishonoring family, neglecting children, and burning food/kitchen problems."[10] Ellsberg and the multi-country study on women's health and domestic violence found that in about one-half of the data collection sites, 50-90% of women agreed that it is acceptable for a man to beat his wife if she fails to obey him, refuses sex, or does not complete the housework.[5,11]

In several countries around the world it is assumed that men are the disciplinarians and that women should be punished for not living up to the expectations of their husbands. In 2009, the author (Cabelus) held a gender-based violence training class for police officers in Kenya. A veteran officer announced to the class that, "Sometimes women need to be hit." In a demonstrative action, he raised his hand to his face. The police officer turned to a male course instructor for validation but did not receive it. Also during this timeframe, in Kenya, a story was widely publicized in the media about a woman who had been hospitalized at Nairobi Women's Hospital after her husband had chopped off her hands when she did not prepare his supper properly.

Research on domestic and sexual violence reveals that in most countries it is culturally acceptable for men to be the disciplinarians of the family unit and for women to be punished for not living up to the expectations of their husbands. Xu et al found that, with current reform initiatives and the development of a "socialist market economy" in China, women are expected to "hold up half of the sky" by striving for economic and political independence.[12] However, the women in Xu's study were not as supportive of gender equality, at least in terms of marital relationships and gender roles, as the new Chinese constitution prescribes. Women adhere to the norms of a male-dominant culture to some degree but also believe that traditional culture and the likelihood of abuse were strongly associated.

Xu et al further report in their study on IPV against Chinese women that battered women were willing to talk about IPV with researchers but believed that family problems should only be addressed within the family.[12] This belief rings true in many parts of the world. As laws against domestic violence are passed, what used to be considered family matters are now transferred to the police for investigation; therefore, the attitude of law enforcement officers must also change. Denmark, a part of Europe that is usually considered very advanced with regard to socio-cultural attitudes, uses the term house disturbance (husspektakler) to describe domestic violence, which implies that the problem is perceived as "not so serious."[1] Law enforcement officers may feel that IPV should be handled in the home, especially when the police officers themselves were raised in a household where battering took place. Anderson and Lo found that officers who work in stressful environments are more likely to be aggressors in an intimate relationship.[13]

For a change in attitude and behavior to occur, researchers must first identify the root cause of the violence. Having a history of family violence has emerged in research findings as a high risk factor for partner aggression by men. Studies in Brazil, Cambodia, Canada, Chile, Colombia, Costa Rica, El Salvador, Indonesia, Nicaragua, Spain, the United States, and Venezuela all found that rates of abuse were higher among women whose husbands had either themselves been beaten as children or had witnessed their mothers being beaten.[14] Most domestic violence involves male anger directed against their partners, and according to the United Nations Population Fund, this gender difference appears to be rooted in the way boys and men are socialized. In Arab nations, boys learn to be strong and dominant, while girls are taught to be weak and submissive.[15,16] If men perceive that their power and privileges are being threatened, they may use violence as a way to restore their dominant status.[16] Learned behavior and cultural belief are often factors that perpetuate the cycle of violence, but not all boys who witness battering in the home become batters themselves. WHO's 2002 report implies that more research could be framed around the theoretical question of what distinguishes those men who are able to form healthy, non-violent relationships despite childhood adversity from those who become abusive.

Chan conducted a study on Chinese males who batter to determine if "face" was a factor in prompting men to inflict violence upon their wives.[17] Face, or mien, as defined for this study means social status, specifically, how the male would be respected by his society and how his intimate partner complies with that level of respect. Losing "face" could result in raised levels of anger and dominance leading to violent acts committed by the man against his wife and children. Chan's study, albeit limited by a small sample of 18 male batterers, found that "the stronger the face orientation, the greater the masculine gender role stress and thus the greater likelihood of using violence against female partners."[17]

Multiple Wives, Polygamy, and Jealousy

While it is an extreme dishonor to a man and his family when a woman has a romantic relationship outside of her marriage, it is common practice in many countries for men to have multiple wives and lovers. In a South African study conducted by Madzimbalale & Khoza, researchers sought to teach nursing students to identify symbols (signs) of battering while counseling patients.[18] One South African study participant, intolerant of her husband's extramarital affair, gives her account of violence:

"Do you want to see? Look at this." The participant took off her clothes and showed her left breast with a burn scar. "My husband threw a kettle with boiling water at me. He was angry with me because I chased his girlfriend away. His girlfriend used to come and visit him every Friday night and leave on Monday morning. So I beat her and chased her away before my husband returned from work. When he returned from work and heard that I had beaten and chased his girlfriend away, he went into a fit. That is why I have sustained this scar of burns." The researcher observed a burn scar on the left breast of the participant. The scar was major because the whole upper part of the breast was burned and the nipple was also affected. The nipple had a dimple. The participant also said, "I have a problem with this scar because I have a small baby whom I am breastfeeding. I cannot breastfeed her on my left breast because of deformity. I reported the matter to the South African police..."[18]

Methods of Intimate Partner Assault

Seager reports that in South Africa 40%-70% of all female murder victims are killed by a husband or boyfriend.[3] The following sections will describe some of the extreme methods by which women are assaulted by intimate partners or family members.

Bride Burning and Acid Throwing

Bride burning is when a woman, usually between the ages of 18-30, is set afire by her husband or in-laws who proclaim the act to be accidental.[19] Also called dowry death, the motive is financial gain and escape from a current marriage so that the husband can marry a new wife.[19] In India, it is estimated that an instance of bride burning takes place every 2 hours to punish a woman for an inadequate dowry or to eliminate her so that a man can remarry.[8] Kristof and WuDunn also report that, in the past decade in the cities of Islamabad and Rawalpindi, approximately 5000 women and girls have been either set afire or seared with acid by family members or in-laws for perceived disobedience and that nothing is done about it.[8] Acid throwing, commonly at the face of the victim, causes severe, disfiguring burns and scarring and can also cause blindness or death.[19] In Bangladesh, an acid throwing incident occurs about every 2 days and about 70% of the attacks are on women.[20]

Honor Killing

In some places, ties between male honor and female chastity put women at risk.[5] In the Eastern Mediterranean, Middle East, and African regions, it is culturally acceptable to link a man's honor to the perceived sexual purity of the women in his family. When a female is "defiled" sexually, either through rape or by engaging voluntarily in sex outside marriage, it is believed she has disgraced family honor.[3,5] Honor killing is the commission of the murder of a woman who has tarnished her family's honor. Honor killings (HK) are commonly practiced in the countries of Pakistan, Jordan, and Saudi Arabia.[3,19] In Jordan, 20-30 women each year fall victim to honor killings.[3]

In Pakistan, HK is a custom of domestic violence in which mostly women and sometimes men are murdered after accusations of alleged sexual infidelity. In Sindh province, HK is referred to as "Karo Kari, where Karo refers to the 'blackened' or dishonored man and Kari to the 'blackened' woman."[21] The Human Rights Commission of Pakistan reported that between 2004-2007 there were 1957 events of HK recorded. The majority of the killings were against adults but 175 persons killed were under 18 years of age. The most common methodology of HK was a firearm, but an axe was used in 220 cases and strangulation in 167 cases.[21] In Egypt, 47% of honor killings between 2000-2006 happened because the woman had been raped.

Virginity Testing

Virginity testers, usually older women, conduct vaginal exams to determine if a female's hymen is intact and to assess other physical features as indicators of "the innocence and purity of the individual tested such as her muscle tone and the firmness of her breasts."[22]

Virginity testing is commonly practiced in African and the Middle Eastern regions and falls short of scientific method. In Zambia, when police conduct an investigation into an alleged rape they frequently require that a medical doctor, sometimes a pathologist, is paid to perform an examination to determine if the victim is a virgin or not. If the doctor deems that penetration into the vagina could not have happened "because the hymen is intact," then rape could not have occurred and the police investigation will not go forward (Personal communication, Zambia Police Services, July 2009). In Afghanistan, virginity tests are conducted by a medical examiner to certify the purity of the woman or bride-to-be (Personal communication, Stephan Schmitt, Physicians for Human Rights, May 24, 2011). Too often, corruption plays a part in the "tests" and doctors can be bribed in exchange for their fictitious reports.

The "Virgin Cure" and Belief that Having Sex with a Virgin Cures AIDS

The unsettling belief that having sexual intercourse with a virgin will cure AIDS is often the reason behind incidents of child rape, especially in sub-Saharan Africa where in 2007 approximately 22.5 million people were infected with HIV.[3,19,23] The myth of the "Virgin Cure" dates back to 16th Century England when it was believed that having sexual intercourse with a virgin would kill sexually transmitted infections, such as syphilis and gonorrhea. Syphilis, like AIDS, could become a terminal disease and soldiers returning home to the eastern cape of South Africa following WWII would desperately seek out a cure.[23] A survey conducted by the University of South Africa at the Daimler Chrysler plant in East London found that 18% of the 498 workers surveyed believed that having sex with a virgin would cure HIV/AIDS.[24] "The idea that having sex with a virgin cleanses you of AIDS does exist, and there have been reported cases of this as a motivating factor for child rape. But evidence suggests that this is infrequently the case," said Dr. Rachel Jewkes, director of the University's Medical Research Council's Gender and Health Research Group.[24] The AIDS virus has wiped out a generation of young parents, which adds to the vulnerability of surviving children and the risk of sexual violence visited upon them. There are 15 000 000 AIDS orphans in the world, 12 000 000 of whom are in Sub-Saharan Africa.[3]

While working as a law enforcement advisor in Kenya, author Nancy Cabelus learned that at Kenyatta National Hospital, Kenya's largest teaching hospital, babies sometimes arrive to the Casualty Department after being so severely raped that they require either extensive surgical repair or hysterectomy or are, in some cases, dead on arrival (Personal communication, Rose Wafubwa, RN, February 9, 2010). Whether the motivation behind these cases is a sought cure for AIDS, an act of pedophilia, or another inflicted form of violence remains unknown because thorough forensic investigations do not take place in Kenya or in most African countries.

Forced Marriage and Widow Cleansing

Human rights come into conflict with traditional practices of early and forced marriage and "widow cleansing." Worldwide, 82 000 000 girls, generally from poor families, will marry before age 18 and will be more susceptible to HIV/AIDS infections than their peers who are not married.[25]

Widow cleansing is a traditional practice in which widows are expected to have sexual relations, often with a relative of their deceased husband.[25] The cleansing process forces the widow to have sex with her husband's brothers and possibly other males relatives, regardless of age, to allow her to continue occupying the land with her children. In some countries, women who are predeceased by their husband are banned from living on the couple's property without being subjected to this practice, especially in countries where women do not have rights to own land. In some instances, men may inherit unmarried women as wives by raping them.[3]

Female Genital Mutilation (FGM)

An estimated 100-140 million women and girls worldwide have undergone female genital mutilation or circumcision (FGM/FGC), and 3 000 000 more girls are at risk each year.[26] FGM is defined by WHO as any procedure that involves the partial or total removal of female genitalia or as injury to the genitals for non-medical reasons. FGM is performed on young girls to ensure their suitability and desirability for marriage and to control their sexual behavior.[3] The cutting is often done with crude instruments such as a sharp stone, piece of glass, a rusty knife, razor, machete, or scissors.[27] This type of assault against girls and women elevates their risk of severe trauma and health consequences, including psychological trauma, bleeding, infection, and susceptibility to STIs; an array of health problems, such as urinary incontinence, and painful intercourse; and obstetrical difficulties, such as vaginal tearing during childbirth and perinatal death.[3,19,27] Vesico-vaginal fistula, a fistula that forms between the urinary bladder and vaginal vault, causing leakage of urine into the vagina, is another complication of FGM.

Some progress made towards banning the practice of FGM in certain developing countries. In some cultures, however, where the ritual is deeply rooted and deemed necessary, there has been a movement to medicalize the procedure.[27] It is perceived by laypersons that if a medical doctor completed the cutting procedure, the risks for infection, complications, and death may be reduced. Education is key to preventing the occurrences altogether. During a training program of police officers in Kenya led by Nancy Cabelus that addressed FGM as a form of gender-based violence, a video called Africa Rising was shown to the class. Equality Now, a non-government organization that condemns FGM, created the video that depicts serious and sometimes fatal outcomes of FGM. After the video, a male police officer courageously stood up in the classroom full of his peers and stated,

"Thank you for helping us to protect our daughters. We did not know." (Personal communication, Anonymous. Kenya Police College, June 2010).

Violence Against Men

Though not as frequently as women, men and boys may also be subjected to domestic or sexual violence occurring in their homes and villages that places them at risk for injury and abuse. A study on the characteristics of callers to the domestic violence helpline for men in the United States investigated 190 calls placed by men. All callers had experienced physical violence and were fearful of their female partners. Complainants also reported that their female abusers had a history of trauma, alcohol or drug problems, mental illness, and homicidal and suicidal ideations.[28]

More commonly, in conflict zones around the world, men are subjected to torture and rape. In the eastern region of the Democratic Republic of Congo, where conflict is ongoing, 22% of all men and 30% of all women have reportedly been raped.[29] According to researcher Lara Stemple of the University of California Law School Health and Human Rights Project, there are 4076 non-government organizations that assist wartime victims of sexual assault, but only 3% of these groups mention male rapes in the literature.[29] Male survivors usually fail to report sexual abuse and torture because of feelings of shame or fear that disclosure will subject them to further abuse.[30]

The following 2 categories of discussion, human trafficking and armed conflict, reach beyond the commonly known framework of intimate partner violence but are mentioned because sexual assault and violence against vulnerable populations is taking place globally in these contexts. Nearly 27 000 000 persons are trafficked globally each year.[31] Many victims are lured into the slave trade by boyfriends-turned-traffickers. In situations of civil war and conflict, refugees flee for shelter and safety in camps for internally displaced persons, known as "IDP camps." The camps are lawless and lack the protection of police services, leaving victims of sexual violence without help. Transnational alliances have become important forces in combatting these forms of violence on the global scale.

Human Trafficking and Sex Tourism

Sex trafficking is a multi-billion dollar industry that is driven by an unlimited supply of victims and a global demand for sex. Trafficking victims are most often deceived by their captors by means of force, fraud, or coercion for the purpose of forced labor or sex work or both.[31,32] Women and girls are often tricked into the sex trade with false promises of employment and better opportunities. Soon after, they are forced into sexual slavery and are no longer free to leave without fear of further harm to themselves, threat of terror to their families, and the risk of being killed. Trafficking survivors are at high risk for long-lasting physical, sexual, and psychological trauma.

Each year, the United States Department of State releases a Trafficking in Persons (TIP) Report that now ranks 183 countries around the world on their efforts to prevent trafficking in persons, prosecute trafficking cases, and protect trafficking survivors. Through global awareness of this serious situation, the rate of detection of cases is on the rise, but conviction rates remain unfortunately low. In 2006, European countries prosecuted 2950 cases of trafficking and obtained convictions in 1821, while North and South America combined prosecuted 443 cases with only 63 resulting in conviction of the offenders.[3]

Armed Conflict and Rape as a Weapon of War

As previously mentioned in this chapter, the rape of a woman or girl brings stigma not only to the female survivor but also dishonor to the male husband or parent, his family, and the community. In regions of civil war and conflict, militant rebels will rape women to degrade a man's social or community status. Also, in regions of conflict, people are often forced from their homes and villages by rebel extremists. Refugees take up temporary living arrangements in tented communities often known as *Internally Displaced Persons* or IDP camps. Internally Displaced Persons (IDPs) "are persons or groups of persons who have been forced or obliged to flee or leave their homes or places of habitual residence, in particular as a result or in order to avoid the effects of armed conflict, situations of generalized violence, violations of human rights, or natural or man-made disasters, and who have not crossed an internationally recognized border."[33] News media reports sometimes expose situations of persons living in IDP camps under deplorable conditions of filth and squalor. To make matters worse, women and children, among the most vulnerable of populations, are frequently sexually assaulted within the camps. Following an episode of sexual violence, the IDP has nowhere to turn to report the complaint and is left powerless. Security officers who guard the camps are primarily responsible for peacekeeping and are not trained to receive or investigate complaints. The need for protection within the camps is growing in tandem with the number and gravity of human rights violations.[34]

In Sudan and in Pakistan the numbers of IDPs are particularly high, with 4-5 million persons displaced in Sudan and nearly 1 000 000 persons affected in Pakistan.[34] The increase in numbers fleeing to camps is due in part to continuous civil unrest and also to severe drought conditions. A 2006 report filed by the Physicians for Human Rights (PHR) entitled "Darfur, Assault on Survival" quoted one Darfurian woman describing being chased into the bush by Janjaweed (armed militia) attackers. The woman overheard an attacker say, "Don't waste the bullet, they've got nothing to eat and will die of hunger."[33] PHR reports that mass rape in war "ruptures family and community structure," and, in a culture like Darfur's, rape is especially devastating. Women most often will not report sexual assault to anyone, including health care workers, for fear of isolation. Persons who choose to report rape and do not come forward with four male witnesses face prosecution for adultery and imprisonment.[33]

According to the United Nations Human Rights Commission, the country of Colombia continues to face a serious displacement crisis despite steps taken by the authorities to meet the challenge. Colombia's IDP population is more than 3 000 000 and is among the highest in the world.[34] Colombians have endured a 40-year civil war between Colombia's government and the leftist terrorist group Revolutionary Armed Forces of Colombia, also known as "the FARC." Citizens are faced with a weak criminal justice system that fails to protect them against violence and crimes of sexual assault. Children from the poorest communities become easy targets on the streets.[35] The UN Global Women's Fund reports that indigenous, rural, and Afro-Colombian women area at greatest risk for violence, assassination, harassment, and displacement due to marginalization.[36] UNHCR reports that it is working to reinforce the capacity of the Colombian government to address internal displacement within the framework of the Colombian Constitution and in line with international law.

HEALTH CONSEQUENCES

Forced sex is linked to a range of reproductive health problems and violence greatly limits married women's ability to use contraceptives.[37] According to the reports released by the United Nations, young women who had their first sexual relationship before age 15 are 3 times more likely to become HIV-infected than men.[2] The U.N. found that there is a relationship between exposure to violence and poor physical, mental, and sexual health status. Not being allowed to report the violence or failure to seek treatment may further complicate health problems. The World Health Organization (2009) has identified health consequences that can result directly from violent acts or from the long-term effects of violence.[37]

GLOBAL POLICY DEVELOPMENT

Research findings have identified sexual assault and intimate partner violence as global public health problems and have prompted the development of both national and international policies to end violence and discrimination against women. Examples of major policies that address sexual and gender-based violence are briefly discussed in the following paragraphs.

CONVENTION ON THE ELIMINATION OF ALL FORMS OF DISCRIMINATION AGAINST WOMEN (CEDAW)

The Convention on the Elimination of All Forms of Discrimination Against Women (CEDAW) is the UN treaty adopted in 1979 to protect the human rights of women internationally. The Convention strives for gender equality between women and men, ensuring equal opportunities for women in political and public life, including education, health, employment, and the right to vote and to stand for election. Further, the Convention is the only human rights treaty that affirms the reproductive rights of women and targets culture and tradition as influential forces shaping gender roles and family relations. Countries that have ratified the Convention are legally responsible to implement its provisions. Ratifying nations are further required to submit national reports at least once every 4 years describing the measures they have taken to comply with their treaty obligations. Hester anticipates that CEDAW will become even more significant in the future for bringing global partners together in the development of stronger policy to ensure the safety of women and children.[1]

MILLENNIUM DEVELOPMENT GOALS (MDG)

The United Nations Millennium Development Goals (MDG) were set to help eradicate poverty by 2015.[39] Of the 8 goals, those that most closely relate to prevention of sexual violence are 3) to promote gender equality and empower women; 5) to improve maternal health and 6) to combat HIV/AIDS, malaria, and other diseases.[39] The MDGs draw attention to the needs of the most vulnerable populations. The UN MDG report states, "Gender equality and the empowerment of women are at the heart of the MDGs and are preconditions for overcoming poverty, hunger, and disease."[39] The UN recognizes that further policy development is necessary to narrow the gaps of inequalities between the rich and the poor, especially those most disadvantaged by geographic locations, sex, age, disability, and ethnicity.

Progress has been slow, but the UN reports that the MDGs are still attainable. "The Millennium Declaration represents the most important promise ever made to the world's most vulnerable people."[39] This commitment strives for an unprecedented level of global partnership in creating healthier lives and safer living environments for billions of people.

POLICY ON INTERNALLY DISPLACED PERSONS

World news reports this year have exposed the gravity of conditions at IDP camps in the Horn of Africa and the millions of desperate persons compelled to seek refuge within the camps. The United Nations Commission on Human Rights (UNHCR) promises to be the link between monitoring and reporting of population movements and protection of IDPs, specifically women, children, youth, the elderly, the disabled, and ethnic minorities.[34] The UN Global Appeal intends to include the participation of IDP communities in an effort to ensure that public policy addresses the situation of IDPs and persons at risk of displacement.[34]

VIOLENCE AGAINST WOMEN ACT (UNITED STATES)

In the US, the Violence Against Women Act (VAWA) is the leading legislation to protect women against domestic violence. This important legislation, authored by then-Senator Joseph Biden and introduced to Congress in 1994, was reauthorized in 2000, 2005, and 2010. The Act provides grant programs for prevention of violence against women, stronger protections to victims of domestic violence, and a national domestic violence hotline. VAWA encourages collaboration of law enforcement agents, legal personnel, and victim service providers for a more unified approach to combating violence.[40] VAWA is funded through the United States Departments of Justice and Health & Human Services. In his FY2011 budget proposal, President Barack Obama requested $649 million in funding for violence against women programs.[40]

The Office on Violence Against Women is located within the Department of Justice and since its inception the Office has provided over $4 000 000 000 in grants and cooperative agreements.[41] US effort is also being made to pass the International Violence Against Women Act into law that would provide foreign aid to address human rights violations such as honor killings, bride burning, acid attacks, and domestic violence.[8]

The Office on Global Women's Issues falls within the auspices of the US Department of State. This Office works to address and combat gender-based violence across the globe. In a press statement made on June 16, 2011, Secretary of State Hillary Rodham Clinton stated that she had deep concern about the "wide-scale rapes in Libya and reports of sexual violence used by governments to intimidate and punish protesters seeking democratic reforms across the Middle East and North Africa. Rape, physical intimidation, sexual harassment, and even so-called 'virginity tests' have taken place in countries throughout the region." Secretary Clinton called these acts "violations of human dignity" and urged "all governments to conduct immediate, transparent investigations into these allegations, and to hold accountable those found responsible."[42]

COUNCIL OF EUROPE CONVENTION ON
PREVENTING AND COMBATING VIOLENCE AGAINST WOMEN

In May of 2011 in Istanbul, Turkey, the Council of Europe Convention on Preventing and Combating Violence Against Women was opened for signature. The country of Turkey was the first signatory on the convention and the treaty extends to 47 additional countries. This landmark legislation prohibits all forms of violence against women, including domestic violence, and could include violence against men and children if State signatories agree to it. This comprehensive legislation contains 81 articles that criminalize sexual harassment and illegal abortions. It also provides extensive services to victims of rape including health care, shelter, and counseling.[43]

Laws intended to protect women from sexual and intimate partner violence have been passed in a moderate number of countries around the world, but often fall short with implementation and enforcement of the laws. In South Africa, legislative action has been taken to "end virginity testing."[22] South Africa's Commission on Gender Equality strives to criminalize all "harmful social, cultural, and religious practices that affect women and girls" but has focused its efforts on eliminating virginity testing and female circumcision.[22] In Kenya, the Sexual Offences Act was passed in 2006 and the Kenyan government has called upon the United States and other international donors to assist with implementation of the Act. Law enforcement training, sensitization programs, and public awareness campaigns have been held, but the impact is limited. When considering the vast population of 39 000 000 and the country's limited resources, it will take several years for the information to reach rural provinces and for the law to be effectively implemented.

LIMITATIONS IN REGIONAL RESEARCH AND POLICY DEVELOPMENT

Awareness of intimate partner violence (IPV) is on the increase globally and has been identified as a problem in many countries in the Middle East and North Africa. Nonetheless, there are regions of the world that remain uncharted by sexual violence researchers. Research by Boy and Kulczycki revealed that a number of studies have been conducted on particular aspects of gender-based violence in the Middle East and North Africa, especially honor killings or female genital mutilation, but otherwise there is very little research in this region on violence against women committed by their intimate partners.[9] The World Health Organization's World Report on Violence and Health in 2002 could cite only 3 studies for the Eastern Mediterranean Region.[9] In countries such as Sudan, Iraq, and Afghanistan, national policies to protect women's rights are non-existent. In fact, in 2009 Afghan legislation was passed that allows Shia men to deprive their wives of food and sustenance should they refuse their husband's sexual demands and also prohibits women from work, education, doctor's visits, and leaving the house without their husband's permission.[44] Despite international calls for policy reform, little progress has been made.

IMPLICATIONS FOR CLINICAL/FORENSIC NURSING PRACTICE

When providing care for survivors of intimate partner violence and sexual assault there are several key implications to consider. Forensic nurses require awareness of various forms of sexual and gender-based violence, must have knowledge of culturally sensitive care, and must know how to assess for injury. Watts and Mayhew recommend that nurses be informed about the types, extent, and underlying causes of violence.[37] It is important that forensic nurses educate themselves on other cultures around the world to provide culturally sensitive care to clients.[45]

Battering, one of the most common forms of violence, involves physical, emotional, and sexual abuse. Forensic nurse examiners are highly qualified to provide comprehensive care to address these concerns.[6] Injuries related to domestic violence, battering, and sexual abuse are often located on the trunk of the body such as the breasts, buttocks, chest, or back where the victim can easily conceal them.[6] Screening for abuse during reproductive health consultations is recommended by Watts and Mayhew, who also advise to support patients emotionally by validating their experiences and by being nonjudgmental and willing to listen.[37] Forensic nurses must keep in mind that opportunities for primary prevention of human rights such as sexual assault, torture, and various physical abuses can happen in the clinical arena.

It may be helpful "for providers to prepare a list of potential indicators of partner violence, such as a history of unexplained injury or maternal bleeding, preterm labor or birth, and fetal injury or death," to have on hand during a health assessment.[37] A South African study by Madzimbalale and Khoza explored the "symbols" of physical violence of women who live with intimate partners.[18] They found that most victims of physical aggression are subjected to multiple acts of violence over time and that victims tend to suffer more than one type of abuse. When screening for IPV, the nurse should always refer to the patient's medical records from previous admissions to check for documentation of prior injuries or incidents of abuse in the patient's history.[46]

Ensuring patient safety is paramount. Following initial treatment, resources for safeguarding the battered patient may be limited and it can be difficult to find safe places where patients can seek refuge. The concepts of shelters as temporary refuge from a battered relationship may either not exist or may be few and far between in undeveloped countries. Historically, shelters for women first opened their doors in Japan and the United Kingdom in the 1970s.[1] In Japan and South Korea, shelters originally served to protect women from sex tourism and trafficking, and it was not until the 1990s that Japan's shelters became safe houses for domestic violence victims.[1] Today, finding safe houses for survivors remains a challenge even in developed countries. Having knowledge of availability of local resources such as shelters, domestic violence, and trafficking in persons hotlines, and legal services could be helpful for nurses when assisting a patient to create a plan for personal safety.

On local, national, regional, and global scales, there is a lot of work to do regarding the issues of sexual assault and intimate partner violence. Forensic nurses may play a key role in prevention of sexual and intimate partner violence through awareness and education. Effective detection of abuse during clinical care can help to break the cycle of violence and also prevent health consequences that may result from violence. Complete and accurate documentation of care and treatment rendered could contribute to effective case outcomes in court, data collection for research studies, and also program monitoring and evaluation. Nurses may also become involved in prevention of violence by collaborating with key partners on multi-sectoral committees and task forces designated to reduce violence against vulnerable populations. Publicly condemning violence is imperative to counter IPV globally.[37] Nurses can assume leadership roles in the prevention of sexual violence by speaking out in public forums, in educational settings, and in the clinical practice to send the message that sexual assault and intimate partner violence must be taken seriously both globally and at home.

CONCLUSION

This chapter provided a brief overview of some of the documented forms of sexual and intimate partner violence inflicted upon vulnerable populations, particularly against women and girls around the world. Violence against women is the most pervasive yet least recognized human rights violation in the world.[14] Violations of women's rights are well-documented on a global scale, but greater public awareness of the issues at hand are needed to engender a strong public health response that focuses on preventing such violence from the grassroots level up. The WHO Multi-Cultural Study uncovered forms and patterns of intimate partner violence across several countries and cultures and documents the consequences of violence for women's health from geographical areas where data had been previously unavailable.[5] The high rates of violence experienced by girls and women globally are problematic, especially in light of the HIV epidemic. Researchers report that in Asia and the Middle East regions, where reports of violence are very high, there are few publications on violence against women found in the literature.

There is a place on the global platform for nurses to become involved with policy making that could impact the status of women around the world. At the 2011 International Council of Nurses Convention in Malta, nursing leadership called upon WHO to involve nurses at the policy making table. ICN President Rosemary Bryant issued a press statement in connection with that organization's biennial meeting in 2011 to state that:

"At this time of health system redesign aiming to enable access and cost efficiency, it doesn't make sense for WHO to advocate for nurses to fully participate in the health care team at the clinical level, yet exclude them from playing their full role at the policy table. As we move to a discussion of the Resolution on Nursing and Midwifery at the upcoming World Health Assembly, we urge member states to add their weight to the call on Dr. Chan to remedy the appalling lack of nursing leadership positions throughout WHO structures, including at headquarters and in the regional offices, beginning with reestablishment of the post of WHO Chief Nurse Scientist."[47]

REFERENCES

1. Hester M. Future trends and developments: violence against women in Europe and East Asia. *Violence Against Women.* 2004;10(12):1431-1448.

2. United Nations. Convention on the elimination of all forms of violence against women (CEDAW). United Nations Web site. http://www.un.org/womenwatch/daw/cedaw/. Accessed August 7, 2011

3. Seager J. *The Penguin Atlas of Women in the World.* 4th ed. New York, NY: Penguin Books; 2009.

4. Fleishmann J. *Gender-Based Violence and HIV: Emerging Lessons from the PEPFAR Initiative in Tanzania.* Center for Strategic and International Studies: Washington, DC; 2012.

5. World Health Organization. Multi-country study on women's health and domestic violence against women. World Health Organization Web site. http://whqlibdoc.who.int/publications/2005/924159358X_eng.pdf. Published 2005. Accessed July 15, 2013.

6. Moynihan B. Domestic violence. In: Lynch VA, ed. *Forensic Nursing.* St. Louis, MO: Mosby; 2005:260-270.

7. Gorea R. Sociocultural crimes: a forensic approach. In Lynch,VA. *Forensic Nursing Science.* 2nd ed. St. Louis, MO: Mosby; 2010:497-511.

8. Kristof N, WuDunn S. *Half the Sky.* New York, NY: Vintage Books; 2009.

9. Rape, Abuse & Incest National Network. Reporting rates. Rape, Abuse & Incest National Network Web site. http://www.rainn.org/get-information/statistics/reporting-rates. Published 2012. Accessed January 23, 2013.

10. Boy A, Kulczycki A. What we know about intimate partner violence in the Middle East and North Africa. *Violence Against Women.* 2008:14(1):53-71.

11. Ellsberg MC. Violence against women: a global public health crisis. *Scand J Public Health.* 2006:34(1);1-4.

12. Xu X, Zhu F, O'Campo P, Koenig M, Mock V, Campbell J. Prevalence of and risk factors for intimate partner violence in China. *J Public Health.* 2005;95(1):78-85.

13. Anderson AS, Lo CC. Intimate partner violence within law enforcement families. *J Interpers Violence.* 2011;26(6):1176-1194.

14. World Health Organization. World report on violence and health. World Health Organization Web site. http://www.who.int/violence_injury_prevention/violence/world_report/en/summary_en.pdf. Published 2002. Accessed July 20, 2011.

15. United Nations Population Fund. Working to end acid attacks in Bangledesh by 2015. United Nations Population Fund Web site. http://www.unfpa.org/public/site/global/lang/en/pid/3917. Published 2009. Accessed June 17, 2011.

16. Haj-Yahia M. Wife abuse and battering in the sociocultural context of Arab society. *Family Process*. 2000:39(2):237-255.

17. Chan KL. The Chinese concept of face and violence against women. *Int Social Work*. 2006;49(1):65-73.

18. Madzimbalale FC, Khoza LB. Experiences of physical violence by women living with intimate partners. *Curatonis*. 2010;33(2):25-33.

19. Lynch VA. Forensic nursing science and the global agenda. *J Forensic Nurs*. 2007;3(3&4):101-111.

20. United Nations Population Fund. Ending widespread violence against women. United Nations Population Fund Web site. http://www.unfpa.org/gender/violence.htm. Published 2010. Accessed July 20, 2011.

21. Nasrullah M, Haqqi S, Cummings K. The epidemiological patterns of honour killing of women in Pakistan. *Eur J Public Health*. 2009;19(2):193-197.

22. George ER. Virginity testing and South Africa's HIV/AIDS crisis: beyond rights universalism and cultural relativism toward health capabilities. *California Law Rev*. 2008;6(8):1447-1519.

23. Taylor ME. HIV: the stats, the virgin cure and child rape. Science in Africa Web site. http://www.scienceinafrica.co.za/2002/april/virgin.htm. Published 2002. Accessed July 20, 2011.

24. Integrated Regional Information Networks Reports. South Africa: focus on the virgin myth and HIV/AIDS. IRIN Web site. http://www.irinnews.org/report.aspx?reportid=39838. Published 2002. Accessed July 20, 2011.

25. Joint United Nations Programme on HIV/AIDS, United Nations Population Fund, United Nations Development Fund for Women. Women and HIV/AIDS: confronting the crisis. A joint report. United Nations Population Fund Web site. http://www.unfpa.org/hiv/women/report/chapter1.html. Published 2004. Accessed August 1, 2011.

26. United Nations Trust Fund to End Violence Against Women. United Nations Development Fund for Women. http://www.unifem.org/materials/item_detail.php?ProductID=127 . Published 2008. Accessed July 20, 2011.

27. Crane PA. Female genital mutilation. In: Lynch VA. *Forensic Nursing Science*. 2nd ed. St. Louis, MO: Mosby; 2010:521-530.

28. Hines D, Brown J, Dunning E. Characteristics of callers to the Domestic Abuse Helpline for Men. *J Fam Violence*. 2007;(22):63-72.

29. Storr W. The rape of men. The Observer Web site. http://www.guardian.co.uk/society/2011/jul/17/the-rape-of-men. Published 2011. August 24, 2011.

30. Oosterhoff P, Zwanikken P, Ketting, E. Sexual torture of men in Croatia and other conflict situations: an open secret. *Reproductive Health Matters*. 2004;12(23):68-77.

31. United States Department of State. Trafficking in persons report. United States Department of State Web site. http://www.state.gov/j/tip/rls/tiprpt/2011. Published 2011. Accessed December 1, 2012.

32. United Nations Office on Drugs and Crime. Global report on trafficking in persons. from http://www.unodc.org/unodc/en/human-trafficking/what-is-human-trafficking.html?ref=menuside. Published 2011. Accessed August 7, 2011.

33. Physicians for Human Rights. *Darfur: Assault On Survival. A Call For Security, Justice, and Restitution.* Washington, DC: Library of Congress; 2006.

34. United Nations Human Rights Commission. Working internally with the displaced. United Nations Human Rights Commission Web site. http://www.unhcr.org/4b0509619.html. Published 2010. Accessed July 20, 2011.

35. Cabelus N, Sheridan G. Forensic investigation of sex crimes in Colombia. *J Forensic Nurs.* 2007;3(3-4):112-116.

36. Rosas EG. Global Fund outreach trip report. Peace Women Web site. http://www.peacewomen.org/assets/file/partpol-colombia-ecuador08.pdf. Published 2008. Accessed July 15, 2013.

37. Watts C, Mayhew S. Reproductive health services and intimate partner violence: shaping a pragmatic response in Sub-Saharan Africa. *Int Family Planning Perspectives.* 2004;30:(4);207-213.

38. World Health Organization. Media centre fact sheet on violence against women. World Health Organization Web site. http://www.who.int/mediacentre/factsheets/fs239/en/. Published 2009. Accessed July 7, 2011.

39. United Nations. Millennium development goals report 2010. United Nations Web site. http://www.un.org/millenniumgoals/pdf/MDG%20Report%202010%20En%20r15%20-low%20res%2020100615%20-.pdf. Published 2010. Accessed July 20, 2011.

40. Laney G. Violence against women act: history and federal funding. ILW Web site. http://www.ilw.com/immigrationdaily/news/2010,0525-crs.pdf. Published 2010. Accessed July 7, 2011.

41. United States Department of Justice. Office on Violence Against Women Web site. http://www.ovw.usdoj.gov/overview.htm. Published 2011. Accessed August 7, 2011.

42. Clinton H. Sexual violence in Libya, the Middle East and North Africa. United States Department of State Web site. http://www.state.gov/secretary/rm/2011/06/166369.htm. Published 2011. Accessed September 7, 2011.

43. Council of Europe convention on preventing and combating violence against women. Council of Europe Web site. https://wcd.coe.int/ViewDoc.jsp?id=1772191&Site=COE&BackColorInternet=DBDCF2&BackColorIntranet=FDC864&BackColorLogged=FDC864. Published 2011. Accessed July 15, 2013.

44. Boone J. Worse than the Taliban: new law rolls back rights for Afghan women. The Guardian Web site. http://www.rawa.org/temp/runews/2009/03/31/and-8216-worse-than-the-talibanand-8217-new-law-rolls-back-rights-for-afghan-women.html. Published 2009. Accessed July 20, 2011.

45. Amar A, Stockbridge J, Bess R. Global voices on gender-based violence. *J Forensic Nurs.* 2008;4(4):182-184.

46. Campbell J, Lynch V. Violence against women. In: Lynch VA. *Forensic Nursing*. St. Louis, MO: Mosby; 2005:52-69.

47. Nursing leaders call on Director General of WHO to change policy about nursing leadership. Global Health Delivery Online Web site. http://www.ghdonline.org/nursing/discussion/nursing-leaders-call-on-director-general-of-who-to. Published 2011. Accessed June 18, 2011.

Chapter 14

STRANGULATION IN THE LIVING IPV PATIENT

Jennifer Pierce-Weeks, RN, SANE-P, SANE-A
Megan Lechner, MSN, RN, CNS, SANE-P, SANE-A

KEY POINTS

1. Studies indicate that between 23% and 68% of women who are victims of intimate partner violence (IPV) will experience at least 1 strangulation-related incident at the hands of their abusive partner.

2. Women who experience a non-fatal strangulation by an intimate partner are 7 times more likely to become a victim of homicide.

3. Physical signs of strangulation may or may not be visible. The health professional should look for other signs and symptoms, including: loss of consciousness, incontinence, bleeding, coughing, headache, vision changes, nausea, lightheadedness, numbness, and irritability.

4. The health professional should take care to make an accurate record of symptoms and injuries utilizing a strangulation assessment tool, as well as ensuring that photographs are taken of any visible injuries.

5. The victim should be referred to a victim advocacy service or community-based crisis center for assistance and support.

INTRODUCTION

Strangulation is a type of asphyxiation characterized by closure of the blood vessels or air passages of the neck as a result of external pressure,[1,2] and accounts for 10% of all violent deaths in the United States.[3] While strangulation can be divided into 4 categories, hanging, ligature, manual, and positional, research indicates that manual strangulation is the most common form of strangulation used in domestic violence cases.[4] Regardless of category, strangulation is also considered a blunt force trauma to the neck. Studies indicate that 23% to 68% of female domestic violence victims will experience at least 1 strangulation-related incident at the hands of their abusive male partner during their lifetime.[5,6] In Brink's study of 1 106 victims of violence and the types of injuries seen in male and female patients, a full 10% of women had experienced a strangulation attempt.[7] Additionally, women who experience intimate partner sexual assault often experience strangulation as a co-occurring issue.[8] Overall, women who experience non-fatal strangulation by an intimate partner have greater than seven-fold odds of becoming a victim of homicide.[9] Kimberg performed a fairly extensive review of the literature regarding IPV and men,[10] and, while it is clear than men sustain injuries inflicted by their intimate partner, clear patterns of injury for male victims have not been well studied,[11] particularly with regard to strangulation.

Strangulation in a living patient, with or without symptoms, warrants a thorough medical evaluation not only because of the immediate risk of death,[12,13] but also because of the potential delayed lethality.[14-17] Life-threatening medical emergencies, and death following manual strangulation has been reported hours to weeks following the event, with diagnoses that include carotid aneurysm or pseudo aneurysm, cerebral artery infarct, post-traumatic arterial thrombosis, and fractured trachea or larynx, to name but a few.[18,19] These diagnoses do not differ dramatically from those found following blunt traumatic injury to the neck when the mechanism involves accidental means.[20-22]

Despite this knowledge, strangulation is routinely under-evaluated in the emergency department setting,[23] and is rarely referred to as blunt traumatic injury to the neck. One of the challenges in educating clinicians about delayed lethality is the limited research on clinical manifestations in surviving victims of strangulation. The vast majority of data in strangulation cases comes from autopsy. Yet, hidden within the research on blunt traumatic injury to the neck is a population of strangulation victims. In their study of blunt carotid arterial injuries, Biffl et al, describe mechanisms of injury that include motor vehicle and motorcycle crashes; pedestrians struck by automobiles; skiing, horseback riding, bicycling, and construction accidents; assault; and near-hangings with a mortality of 15% and severe neurologic morbidity in 16% of survivors.[24]

ASSESSMENT OF STRANGULATION

For many years, providers have been encouraged to routinely assess their patients for the presence of IPV.[25] The recommendations regarding this assessment have begun to reflect the inclusion of assessing for strangulation in the context of abuse. Laughon et al describe purposeful modification of the Abuse Assessment Screen to include strangulation as a result of emerging data regarding its co-occurrence with IPV.[26] In living victims, physical signs and symptoms may or may not be present. McClane et al found that 50% of nonfatal strangulation victims had visible injury,[23] while Shields et al describe 85% of the victims evaluated having neck injuries.[8] In fact, signs and symptoms differ depending on many variables, including the type of strangulation, the force used, the duration of the strangulation, and the possibility that multiple strangulation attempts took place during the assault.

Because the clinical picture can vary so dramatically from patient to patient, and because the patient may not think to mention the strangulation component of the assault, asking about strangulation directly is the critical first step in a proper assessment. The patient may refer to the strangulation event as being "choked," so it is helpful when asking about strangulation to use language with which the patient is familiar; however, the provider should recognize that the mechanism of injury in choking, a foreign body airway obstruction, is significantly different than the mechanism in strangulation. Strangulation or blunt traumatic injury to the neck is the terminology that should be used throughout the medical record except in cases where the clinician is actually quoting the patient's use of the word "choke."

The provider should ask the patient for a description of the event, and should document that description using the patient's own words in quotation marks. Typically, ligature and hanging are uncommon forms of strangulation in IPV events; however, clinicians must consider the risks commonly associated with hanging when the patients report the use of a ligature or indicate that they were lifted partially or completely off the ground during a strangulation event. When hanging or ligature use is present, it is not uncommon to find obvious ligature marks on the patient's neck (**Figure 14-1**). Additionally, the patient is at greater risk of hyoid bone and thyroid cartilage fractures.[27]

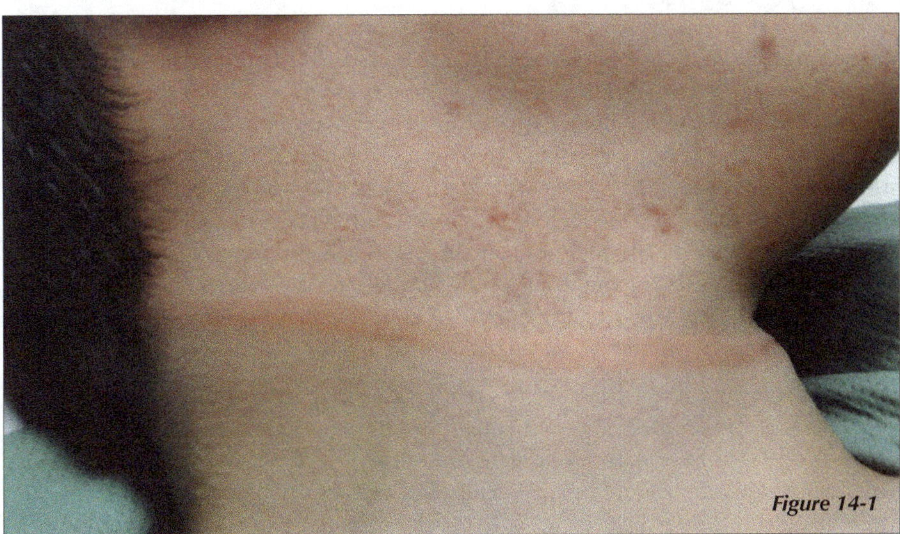

Figure 14-1.
Ligature mark.

Nichols et al found a mortality rate of 14.9% in their study of near-hanging victims, with injuries including hyoid bone and thyroid cartilage fractures, carotid occlusions, cervical spine subluxation, and spinal cord contusions.[28] While their patient population was composed entirely of individuals having attempted suicide, it is important to recognize that the mechanism of injury is the same, and the results can shed light on potential signs of IPV-related ligature strangulation.

It can also be helpful to inquire and document the patient's thought process during the attack. McClane et al describe a consistent stream of consciousness in strangulation victims that includes a 4-step process from beginning of strangulation to loss of consciousness (see **Table 14-1**).[23]

In denial, the patient describes not believing that this is happening. During realization, the patient describes suddenly understanding what is happening. In the primal phase, the patient describes fighting for her life, and, in resignation, just prior to loss of consciousness, an understanding that the perpetrator is going to kill her. Clinicians must recognize that not all patients will be able to fully describe these 4 phases. What is most important is obtaining clinical information about the patient's mindset at the time of the strangulation assault. This provides context for presenting symptoms such as acute stress reactions seen in patients who have survived a life-threatening event or self-inflicted injuries to the face and neck, which may occur during patients' struggles to stay alive.

Documentation of the patient's mental status upon arrival, particularly if there has been no delay in seeking treatment, is important. The patient may appear to be

Table 14-1. Subjective Process of Strangulation in Victims
1. Denial
2. Realization
3. Primal
4. Resignation

having a panic attack, when, in fact, she is trying to recover from an episode of oxygen deprivation; she may initially appear postictal from loss of consciousness and possible seizure activity, or she may appear drunken or psychotic. It is important that staff avoid assumptions regarding the patient's behavior and evaluate fully for the possibility that such behavior is the result of strangulation or other trauma. Other signs and symptoms strangulation patients may present with include: loss of consciousness, incontinence of bladder or bowel, bleeding, coughing, dyspnea, headache, otorrhagia, neck tenderness, vision changes, throat pain, lightheadedness, voice changes, memory loss, numbness or tingling of extremities, odynophagia or dysphagia, crepitus, nausea or vomiting, and irritability. These are some of the more common signs and symptoms, though each patient may present differently.

Patients presenting with a history of strangulation require a thorough and detailed assessment. It is common for the patient who has experienced strangulation in the context of IPV to have received other assault-related injuries. A complete head-to-toe physical examination should be conducted. The provider will want to look closely for any signs of injury on the patient. It is equally important to ask about co-occurring factors, such as use of a ligature to strangle, or use of a smothering device.

Specific to strangulation injuries, the provider will want to carefully assess the heads and necks of these patients, looking closely for the signs and symptoms previously described, as injuries may be subtle. The patient's eyes, ears, nose, mouth, and throat require a detailed examination. When neck injuries are seen, they commonly include abrasion (**Figure 14-2**), mild to extreme bruising (**Figures 14-3 to 14-5**), hematomas (**Figure 14-6**), and petechiae (**Figure 14-7**). Palpating the patient's neck, shoulders, and upper chest for crepitus or subcutaneous emphysema is important in identifying tracheal and thorax injuries, as well as recognizing soft tissue injuries when palpated. Special attention will need to be paid in assessing the patients' tympanic membranes, oral cavity, skin, and scalp for petechiae, as this is a common finding resulting from the venous congestion that occurs during strangulation (**Figure 14-8**). Carefully inspect behind the ears as co-occurring injury is frequently found in this location (**Figures 14-9** and **14-10**). Additionally, a close-up inspection of the eyelids (outer and inner), conjunctiva, and sclera for the presence of petechiae is critical. Subconjunctival hemorrhage or hyphema may also be present (**Figure 14-11**). Cranial nerve assessment and auscultation of the heart, lungs, and carotid arteries should be performed to identify any abnormalities.

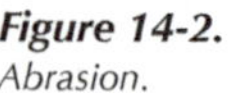

Figure 14-2.
Abrasion.

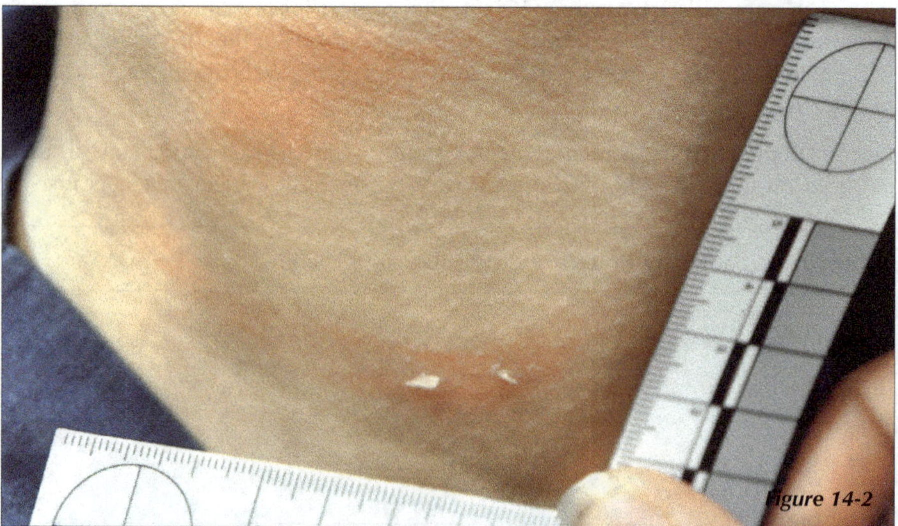

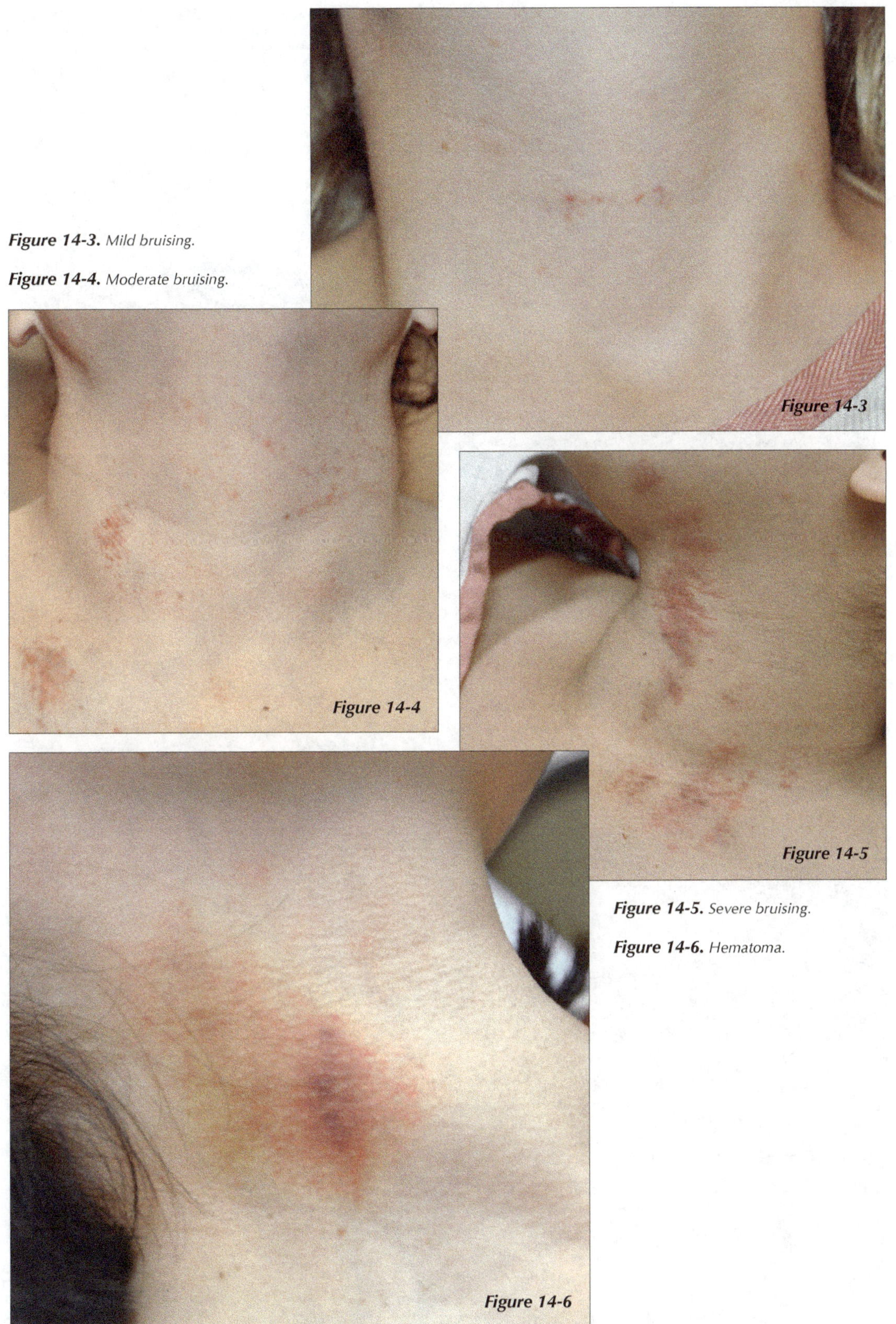

Figure 14-3. Mild bruising.

Figure 14-4. Moderate bruising.

Figure 14-3

Figure 14-4

Figure 14-5

Figure 14-5. Severe bruising.

Figure 14-6. Hematoma.

Figure 14-6

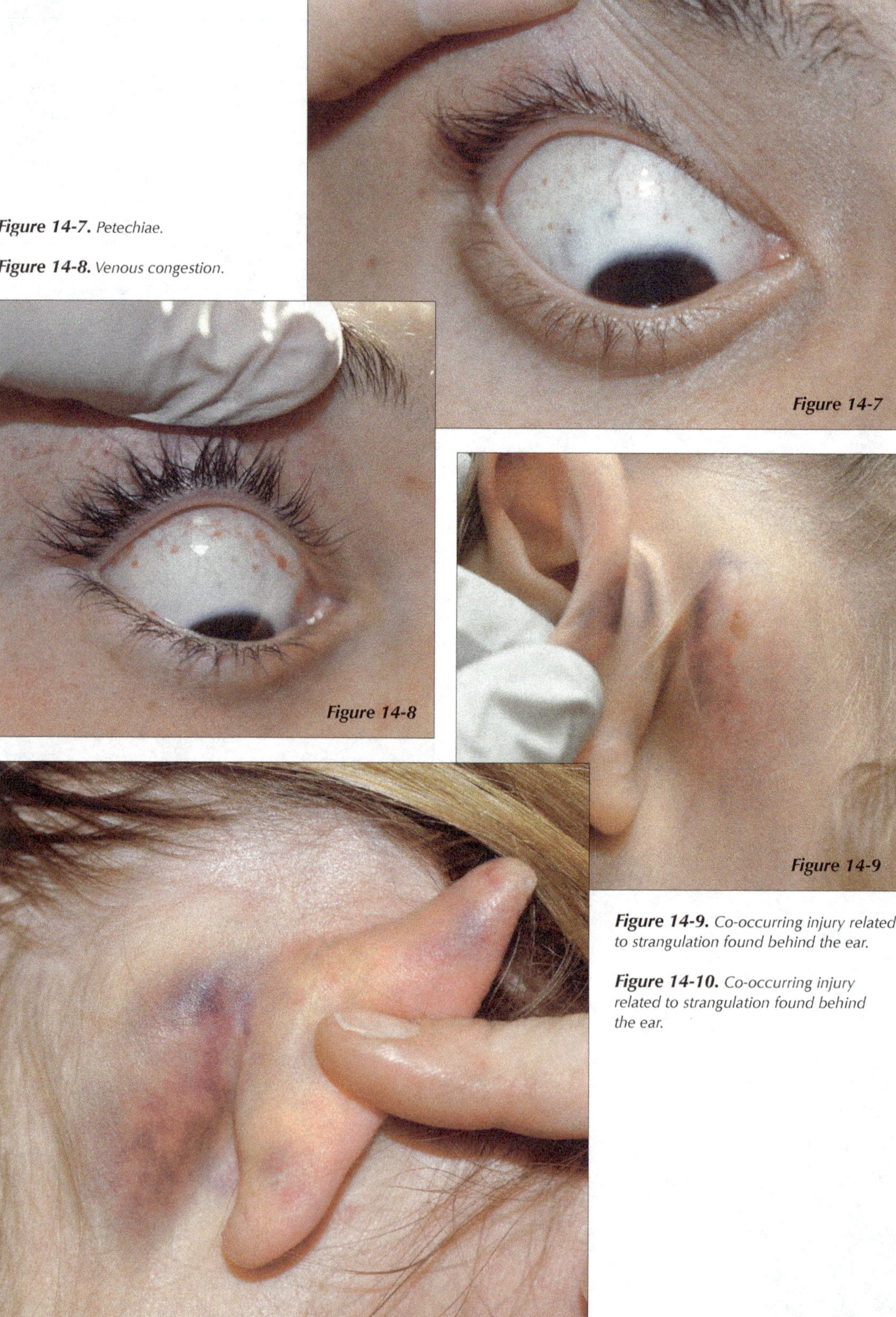

Figure 14-7. *Petechiae.*

Figure 14-8. *Venous congestion.*

Figure 14-7

Figure 14-8

Figure 14-9

Figure 14-9. *Co-occurring injury related to strangulation found behind the ear.*

Figure 14-10. *Co-occurring injury related to strangulation found behind the ear.*

Figure 14-10

Vital signs and oxygenation saturation (SaO2) levels should also be obtained upon arrival and at intervals throughout the patient's stay.

Assessment and documentation of a strangulation patient's objective and subjective signs and symptoms is of vital importance. This can easily be done utilizing a strangulation assessment form or tool (see **Appendix 14-1**). There are a variety of forms available, or one can be created to meet the needs of the provider or institution. Typically these forms will include sections to document (in the patient's own words) a history of the strangulation event, the method or manner of strangulation (eg, manual, 1 or 2 hands, or ligature), whether there were multiple strangulation attempts, and signs and symptoms present during and after the assault. The tool should also have a place to document the patient's description of the amount of pressure or pain the assailant inflicted during the strangulation, using an appropriate scale (eg, numerical, Wong-Baker Faces, etc.).

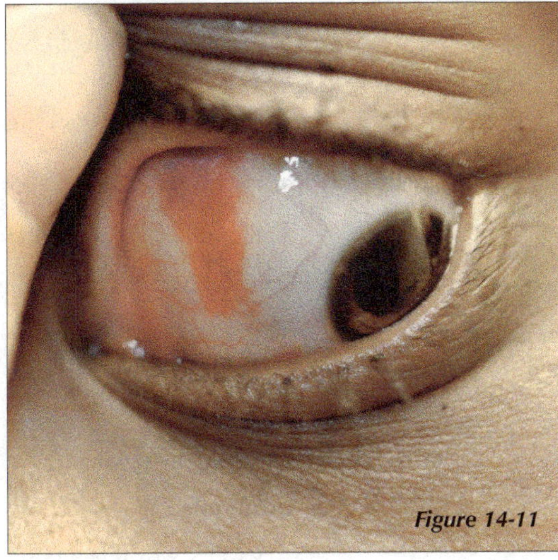

Figure 14-11

Figure 14-11. *Subconjunctival hemorrhage.*

The tool should further allow for documentation of the physical assessment, including Glasgow Coma Scale, documentation of heart and lung sounds, initial and follow-up SaO2 levels, and a head and neck diagram for the provider to document any physical findings. These diagrams should include magnified body maps for the eyes, eyelids, ears, and mouth. The findings should be described, measured, and photographed whenever possible. See **Table 14-2** for a recommended list of what should be included in the strangulation assessment.

Lastly, consideration should be given to the collection of evidence from the patient's body that could corroborate the description of the strangulation event and prove beneficial in prosecution. More than 30 states have felony strangulation laws, and those without felony strangulation laws have begun filing charges such as attempted murder to better legally address the lethal implications of this act.[29,30] Additionally, studies have shown both low- and high-yield collection of assailant epithelial cell DNA from the necks of strangulation victims.[31-33] Future research should be directed at larger scale studies that can better show the usefulness or lack of usefulness of this approach in the clinical setting.

Case Study 14-1.

Verbatim history given by patient and recorded in medical record:

"I told him he had to leave because he was getting out of hand. He left, but came back 5 or 10 minutes later. He asked why and I said, 'because we are not together.' And that's when he grabbed me by the neck and carried me from the kitchen to the living room. He was laughing and telling me to beg for my life. I begged, but he just laughed and said, 'That's not gonna happen.' I passed out again, and when I woke up, I ran to my neighbor's house, but they said they didn't have a phone, so I waved down some people on the street and used their phone to call 911."

Diagnostic Testing

As previously stated, living strangulation victims are frequently underevaluated by health care professionals. There are many hypotheses as to the underevaluation, ranging from a lack of visible injury to the fact that the patient is an IPV victim. Regardless, there remains a great need for medical guidelines and protocols for evaluation of these patients. In an attempt to address the need for standardized protocols, McClane et al offered some guidance regarding assessment tools and studies health care providers can

<table>
<tr><td>

Table 14-2. Recommended Strangulation Assessment Elements

— A description of the strangulation(s) in the patient's own words, using quotations

— A rating of the pressure or pain of each strangulation event on a developmentally appropriate assessment scale (0-10, Wong-Baker Faces, etc.)

— Date and time of the strangulation(s)

— Method or manner of strangulation;

    — One or two hands, ligature, chokehold, approach (front or behind), lifted off ground

    — Multiple strangulations

    — Smothering

    — Jewelry worn by victim or assailant

— Symptoms during strangulation and symptoms since strangulation to include:

    — Loss of consciousness

    — Incontinence of urine or stool

    — Bleeding (describe)

    — Coughing or dyspnea

    — Dysphagia or odynophagia

    — Lightheadedness, dizziness, or headache

    — Nose, neck, or throat pain

    — Nausea or vomiting

    — Neck swelling

    — Drooling

    — Uncontrolled shaking

    — Voice or vision changes

    — Combativeness, irritability, or restlessness

    — Numbness or tingling of the extremities

    — Memory loss

    — Bleeding

— Physical assessment documentation

— Full review of systems, including palpation for tenderness, abnormal carotid pulse, and crepitus

— SaO2 levels, minimum of two intervals

— Injury documentation using body diagrams and photographs

— Evidence collection when appropriate

</td></tr>
</table>

use to adequately evaluate the strangulation patient. **Table 14-3** combines McClane's recommendations with typical testing found following blunt carotid injury.

PHOTOGRAPHY

Photographs are a form of documentation and can assume the status of evidence.[34] Whenever possible, photographs of all injuries should be taken. Photographs are in no way a replacement for written documentation or diagramming of injuries, but are an extremely helpful addition to documentation. In the event photography cannot be utilized, detailed body maps and diagrams are critical for injury documentation.

Ideally, informed consent should be obtained prior to photographing injuries. If a patient provides the proper consent, copies of the photographs and record can be released to investigation agencies, or used for educational purposes. Informed consent may be waived if the person is unable to provide it, such as in cases of a trauma, or if the patient is a minor, such as in cases of child abuse. Depending on the institution, consent for photography may be included in the general consent signed during hospital registration. It is vitally important that the clinician understand his or her local policies regarding photography.

Once informed consent has been obtained, begin the process by first photographing the patient's identifying information. This includes the patient's name, date of birth, age, sex, medical record number, and date of service. All too often, there is no information identifying the patient in the photograph, making it impossible on case or peer review to say with certainty that the photographs being visualized are those of the patient. This is particularly true with photographs that are limited to the area of specific injuries and do not include a patient's face or identifying features.

Table 14-3. Strangulation-Related Uses of Various Assessment Tools and Tests	
TEST	RATIONALE
Pulse oximetry	Evaluation of oxygen status
Soft tissue of the neck X-ray	Evaluation of subcutaneous emphysema Identification of tracheal deviation, edema, hematoma
Cervical spine X-ray	Identification of a fractured hyoid bone
Computed axial tomography (CT) scan	Detailed evaluation of neck structures
Carotid doppler ultrasound	Identification of carotid artery dissection
Computed axial tomography (CT) scan with angiogram	Detailed evaluation of neck structures including the vessels
Chest X-ray	Identification of pulmonary edema, aspiration or pneumonia
Magnetic resonance imaging	Comprehensive evaluation of the neck structures
Pharyngoscopy	Identification of pharyngeal petecchia, edema, and other injury
Fiberoptic laryngobronchoscopy	Evaluation of the vocal cords and trachea

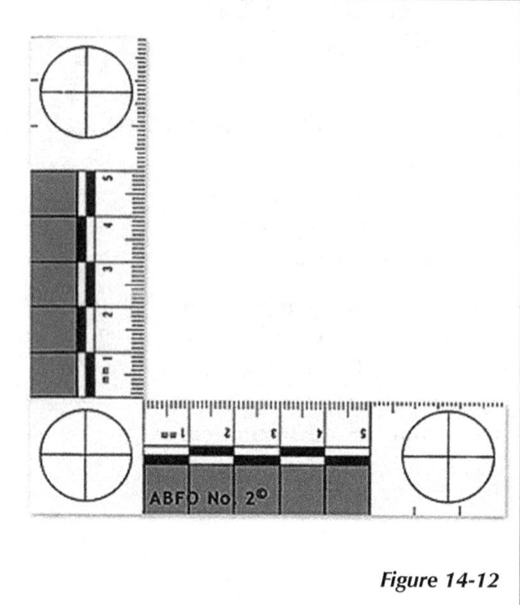

Figure 14-12

A full-length orientation photograph of the patient should start the photo series. Once obtained, images of each injury can be captured. Each injury should be photographed a minimum of three times. This includes a mid-distance photograph for orientation purposes, a close-up of the injury, and a close-up of the injury with a standard, such as an American Board of Forensic Odontology (ABFO) No. 2 reference scale (**Figure 14-12**). This standard provides accurate size and color documentation, while the photograph without the standard demonstrates that nothing has been hidden by its use.

All photographs should be taken with the camera at a 90-degree angle to the injury to avoid distortion of the wound. This provides the most accurate capture of the injury shape and size. The ABFO No. 2 reference scale also serves as a guide for this; the circles on the scale should appear as such, not as ellipticals, when photographed properly.

DISPOSITION

It has been suggested that, for the purposes of adequate observation, the living strangulation patient be admitted for observation if seen acutely within the first 24-48 hours of injury.[35] However, the lack of accumulated evidence and of provider education regarding strangulation and its potential lethality often make this suggestion difficult to implement. In either case, detailed and thorough discharge instructions are imperative and should be tailored to the individual patient's particular constellation of signs and symptoms.

If the patient is being discharged to home within the first 48-72 hours of the strangulation event, care should be taken to give the patient detailed instructions of symptoms that warrant the patient's return to the emergency department (see **Table 14-4**).

When available, community-based crisis center advocates should be called and brought in to assist patients with understanding the availability of community resources and ongoing support, accessing services such as restraining orders and counseling, and completing a formal safety plan whether the patient is choosing to remain in the relationship or leave.

Table 14-4. Symptoms Warranting Return for Immediate Evaluation

— Increasing or severe headache pain

— Increasing neck pain

— Drooping eyelid

— Difficulty speaking or understanding speech

— Difficulty walking

— Difficulty breathing

— Dizziness or lightheadedness

(continued)

Table 14-4. Symptoms Warranting Return for Immediate Evaluation *(continued)*

— Numbness, paralysis, or weakness, usually on one side of the body

— Seizure

— Sudden confusion

— Sudden decrease in the level of consciousness

— Sudden loss of balance or coordination

— Sudden vision problems (e.g., blurry vision, blindness in one eye)

— Vomiting

— Vaginal bleeding (if you are pregnant)

— Thoughts of suicide

SYMPTOMS WARRANTING RETURN FOR DOCUMENTATION

— Pinpoint red or purple dots on your face or neck

— Bruises on your face, neck or body

— Burst blood vessels in your eye

— Swelling of your face or neck

APPENDIX 14-1: STRANGULATION EVALUATION TOOL

STRANGULATION EVALUATION TOOL

Exam Date   Exam Time
Strangulation Date   Strangulation Time

Glascow Coma Scale (Circle the appropriate score for each, complete the total at the bottom)

Eye Opening	Score
Spontaneous	4
To speech	3
To pain	2
None	1

Verbal Response	Score
Oriented	5
Confused	4
Inappropriate	3
Incomprehensible	2
None	1

Motor Response	Score
Obeys commands	6
Localizes to pain	5
Withdraws from pain	4
Flexion to pain (decorticate)	3
Extension to pain (decerebrate)	2
None	1
Total Score (enter)	

Description of strangulation event(s) in patient's own words:_______________

____

____

____

____

____

____

____

Signature_______________________________ Date_____________ - 1 -

STRANGULATION EVALUATION TOOL

Method/Manner of Strangulation:

☐ One hand   Estimated length of time: ______seconds ______minutes

☐ Two hands   Estimated length of time: ______seconds ______minutes

☐ "Chokehold"   Estimated length of time: ______seconds ______minutes

☐ Approached from the front

☐ Approached from behind

☐ Multiple strangulation attempts during incident (how many)________________

☐ Jewelry on patient's neck during strangulation

☐ Jewelry on suspect's hands/wrist during strangulation

☐ Ligature used (describe if possible)________________

☐ Smothering attempt (describe)________________

☐ Other (describe)________________

During strangulation did the patient note any of the following:

☐ Loss of consciousness/blacking out/passing out

______________Number of times

☐ Incontinence of Urine

☐ Incontinence of Stool

☐ Bleeding (describe)________________

☐ Patient's feet were lifted off the ground

☐ S/he was smothered in addition to strangled (with what)________________

Since the strangulation, has the patient noted any of the following symptoms:

☐ Coughing	☐ Drooling	☐ Dyspnea
☐ Dysphagia	☐ Odynophagia	☐ Headache
☐ Lightheadedness	☐ Neck Pain	☐ Neck swelling
☐ Nose Pain	☐ Nausea	☐ Vomiting
☐ Sore throat	☐ Crepitus/Subcutaneous emphysema	
☐ Uncontrolled shaking	☐ Combativeness/irritability/restlessness	

☐ Voice changes (describe)________________

☐ Vision changes (describe)________________

☐ Loss of memory (describe)________________

☐ Bleeding (describe)________________

☐ Weakness/numbness of extremities (describe)________________

Signature_______________________________ Date_____________ - 2 -

STRANGULATION EVALUATION TOOL

On a scale of zero (0) meaning no pressure and ten (10) meaning the worst pressure you can imagine, how hard was the suspect's grip or pressure (circle the one that applies):

0   1   2   3   4   5   6   7   8   9   10

☐ Wong-Baker FACES Scale used (insert score)________

Examination:
Patient Pregnant: ☐ No   ☐ Yes   Number of weeks____
Fetal Heart Rate _____
Pregnancy related symptoms during or since strangulation:

____
____

O2 Saturation:
    Time:________ Level:____________
    Time:________ Level:____________
Lung Sounds:_______________________________________
Heart Sounds:______________________________________
☐ Abnormal carotid pulse (describe)__________________________

☐ Petechiae   ☐ Facial_____________________
                     ☐ Ears______________________
                     ☐ Eyes______________________
                     ☐ Conjunctival________________
☐ Tongue injury   _____________________________
☐ Oral cavity injuries ___________________________
☐ Subconjunctival hemorrhage______________________
☐ Neurologic findings: ☐ Ptosis   ☐ Facial droop   ☐ Unilateral weakness
                           ☐ Paralysis   ☐ Loss of sensation
☐ Absence of normal crepitus felt during manipulation of cricoid cartilage
☐ Visible Injury (described on body maps below)
☐ Digital photographs taken

Signature____Date________________   - 3 -

STRANGULATION EVALUATION TOOL

Cranial Nerve Assessment

CN I	
CN II	
CN III	
CN IV	
CN V	
CN VI	
CN VII	
CN VIII	
CN IX	
CN X	
CN XI	
CN XII	

Signature____Date________________   - 4 -

STRANGULATION EVALUATION TOOL

Right Eye

____
____
____

Left Eye

____
____
____
____

Signature____Date________________   - 5 -

STRANGULATION EVALUATION TOOL

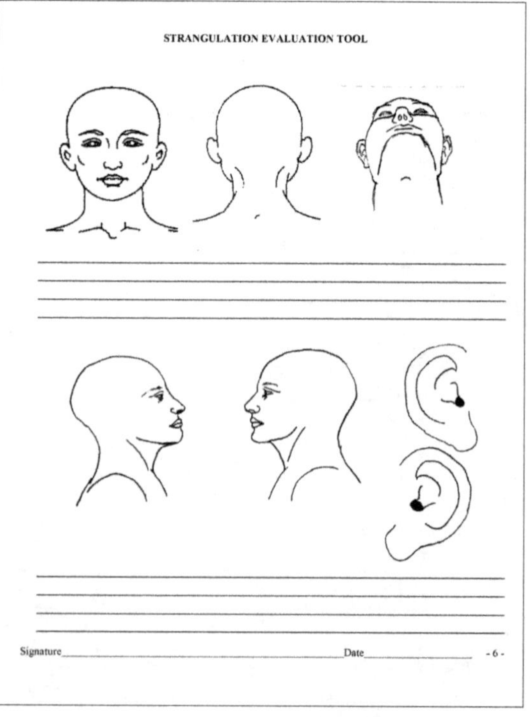

____
____
____

____
____
____
____

Signature____Date________________   - 6 -

APPENDIX 14-2: COMPLETED STRANGULATION EVALUATION TOOL

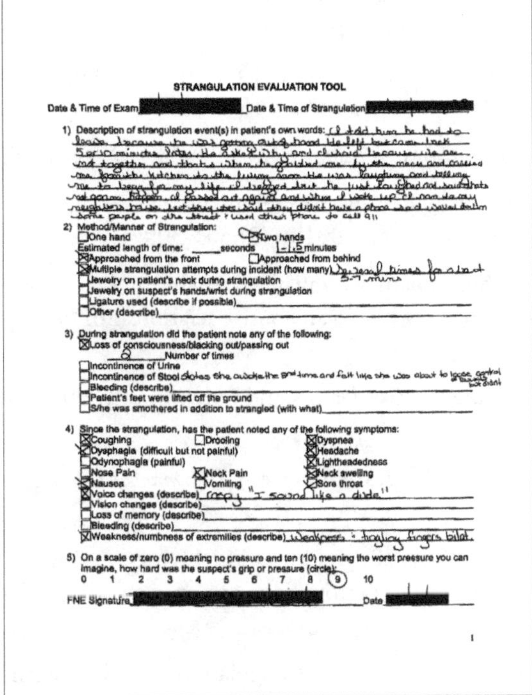

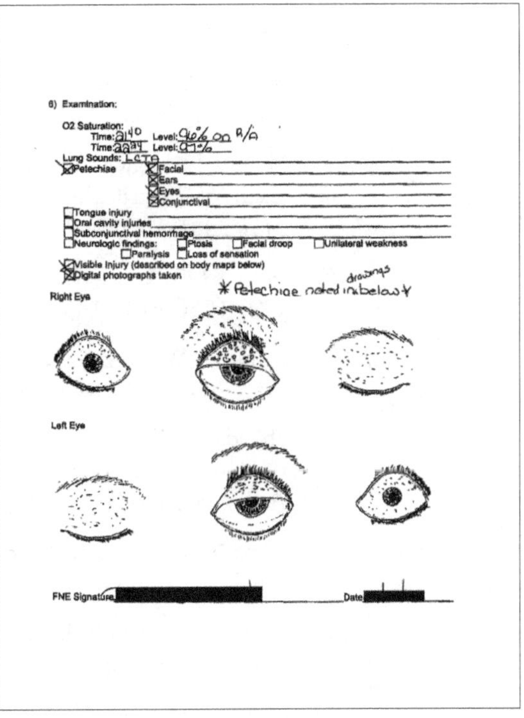

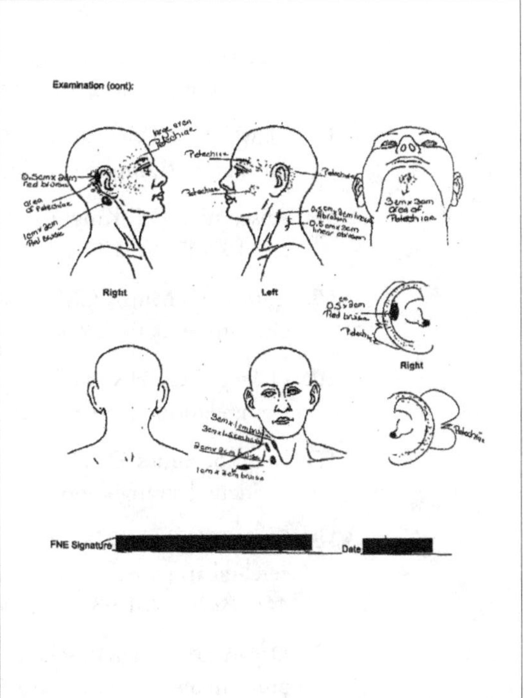

REFERENCES

1. Iserson KV. Strangulation: a review of ligature, manual, and postural neck compression injuries. *Ann Emerg Med.* 1984;13(3):179-185.

2. Line WS Jr, Stanley RB Jr, Choi JH. Strangulation: a full spectrum of blunt neck trauma. *Ann Otol Rhino Laryngo.* 1985;94(6 pt 1):542-546.

3. Funk M, Schuppel J. Strangulation injuries. *Wisconsin Med J.* 2003;102(3):41-45.

4. Strack GB, McClane GE, Hawley D. A Review of 300 attempted strangulation cases, part I: criminal legal issues. *J Emerg Med.* 2001:21(3);303-309.

5. Wilbur L, Higley M, Hatfield J, Surprenant Z, Taliaferro E, Smith DJ. Survey results of women who have been strangled while in an abusive relationship. *J Emerg Med.* 2001;21(3):297-302.

6. Berrios DC, Grady D. Domestic violence: risk factors and outcomes. *West J Med.* 1991;155(2):133-135.

7. Brink O. When violence strikes the head, neck, and face. *J Trauma Inj Infect Crit Care.* 2009;67(1):147-151.

8. Shields LBE, Corey TS, Weakley-Jones B, Stewart D. Living victims of strangulation: a 10-year review of cases in a metropolitan community. *Am J Med Pathol.* 2010;31(4):320-325.

9. Glass N, Laughon K, Campbell J, et al. Non-fatal strangulation is an important risk factor for homicide of women. *J Emerg Med.* 2008;35(3):329-335.

10. Kimberg LS. Addressing intimate partner violence with male patients: a review and introduction of pilot guidelines. *J Gen Intern Med.* 2008;23(12):2071-2078.

11. Sheridan D, Nash K. Acute injury patterns of intimate partner violence victims. *Trauma Violence Abuse.* 2007;8(3):281-289.

12. Di Maio VJM, Dana SE. *Handbook of Forensic Pathology.* New Delhi, India: Viva Books Private Limited; 1999:139-140.

13. Hawley DA, McClane GE, Strack GB. A review of 300 attempted strangulation cases part III: injuries in fatal cases. *J Emerg Med.* 2001;21(3):317-322.

14. Anscombe AM, Knight BH. Delayed death after pressure on the neck. *Forensic Sci Int.* 1996;78(3):193-197.

15. Lumb PD, Milroy CM, Whitwell HL. Neuropathological changes in delayed death after strangulation. *Emerg Med News.* 2002;24(5):1-42.

16. Helwig FC. Histopathologic studies of the brain in delayed death following strangulation. *Am J Forensic Med Pathol.* 1989;10(3):266-267.

17. Kiani S, Simes D. Delayed bilateral internal carotid artery thrombosis following accidental strangulation. *Br J Anaesthesia.* 2000:84(4):521-524.

18. Sethi PK, Sethi NK, Torgovnick J, Arsura E. Delayed left anterior and middle cerebral artery hemorrhagic infarctions after attempted strangulation. *Am J Forensic Med Pathol.* 2012;33(1):105-106.

19. Dayapala A, Samarasekera A, Jayasena A. An uncommon delayed sequela after pressure on the neck. *Am J Forensic Med Pathology.* 2012;33(1):80-82.

20. Assimikopolous D, Tsirves G. Blunt trauma of the larynx and pneumomediastinum. *Otolaryngology–Head and Neck Surgery.* 2009;141(6):788-789.

21. McKevitt EC, Kirkpatrick AW, Vertesi L, Granger R, Simons RK. Blunt vascular neck injuries: diagnosis and outcomes of extracranial vessel injury. *J Trauma Inj Infect Crit Care.* 2002;53(3): 472-476.

22. Fabian TC, Patton JH Jr, Croce MA, Minard G, Kudsk KA, Pritchard FE. Blunt carotid injury: importance of early diagnosis and anticoagulant therapy. *Ann Surg.* 1996;223(5):513-525.

23. McClane GE, Strack GB, Hawley D. A review of 300 attempted strangulation cases part II: clinical evaluation of the surviving victim. *J Emerg Med.* 2001;21(3):311-315.

24. Biffle WL, Moore EE, Ryu RK, et al. The unrecognized epidemic of blunt carotid arterial injuries early diagnosis improves neurologic outcome. *Ann Surg.* 1998;28(4):462-470.

25. Family Violence Prevention Fund. The national consensus guidelines on identifying and responding to domestic violence victimization, 2004. San Francisco, CA: San Francisco Family Violence Prevention Fund; 2004. Futures Without Violence Web site. http://www.futureswithoutviolence.org/userfiles/file/HealthCare/consensus. pdf. Accessed February 11, 2013.

26. Laughon K, Renker P, Glass N, Parker B. Revision of the abuse assessment screen to address nonlethal strangulation. *J Obstet Gynecol Neonatal Nur.* 2008:37(4);502-507.

27. Azmak D. Asphyxial deaths: a retrospective study and review of the literature. *Am J Forensic Med Pathol.* (2006);27(2):134-144.

28. Nichols SD, McCarthy MC, Ekeh AP, Woods RJ, Walusimbi MS, Saxe JM. Outcome of cervical near-hanging injuries. *J Trauma Inj Infect Crit Care.* 2009;66(1):174-178.

29. Laughon K, Glass N, Worrell C. Review and analysis of laws related to strangulation in 50 states. *Eval Rev.* 2009;33(4):358-369.

30. Turkel A; National Center for the Prosecution of Violence Against Women. And then he choked me: understanding, investigating and prosecuting strangulation cases. *The Voice.* 2007;2(1):1-4. National District Attorneys Association Web site. http://www.ndaa.org/pdf/the_voice_vol_2_no_1_08.pdf. Accessed February 11, 2013.

31. Wiegand P, Kleiber M. DNA typing of epithelia cells after strangulation. *Int J Legal Med.* 1997;10(4):181-183.

32. Graham EAM, Rutty GN. Investigation into "normal" background DNA on adult necks: implications for DNA profiling of manual strangulation victims. *J Forensic Sci.* 2008;53(5):1074-1082.

33. Rutty GN. An investigation into the transference and survivability of human DNA following simulated manual strangulation with consideration of the problem of third party contamination. *Int J Legal Med.* 2002;116(3):170-173.

34. Banks M. Visual methods in social research. London, UK: Sage Publications; 2001.

35. Mitchell C, Anglin D. *Intimate Partner Violence: A Health-based Perspective.* New York, NY: Oxford University Press; 2009.

Chapter 15

STALKING

Catherine Mortiere, PhD
Richard Sochor, MA

KEY POINTS

1. Stalking can be described as the pernicious, unwanted attention of one individual toward another. Behaviors can include following victims; contacting victims through unsolicited phone calls, letters, or emails; threatening victims; and vandalizing property.

2. The first anti-stalking law was passed in 1990, in California. By 1995, all states, including the District of Columbia, had passed some version of an anti-stalking law.

3. It has been suggested that between 2% and 13% of males and 8% to 12% of females will be victimized by a stalker at some point in their adult life.

4. There are over 20 different stalker typologies that fit into 3 categories: typologies that classify based on mental disorders, typologies that classify based on the relationship of the perpetrator to the victim, and typologies that classify according to the motivation for stalking.

5. Stalking behavior has negative effects on the victim. Those effects can sometimes result in severe psychological issues, and in extreme cases stalking can result in bodily harm or death.

6. Cyberstalking, as well as the use of electronic monitoring devices, have become increasingly more common. Many states have yet to include cyberstalking in their definitions of stalking.

INTRODUCTION

The meaning of the term "stalking" in its modern colloquial usage is relatively new compared to its historical meaning. The term stalking was previously associated with hunting animals. For example, a person who hunted deer was customarily referred to as a deer-stalker. It wasn't until the late 20th century that the definition of the word was expanded to include people as victim prey, and the pattern of behaviors that define stalking as a criminal act.[1,2] Within the context of intimate partner violence (IPV), stalking is not only more common than ever before but has become easier to execute and more clandestine given our growing technology. Our current system is working toward becoming more equipped to handle stalking at the judicial, legislative and executive levels of government.

Stalking, in the current context, refers to the sociopathological entity of pernicious unwanted attention of one individual toward another. This has captured public interest and has been memorably portrayed in such Hollywood movies as *Single White Female, Fatal Attraction, One Hour Photo*, and, more recently, *The Roommate*. Behavior considered to be stalking has been defined as the "willful, malicious, and repeated following and harassing of another person that threatens his or her safety."[3] Another definition, presented by Pathé and Mullen, is "a constellation of behaviors in which 1 individual inflicts on another repeated unwanted intrusions and communications."[4] However, stalking is ultimately defined, as most experts and statutes typically emphasize, as a course of conduct involving repeated actions, which must occur on more than one occasion.[2] Some examples of stalking behaviors include:

— Following victims

— Loitering near victims' homes and workplaces

— Giving gifts

— Sending letters

— Transmitting e-mails

— Making phone calls

— Vandalizing property (car or home, for example)

— Photographing the victims or their families

— Making threats

— Approaching or confronting the victims in public places or near the victims' homes or workplaces

— Physical and/or sexual assaults[1]

The most significant problem often lies in determining an appropriate threshold for behavior to be considered merely an annoyance or irritation, from what is potentially dangerous, and therefore regarded as "stalking."[2] "Many of the stalking behaviors are not illegal and are even innocuous, but the pattern and the purpose of the actions characterize them as stalking."[1]

Although the meaning of the word stalking has expanded, there is no reason to believe that stalking (by modern definition) is an entirely recent phenomenon.[5] One of the first accounts of what we would call today a "celebrity stalker" is described in the book *Queen Victoria's Stalker: The Strange Case of the Boy Jones*,[6] which depicts events following the 1838 coronation of Queen Victoria and the difficulties that she confronted with a young stalker, nicknamed the Boy Jones who on a number of occasions managed to sneak into Buckingham Palace. On 2 of these instances he was found hiding in the Queen's dressing room and even stealing her underwear. Due to the fact that "simple trespass" was not at that time a criminal offense (even in Buckingham Palace), he continued to be a problem. Ultimately, as a last resort and in fear for the safety of the Queen, Boy Jones was kidnapped by government men who forced him to serve as a sailor in the Royal Navy for more than 5 years without charge or trial.

Today's perpetual media coverage of stories such as these would have many believe that this behavior is more common than ever. Some consider that this may stand as a reflection of changes in modern society. For example, Mullen et al theorize that "[m]odern man, wrapped up in his individual rights, fed on expectations, is all too vulnerable to disappointed expectations which can on occasion breed the rancor and resentment that explodes in stalking."[2] They go on to suggest that perhaps "…more importantly the changing role of women in the domestic, work, and public spheres has created, particularly for the unregenerate male, challenges and temptations that some are ill equipped to manage."[2]

Whatever the history of stalking may be, what is new, however, is that this pattern of behaviors identified as stalking is now an explicit, criminal offense. The first anti-stalking law in the United States was passed in 1990, by the state of California, in reaction to a number of highly publicized cases.[2] One well-known case was of the young actress Rebecca Schaeffer, who in 1989, was murdered at her door by Robert Bardo, who stalked her for 3 years prior to this finite murderous act. Robert Bardo was a diagnosed schizophrenic (paranoid type) young man who "fell in love" with Schaeffer after seeing her on television. However, Bardo's adoration turned to anger when he saw a movie in which Schaeffer acted in a bedroom scene. This ruined his perception of Schaeffer as the perfect woman. He became convinced that she had become another "Hollywood tramp" and that she had to be punished. Bardo hired a private detective who obtained her address from California's motor vehicle records. He then went to Schaeffer's apartment, rang the bell, and fatally shot her when she came to the door.[7]

Within just 1 year, 4 more women were killed in Orange County, California, all by separate stalkers. Another infamous case occurred in 1982, several years prior. Theresa Saldana, another actress, had been stabbed 10 times by her stalker, but survived because her screams were heard by a nearby delivery man who restrained the stalker.[1] The media attention dedicated to these horrific events brought the issue of stalking to the public's attention. It became evident that the early identification and prosecution of stalking behavior could have altered the tragic conclusions to such cases. The macabre events served as a catalytic force that directed the California legislation to pass the very first laws criminalizing stalking.

Shortly after California passed its anti-stalking laws, other states enacted similar legislation. By 1995, all states, including the District of Columbia, had legislated some version of an anti-stalking law. A federal law (18 USC § 2261A) was enacted in 1996, prohibiting stalkers from traveling across state lines with the intent to injure or harass another person or placing such person in reasonable fear of death or bodily injury as a result of, or in the course of, such travel.[8,9]

Despite the fact that all 50 states and the Federal Government enacted statutes regarding stalking, the legal definition for stalking varies across jurisdictions. As pointed out by Baum et al:

State laws vary regarding the element of victim fear and emotional distress, as well as the requisite intent of the stalker. Some state laws specify that the victim must have been frightened by the stalking, while others require only that the stalking behavior would have caused a reasonable person to experience fear. In addition, states vary regarding what level of fear is required. Some state laws require prosecutors to establish fear of death or serious bodily harm, while others require only that prosecutors establish that the victim suffered emotional distress.[10]

For specific information regarding stalking laws by state visit The National Center for Victims of Crime: Stalking resource center web site on stalking laws at: http://www.ncvc.org/src/main.aspx?dbID=DB_Register204

Non-uniformity and glaring variability in the fundamental definition of stalking as a criminal offense has the potential to create problems and confusion. What one state considers stalking behavior, or in other words wrongful behavior, may be acceptable (at least legally) in others. The general public desires consistency in how we define what is lawful or unlawful. Consistency in legislation helps build confidence in the general public and potential victims who feel they need to protect themselves. Perpetrators often know the particulars of the law better than some of the law officers sworn to enforce it. This is akin to the wiles of some pedophiles who are keenly aware of the age-of-consent-laws in various states. Consequently, stalkers are commonly aware of what states they can get away with certain behavior without being arrested, and/or what laws the local police may enforce more than others.

STATISTICS

Given the fact that definitions of stalking often vary widely, so too do estimates regarding the prevalence of stalking behavior. Large-scale, representative, international studies of stalking behavior indicate that between 2%–13% of males and 8%–32% of females at some point in their adult lives will be victimized by a stalker.[11-20] "Most of these studies have attempted to use definitions that translated legal criteria into everyday language."[21]

In an early study, commissioned by the United States National Institute of Justice (USNIJ), Tjaden and Thoennes[20] examined the results of a nationally representative telephone survey of 8000 women and 8000 men that targeted their experiences with stalking. This survey became one aspect of the larger National Violence Against Women Survey. The USNIJ study did not use the word stalking in screening questions in order to avoid preconceived notions regarding its definition. They instead posed questions to respondents in behavioral terms. For example, one question asked, "Not including bill collectors, telephone solicitors, or other sales people, has anyone, male or female, ever..." The choices given were: (1) followed or spied on you; (2) sent you unsolicited letters or written correspondence; (3) made unsolicited phone calls to you; (4) stood outside your home, school, or workplace; (5) showed up at places you were, even though he or she had no business being there; (6) left unwanted items for you to find; (7) tried to communicate in other ways against your will; (8) vandalized your property or destroyed something you loved."[20] If respondents answered "yes" to 1 or more of these questions, they were subsequently asked whether they had ever been victim to any of these things on more than 1 occasion; thus highlighting the concept that stalking involves a series of behaviors. If respondents did report being victimized on more than 1 occasion, they were finally asked how frightened the behavior made them feel and whether they feared their assailants would seriously harm them or people close to them. Only if respondents reported that they were very frightened or feared bodily harm, were they counted as stalking victims for this study.[20]

According to the above criteria, Tjaden and Thoennes' analysis found that 8% of women and 2% of men in the United States (US) had experienced stalking at some time in their lives.[20] However, when the criteria were loosened to include respondents answering that they were only a little or somewhat frightened, the prevalence increased significantly to 12% of women and 4% of men. This adjustment emphasizes how important it is to carefully define these measures and how easily the results can be affected.

Other notable results from this sample (using the more stringent criteria) include the finding that 78% of reported stalking victims were female and 87% of stalking perpetrators were male. Within the entire sample of victims of stalking, 52% were between the ages of 18 and 29 years old. In most stalking cases, the victim and perpetrator were acquainted, and women were stalked by strangers 23% of the time, and males 36% of the time. Women were more likely to be stalked by an intimate partner (59%) than men (30%), about one-half of which occurred while the relationship was still intact. Stalking was also associated with other violent behaviors. In intimate relationships, 81% of women who were stalked by a current or former partner were also physically assaulted by that partner, and 31% of those were also sexually assaulted. Though fewer than half of all victims received direct threats by their stalkers, the victims did experience intense fear. All stalking cases lasted for an average of 1.8 years.[20]

A more recent analysis by Baum et al[10] published by the United States Department of Justice (USDOJ), utilized data from The Supplemental Victimization Survey (SVS), an accompanying survey added to the National Crime Victimization Survey (NCVS).

Approximately 65 270 individuals participated in the SVS. The SVS utilized a similar method to Tjaden and Theonnes'[20] study. In addition to not explicitly mentioning the word stalking, the SVS used many of the same, though often more detailed, questions, and had the same emphasis on repeated incidences and level of perceived fear; however, the questions in the SVS were more structured and utilized a fuller multiple-choice structure.

For a 12-month period, the SVS study (2006) gathered data and found:

An estimated 14 in every 1000 persons age 18 or older were victims of stalking. About half (46%) of stalking victims experienced at least 1 unwanted contact per week, and 11% of victims said they had been stalked for 5 years or more. The risk of stalking victimization was highest for individuals who were divorced or separated—34 per 1000 individuals. Women were at greater risk than men for stalking victimization; however, women and men were equally likely to experience harassment. Male (37%) and female (41%) stalking victimizations were equally likely to be reported to the police. Approximately 1 in 4 stalking victims reported some form of cyber stalking, i.e., e-mail (83%) or instant messaging (35%), and 46% of stalking victims felt fear of not knowing what would happen next. Nearly 3 in 4 stalking victims knew their offender in some capacity.[10]

Although much is being learned regarding stalking behavior and its prevalence, the body of research is still relatively young, and often inconsistent, in part, due to the difficulties involved in properly defining stalking. Unlike other crimes, such as physical assault, the perception and emotional reaction to stalking are extremely subjective. The majority of behaviors that constitute stalking are not necessarily illegal, in many instances are quite normal in contemporary social contexts, and are often welcome. A friend or partner that shows up unexpectedly or leaves a gift would not necessarily evoke fear in the same way that a stalker would. When a friend or partner does something like this, it is generally considered a kind or caring gesture. The difference with a stalker, on the other hand, lays in the intended message of such a gesture, ie, "I know where you are." One would have to examine the meaning of seemingly caring gestures in order to determine the motivation of a stalker's behavior. Unfortunately, the threatening subtext of such messages is often lost when divorced from the context of repeated, unwanted intrusions, and from a legal perspective, this claim is often difficult to support.

Fox et al[22] draws attention to the way in which the inconsistencies with defining stalking have led researchers to measure the phenomenon using a variety of different methods. They posit the argument that although "measuring stalking with a variety of methods facilitates a deeper understanding of the crime, methodological inconsistencies within each of these various measurement methods have largely omitted discussions about the validity and reliability of measurement and the generalizability of published results."[22] Hence, unifying data on stalking is certainly an essential, yet complicated, endeavor for the field of research and legislation to surmount. A consensus on defining stalking would further improve the way in which this problem is approached by all branches of government.

STALKING TYPOLOGIES

Stalking in its essence encompasses a wide range of assorted behaviors ranging from the seemingly mundane to the violent and potentially fatal. When studying a complex phenomenon such as this, it is important to distinguish between different varieties of the phenomenon. This is important not only for purposes of describing and explaining the phenomena, but also for purposes of dangerousness and risk assessment. It is important for experts to be able to make more informed predictions in regard to which types of stalkers have the most potential for violence. As Mullen et al advocates,

"Classifications should not simply facilitate communication by giving names to items in a previously undistinguished landscape, but should both articulate relationships between conceptually similar groups and tell us something about what can be expected of each class."[2]

The way in which stalkers are classified often varies according to the particular needs and concerns of the group utilizing the classification system. For example, law enforcement officers, mental health professionals, and victim advocates all have differing, yet appropriate concerns in regard to stalkers. These institutions have each developed and embraced different classifications, which address specific issues and concerns for their area of expertise, all while preserving the technical terminology that is often specific within a particular domain.[2]

With the lack of any complete explanatory theory of stalking, a large number of typologies have been offered. In their 2007 review, Spitzburg and Cupach[21] identified over 20 different stalker typologies. The majority of these different typologies can fit into 3 general categories, "those that classify according to an underlying mental disorder; those that classify according to the stalker's prior relationship with the victim; and those that classify according to the primary motivation for stalking."[2] These 3 general categories are useful in contextualizing stalking behavior in order to gain a better understanding of a stalker's motivation.

Underlying Mental Disorder

Following the highly publicized events of the 1980s, such as the murder of actress Rebecca Schaeffer, the Los Angeles Police Department created the Threat Management Unit (TMU) for the purpose of becoming more proactive in the intervention of stalking cases before they end in fatalities. Based on the stalking cases encountered in the TMU, Zona et al[23] proposed the first stalker classification structure. They believed that understanding stalkers purely in terms of the established diagnostic categories, as in the Diagnostic and Statistical Manual for Mental Disorders (DSM), is useful, but can also pose limitations.

As they found, many stalkers do not fit exclusively into 1 diagnostic category. They suggest that cases are best understood when taking into account the nature of the subject's preoccupation and prior relationship with their victim. They believe, "It is the relationship between the 2 parties, real or imagined, that best informs our understanding of stalkers and their motivations. From this frame of reference, the various stalker and victim types were developed."[23] The 3 types of stalkers the authors identified were termed simple obsessional, love obsessional, and erotomanic.

Simple Obsessional

The *simple obsessional* type is the name given in cases where the victim and perpetrator have some prior knowledge of one another. These include relationships such as ex-significant partners, casual acquaintances, business associates, professional contacts, as well as friends and neighbors. They found these to be the most common and often most dangerous cases.[23]

Although not always, the authors found that a significant number of simple obsessional cases originate from the outgrowth of an intimate relationship. These cases often occur after an individual breaks away from a domestic violence situation "only to have his or her ex-partner initiate a campaign of harassment, intimidation, and mental terrorism."[23] The motive in such cases may be either to coerce the victim back into a relationship, or simply to seek revenge by making the victim's life miserable.

In some relationships involving the simple obsessional type, there is nothing more than a brief period of dating that may end with one partner deciding not to continue the relationship. According to Zona et al,[23] "In certain situations, however, one partner may have an unrealistically high degree of emotional investment in the relationship and becomes angered as a result of a loss of control, an attack on his self-image, or a sense of mistreatment." They found that individuals with personality disorders, ie, borderline personality disorder or narcissistic personality disorder, were more likely to engage in stalking behavior following the development of this type of reaction.

Simple obsessional cases can also occur in the context of non-intimate relationships, ie, within the workplace. A typical example of such a scenario would be a "suspended or terminated employee who perceives that one particular supervisor is the direct cause of his troubles and initiates a pattern of stalking behavior designed to terrorize this person."[23] This type of situation may escalate to the point of direct confrontation and violence. Another common workplace scenario may occur when an employee, frequently male, attempts to establish a personal relationship with a co-worker and is rejected. In most cases, however, the authors found that non-intimate simple obsessional stalking involves people who had some prior form of professional relationship, such as physician-patient, psychotherapist-client, teacher-student, business partners, or similar relations.[23]

Love Obsessional

The category they termed *love obsessional* is the name given in cases characterized by the absence of an existing relationship between the perpetrator and victim. The victims in love obsessional cases are often celebrities or public figures known to the stalker only through media, such as radio, movies, and television. Although media celebrities are the most frequent, ordinary individuals are also vulnerable to this type of stalking. Many stalkers of this type are found to suffer from schizophrenia, a psychotic disorder, or bipolar disorder, which can have psychotic features. Additionally, they were frequently socially maladjusted and have seldom, if ever, been involved in a meaningful intimate relationship. Though these behaviors may seem to be strange or disturbing, the authors found that those that fit into this category are usually less dangerous than the simple obsessional stalker type.[23] The Bardo case discussed above would fit into this category. He suffered from schizophrenia and believed he was in love with his victim, Rebecca Schaeffer, though they had never met.

Erotomanic

Lastly, the category termed *erotomanic* is unique in the finding that in such cases the perpetrator holds the delusional belief not only that they are in love with the victim, but also that the victim loves them in return. Similar to those in the love obsessional category, perpetrators that fit into the erotomanic category typically have no prior relationship with the victim. Again, public figures and celebrities are often, but not exclusively, the victims of such behavior. At the time of the study, this group met DSM III R criteria for delusional (paranoid) disorder, erotomanic type.[2] In the population studied, the authors found that the most unique feature of erotomanic stalking cases was that the majority of suspects were female. Additionally, the victims were often older men of higher socioeconomic status.[23]

Case Study

Chief Judge Solomon Wachtler (Sol), who served on the New York State Supreme Court and the Court of Appeals for nearly 20 years and was a protégé of Nelson Rockefeller, was known for the remark, "A marriage license should not be viewed as a license for a husband to forcibly rape his wife with impunity."[24] He was also a key figure in the crafting of legislation that made spousal rape a criminal offense. In 1985 he found himself involved with a woman named Joy. He was married at the time with grown children, and told Joy that he did not want to engage in adultery; however, she continued to pursue him. She made 7-10 telephone calls to the bench daily, and bought him expensive gifts and dinners. She sought political advice from Sol and used him for his guidance and connections to get her an ambassadorship, run for public office, and visit the White House. He began having an affair with her in 1988. In a desperate attempt to be with Sol, Joy took him to her therapist in order to convince him to leave his wife. She also befriended his oldest daughter, and was careful about public appearances because she aspired to run for public office. When none of her attempts worked, Joy became involved with another prominent public figure named David, and ended her relationship with Sol.

At the point when Joy ended her relationship with Sol, she no longer consented to any continuation of intimate contact. Additionally, she made her decision even more clear when she became involved with another man. As in many cases of IPV, the perpetrator refuses to accept that the relationship that may once have existed must end. No matter how a perpetrator may want to place blame upon a victim with whom he was once involved, the responsibility lies solely with the stalker. It was very difficult for Sol to cope with Joy being romantically involved with David, and he began using his connections on the bench to investigate him. In the course of his investigation Sol learned that David was married. Sol disguised his voice, called David's wife, and told her he was a private investigator (PI) and had photographs of her husband with Joy. Unfortunately for Sol, his wife did not care that her husband was having an affair. Sol's anger and frustration continued to grow. He began making hang-up calls, sending Hallmark cards with sexual content to her from this fictitious PI, and even dressed as a cowboy and went to her Park Avenue apartment to leave a message for her from the PI. The number of cards sent to Joy increased, with one threatening to kidnap her 14-year-old daughter.

With the threat to her daughter, Joy called the Federal Bureau of Investigation (FBI). While the case was being investigated by the FBI, Sol sent a card threatening to kill Joy and asked for money in exchange for audiotapes of her with David, as well as photographs of them together. A female undercover FBI agent met with Sol to deliver the $20 000 ransom, and Sol was arrested. He was charged with extortion, racketeering, and blackmail.

Sol surrendered his law license and was giving speeches at law schools and television stations. While the investigation ensued, he purported to be "insane." During this time Sol called Joy and told her that he was having brain surgery and was leaving money to her. He also said he was having an affair with another woman, all of which were untrue.

Sol had an underlying mental illness called bipolar disorder. He was also diagnosed with obsessional disorder and narcissistic personality traits. He avoided going to trial and accepted a plea bargain of 18 months in federal prison. Sol faked being the victim of an assault while in prison and was able to serve the remainder of his sentence in a federal medical center. He began writing his memoirs and managed to remain married to his wife, who stuck by him through his political and personal tribulations.

Sol published his memoir, *After the Madness, A Judge's Own Personal Memoir,*[25] and a book of fiction, *Blood Brothers.*[26] He also made contributions to the book *Serving Mentally Ill Defendants.*[27] He is a Law Professor at Touro Law School and Chairman of the Law and Psychiatry Institute of North Shore Long Island Jewish Hospital. He advocates for the mentally ill and has received several awards for his work. He was reinstated to the New York State bar in 2007.[25]

Prior Relationship/Motivation

Another typology of growing popularity was introduced by Mohandie et al,[28] who argued that "the mixing of mental health labels and typological categories seems to complicate research into the relationship between stalking behavior and mental disorders, as well as to introduce the weakness of redundancy,"[28] such as those found in the Zona et al typology. They reasoned that any useful typology of stalkers needed to be parsimonious, in order to avoid unnecessary confusion or overlap between groupings; stable in terms of inter-rater and temporal reliability; and behaviorally based. They added that it must be applicable to a variety of audiences, including mental health, law enforcement, criminal justice professionals, victims' rights activists, and researchers contributing to the field.[2,28]

Based upon the above concerns, Mohandie et al[28] developed what they termed the RE-CON typology. The acronym RECON refers to 2 axes upon which the typology is based. The first axis, RE, addresses the perpetrator's relationship, or the lack thereof, with the victim, and the second axis, CON, addresses the context of the pursuit (private vs. public figures). This typology identifies 2 types of stalking, each with 2 subcategories, that yield 4 stalker categories in total. Type I signifies a previous relationship between the stalker and victim. The nature of this relationship is then subcategorized as either intimate or acquaintance. Type II indicates no contact, or very limited, with the victim. This type is then subcategorized on the basis of the victim being either a public figure or a private stranger.[2,28]

The authors attest that this typology makes it easy to categorize cases, and that it exhibits some theoretical consistency with previous models. They also argue that this typology provides a unifying platform on which it is possible to organize prior data and research from other models.[28] Mullen and colleagues point out that although this typology meets its purpose of being a relatively uncomplicated method of classification with adequate validity, "the results are generalizable only to stalkers who come into contact with law enforcement or private security companies."[2] In regard to mental health professionals and victims' rights activists, the applicability of the RECON typology is more questionable. As they point out, "[t]he major limitation of the RECON is the decision to exclude any consideration of the stalker's motivation for the pursuit, on the basis that this is too dynamic a factor to usefully inform any typology."[2(p63)]

PRIMARY MOTIVATION FOR STALKING

Alternatively, Mullen et al[2,29] offer their own version of a stalker typology that adds the dimension of motivation of pursuit. Their categorizations were developed from their experiences with stalkers in a clinical setting. Most of the stalkers were referred through the courts, as the clinic had a known interest in stalkers.[30] The clinic also provided services to stalking victims. They argue that this classification system is capable of serving both forensic and mental health purposes.

The primary types of stalkers proposed by these authors were: the rejected, the resentful, the intimacy seeker, the incompetent suitor, and the predatory. These categories attempt to take into account the primary motivation behind the behavior of the stalker, which the authors identify as the first of 3 axes. "The stalking behaviors have a meaning for the stalker which relates in some way to their goals. Equally, for the stalker to persist in such apparently destructive behaviors there must be results from their actions which are sufficiently rewarding to maintain the behavior."[2] They posit that the context in which the stalking arises is also of relevance. The context helps to explain the stalker's ultimate goals and the manner in which these goals may be achieved. The authors emphasize that this information is relevant whether or not the perpetrator's judgments are distorted or even delusional.

The intimacy seekers are responding to loneliness by attempting to establish a close relationship. The rejected are responding to an unwelcome end to a close relationship by actions intended to lead to reconciliation, extract reparation, or both. The resentful are responding to a perceived insult or injury by actions aimed not just at revenge but at vindication. The predatory are pursuing their desires for sexual gratification and control both in and through the stalking. The incompetents are would be suitors seeking a partner by methods that are likely to be, at best, counterproductive and, at worst, terrifying for their target.[2]

Their second axis is determined by the stalker's relationship to the victim. This is separated into categories[2]:

— Prior intimate partners

— Professional contacts

— Work-related contacts

— Casual acquaintances and friends

— The famous

— Strangers who had had no contact prior to the onset of the stalking

Lastly, the authors identify a third axis which relates to the psychiatric condition of the stalker. This is divided into psychotic, which includes schizophrenia, delusional disorders, affective psychosis and organic psychosis, and non-psychotic, being predominantly personality disorders, but may also contain both depressive and anxiety disorders, though they are less common.[2]

Again, an understanding of stalker types can offer important information regarding subsequent risk assessment and management, and facilitates grouping the assorted stalking population into more manageable subtypes. These differing typologies have their own strengths and weaknesses, and in different arenas, some may prove more useful, depending on the circumstances and available information. Although they offer no unifying theory of stalking, typologies can provide a general guide to the expected course and duration of harassment and the probability of violence, and could provide insight into the most appropriate intervention strategies and treatments for a given stalker type.[31]

STALKING RISK ASSESSMENT

In determining one's risk, it is not only important to examine static factors, ie, age, sex, race, history of arrests, and psychiatric history, in order to determine what level of risk a stalker may be but to also look at what is often referred to as the dynamic factors. Static factors may tell an evaluator if a stalker fits into a particular category of risk based on statistical probabilities, but 'dynamic factors' offer an entire picture. Dynamic factors include things such as current mental status, motivation, relationship status, system of support, etc. It is also important to know if a stalker has a current obsession with someone and what course that has taken over time, ie, escalation or de-escalation. If there are unreasonable expectations of a potential victim of stalking, an evaluator should explore the quality of those expectations. It is also important to know if a stalker is offended by the victim's behavior in some way.

CONSEQUENCES TO THE VICTIM

While the principal concern for victims of stalking is frequently the potentially dangerous nature of their pursuers, there are many additional consequences that victims are likely to experience, many of which may last long after the stalking behavior resolves.[32] "Victims of stalking typically describe feelings of violation, a profound sense of loss of control over their lives, and a pervasive mistrust of others. They commonly employ terms such as 'emotional rape' and 'psychological terrorism' in defining their ordeal."[2]

Clinical studies frequently report high rates of post-traumatic stress, anxiety, depression, and suicidality among victims presenting for services.[4,33,34] In addition, these victims experience significant disruption in their social and work lives, and frequently report having to change or cease employment and move from their homes as a result of stalking behavior.[4] Concomitantly, other individuals, such as the victim's friends, family, coworkers, neighbors, and community, may also suffer negative psychosocial effects from the disruptive actions of a stalker.

In one study,[32] victims who had been threatened by a perpetrator were 3 times more likely to report significant post-trauma symptoms than those who were not; however, in cases where the victim experienced actual physical assaults, no reliable correlation was found between abuse and post-traumatic symptomatology, suggesting that threats of violence may be more emotionally damaging to victims than the reality of physical harm. Although there is currently no established association between the severity of psychological symptoms and either the nature of the prior victim-stalker relationship, methods of pursuit, or the use of violence, there is evidence that the longer the harassment continues, the more harmful its effects may be.[31,32] A case study from Mullen and colleagues[2] powerfully illustrates the degree to which a stalker's actions can impact a victim's life:

Jane, a 45-year-old, was stalked for 6 years by a former boyfriend. Her two-year relationship with the 40-year-old was characterized by his alcohol and marijuana abuse, physical assaultiveness, and jealous rages. He assumed control over most aspects of her life, progressively destroying her existing support network by denigrating and preventing contact with them. He sabotaged the job she had held for 15 years and prevented her from pursuing further employment. He threatened male acquaintances, damaging the car of one who drove her home. He controlled her bank account, wardrobe, choice of medical practitioners and hairdresser, and even her diet. Jane made multiple attempts to end the relationship, but he pledged his undying devotion and begged her to reconsider. The more determined her resistance, the more retaliation, which included dousing her car with acid, slashing her tires, and collecting and shredding her dry cleaning. Although Jane succeeded in obtaining a restraining order, the harassment escalated and there was little Jane could say or do that brought any assertive action from the police.

When her stalker confronted her with a machete and attempted to drag her into his car, the police and courts were persuaded of the gravity of the situation, and the perpetrator was arrested. He subsequently received a 3-year prison term for stalking. Although the threat was removed, Jane's stalker had become a part of her inner life, and she remained preoccupied with him. She assumed responsibility for his imprisonment and all the suffering she imagined he would have to endure. She claimed her life felt strangely incomplete without him, likening him to a 'phantom limb.'

Therapy is gradually helping Jane to reconstitute social ties, enhance her debased self-image, and recover some initiative. Jane admits that she still frequently thinks about her stalker and wonders how he is faring, but he no longer monopolizes her attention.[2]

Jane's reaction to her stalker is not uncommon. Much like other forms of abuse, the victim may feel that in some way he or she caused the stalking behavior. In addition to guilty feelings that may exist, there are coping mechanisms that come into play that can often become unhealthy. In Jane's case, unhealthy coping caused her to try and please her stalker in order to reduce the likelihood of violence. She was also hyper-vigilant and attended to his intrusive presence, which caused her to become preoccupied to the point where she became co-dependent upon him psychologically. Much like a kidnap victim who feels completely controlled, a stalking victim may choose to remain close and friendly toward her aggressor in order to mitigate potential violence. Even after he finally became violent and was arrested, Jane could not find relief in that safety. Again, she felt guilt over his imprisonment, and did not know what to do without the feeling of being completely controlled by her stalker. The powerlessness she felt at the hands of her stalker continued after he was imprisoned, but had been internalized to the point that she required therapy in order to return to a state of being productive. The psychological effects of stalking in Jane's case are common to many victims.

The probability of violence accompanying stalking behavior is of the utmost concern to all who confront this phenomenon. In a 2004 meta-analysis by Rosenfeld,[35] he found that violence occurred often in cases involving stalking (between 30% and 50% of cases); however, severe violence was reported much less frequently. A study examining instances of violence by Rosenfeld and Harmon[36] found cases of severe violence to be relatively infrequent (12 of 204 cases, or 6%). The authors posit that "high-profile cases of stalking-related homicide may fuel public concerns, but these cases appear to be relatively atypical in the spectrum of stalking cases."[35(p31)]

TECHNOLOGY AND STALKING

With the rapid and continuous advancement in modern technology, stalkers are increasingly gaining access to a whole new arsenal of tools with which to pursue, harass, control, violate, and invoke fear in their victims. Unfortunately, it seems that our laws and the empirical research regarding stalking have been unable to maintain an equal pace with contemporary innovations, leaving many at risk. Computers; the Internet; and other technology, such as cell phones, have forever altered the scope, context, and way in which we manage our personal information and, in many ways, have made us more vulnerable. No matter how carefully information is managed, there are still ways in which new technology can be exploited for purposes of stalking and victimizing.

CYBERSTALKING

Cyberstalking can be defined as a pattern of threatening behavior or unwanted advances directed at another, using computers, the Internet, e-mail, and other forms of electronic communication. The use of computers, cell telephones and other electronic devices may, in fact, be the easiest method of stalking, and is quickly becoming the most widespread. These can all be used without much effort or having any direct contact with a victim, and are often untraceable. Stalkers can also be in other states or countries when committing these illegal acts.

In one study, Sheridan and Grant[37] examined the difference between cyberstalking and other forms of stalking in order to understand if they should be regarded as distinctive phenomena, or if cyberstalking was just another tool in the stalker's arsenal. They concluded that cyberstalking and offline stalking were more similar than different. They also argued that cyberstalking is essentially one more invasive technique available to stalkers. Some typical examples of cyberstalking techniques include:

— Seeking and compiling information on the victim in order to harass, threaten, and intimidate the victim online or off-line

— Repeated unsolicited e-mailing and instant messaging (IM)

— Electronic sabotage, such as spamming and sending viruses to the target

— Identity theft

— Subscribing the victim to services

— Purchasing goods and services in the victim's name

— Impersonating another online

— Sending or posting hostile material, misinformation and false messages, ie, to Usenet groups

— Tricking other Internet users into harassing or threatening a victim, ie, by posting the victim's personal details on a bulletin board along with a controversial invitation[37]

Although there are many similarities to offline stalking, there are some important and notable features that characterize cyberstalking. For one, cyberstalkers can use the Internet to instantly harass their victims in a larger, more public forum than any conventional form of offline stalking, and it can be done inexpensively and efficiently. For example, rather than making individual phone calls, an offender can repeatedly send thousands of harassing e-mail messages through scheduled automated programs, sometimes called e-mail bombing. Additionally, cyberstalkers have the ability to act while being physically far removed from their victims. This makes escaping the reach of the perpetrator a nearly impossible task, but also adds a terrifying element of uncertainty to the victim, who never can be sure of the physical location of her offender. This may also present legal issues regarding jurisdiction. Since cyberstalking can take place across state lines, prosecutors often run into difficulty when enforcing state laws. Furthermore, cyberstalkers have the capability of remaining virtually anonymous. This frequently allows otherwise shy or unassertive individuals to overcome their personal inhibitions, or any hesitation when confronting a victim in person. Also very unique to cyberstalking is that online offenders can easily impersonate their victims. This is often used to tarnish a victim's reputation and usually to align other individuals against the victim. Finally, cyberstalkers can incite others to harass their victims. This is often referred to as *stalker by proxy*.[38]

One of the first men to be charged under a states' computer stalking laws, an example of stalking by proxy, was in 1999: a 50-year-old Californian named Gary Dellapenta. After being rejected by his victim, the offender, a security guard, used the Internet to impersonate his victim on websites and chatrooms. While impersonating his victim, he expressed interest in rape fantasies and provided her home address in order to lure men to her apartment to satisfy this spurious wish. Although the woman was not harmed, six men did show up to her North Hollywood apartment on separate occasions, in response to these bogus ads. Mr. Dellapenta was eventually tracked down and was sentenced to 6 years in prison under California's then-new cyberstalking law.[39] In addition to demonstrating the terrifying acts that a cyberstalker is capable of, this case also illuminates the fact that a victim does not even need to own a computer in order to fall prey to the offender's computer-generated behaviors.

Cyberstalking uses computers to potentially provoke and incite others against a victim without having to be physically present. As discussed above in the case of Jane, this serves not only to harass and intimidate a victim, but also to isolate a victim from others, which facilitates stalking behavior and creates a feeling of vulnerability and fear in the victim.

ELECTRONIC MONITORING DEVICES

Some of these techniques that stalkers and cyberstalkers employ allow them to obtain information from afar, while other technologies require the offender to have, at least temporarily, a close proximity to the victim. Several of these technologies, or a combination thereof, can infiltrate nearly every aspect of a victim's personal life, making them extremely vulnerable. Many individuals do not even know most of these technologies exist, and often-times the perpetrator is someone they know closely, such as a suspicious partner.

Many stalkers, at some point in their offending, utilize a telephone to violate their victim in a particular manner. They will often use prepaid calling cards to make their calls difficult to trace. Also, if a victim uses a cordless telephone in her home, a perpetrator has the potential to listen in on conversations with the simplest devices, such as a baby monitor, walkie-talkie, or radio scanner.[40] Most individuals are familiar with caller identification (caller ID); what many do not suspect is that there are techniques that perpetrators can easily employ to either conceal the number they are calling from, or make it appear that they are calling from any number of their choosing, ie, a victim's family member, friend, co-worker, or boss. This specific type of stalking behavior is called caller ID spoofing. They can also use this technique to call straight to a victim's digital voicemail, bypassing the ring altogether, in order to leave harassing messages without the victim having the chance to hang up. Spoofing can also be achieved with e-mail accounts in much the same manner, by disguising the stalker's incoming e-mail to one of their choosing.

Modern cellular phones and smart-phones, with all their useful features, create a wealth of new vulnerabilities to potential victims. If an offender is able to gain temporary physical access to a victim's cellular phone, he can install an undetectable suite of software to monitor all aspects of the victim's life. These services, which are easily available online, make it possible for the offender to listen in on phone calls from anywhere, while even alerting the stalker when calls are being made. This also gives the ability to check text messages, e-mails, contact lists, and call history. Furthermore, the offender can also have the ability to remotely turn on the telephone's microphone while the device is not in use in order to listen in on the telephone's surroundings, essentially turning it into a room bug. Perhaps most frighteningly, the software can also give information from the global positioning system (GPS), available in many new smart phones, in order to give nearly exact coordinates of the victim's physical location at any time. In one news article, journalist Ben Goldacre[41] investigated just how easy this was to set up (with his girlfriend's permission). He recalled:

First I had to get hold of her phone. It wasn't difficult. We live together and she has no reason not to trust me, so she often leaves it lying around. And, after all, I only needed it for 5 minutes. I unplugged her phone and took it upstairs to register it on a website I had been told about... Almost immediately, my girlfriend's phone vibrated with a new text message. "Ben Goldacre has requested to add you to their Buddy List! To accept, simply reply to this message with 'LOCATE'." I sent the requested reply. The phone vibrated again. A second text arrived: "WARNING: [this service] allows other people to know where you are. For your own safety make sure that you know who is locating you." I deleted both these text messages.

The feature of cellular GPS tracking is also a service that many telephone companies offer right in their own plans in order for parents to keep track of their children. However, the service of GPS tracking is also abused for illicit purposes. Kathleen Krenek, director of the Next Door Solutions for Battered Women shelter in San Jose, expresses that in such cases, "[t]he abuser is usually tracking a victim's cell telephone. That comes as a shock to many stalking victims, who often believe that carrying a phone makes them safer because they can call 911 if they're attacked."[42]

Another way stalkers can easily and cheaply monitor a victim's behavior is by simply placing standalone GPS devices onto a target's car. These devices are manufactured so they can easily and secretly be attached to the outside of a vehicle or, if access is permitted, hidden inside somewhere, eg., in the dashboard, trunk, or under seats. These devices can monitor, in real time, the location of a target and can be installed very quickly, anytime the victim's vehicle is unattended. Many other devices not mentioned in detail here, such as hidden video cameras and audio recorders, also exist, and as technology advances, novel ways to intrude on the privacy of others will evolve in parallel fashion.

In modern times it is important to remain aware of where personal information is located, and who is in charge of keeping it secure. It is important to remember never to give away passwords or any other information that might compromise your privacy or security and make it easy to become a victim. The persistent offender can always find some way to compromise an individual's security. If an offender appears to be following too closely, or is too knowledgeable of a victim's whereabouts or personal information, one must suspect technology in the employ of stalking.

Cyberstalking and Electronic Monitoring Statistics

Very little research has been conducted concerning the prevalence of cyberstalking, and the statistics that do exist are inconsistent; however, the organization Working to Halt Online Abuse (WHOA), founded in 1997 to help fight online harassment, has been gathering demographic and statistical information from victims of cyberstalking statistics since 2000. In the review of their 2010 statistics,[43] they noted that compared to prior years, the gap between male and female harassers was shrinking, with 2010 statistics being almost even compared to the year 2000, when 68% of offenders were male. Not surprisingly, the primary targets were aged 18 to 30, while the next largest victim age group was 41 and up.

The majority of victims were single (45.5%), followed by married (28.25%), divorced (11.5%), separated (4.25%), and life partners (2.5%), with the remaining 8% unknown. Most of the victims who sought help were Caucasian (66.5%). Of all the victims, 47% acknowledged having a prior relationship with their harasser. In cases where the victim knew his or her harasser, 55% were primarily an ex–intimate partner or the girlfriend or wife of an ex-, though not a boyfriend or husband, followed by online acquaintance; work associate; friend or ex-friend; family member; and school connection, usually a fellow student.

According to their statistics,[43] the primary way harassment began, regardless of the nature of the relationship (or lack thereof), was by e-mail (34%). In 2010, for the first time, e-mail was followed by the social networking site Facebook (16.5%), then message boards, telephone, IM, and web sites created to specifically harass the victim. Approximately 80% of cases escalated online, following the initial harassment. This was primarily by e-mail (18%), followed closely by Facebook (15%), either by wall posts or profiles forged in the victim's name; telephone (12%); and texting (11%). Of all victims, 26% reported offline physical violence or threats.

By state, California had the highest reported number of victims (9.75%), followed by New York, Florida, Texas, Pennsylvania, North Carolina, Canada, Massachusetts, Washington State, and Maryland. Harassers were primarily from Texas, followed by California, New York, Canada, Florida, Illinois, England, Washington State, Tennessee, and Pennsylvania. Only 34.5% of victims lived in the same state or country as their harasser.[43,44]

According to another report utilizing data from the 2006 Supplemental Victimization Survey (SVS), Baum and colleagues[10] found that more than 1 in 4 stalking victims reported that some form of cyberstalking was used, such as e-mail (83%) or IM (35%). Additionally, electronic monitoring devices were used to stalk 1 in 13 victims. Devices such as video or digital cameras (46%) were nearly as likely as listening devices or bugs (42%) to monitor victims. GPS technology comprised about one-tenth of the electronic monitoring of stalking victims. This monitoring can be in the form of GPS devices on cell phones, tracker devices attached to vehicles, or other devices somehow placed on a person's belongings to track their whereabouts.

There are inconsistencies and gaps in the current literature regarding cyberstalking. It is plausible that cyber technology will continue to advance and become widespread tools for stalking; therefore, extra precautionary measures and legislation will be necessary to confront and deter the problem of stalking as a possible "cyber" crime. As Fox et al point out, "[t]he majority of states have not included cyberstalking as part of their legal definition of stalking; however, lawmakers are increasingly becoming sensitive to its novel and emerging forms."[22] They continue to argue "[w]hile state stalking statutes offer similar descriptions of stalking-related behavior, i.e., unwanted behaviors committed repeatedly, they vary considerably regarding the specific types of behaviors that characterize stalking, ie, method of communication, cyberstalking. The variation among stalking statutes contributes to the challenges researchers experience when defining and operationalizing stalking victimization and perpetration."[22] In terms of developing a thorough body of empirical research, specific cyberstalking measures often remain absent from many studies' scales.[22]

CONCLUSION

As discussed in this chapter, stalking is a serious crime facing society today. It is a crime that serves to isolate and terrorize victims, often for years on end. Within the realm of IPV, it is an important area to address as it is often the precursor to a violent outcome.

With growing technology, stalking has evolved in ways that current statutes still need to address. These technological advances have made it increasingly more difficult to monitor and thwart unwanted intrusions by stalkers. As pointed out in detail, there is great need for agreement in defining the term and elements of stalking in order to have uniformity within and between states when creating statutes appropriate to deal with this issue. As is the key with deterrence for any type of crime, education and awareness are at the forefront.

REFERENCES

1. Jackson NA. *Encyclopedia of Domestic Violence.* Boca Raton, FL: CRC Press; 2007.

2. Mullen PE, Pathé M, Purcell R. *Stalkers and Their Victims.* Cambridge: Cambridge University Press; 2009.

3. Meloy JR, Gothard S. Demographic and clinical comparison of obsessional followers and offenders with mental disorders. *Am J Psychiatry.* 1995;152(2):258-263.

4. Pathe M, Mullen PE. The impact of stalkers on their victims. *Br J Psychiatry.* 1997;170(1):12-17.

5. Meloy JR. Stalking: an old behavior, a new crime. *Psychiatr Clin North Am.* 1999;22(1):85–99.

6. Bondeson J. *Queen Victoria's Stalker: The Strange Case of the Boy Jones.* Kent, Ohio: Kent State University Press; 2011.

7. Meloy J, Sheridan L, Hoffman J. *Stalking, Threatening, and Attacking Public Figures: A Psychological and Behavioral Analysis.* New York, NY: Oxford University Press; 2008.

8. Davis KE, Frieze IH, Maiuro RD. *Stalking: Perspectives on Victims and Perpetrators.* New York, NY: Springer Publishing Company; 2004.

9. United States Department of Justice Office on Violence Against Women; National Institute of Justice. *Stalking and Domestic Violence: The Third Annual Report to Congress Under the Violence Against Women Act.* Washington, DC: United States Department of Justice; 1998.

10. Baum K, Catalano S, Rand M, Rose K. *Stalking Victimization in the United States.* Washington, DC: Bureau of Justice Statistics; 2009.

11. Budd T, Mattinson J. *Stalking: Findings from the 1998 British crime survey. Home Office Research, Research Findings No. 129.* London, England: Research Development and Statistics Directorate; 2000.

12. Elliott L, Brantley C. *Sex on Campus: The Naked Truth About the Real Sex Lives of College Students.* New York, NY: Random House; 1997.

13. Fisher BS, Cullen FT, Turner MG. *The Sexual Victimization of College Women.* Washington, DC: National Institute of Justice, Bureau of Justice Statistics, Department of Justice; 2000.

14. Hackett K. Criminal harassment. *Juristat.* 2000;20(11):1-16.

15. Kohn M, Flood H, Chase J, McMahon PM. Prevalence and health consequences of stalking—Louisiana, 1998–1999. *Morbidity and Mortality Weekly Report.* 2000;49(29):653-655.

16. Kong R. Criminal harassment. *Juristat.* 1996;16(12):1-13.

17. McLennan W. *Crimes Family Violence Act. 1995/96 monitoring report.* Victoria, Australia: Magistrates' and Children's Courts; 1996.

18. McLennan W. *Women's Safety.* Canberra, Australia: Australian Bureau of Statistics; 1996.

19. Purcell R, Pathé M, Mullen PE. The prevalence and nature of stalking in the Australian community. *Aust N Z J Psychiatry.* 2002;36(1):114–120.

20. Tjaden P, Thoennes N. *Stalking in America: Findings from the National Violence Against Women Survey.* Washington, DC: United States Department of Justice; 1998.

21. Spitzberg B, Cupach W. The state of the art of stalking: taking stock of the emerging literature. *Aggression Violent Behav.* 2007;12(1):64-86.

22. Fox KA, Nobles MR, Fisher BS. Method behind the madness: an examination of stalking measurements. *Aggression Violent Behav.* 2011;16(1):74-84.

23. Zona MA, Palarea RE, Lane JC. Psychiatric diagnosis and the offender-victim typology of stalking. In: Meloy JR, ed. *The Psychology of Stalking: Clinical and Forensic Perspectives.* San Diego, CA: Academic Press; 1998:69-84.

24. *People v Liberta,* 64 NY2d 152, 474 NE2d 567 (1984), cert, denied, 471 US 1020 (1985).

25. Wachtler S. *After the Madness.* New York, NY: e-reads.com; 2003.

26. Wachtler S, Gould D. *Blood Brothers.* Milwaukee, WI: New Millennium Publishing; 2003.

27. Lansberg G, Rock M, Berg L. *Serving Mentally Ill Offenders: Challenges and Opportunities for Mental Health Professionals.* New York, NY: Springer Publishing; 2002.

28. Mohandie K, Meloy JUR, Green McGowan M, Williams J. The RECON typology of stalking: reliability and validity based upon a large sample of North American stalkers. *J Forensic Sci.* 2006;51(1):147-155.

29. Mullen PE, Pathé M, Purcell R, Stuart GW. Study of stalkers. *Am J Psychiatry.* 1999;156(8):1244–1249.

30. Warren LJ, MacKenzie R, Mullen PE, Ogloff JR. The problem behavior model: the development of a stalkers clinic and a threateners clinic. *Behav Sci Law.* 2005;23(3):387–97.

31. McEwan TE, Pathé M, Ogloff JRP. Advances in stalking risk assessment. *Behav Sci Law.* 2011;29(2):180-201.

32. Purcell R, Pathé M, Mullen PE. Association between stalking victimization and psychiatric morbidity in a random community sample. *Br J Psychiatry.* 2005;187:416-420.

33. Kamphuis JH, Emmelkamp PMG. Traumatic distress among support-seeking female victims of stalking. *Am J Psychiatry.* 2001;158:795-798.

34. Blaauw E, Winkel FW, Arensman E, Sheridan L, Freeve A. The toll of stalking: the relationship between features of stalking and psychopathology of victims. *J Interpers Violence.* 2002;17(1):50-63.

35. Rosenfeld B. Violence risk factors in stalking and obsessional harassment: a review and preliminary meta-analysis. *Crim Justice Behav.* 2004;31(1):9-36.

36. Rosenfield B, Harmon R. Factors associated with violence in stalking and obsessional harassment cases. *Crim Justice Behav.* 2002;29:671-691. Cited by: Rosenfield B. Violence risk factors in stalking and obsessional harassment: a review and preliminary meta-analysis. *Crim Justice Behav.* 2004;31(1):9-36.

37. Sheridan LP, Grant TD. Is cyberstalking different? *Psychol Crime Law.* 2007;13(6):627-640.

38. Goodno NH. Cyberstalking, a new crime: evaluating the effectiveness of current state and federal laws. *Mo Law Rev.* 2006;72:125-197.

39. Zeller T. A sinister web entraps victims of cyberstalkers. *The New York Times.* April 17, 2006. New York Times Web site. http://www.nytimes.com/2006/04/17/technology/17stalk.html. Accessed July 16, 2013.

40. Southworth C, Finn J, Dawson S, Fraser C, Tucker S. Intimate partner violence, technology, and stalking. *Violence Against Women.* 2007;13(8):842-856.

41. Goldacre B. How I stalked my girlfriend. *The Guardian.* January 31, 2006. Guardian Web site. http://www.theguardian.com/technology/2006/feb/01/news.g2?INTCMP=SRCH. Accessed July 16, 2013.

42. Scheck J. Stalkers exploit cell phone GPS. *The Wall Street Journal.* August 5, 2010. Wall Street Journal Web site. http://online.wsj.com/article/SB10001424052748703467304575383522318244234.html. Accessed July 16, 2013.

43. Working to Halt Online Abuse (WHOA). 2010 cyberstalking statistics. Halt Abuse Web site. http://www.haltabuse.org/resources/stats/2010Statistics.pdf. Published 2011. Accessed July 16, 2013.

44. Hitchcock J. WHOA releases 2010 cyberstalking statistics. March 3, 2011. *Net Crimes & Misdemeanors.* LiveJournal Web site. http://netcrimes.livejournal.com/209138.html. Accessed July 16, 2013.

FATAL INTIMATE PARTNER VIOLENCE

Jonel Thaller, MSW
Jill Messing, MSW, PhD
Kathryn Laughon, PhD, RN, FAAN
Jackie Campbell, PhD, RN, FAAN

KEY POINTS

1. Intimate partner violence (IPV) accounts for 2300 deaths in the US each year. Women are 2.5 times more likely than men to be murdered by an intimate partner. Nearly one-half of all murdered women are killed by an intimate partner.

2. Health care professionals have an important role to play, as many victims of intimate partner (IP) homicide or attempted murder had been seen in the health care system in the year prior to the incident. Health care, mental health, and social service professionals should screen for IPV.

3. The Danger Assessment (DA) is a screening tool that can help health care, mental health, and social service professionals assess the risk of fatal IPV.

4. An abusive partner's employment status can influence the level of risk for fatal IPV. Other risk factors include previous IPV-related events, non-fatal strangulation, access to firearms, substance abuse, mental illness, and recent separation.

5. A short version of the Danger Assessment, called the Lethality Assessment, has been developed to help law enforcement quickly assess the risk of lethality in cases of IPV.

INTRODUCTION

Intimate partner violence (IPV) accounts for at least 2300 adult deaths in the United States each year, with women at least 2 1/2 times more likely than men to be murdered by an intimate partner.[1] Though the public may believe that a woman is more at risk of death from a stranger than someone she knows, nearly one-half of all murdered women are killed by an intimate or formerly intimate partner,[2-5] compared with 5% to 7% of murdered men.[6,7] Over the past 4 decades, broader acknowledgement of domestic violence as a crime, rather than a private family matter, has increased demand for legal sanctions against perpetrators and services for victims, and this response may account for the 40% decrease in intimate partner (IP) homicide between 1970 and 2000.[8] However, it is important to note that the decline in fatal IPV is nearly twice the rate for male victims as for female victims,[9] which supports the claim that a majority of female perpetrators act in self-defense. If women are less likely to kill their abusive partners when resources for survivors of IPV are available,[10,11]it comes as no surprise that states with the most comprehensive domestic violence resources and laws have reported the largest decrease in rates of IP homicide against men.[12]

Although developments in legislation and available services may have facilitated the decrease in IP homicides,[10,13] myths about this phenomenon continue to prevail and may hinder detection of those at risk. Contrary to the common belief that men who inflict fatal IPV are psychopaths or career criminals of low socio-economic status, men at risk of perpetrating severe IPV come from all strata of society and may have no prior criminal record.[14,15] For many abusers, their intimate partner has been the sole recipient of their violent behavior and has endured a history of coercion and abuse that may not be perceptible to those outside of the relationship, especially if the victim has become isolated.[16] Many batterers are adept at maintaining a positive image and might even be described by others as "charming" while concealing abuse from health care providers, therapists, case workers, co-workers, friends, and even family members.[14] The difficulty of identifying those most at risk of fatal IPV underscores the need for tools to assist in the regular assessment of IPV and risk for IP homicide.

THE ROLE OF HEALTH CARE, MENTAL HEALTH, AND SOCIAL SERVICE PROFESSIONALS IN ASSESSING FOR FATAL IPV

Recognition of IPV as a public health issue has led to increased opportunities for intervention. The last 20 years has seen the creation of hotlines and emergency shelters for survivors of IPV as well as advocacy programs in family and criminal courts and counseling programs in virtually every community. In a more recent development, child welfare programs are beginning to take domestic violence into account and to offer services to mothers as an integral component of child safety. Early detection of IPV is crucial because violence may escalate without intervention. Yet, risk assessment for IPV recidivism and lethality appear to be lacking in many social service and health care arenas.

Based on data from a study of female IP homicides and attempted murders of women in 11 US cities, Sharps, Koziol-McLain, et al[17] found that 42% of the victims had been seen in the health care system for some ailment during the year before the incident. Of those, 74% of the murdered women and 88% of the survivors of attempted murder had previously sought help for injuries from their abusive partners in hospital emergency departments, hospital inpatient units, or ambulatory care settings. More recently, there has been a salient push for IPV screening in emergency departments and prenatal settings, and many hospitals have established advocacy and counseling programs to help victims of IPV. In hospital emergency departments, directly questioning women about abuse leads to an increase in reporting, from 0.4% to 14.2%.[18]

Mental health and social service professionals are also in a position to assess clients for IPV but may neglect to do so. Only 4% of marital counselors from the American Association for Marriage and Family Therapy reported consistently assessing clients for IPV.[19] In another study, although IPV was present for up to 60% of couples in counseling, only 6% disclosed this information without prompting.[20] In the case of family violence, Shlonsky and Friend[21] noted that child welfare workers assessed households under investigation for child abuse but not for IPV, though child abuse and IPV often co-occur. Likewise, in a study by Lindhorst, Casey, and Meyers,[22] caseworkers for welfare recipients were required to assess for IPV but rarely did. These findings indicate that IPV screening is under-utilized across a variety of professional settings though opportunities for identification and intervention exist.

ASSESSING RISK OF FATAL IPV
THE DANGER ASSESSMENT
The ***Danger Assessment*** (DA) is the only clinical research instrument designed specifically to aid women in abusive relationships in assessing their danger of being murdered

by their intimate partners (see **Figure 16-1**). This instrument was first developed in collaboration with various experts on IPV, including women in abusive relationships, advocates, and representatives of the criminal justice system.[23] Original DA items were selected based upon data from existing studies of IP homicide or serious injury.[24-27] The assessment is currently available in English, Spanish, Portuguese, and French *(www. dangerassessment.org)* and has been used to evaluate danger among African American, Caucasian, and Hispanic women.[23,28]

For the first portion of the DA, the woman is presented with a calendar of the previous year, a tool intended to assist her in recalling the severity and frequency of physical abuse. She is asked to mark the approximate days when abusive incidents occurred, and to rank the severity of each incident on a 1-to-5 scale (1, slaping, pushing, no injuries and/or lasting pain, through 5, use of a weapon and/or wounds from weapon). Use of the calendar in this and other contexts has been shown to raise consciousness and improve the accuracy of women's recall, while reducing minimization of serious incidents.[23,29,30] During development of this measure, 38% of women who initially reported no increase in severity and frequency of violence

DANGER ASSESSMENT

Jacquelyn C. Campbell, Ph.D., R.N.
Copyright, 2003; www.dangerassessment.com

Several risk factors have been associated with increased risk of homicides (murders) of women and men in violent relationships. We cannot predict what will happen in your case, but we would like you to be aware of the danger of homicide in situations of abuse and for you to see how many of the risk factors apply to your situation.

Using the calendar, please mark the approximate dates during the past year when you were abused by your partner or ex partner. Write on that date how bad the incident was according to the following scale:

1. Slapping, pushing; no injuries and/or lasting pain
2. Punching, kicking; bruises, cuts, and/or continuing pain
3. "Beating up"; severe contusions, burns, broken bones
4. Threat to use weapon; head injury, internal injury, permanent injury
5. Use of weapon; wounds from weapon

(If **any** of the descriptions for the higher number apply, use the higher number.)

Mark **Yes** or **No** for each of the following. ("He" refers to your husband, partner, ex-husband, ex-partner, or whoever is currently physically hurting you.)

___ 1. Has the physical violence increased in severity or frequency over the past year?
___ 2. Does he own a gun?
___ 3. Have you left him after living together during the past year?
      3a. (If have *never* lived with him, check here___)
___ 4. Is he unemployed?
___ 5. Has he ever used a weapon against you or threatened you with a lethal weapon?
      (If yes, was the weapon a gun?___)
___ 6. Does he threaten to kill you?
___ 7. Has he avoided being arrested for domestic violence?
___ 8. Do you have a child that is not his?
___ 9. Has he ever forced you to have sex when you did not wish to do so?
___ 10. Does he ever try to choke you?
___ 11. Does he use illegal drugs? By drugs, I mean "uppers" or amphetamines, "meth", speed, angel dust, cocaine, "crack", street drugs or mixtures.
___ 12. Is he an alcoholic or problem drinker?
___ 13. Does he control most or all of your daily activities? For instance: does he tell you who you can be friends with, when you can see your family, how much money you can use, or when you can take the car? (If he tries, but you do not let him, check here: ___)
___ 14. Is he violently and constantly jealous of you? (For instance, does he say "If I can't have you, no one can.")
___ 15. Have you ever been beaten by him while you were pregnant? (If you have never been pregnant by him, check here: ___)
___ 16. Has he ever threatened or tried to commit suicide?
___ 17. Does he threaten to harm your children?
___ 18. Do you believe he is capable of killing you?
___ 19. Does he follow or spy on you, leave threatening notes or messages, destroy your property, or call you when you don't want him to?
___ 20. Have you ever threatened or tried to commit suicide?
___ Total "Yes" Answers

Thank you. Please talk to your nurse, advocate or counselor about what the Danger Assessment means in terms of your situation.

Figure 16-1

Figure 16-1.
Danger Assessment Form

in the prior year changed their response after filling in the calendar.[23,29] The second portion of the DA is currently comprised of 20 dichotomous (yes/no) items reflecting risk factors for IP homicide. This portion of the DA was originally only comprised of 15 items, but has been expanded to the current 20 based on findings from a study on female IP homicides and attempted homicides.[3,4]

Approximately 20 minutes are needed to complete each part of the assessment. Although a woman can complete the instrument alone, interpretation of the score is best conducted in collaboration with a knowledgeable health professional, victim advocate, or criminal justice practitioner who can assist the woman in examining the results of the DA in the context of her current situation and to formulate appropriate safety strategies. There are 2 ways of scoring the DA. Users can simply tally the number of "yes" responses, with a higher number indicating more risk factors for IP homicide; however, a more accurate weighed scoring scheme was developed using analysis of findings from the 11-city IP homicide study.[4,31,32] The revised DA and information about how to receive training for weighted scoring can be accessed on the DA website.

Recent independent studies of predictive validity also support the DA's utility in assessing for risk of future incidents of non-lethal assault.[33,34] In a separate study, RAVE, the DA was found to be more predictive than 3 other risk assessment instruments – the Domestic Violence Screening Instrument (DVSI),[35] the Kingston Screening Instrument for Domestic Violence (K-SID),[36] and Domestic Violence MOSAIC (DV-MOSAIC), as well as women's personal perception of risk.[37] The DA is becoming more specialized as research is able to tailor the risk assessment to various populations. Glass and colleagues[38] have revised the DA for use in predicting lethal abuse in same-sex female couples. The resulting DA-R is comprised of 18 dichotomous questions, 8 of which are from the original DA. The remaining 10 questions are similar to those from the DA but have been reworded or revised to fit the population. Similarly, a version of the DA for immigrant women has been developed;[39] this version of the DA retains 14 of the original DA items and adds 11 items specific to the experiences of women who have immigrated to the US. Both revised versions of the DA are intended for administration with the survey administrator working in collaboration with the victim.

In summary, the DA is intended to be a collaborative effort between an abused woman and a knowledgeable professional, such as a health care worker, domestic violence advocate, or member of the criminal justice system. It is meant to provide information about a woman's risk of lethal violence, in conjunction with her own perception of risk, as the basis for safety planning within her current situation.[33,34,40,41] Other risk assessment instruments have been introduced to assess risk of IPV recidivism, but the DA is the only instrument designed specifically for determining risk of IP homicide.[31]

HELP SEEKING AMONG VICTIMS OF IPV

In contrast with earlier misconceptions of survivors of IPV as helpless, women in violent relationships are often actively engaged in the process of keeping themselves and their children safe, including safety behaviors that could be described as either formal or informal help seeking as well as placating or resisting their partners.[42,43] Abused women in a study by Glass et al[44] reported sharing their concerns about safety with a friend (64%), family member (49%), spiritual advisor or clergy member (34%), school staff (28%), or health care professional (26%), and more than half had created a safety plan. The majority of abused women eventually leave or otherwise manage to end their violent relationships,[45] but this process takes time and may involve complex issues such as child custody and access to affordable housing and a living wage.

Calling the police is one of the most commonly employed help seeking strategies by women in abusive relationships.[46] The percentage of female IPV victims who reported their victimization to the police was approximately 60% in 1998, a significant increase from 1993.[47] When the victim identifies IPV as a crime, domestic violence is reported to the police at rates equal to the reporting of other crimes.[48] Furthermore, as the severity or frequency of abuse increases, so do calls to the police.[49,50] Just over one-half of the abused women killed in the 11-city study of IP homicides, for example, had called the police before the fatal incident.[17] Accessing domestic violence services, such as obtaining counseling or staying at a shelter, occurs much less often. Only 4% of the IP homicide victims in the 11-city study had accessed shelter services.[17]

SERVICE DELIVERY: THE OPEN WINDOW THEORY

Curnow's *open window theory*[51] posits that the best time to intervene in cases of IPV is directly after a violent incident, during the "open window phase." While it is characteristic for a victim of IPV to minimize, deny, excuse, and blame herself for her partner's behavior, these defenses may temporarily subside during that time. When cognitive awareness of the abuse sets in, some women describe the feeling as "waking up,"[51] and this awareness then leads to help-seeking behavior, which may include calling the police or seeking shelter services. With appropriate intervention during this open window phase, it is more likely that the victim of abuse will seek services and employ strategies toward safety. An experimental intervention found that providing safety planning services to victims while in a hospital setting decreased violence and increased safety behaviors at 6-, 12-, 18-, and 24-months follow-up.[52]

SAFETY PLANNING

Safety planning is the foundation of advocacy interventions for abused women, and plans for safety need to be individualized according to a woman's level of risk and within the context of her current situation. Strategies may differ dramatically depending on whether a woman is determined to leave, has already left, or has decided to stay in an abusive relationship. Practitioners who work with women who are being abused recognize that these choices may change over time, and that oscillating among choices is a normal part of the process of dealing with the violence and testing different strategies to end it. Minimization of violence can be interpreted as an adaptive coping mechanism that allows victims to reduce distressing symptoms of trauma and continue to invest in their relationships.[45] Moreover, many women are acutely aware that any attempt to leave their relationships might cause the violence to escalate,[37,41] and many are mindful that legal attempts to protect themselves from violence, such as pursuing an order of protection or calling the police, cannot guarantee safety.[14,53] The challenge to practitioners, advocates, and researchers is to help women stay safe during this time of planning and decision making. Using the DA to conduct a risk assessment may assist a woman in developing a more realistic understanding of the danger in her situation and facilitate planning for her and her children's safety.

DEMOGRAPHIC CHARACTERISTICS ASSOCIATED WITH IP HOMICIDE

Similar to perpetrators of other homicides, male perpetrators of IP homicides in the United States are disproportionately young, poor, and African American, with a history of other violence as well as substance abuse.[54] In the 11-city study of female IP homicides,[4] unemployment was the most significant demographic characteristic and subsumed the risk associated with race and low levels of education. Because demographic variables are often associated, the increased risk of IP homicides of women often attributed to race might actually be due to unemployment, as African American men in the United States are more likely to be unemployed or underemployed. From a sociological perspective, the *resource theory* of intimate partner violence may offer a partial explanation for why unemployment is such a salient risk factor. This theory suggests that a man may use violence toward a female partner when his personal resources, such as education, income, job prestige, and community standing, are lower than hers in an effort to decrease the perceived status difference.[55,56]

DEMOGRAPHIC CHARACTERISTICS OF WOMEN AT RISK OF IP HOMICIDE

There are clear race and ethnicity disparities in rates of IP homicide, with Native American and African American women most at risk.[57,58] Although a significant proportion of this variation can be explained by increased rates of unemployment among Native American and African American men,[3] few investigations have tried to delineate what accounts for these discrepancies. In the 11-city study, prior arrest of the perpetrator was found to be strongly protective against IP homicide for white and mixed-race couples but not protective for African American and Hispanic couples. When looking at the data more closely, this was related to the finding that males in ethnic minority groups who killed their partners were more frequently arrested than the white male killers. Pregnancy-associated homicide is another important source of health disparity, as African American women are 3 to 7 times more likely to experience pregnancy-associated IP homicide when compared with white women.[59,60] Moreover, Krulewitch et al[61] reported that pregnant homicide victims were 3 times more likely to be adolescents than non-pregnant victims.

Although rates of IP homicide are decreasing, they are not decreasing uniformly. Between 1976 and 2005, the decline in victimization through IP homicide was 6% for white females, in contrast to 52% for African American females, 61% for white males, and 83% for African American males.[9] Though differences exist, most research has not examined risk factors for IP homicide by racial group. Dugan et al,[10,13] a notable exception, has found that increased levels of education operate differently for African American and white women. For African American women, increased levels of education are linked to increased rates of IP homicide, whereas for white women, higher levels of education are associated with decreases in IP homicide. This result can be attributed to gender status inconsistency, a factor that has been found to be associated with IPV. One theory is that for white women in relationships with white men, increasing levels of education has resulted in gender parity whereas for African American women in relationships with African American men, an increase in education has resulted in women becoming more educated than their partners.[62] The same connection might also be made for race and employment status.

TYPOLOGIES OF MEN WHO KILL WOMEN

Although the population of men who murder their female partners is fairly heterogeneous, some researchers have attempted to categorize these men into specific types of abusers in order to better understand their motivations and to predict when the most extreme violence is likely to occur.

PIT BULLS VS COBRAS

One commonly referenced typology of male batterers was described by Jacobson and Gottman.[63] Within this particular typology, male batterers are classified as either a *pit bull* or a *cobra*. Men who fit the pit bull description are typically emotionally dependent on and loyal to their female partners, though they will blame their partners for the abuse that they perpetrate. Pit bulls often fear abandonment and have a poor sense of self-worth. As such, they depend upon their partners to meet their emotional needs. They are prone to emotional outbursts as well as extreme jealousy and possessiveness, and their violent behaviors will escalate if their partner leaves or threatens to leave the relationship. The extent of coercion and abuse in this relationship can be severe, but evidence has demonstrated that some pit bulls do respond well to batterer treatment programs.

Cobras, on the other hand, are more likely to display characteristics of an antisocial personality and often do not respond well to treatment. They are more likely to have a history of childhood trauma, violence, and criminality in their lives. As a coping mechanism, many have developed a grandiose sense of self and expect their female partners to comply with their every demand. Cobras are more coldly detached from their partners and may even show contempt for them. Their violence, rather than stemming from emotion, is more often instrumental. Women in this type of relationship may find it difficult to leave their abusers initially, but may not experience the same type of long-term abuse after leaving as those women who have attempted to leave men classified as pit bulls. In both cases, the men have learned to manipulate others to meet their needs and can appear quite charming or convincing to those who are otherwise unaware of their abusive history.

MEN INCARCERATED FOR IP HOMICIDE: FIVE PROFILES

Adams[14] has specifically examined the characteristics of men who have killed, or attempted to kill, their female intimate partners. Based on interviews with 31 such men after the crime, Adams categorized them into 5 broad and sometimes overlapping types: the *jealous type*, the *substance-abusing type*, the *materially motivated type*, the *suicidal type*, and the *career criminal type*.

The jealous type of perpetrator was most common (71%) and was typically obsessed with the idea that his partner was having an affair or was interested in another person sexually. In one case, the jealousy was so extreme that the batterer accused her of having sexual intentions toward a family member. These jealous fantasies inevitably led to monitoring and stalking behaviors that were often extreme and interfered with other aspects of life. This type of abuser was enraged when his partner left him or threatened to leave him, and this was often the impetus for the final act of violence. In some cases, the abuser might have also inflicted physical harm on the perceived object of his partner's affection. In the Adams study, most of these men claimed to kill while in "a jealous rage," but, in a majority of the cases, juries had determined the murders were premeditated.

The substance-abusing type tended to fit the definition of an alcoholic or drug addict. These men were more likely than the others to be young, unmarried, and unemployed. Violence toward their partners, even when non-lethal, was likely to be more severe, especially if the abuser was drunk or high at the time of the incident. Although women who experience violence in this type of relationship may blame their partners' alcohol or drug use for the abuse, some evidence suggests that this type of abuser intentionally uses alcohol and drugs as an excuse for violent behavior. Because many alcoholics and substance abusers have an unstable history of employment, this type of abuser tended to depend on female partners for financial support, and this was often a point of conflict.

The materially motivated type was characterized by dependence on the female partner for material benefits, such as financial and emotional support, sex, housework, and childcare. This type of killer was characterized by a lack of jealousy toward his partner and often had contempt for women in general. Although he may not have been jealous, he was likely possessive, for he had invested in the material benefits his partner provided for him. These men were likely to have had numerous affairs and to become agitated if their partners complained about their infidelity. They were rarely, if at all, apologetic for their abuse and saw themselves as deserving of a certain standard of living because of their male status.

Adams was also able to interview a limited number of incarcerated men who had killed their partners and then attempted, unsuccessfully, to kill themselves, and he referred to these abusive men as the suicidal type. These men tended to be older than other perpetrators of IP homicide and were generally older, by an average of 6 years, than their female partners. These men were more likely than other types of abusers to be married to their intimate partners and have children living in the home with them. Many men classified as this type had a history of depression and may have been more likely than non-suicidal perpetrators of fatal IPV to use alcohol at the time of the homicide, though they may not have been problem drinkers. According to Adams, these men were most similar to the jealous type in that violence was likely to escalate when their partner left them or threatened to leave them. The suicidal type may also be motivated toward extreme violence if they have lost their jobs and are no longer able to provide for their families. One theory is that this abuser perceives his family as an extension of himself, and he determines that if he must die they should also die. In 70% of fatal IP homicide-suicide cases, Koziol-McLain and colleagues[64] found that there had been prior violence toward the female victim.

The career criminal type, which accounted for 21% of Adams' sample, may be most similar to the materially motivated type in that this perpetrator demonstrated little regard for his partner and displayed characteristics similar to antisocial personality. He tended to be impulsive, manipulative, and lacking in empathy for others or remorse for his actions. This type of abuser typically had a long history of criminal and violent behavior and was motivated to violence by seemingly mundane arguments for which he was likely to blame his victim.

Within the Adams study, the most common overlap in all 5 of these profiles was the substance-abusing and jealous types, with approximately two-thirds of the substance-abusing type also meeting criteria for the jealous type. This combination can be doubly dangerous because alcohol and substance use exacerbates the jealousy and paranoia. However, other profiles in combination were similarly dangerous, as all the men interviewed for this study had eventually killed their partners. The case studies that follow provide examples of overlapping profiles.

Case Study 16-1.

Freddie and Rayanna began dating in high school and were married soon after graduation. Shortly thereafter, Freddie began to accuse Rayanna of having affairs, even when she was just having dinner with relatives or co-workers. Close friends and relatives of the couple described Freddie as a sometimes paranoid, jealous man with a history of marijuana use. When the couple would fight, Freddie would often fly into a rage and threaten to commit suicide. He often wondered out loud if anyone could survive a fall from the beach cliffs near their home. Freddie was arrested for domestic violence when, he claimed, Rayanna had accidentally fallen through a glass door during a fight. A few months later, Rayanna moved out of their home, and Freddie threatened to burn down the house where she was staying. When Rayanna became pregnant with their second child, Freddie refused to believe the child was his. One day, as the couple was fighting, he ordered Rayanna to take their 4-year-old daughter out of the car. Rayanna refused, believing that if she and her daughter stayed in the car, Freddie would not kill himself as he had frequently threatened. But Freddie proceeded with his plan and drove the entire family over a cliff and 150 feet into the ocean. Though Freddie survived the crash, Rayanna and his two daughters were killed, with DNA tests later proving that the unborn child was his. Tests also revealed that traces of marijuana, Valium, and methamphetamine were in Freddie's blood at the time of the incident. At his trial, Freddie's long-time employers described him as a kind, hard-working man with "a heart of gold."

Case Study16-2.

Reginald had an extensive criminal record, including robbery and sexual assault, by the time he met Donna. He had rarely been held accountable for these crimes, however, because of a lack of evidence or glitches in the criminal justice system. Reginald also had a history of alcohol and substance abuse and rarely held a job for more than a few months at a time. Reginald was 26 years old when he met Donna, and they quickly moved in together. At this time, Donna says she was unaware of Reginald's criminal record. However, during the course of their relationship, Reginald would be implicated in a variety of crimes against her, including aggravated assault, burglary, and violation of court orders. At one point, Reginald beat Donna so badly that she was hospitalized for a fractured jaw and other broken bones. Donna also disclosed to friends that Reginald demanded daily sex and would "take it" whether or not she was in the mood. Reginald and Donna had one child together, but only lived in the same home for a short time. The rest of their relationship was characterized by periods when Donna would allow Reginald to visit their child and periods when the couple would fight and Donna would not allow the visitations. One day, after fighting and making up, Donna arranged to meet Reginald in the parking lot of their daughter's daycare so that he could see his child. At this point, Reginald removed a gun from his jacket and shot Donna in the face at close range while the car was still running.

Case Study 16-3.

James was a successful money manager living in a suburban neighborhood with his wife Julie and her 18-year-old daughter Lacey, who was mildly disabled. Julie and James were both divorced and had met over the Internet. Julie felt sorry for James because his ex-wife had moved away within the past year and refused to let him see his children. Julie and James had only known each other for 2 months when they decided to get married and move in together. Since that time, James had grown jealous of the close relationship between Julie and Lacey and often suggested that Lacey should move out and attempt to live on her own. Julie disagreed that this was something Lacey could do and frequently argued this point with James. At first, their arguments would escalate to the point where James would shove Julie against the wall or slap her across the face, but eventually he began to hit Julie with a closed fist and threatened to empty all their bank accounts if Lacey did not move out. James had also begun to threaten Lacey with violence, so Julie sent her to live with an out-of-state relative. Julie had assumed James would become less violent at this point, but he found other reasons to argue with her. During one argument, James accused Julie of spending too much money while shopping with friends and pulled her around the house by her hair until she begged him to stop. Several days later, James overheard Julie talking with someone on the phone and became convinced she was talking about him. A fight ensued, and James beat Julie until she became unconscious. She died from brain injuries 2 days later while in the hospital.

RISK FACTORS ASSOCIATED WITH IP HOMICIDE

There is a need to examine existing research on fatal IPV to determine salient risk factors in order to assist professionals in identifying and better serving those in greatest danger.

PREVIOUS IPV IN THE RELATIONSHIP

Prior domestic violence against a female is the number-one risk factor of IP homicide, whether the victim of homicide is the male or female partner. A history of IPV against the female partner precedes approximately 67% to 75% of fatal IPV cases.[4,65-70] The 11-city study of female IP homicide documented that 72% of the IP homicides and attempted homicides were preceded by physical violence from the male partner.[4] Moreover, 2 US studies from different jurisdictions (Ohio and North Carolina) found a documented history of abuse against the female in two-thirds of IP homicides. IP homicides against men by women were characterized by a history of IPV against the female perpetrator in up to 75% of cases.[66,71] As illustrated in the following case study, female-perpetrated IP homicide is often initiated by the woman's self-defense against IPV.[12,66,70,72-76]

Case Study 16-4.

Amber and her boyfriend Joseph were IV drug users who had been living together on and off for almost a year. Both loved to go out and "party" with mutual friends, and Amber had become accustomed to Joseph's violent behavior toward her, which would often escalate when he was high. Amber would frequently fight back when Joseph accused her of stealing money from him or looking at other men. If Joseph pushed her, she would push him back, and he would often respond by beating her. At times, he would threaten to kill her. On one particular night, Joseph and Amber were fighting in a parking lot outside of a bar when Joseph pushed her down and began choking her. Amber became terrified and thought he would kill her, but Joseph stopped choking her when a car pulled into the parking lot. At this point, Amber ran back into the bar and went home with a friend because she was afraid to go home to Joseph. The couple eventually reconciled their relationship and started getting high together again, but Joseph made sure to show Amber a gun he had stolen from his brother. To Amber, this was Joseph's way of keeping her in line, and she began to respond less forcefully to his arguments. However, during one particular night when they were using drugs, their fighting escalated to a point that Amber was convinced Joseph would kill her. She got to the stolen gun before he could and pulled the trigger just as he was lunging at her. Joseph died at the hospital that night from a gunshot to the chest.

STALKING

Stalking, defined as repeated visual or physical proximity, nonconsensual communication, or implied threats,[77] by current or former intimate partners may be an even more common risk factor for IP homicide than previous abuse, especially for offenders who can be considered the jealous type.[14] Though research in this area is limited, McFarlane et al[67] reported that stalking and harassment occurred in 70% to 90% of 200 actual and attempted homicides of women in 11 US cities. The types of stalking most strongly correlated with female IP homicide were following the victim to work or school, destruction of the victim's property, and leaving threatening messages by voicemail.[4] Some jealous types reported an obsession with tracking every move of their partner, or ex-partner, to the extent that they had quit their jobs in order to devote more time to following them.[14] Stalking was associated with victims who had been estranged from their partners as well as those who were still living in intact, physically abusive relationships.[4]

RECENT ESTRANGEMENT

Studies have found a consistent association between IP homicide and married couples with a history of estrangement, a condition that can be characterized by physically leaving the relationship or beginning the steps toward legal separation.[71,78-80] While estrangement may be equally risky for unmarried women in abusive relationships, this has been difficult to determine because the proportion of separated to intact couples at the time of the incident is typically not known. In an analysis of spousal homicide data from the United States, Canada, and the United Kingdom, Wilson and Daly[79] found that the combination of physical and legal separation posed the greatest risk for murder by an intimate partner. In the 11-city study, 55% of female IP homicide victims had separated from their partners at least once during the year prior to the murder.[4] Wilson and Daly[79] and Wilson et al[80] found that the time of greatest risk was the first 3 months after separation. The majority of abused women eventually leave their partners,[47,81] and only a small proportion are killed, but those who experience fatal IPV are usually killed within the first year after separation.

From these studies and clinical experience with women in abusive relationships, it has been theorized that male partners experience a loss of control when their female partners decide to leave the relationship, and some men will increase their violent behavior in an effort to reclaim control. In the 11-city study, women estranged from their abusive partners within a year prior to the study were at nearly 4 times the risk of IP homicide than other abused women. When the abusive partner had been highly controlling, the woman was at nearly 6 times the risk.[4] Although risk of violence increases in the period following separation, this danger has not been compared with the risk of staying in an abusive relationship.

NON-FATAL STRANGULATION

Studies have recently demonstrated that non-fatal strangulation, or being choked, is a common form of abuse leading up to IP homicide. In the 11-city study, nonfatal strangulation prior to IP homicide was reported in 43% (n = 89) of cases.[82] Women who had experienced prior non-fatal strangulation as a form of abuse were more than 7 times more at risk of IP homicide than other abused women, and this risk was even stronger for women almost killed by their partners.[82] Although Block et al[83] did not find that non-fatal strangulation presented an increased risk for IP homicide, they found that strangulation during a specific incident increased the odds of that incident being fatal. Women who were strangled by an intimate partner in a specific incident were more likely to die as a result of that incident than incidents in which other types of violence were used, though this finding was not significant for women abused by a same-sex partner. This research, conducted in Chicago, examining all women killed by an intimate partner during a 2-year period, found that nearly one-fourth were killed by strangulation.

ACCESS TO FIREARMS AND GUN USE

Guns are the most frequent means of killing an intimate partner, with percentages varying according to gender and marital status.[9] During the period from 1990 to 2002, ex-husbands and ex-wives were most frequently killed with guns (87% and 78%, respectively), followed by husbands (70%) and wives (68%). Boyfriends (46%) and girlfriends (57%) were least often killed with guns. Availability of firearms in the United States greatly increases the risk of homicide in general, as well as the risk of IP homicide.[84] Prior IPV and gun ownership have been strongly associated with female homicide in the home.[65] In the 11-city study of female IP homicide,[4] a woman whose abusive partner had access to a gun was at 5 times the risk of IP homicide than other abused women. Moreover, use of a gun dramatically increased the risk of fatality when taking other significant variables into consideration, multiplying it by more than 40 times. Studies have also associated the use of guns and substance abuse, both drugs and alcohol, with IP homicide.[12,29]

DRUG OR ALCOHOL USE

Studies have noted some association between alcohol or drug use and IP homicide, though more powerful predictors, such as gun use, often subsume this factor. Moreover, it is generally difficult to determine with certainty perpetrators' substance abuse at the time of the homicide unless they have committed suicide or have volunteered samples for testing. In the 11-city female IP homicide investigation, a notable 70% of male perpetrators were using drugs or alcohol at the time of the incident, and 33% had been in previous contact with an alcohol or drug treatment program.[4,85] In his study of incarcerated IP homicide offenders, Adams[14] found that approximately 60% had been alcohol or drug abusers and that one-half of all the killers in his study had been drunk or high at the time of the crime. Other studies have found that daily use of drugs and alcohol is more closely associated with extreme partner violence than occasional use. The typology of abuser described by Adams[14] as the substance-abusing type was more likely to have inflicted severe injury on his female partner prior to the lethal incident.

MENTAL ILLNESS

Some association between a perpetrator's mental health and IP homicide have been found although further research is needed to explicate this link; most studies have not been able to accurately measure the extent of an offender's mental state, as mental health diagnosis often requires sufficient time and expertise. An analysis of IP homicides (n = 540) across the United States found that 13% of perpetrators, including both male and female, had a history of mental illness, compared to 3% of homicide offenders who did not kill an intimate partner.[86] Approximately one-third of the 200 male perpetrators in the 11-city study of IP homicides of women were described as being in poor mental health.[17] In addition, 46% of male perpetrators had had at least one contact with a mental health professional, as compared to 29% of the victims of attempted or actual homicides. Adams[14] found that one-half of all the killers he interviewed reported having been depressed over a significant period of time. A stronger association between the perpetrator's mental health and fatal IPV is found in studies of IP homicide-suicide.[64]

SHORT COURTSHIP

Some evidence has found an association between short courtships, that is, relationships having a short time between when a couple meets and when they move in together, and IP homicides. In the Adams[14] study, half of the relationships that had culminated in fatal IPV had begun with a courtship of 3 months or less. He found that relationships with short courtships were generally more unstable and more violent and that many of the victims had not known of their abusers' criminal history or history of IPV before moving in. In this type of case, the victim is murdered when she decides to leave the relationship, which is often because she has become fed up with repeated incidents of physical abuse.

ABUSE DURING PREGNANCY

Abuse during pregnancy has been identified as a specific risk factor for fatal IPV. Specifically, women who are abused while pregnant are at nearly 3 times the risk for serious injury and IP homicide than other abused women.[60,61,87] In the 11-city study of female IP homicide, 25.8% of the women who had been killed or almost killed by their male partners had been abused by them during pregnancy, and at least 4.2% were murdered while pregnant. IP homicide is a common cause of maternal death during pregnancy in the United States[60,61,88] and has been the leading cause of maternal mortality in several US cities and the entire state of Maryland, accounting for up to 20% of maternal deaths.[89]

FORCED SEX AND THE PRESENCE OF STEPCHILDREN

IP homicide has also been associated with forced sex.[23,90-92] In the 11-city study, women who had been sexually assaulted by their abusive partners were found to be at twice the risk for IP homicide. The presence of stepchildren in the home was also associated with increased risk of IP homicide, especially for male perpetrators with extreme sexual jealousy.[93] In the 11-city study of female IP homicide, the victim was at twice the risk of being killed if she had a child that was not biologically related to her abusive male partner. Stepchildren are also more likely to be murdered during male-perpetrated familicides than biological offspring.[94]

IP HOMICIDE-SUICIDE

Homicide-suicide, where a perpetrator kills his partner and then himself, represents a significant proportion of intimate partner homicides, up to 30% by some estimates.[37,64] A study of intimate partner homicide-suicides in 17 states indicated that IP homicide places more than just intimate partners at risk, as nearly 10% of these murders also involved the murder of people other than the intimate partner. Two-thirds of other victims were children, whereas another one-third were other family members, friends, babysitters, or strangers.[95,96] For male perpetrators of homicide-suicide where there had been a history of relationship violence, an estimated 40% were believed to have been responding to a recent break-up or divorce request, and another 18% were currently undergoing legal proceedings for divorce or custody issues or had recently been issued a restraining order. By some estimates, approximately 4000 children in the United States lose both of their parents to IPV each year.[97]

Risk factors for the perpetration of IP homicide-suicide are similar to those for IP homicide and include gender (male perpetrator), jealousy, current or past depression, a longstanding relationship with the victim, a history of physical abuse, a history of separation-reunion episodes, personality disorder, and alcohol abuse.[58,98] In a North Carolina study, 45% of IP homicide-suicide perpetrators were estranged from their victim; 15% had received mental health services in the year prior to the incident; and 38% had ingested alcohol before death, a slightly lower percentage than for IP homicides without suicide.[58,98] In the 11-city study of attempted and actual female IP homicide, 32% of homicides were homicide-suicides. Similar to IP homicides without suicide, prior abuse, estrangement, and the presence of a stepchild in the home were identified as risk factors. Perpetrator threats of suicide and a history of poor mental health were additional prominent predictors of IP homicide-suicides.[64]

Demographic characteristics of perpetrators of IP homicide-suicides differ slightly from perpetrators of other IP homicides, with perpetrators more likely to be married, white, unemployed, and significantly older than their victims.[4,70,98] Perpetrators of this type of murder were also more likely to reside in Southern and Western regions of the US than in the Northern, Central, or Eastern states.[4] The most common profile of a perpetrator of IP homicide-suicide is an abusive husband who has never been arrested for domestic violence but has seen a mental health professional for depression or thoughts of suicide in the year prior to the incident. Typically, this type of perpetrator is distraught because he has lost a job or his wife has decided to end the relationship.

EFFECTS OF IP HOMICIDE ON CHILD SURVIVORS

Approximately 4000 children are orphaned each year through IP homicide, more than those that experience childhood leukemia[99] or Sudden Infant Death Syndrome (SIDS).[100] According to 5 small but relevant preliminary studies,[97,101-105] the lives of children orphaned by IP homicide are significantly disrupted by psychological after effects, such as post-traumatic stress disorder (PTSD), attachment disorders, and behavior problems at school.[102-104,106] Children have reported complicated emotional responses when the killer was their parent as opposed to either a stranger, stepfather, or dating partner of the murdered parent.[105] These children found it more difficult to be angry with a loved one, and they felt guilt or self-blame for their own inability to prevent the murder. Later in life, the adult survivors often had to address the added complication of deciding whether or not to care for the perpetrator when released from prison.

SAME-SEX IP HOMICIDE

Intimate partner homicide in same-sex relationships has not been studied extensively; however, based on data from the SHR from 1981 to 1998, an estimated 6.2% of the total murder rate of men in the US was perpetrated by male same-sex partners, whereas female same-sex partners perpetrated approximately 0.5% of the total murder rate of women. Thus, the male proportion of same-sex IP homicide is over 12 times the female rate; however, there have been no studies to date of male same-sex partner homicides and only 1 study of female same-sex partner homicides or attempted homicides.[82] Prior IPV, estrangement, jealousy, and substance abuse were present prior to the incident, similar to risk factors found in heterosexual couples; however, because of the small subsample (n = 9) for this study, definitive conclusions cannot be drawn. Moreover, the measure used to identify risk factors in the same-sex sample was developed for the study of male-to-female intimate partner violence. As such, critical factors specific to cases of same-sex IPV may have been overlooked.[107]

MOVING FORWARD: FUTURE STEPS TOWARD PREVENTION

From interviews with incarcerated men convicted of murdering a female intimate partner, Adams[14] found that a majority of men stated the greatest deterrent to their crimes would have been more extensive surveillance or punishment by law enforcement. Similarly, studies have shown that attendance in batterer's treatment programs and cessation of violence most often occurs when mandated by law. In the past 25 years, mandatory arrest and "no drop" policies have been widely adopted and are intended to counteract traditional police hesitancy to intervene in domestic affairs,[108,109] yet gaps exist. Fifty-one percent of the perpetrators of homicide or attempted homicide had been previously arrested by police, and 44% were arrested for prior domestic abuse incidents, 37% for other violent crimes, and 58% for other nonviolent crimes.[17] Continued research is needed to identify which policy initiatives truly provide protection against IP homicide and which do not.

GUN OWNERSHIP RESTRICTION FOR KNOWN BATTERERS

One key area for legal intervention is related to gun possession, as firearms are the weapons most frequently used in IP homicide. In a study of men incarcerated for the murder or attempted murder of an intimate female partner, 78% said they would not have killed their partner if they had not had access to a firearm.[14] There is a need for more consistent application of current policies that support removal of guns from the home through training of police officers, judges, and magistrates, but all too often the policies related to enforcement of gun removal are overlooked or not strictly enforced.[110] In the Adams[14] study, more than one-half of the incarcerated men reported that they had obtained their guns illegally. One-third of these men had protective orders against them at the time of the murder and, as such, were prohibited from owning a firearm yet had failed to surrender the firearm to authorities or had gained access to the weapon by other means. Similarly, in the 11-city study, approximately one-third of the perpetrators who possessed guns had been prohibited from gun possession.[4]

Frattaroli and Vernick[111] demonstrated that there are a myriad of different state statutes applying to gun access restrictions for IPV perpetrators. Frattaroli and Teret[112] in Maryland and Seave[113] in California found an inconsistency in the implementation of these statutes; however, Vigdor and Mercy[114] were able to demonstrate a significant 10% decrease in IP homicide overall and 13% decrease of female IP homicide where orders of protection prohibited firearm possession. They found a 7% reduction in IP homicides in states with gun prohibitions related to IPV restraining orders, though it was unclear how effectively the prohibitions had been enforced. According to Bridges et al,[115] family homicide rates have also consistently decreased with the introduction of gun restrictions for known abusers.

THE LETHALITY ASSESSMENT PROGRAM: A COORDINATED EFFORT

Lack of awareness of resources as well as difficulties in accessing services are factors associated with remaining in an abusive relationship.[116] The Lethality Assessment Program (LAP), developed by the Maryland Network Against Domestic Violence (www.mnadv.org), is an innovative effort that facilitates collaboration between law enforcement and social service agencies in informing IPV victims of the resources available to them. Curnow's[51] open window theory suggests that frontline police officers have an ideal opportunity to intervene with victims at the scene of the IPV incident, but police officers face several challenges when attempting to protect victims of IPV. Police officers are responsible for a large number of cases, and it is not always clear if the perpetrator poses a lethal threat to his victim. Even when officers believe a case is high-risk, victims are not always convinced and will not seek services after the incident.[117] In the 11-city female IP homicide study, only about one-half of the women who were killed or almost killed accurately assessed their risk.[4] However, in a study of severely abused women, those who perceived themselves at higher risk took more protective actions.[37] The LAP seeks to increase the victim's perception of risk while providing awareness of and access to services.

Key to this program is the 11-item *Lethality Screen*, a shortened version of the DA that can easily be administered and scored by frontline officers. As the first step in this intervention, police at the scene of an IPV incident assess the victim's risk for homicide by completing the Lethality Screen. If the victim is determined to be at high risk, the responding officer advises her of the results of the assessment, calls a participating local 24-hour hotline, and encourages the victim to speak with an advocate. If the victim agrees, the advocate discusses immediate safety planning measures with the victim and encourages the victim to seek services. The officer then helps to implement any immediate safety plans that have been put in place, such as transporting the victim to a shelter. If the victim declines to speak with the advocate, the officer obtains guidance from the advocate for how to provide the victim with safety steps. If the situation is not deemed highly dangerous, the officer advises the victim that IPV is dangerous and sometimes fatal, warns her to watch for the signs listed in the Lethality Screen, and provides appropriate resources.

Feasibility of this program has been demonstrated with adoption by the LAP in 45 police jurisdictions across the state of Maryland, and other jurisdictions across Delaware, Florida, Georgia, Indiana, Minnesota, Missouri, Nevada, New Hampshire, Oklahoma, Oregon, and Vermont. Pilot research has reported improved communication between law enforcement and service providers. Both police officers and advocates reported that the intervention was easy to administer, and officers reported more confidence about what to do when they encountered a victim who appeared to be in danger. Social Service programs experienced higher numbers of calls and higher demands for shelter, but they reported that the demands were manageable. The LAP is currently being evaluated through a research study funded by the National Institute of Justice.

CONCLUSION

Though IP homicide is a relatively rare event, it continues to be a major threat to women's safety and health. Prior IPV against a female partner is a major risk factor for IP homicide, whether the victim is male or female. Other significant risk factors for fatal IPV are estrangement, perpetrator's ownership of a gun, perpetrator unemployment, threats to kill, threats to harm the victim with a weapon or use of a weapon, forced sex, a highly controlling abuser, abuse during pregnancy, attempted strangulation, the presence a stepchild in the home, and the perpetrator avoiding arrest for domestic violence.

Despite a fairly extensive body of literature related to IP homicide, additional research is necessary to learn more about fatal IPV in same-sex intimate relationships, rural communities, and during pregnancy or the first year after delivery. Additional research is needed to identify causes for significant racial and ethnic disparities in IP homicide, particularly of Native American and African American women. Moreover, additional work is needed to measure the predictive validity of risk assessment as part of the safety planning process. Further research might also test interventions to see which truly work to prevent or decrease IPV and homicide for a variety of populations in health, mental health, social service, and even criminal justice settings.

Whenever women and children enter into a social service or health care setting, there is an opportunity for professionals to assess and intervene. Comprehensive assessment includes identifying previous or current IPV, assessing for injuries or other symptoms, identifying alcohol or substance use, and assessing the risk of lethality. Professionals may need to administer appropriate resources and engage the woman in safety planning that also includes her children, if relevant. Social service and health care home visitors should be alert for signs of IPV, especially if there are children in the home. Policies are needed to support training for social service and health care professionals so that they understand the risk factors for fatal IPV and know how to assess for risk of lethality. Other policies are needed that address the removal of guns from the home, specifically in homes where there is a history of or prior arrest for IPV or active protective orders, and these policies must be enforced as indicated under the federal Violence Against Women Act (VAWA) and according to individual state laws where they exist. Finally, mandated batterer intervention programs that include job readiness training and job placement services, in addition to mental health and substance abuse services, might make a significant impact on the safety of women who are most at risk for fatal IPV.

REFERENCES

1. Catalano S, Smith E, Snyder H, Rand, M. *Female Victims of Violence*. Washington, DC: United States Department of Justice; 2009.

2. Brock K. *When Men Murder Women: An Analysis of 2001 Homicide Data*. Washington, DC: Violence Policy Center Publications; 2003.

3. Campbell JC, Webster D, Koziol-McLain J, et al. Assessing risk factors for intimate partner homicide. *Natl Institute Justice J*. 2003;250:14-19.

4. Campbell JC, Webster D, Koziol-McLain J, et al. Risk factors for femicide in abusive relationships: results from a multisite case control study. *Am J Public Health*. 2003;93(7):1089-1097.

5. Frye V, Hosein V, Waltermaurer E, Blaney S, Wilt S. Femicide in New York City: 1990 to 1999. *Homicide Studies*. 2005;9(3):204-228.

6. Fox JA. Uniform crime reports [United States]: Supplementary homicide reports, 1976-2002 [Computer file] (ICPSR ed). Ann Arbor, MI: Inter-University Consortium for Political and Social Research; 2005.

7. Lattimore PK, Trudeau J, Riley J, Leiter J, Edwards S. *Homicide in Eight Cities: Trends, Context and Policy Implications*. Washington, DC: US Department of Justice, Bureau of Justice Statistics; 1997.

8. Rennison CM. *Intimate Partner Violence, 1993-2001*. Washington, DC: US Department of Justice; 2003.

9. Fox JA, Zawitz MW. *Homicide trends in the US*. Washington, DC: Bureau of Justice Statistics; 1999. Bureau of Justice Statistics Web site. http://www.bjs.gov/content/pub/pdf/htiuscdb.pdf Accessed July 18, 2013.

10. Dugan L, Nagin D, Rosenfeld R. Do domestic violence services save lives? *Natl Inst Justice J*. 2003;250:20-25.

11. Rosenfeld R. Changing relationships between men and women. a note on the decline of intimate partner homicide. *Homicide Stud*. 1997;1(1):72-83.

12. Browne A, Williams KR, Dutton DC. Homicide between intimate partners. In: Smith MD, Zahn M, eds. *Homicide: A Sourcebook of Social Research*. Thousand Oaks, CA: Sage; 1999:149-164.

13. Dugan L, Nagin D, Rosenfeld R. Exposure reduction or retaliation? the effects of domestic violence resources on intimate-partner homicide. *Law Soc Rev*. 2003;37(1):169-198.

14. Adams D. *Why do they Kill? Men who Murder their Intimate Partners*. Nashville, TN: Vanderbilt University Press; 2007.

15. Dobash RE, Dobash RP, Cavanagh K. "Out of the blue:" men who murder an intimate partner. *Fem Criminology.* 2009;4(3):194-225.

16. Stark E. *Coercive Control: How Men Entrap Women in Personal Life.* New York, NY: Oxford University Press; 2007.

17. Sharps PW, Koziol-McLain J, Campbell JC, McFarlane J, Sachs CJ, Xu, X. Health care provider's missed opportunities for preventing femicide. *Prev Med.* 2001;33(5):373-380.

18. Morrison LJ, Allan R, Grunfeld A. Improving the emergency department detection rate of domestic violence using direct questioning. *J Emerg Med.* 2000;19(2):117-124.

19. Schacht RL, Dimidjian S, George WH, Berns SB. Domestic violence assessment procedures among couples therapists. *J Marital Fam Ther.* 2009;35(1):47-59.

20. O'Leary KD, Malone J, Tyree A. Physical aggression in early marriage: prerelationship and relationship effects. *J Consult Clin Psych.* 1994;62(3):594-602.

21. Shlonsky A, Friend C. Double jeopardy: risk assessment in the context of child maltreatment and domestic violence. *Brief Treatment and Crisis Intervention.* 2007;7(4):253-274.

22. Lindhorst T, Casey E, Meyers M. Frontline worker responses to domestic violence disclosure in public welfare offices. *Social Work.* 2010:55(3);235–243.

23. Campbell JC. Nursing assessment of risk of homicide for battered women. *Adv Nurs Sci.* 1986;8(4):36-51.

24. Berk RA, Berk S, Loseke DR, Rauma, D. Mutual combat and other family violence myths. In: Finkelhor D, Gelles RJ, Hotaling GT, Straus MA, eds. *The Dark Side of Families.* Beverly Hills, CA: Sage; 1983:197-212.

25. Browne A. *Battered Women Who Kill.* New York, NY: Free Press; 1987.

26. Campbell JC. Misogyny and homicide of women. *Adv Nurs Sci.* 1981;3(2):67-85.

27. Fagan J, Stewart DE, Hansen K. Violent men or violent husbands? Background factors and situational correlates. In: Gelles RJ, Hotaling G, Straus MA, Finkelhor D, eds. *The Dark Side of Families.* Beverly Hills, CA: Sage;1983:49-68.

28. Campbell JC. *Assessing Dangerousness.* Newbury Park, CA: Sage; 1995.

29. Campbell JC. Prediction of homicide of and by battered women. In: Campbell, JC, ed. *Assessing the Risk of Dangerousness: Potential for Further Violence of Sexual Offenders, Batterers, and Child Abusers.* Thousand Oaks, CA: Sage; 1995:96-113.

30. Ferraro KJ, Johnson JM. How women experience battering: the process of victimization. *Soc Probl.* 1983;30(3):325-339.

31. Campbell JC. Lethality assessment approaches: reflections on their use and ways forward. *Violence Against Women.* 2005;11:1206-1213.

32. Campbell JC, Webster D, Glass NE; Johns Hopkins University. The danger assessment: validation of a lethality risk assessment instrument for intimate partner femicide. *J Interpers Violence.* 2009;24(4):653-674.

33. Goodman L, Dutton MA, Bennett L. Predicting repeat abuse among arrested batterers: use of the Danger Assessment Scale in the criminal justice system. *J Interpers Violence.* 2000;15(1):63-74.

34. Heckert DA, Gondolf EW. Battered women's perceptions of risk versus risk factors and instruments in predicting repeat reassault. *J Interpers Violence.* 2004;19(7):778-800.

35. Williams KR, Houghton AB. Assessing the risk of domestic violence re-offending: a validation study. *Law Human Behav.* 2004;28(4):437-455.

36. Gelles R. Lethality and risk assessment for family violence cases. Paper presented at the 4th International Conference on Children Exposed to Family Violence, San Diego, CA; 1998.

37. Campbell JC, O'Sullivan C, Roehl J, et al. *Intimate Partner Violence Risk Assessment Validation Study: The RAVE Study Practitioner Summary and Recommendations: Validation of Tools for Assessing Risk from Violent Intimate Partners.* Washington, DC: United States Department of Justice; 2005. National Criminal Justice Reference Web site. https://www.ncjrs.gov/pdffiles1/nij/grants/209732.pdf. Accessed July 18, 2013.

38. Glass N, Perrin N, Hanson G, Bloom T, Gardner E, Campbell JC. Risk for reassault in abusive female same-sex relationships. *Am J of Public Health.* 2008;98(6):1021-1027.

39. Messing JT, Amanor-Boadu Y, Cavanaugh CE, Glass N, Campbell JC. Culturally competent intimate partner violence risk assessment: adapting the Danger Assessment for immigrant women. *Soc Work Res.* 2013;37(3).

40. Pinard GF, Pagani L, eds. *Clinical Assessment of Dangerousness: Empirical Contributions.* New York, NY: Cambridge University Press; 2000.

41. Weisz A, Tolman R, Saunders DG. Assessing the risk of severe domestic violence. *J Interpers Violence.* 2000;15(1):75-90.

42. Goodkind JR, Sullivan CS, Bybee DI. A contextual analysis of battered women's safety planning. *Violence Against Women.* 2004;10(5):514-533.

43. Goodman L, Dutton MA, Vankos N, Weinfurt K. Women's resources and use of strategies as risk and protective factors for reabuse over time. *Violence Against Women.* 2005;11(3):311-336.

44. Glass NE, Eden KB, Bloom T, Perrin N. Computerized safety aid improves safety decision process for survivors of intimate partner violence. *J Interpers Violence.* 2010;25(11):1947-1964.

45. Campbell JC, Rose LE, Kub J, Nedd D. Voices of strength and resistance: a contextual and longitudinal analysis of women's responses to battering. *J Interpers Violence.* 1998;13(6):743-762.

46. Hutchinson IW, Hirschel JD. Abused women: help seeking strategies and police utilization. *Violence Against Women.* 1998;4(4):436-456.

47. Rennisen CM, Welchans S. *Intimate partner violence.* Washington, DC: United States Department of Justice; 2000.

48. Felson RB, Messner SF, Hoskin AW, Deane G. Reasons for reporting and not reporting domestic violence to the police. *Criminology.* 2002;40(3):617-648.

49. Bonomi AE, Holt VL, Martin DP, Thompson RS. Severity of intimate partner violence and frequency of police calls. *J Interpers Violence.* 2006;21(10):1354-1364.

50. Johnson IM. A loglinear analysis of wives' decisions to call police in domestic violence disputes. *J Crim Just.* 1990;18:147-159.

51. Curnow SAM. The open window phase: helpseeking and reality behaviors by battered women. *Appl Nurs Res.* 1997;10(3):128-135.

52. McFarlane JM, Groff JY, O'Brien JA, Watson K. Secondary prevention of intimate partner violence: a controlled trial. *Nurs Res.* 2006;55(1):52-61.

53. Webster DW, Frattaroli S, Vernick JS, O'Sullivan C, Roehl J, Campbell JC. Women with protective orders report failure to remove firearms from their abusive partners: results from an exploratory study. *J Womens Health.* 2010;19(1):93-98.

54. Weiner NA, Zahn MA, Sagi RJ, Merton RK. *Violence: Patterns, Causes, Public Policy.* Belmont, CA: Wadsworth; 1990.

55. Howard M. Husband-wife homicide: an essay from a family law perspective. *Law Contemp Probl.* 1986;49(1):63-88.

56. Walker LE. *The Battered Woman Syndrome.* New York, NY: Springer; 1984.

57. Mercy JA, Saltzman LE. Fatal violence among spouses in the United States 1976-85. *Am J Public Health.* 1989;79(5):595-599.

58. Morton E, Runyan CW, Moracco KE, Butts J. Partner homicide victims: a population-based study in North Carolina, 1988-1992. *Violence and Victims.* 1998;13(2):91-106.

59. Chang J, Berg CJ, Saltzman LE, Herndon J. Homicide: a leading cause of injury deaths among pregnant and postpartum women in the United States, 1991-1999. *Am J Public Health.* 2005;95(3):471-477.

60. McFarlane J, Campbell JC, Sharps PW, Watson K. Abuse during pregnancy and femicide: urgent implications for women's health. *Obstet Gynecol.* 2002;100(1):27-36.

61. Krulewitch CJ, Roberts DW, Thompson LS. Adolescent pregnancy and homicide: findings for the Maryland Office of the Chief Medical Examiner, 1994-1998. *Child Maltreatment.* 2003;8(2):122-128.

62. Vest JR, Catlin TK, Chen JJ, Brownson RC. Multistate analysis of factors associated with intimate partner violence. *Am J Prev Med.* 2002;22(3):156-164.

63. Jacobson NS, Gottman JM. *When men batter women: new insights into ending abusive relationships.* New York: Simon & Schuster; 1998.

64. Koziol-McLain J, Webster D, McFarlane J, et al. Risk factors for femicide-suicide in abusive relationships: results from a multi-site case control study. *Violence Vict.* 2006;21(1):3-21.

65. Bailey JE, Kellermann AL, Somes GW, Banton JG, Rivara FP, Rushford NP. Risk factors for violent death of women in the home. *Arch Intern Med.* 1997; 157(7): 777-782.

66. Campbell JC, Webster D, Koziol-McLain J, et al. Risk factors for femicide in abusive relationships: results from a multisite case control study. *Am J Public Health.* 2003;93(7):1089-1097.

67. McFarlane J, Campbell JC, Wilt S, Sachs C, Ulrich Y, Xu X. Stalking and intimate partner femicide. *Homicide Stud.* 1999;3(4):300-316.

68. Moracco KE, Runyan CW, Butts J. Femicide in North Carolina. *Homicide Stud.* 1998;2:422-446.

69. Pataki G. *Intimate Partner Homicides in New York State.* Albany, NY: State of New York; 1998.

70. Websdale N. *Understanding Domestic Homicide.* Boston, MA: Northeastern University Press; 1999.

71. Hall-Smith P, Moracco KE, Butts J. Partner homicide in context. *Homicide Studies.* 1998;2(4):400-421.

72. Block CR, Christakos A. Intimate partner homicide in Chicago over 29 years. *Crime Delinquency.* 1995;41(4):496-526.

73. Crawford M, Gartner R. *Woman Killing: Intimate Femicide in Ontario: 1974-1990.* Ontario, Canada: Women We Honor Action Committee; 1992.

74. Jurik NC, Winn R. Gender and homicide: a comparison of men and women who kill. *Violence Vict.* 1990;5(4):227-242.

75. Smith PH, Moracco KE, Butts J. Partner homicide in context: a population based perspective. *Homicide Stud.* 1998;2(4):400-421.

76. Wolfgang ME. *Patterns in Criminal Homicide.* Philadelphia, PA: University of Pennsylvania Press; 1958.

77. Tjaden P, Thoennes N. *Stalking in America: Findings from the National Violence Against Women Survey.* Washington, DC: United States Department of Justice; 1998.

78. Dawson R, Gartner R. Differences in the characteristics of intimate femicides: the role of relationship state and relationship status. *Homicide Stud.* 1998;2(4):378-399.

79. Wilson M, Daly M. Spousal homicide risk and estrangement. *Violence Vict.* 1993;8(1):3-15.

80. Wilson M, Johnson H, Daly M. Lethal and nonlethal violence against wives. *Can J Criminol.* 1995;37:331-362.

81. Campbell JC, Soeken K. Women's responses to battering over time: an analysis of change. *J Interpers Violence.* 1999;14(1):21-40.

82. Glass NE, Koziol-McLain J, Campbell JC, Block CR. Female-perpetrated femicide and attempted femicide. *Violence Against Women.* 2004;10(6):606-625.

83. Block CR, Devitt CO, Fonda D, et al. *The Chicago Women's Health Study: Risk of Serious Injury or Death in Intimate Violence: A Collaborative Research Project.* Washington, DC: United States Department of Justice; 2000. National Institute of Justice Web site. www.icjia.state.il.us/public/pdf/cwhrs/cwhrs.pdf. Accessed January 31, 2013.

84. Kellerman AL, Rivara FP, Rushforth NB. Gun ownership as a risk factor for homicide in the home. *New Engl J Med.* 1993;329:1084-1091.

85. Sharps PW, Campbell JC, Campbell DW, Gary FA, Webster DW. Risky mix: drinking, drug use, and homicide. *Natl Inst Justice J.* 2003;250:8-13.

86. Zawitz MW. *Violence Between Intimates.* Washington, DC: Bureau of Justice Statistics; 1994.

87. McFarlane J, Parker B, Soeken K. Abuse during pregnancy: frequency, severity, perpetrator, and risk factors of homicide. *Public Health Nurs.* 1995;12(5):284-289.

88. Parsons LH, Harper MA. Violent maternal deaths in North Carolina. *Obstet Gynecol.* 1999;94(6):990-993.

89. Horon IL, Cheng D. Enhanced surveillance for pregnancy-associated mortality—Maryland, 1993-1998. *JAMA.* 2001;285:1455-1459.

90. Campbell JC. *Empowering Survivors of Abuse: Health Care for Battered Women and Their Children.* Thousand Oaks, CA: Sage; 1998.

91. Campbell JC, Soeken K. Forced sex and intimate partner violence: effects on women's health. *Violence Against Women.* 1999;5(9):1017-1035.

92. McFarlane J, Soeken K, Campbell JC, Parker B, Reel S, Silva C. Severity of abuse to pregnant women and associated gun access of the perpetrator. *Public Health Nur.* 1998;15(3):201-206.

93. Brewer VE, Paulsen DJ. A comparison of US and Canadian findings on uxorcide risk for women with children sired by previous partners. *Homicide Stud.* 1999;3(4):317-332.

94. Daly M, Wiseman KA, Wilson M. Women with children sired by previous partners incur excess risk of uxoricide. *Homicide Stud.* 1997;1(1):61-71.

95. Dobash RE, Dobash RP. Who died? The murder of collaterals related to intimate partner conflict. *Violence Against Women.* 2012;18(6):662-671.

96. Logan J, Hill HA, Black ML, Karch DL, Barnes JD, Lubell KM. Characteristics of perpetrators in homicide-followed-by-suicide incidents: National Violent Death Reporting System—17 US States, 2003-2005. *J Am Epidemiol.* 2008;168(9):1056-1064.

97. Steeves RH, Parker B. Adult perspectives on growing up following uxoricide. *J Interpers Violence.* 2007;22(10):1270-1284.

98. Buteau J, Lesage AD, Kiely MC. Homicide followed by suicide: a Quebec case series, 1988-1990. *Can J Psychiat.* 1993;38(8):552-556.

99. American Cancer Society. *Cancer Facts and Figures 2002.* Atlanta, GA: American Cancer Society; 2002. Universal Healthcare Management Systems, Inc. Web site. www.uhmsi.com/docs/CancerFacts&Figures2002.pdf. Accessed July 17, 2013.

100. Minino AM, Heron MP, Smith BL. *Deaths: Preliminary Data for 2004.* Hyattsville, MD: National Center for Health Statistics; 2006.

101. Black D, Kaplan T. Father kills mother: issues and problems encountered by a child psychiatric team. *Br J Psychiatry.* 1988;153:624-630.

102. Clements P, Burgess A. Children's responses to family member homicide. *Community Health.* 2002;25(1):32-42.

103. Eth S, Pynoos RS. Children who witness the homicide of a parent. *Psychiatry.* 1994;57(4):287-306.

104. Hardesty JL, Campbell JC, McFarlane JM, Lewandowski LA. How children and their caregivers adjust after intimate partner femicide. *J Fam Issues.* 2008;29(1):100-124.

105. Laughon K, Steeves R, Parker B, Sawin E, Knopp A. Forgiveness, and other themes, in women whose fathers killed their mothers. *Adv Nurs Sci;* 2008;31(2):153-163.

106. Kaplan T, Black D, Hyman P, Knox J. Outcome of children seen after one parent killed the other. *Clin Child Psychol Psychiatry.* 2001;6(1):9-22.

107. Glass NE, Laughon K, Campbell JC, et al. Non-fatal strangulation is an important risk factor for attempted and completed femicides. *J Emerg Med.* 2008;35(3):329-335.

108. Hirschel D, Buzawa E. Understanding the context of dual arrest with directions for future research. *Violence Against Women.* 2002;8(12):1449-1473.

109. Roberts AR, Kurst-Swanger K. Court responses to battered women and their children. In: Roberts AR, ed. *Handbook of Domestic Violence Intervention Strategies: Policies, Programs, and Legal Remedies.* New York, NY: Oxford University Press; 2002.

110. Zeoli AM, Webster DW. Effects of domestic violence policies, alcohol taxes and police staffing levels on intimate partner homicide in large US cities. *Inj Prev.* 2010;16:90-95.

111. Frattaroli S, Vernick J. Separating batterers and guns: a review and analysis of gun removal laws in 50 states. *Eval Rev.* 2006;30(3):296-312.

112. Frattaroli S, Teret S. Understanding and informing policy implementation: a case study of the domestic violence provisions of the Maryland Gun Violence Act. *Eval Rev.* 2006;30(3):347-360

113. Seave PL. Disarming batterers through restraining orders: the promise and the reality in California. *Eval Rev.* 2006;30(3):245-265.

114. Vigdor ER, Mercy JA. Do laws restricting access to firearms by domestic violence offenders prevent intimate partner homicide? *Evaluation Rev.* 2006;30(3):313-346.

115. Bridges FS, Tatum KM, Kunselman JC. Domestic violence statutes and rates of intimate partner and family homicide: a research note. *Criminal Justice Policy Rev.* 1998;19(1):117-130.

116. Patzel B. What blocked heterosexual women and lesbians in leaving their abusive relationships. *J Am Psychiat Nurs Assoc.* 2006;12(4):208-215.

117. Messing JT. *Assessing the Risk: What Police Reports Reveal About Domestic Violence Escalation* [dissertation]. Berkeley, CA: University of California, Berkeley; 2007.

Chapter 17

SEX-RELATED HOMICIDE

Tara Henry, MSN, FNP-C, SANE-A, SANE-P

KEY POINTS

1. Sex-related homicides make up 1% to 4% of all homicide cases.

2. In many cases of sex-related homicide, the offender was an acquaintance of the victim or had some prior contact with the victim.

3. There is a high prevalence of sexual assault present in many cases of intimate partner violence. Because of this high prevalence, all intimate partner homicides should be evaluated for possible sexual assault and, when identified, should be coded as a sex-homicide.

4. Cause of death in sex-related homicides is most frequently from strangulation, stabbing, or blunt force trauma.

5. Collaboration between forensic pathologists and forensic nurses who specialize in providing medical care to living victims of sexual assault has improved the standard of care for victims of intimate partner homicide and of sex-related homicide.

INTRODUCTION

Sex-related homicide, also known as *sexual homicide,* is the killing of a person with sexual behavior occurring just before, during, or after the event.[1,2] A significant amount of attention is given to this type of crime by the media, particularly in crime fiction and investigative dramas. Historically, there has been a paucity of research on sex-related homicides. Available research and publications are primarily from the law enforcement and psychology professions, with little attention from medical researchers.[1,3,4] Chan and Heide[5] suggest the lack of research connected to sex-related homicides may be related to the unavailability of valid and reliable national crime statistics on sex-related homicide and evolving definitions and terms of sex-related homicide which has resulted in the lack of a standardized definition. Currently, the data available estimates sex-related homicides to be 1% to 4% of all homicides,[2,5,6] indicating this severe crime is a rare event. Henry[1] suggests that it is unrealistic for sex-related homicides to account for less than 4% of all homicides, as national crime data implies and proposes instead that these crimes are going unrecognized.

UNDERSTANDING SEX-RELATED HOMICIDE

Over the years, several offender typologies or profiles have been suggested by law enforcement and psychologists in an attempt to understand the type of offender who sexually assaults and murders. Early seminal publications focusing on sex-related homicide indicated that offenders targeted strangers, were often driven by sadistic fantasies, and engaged in multiple paraphilic behaviors. This framework has been the foundation of much later research; however, the continuation of a narrow research focus may be contributing both to the problem of unrecognized or unreported sex-related homicides and to the difficulty of categorizing this crime in a way that provides for a more accurate representation of its prevalence and context. More recent research has found that adult victims of sex-related homicides are often acquaintances of or have at least had some prior contact with the offender.[1,7-9] As law enforcement, psychologists, and medical providers expand the research on sex-related homicides and strive to obtain more valid statistics, they should begin investigating sex-related homicides that occur in the context of a domestic violence/intimate partner homicide. Doing so is likely to identify a large number of sex-related homicides that currently go unrecognized.

In 2008, men murdered 1817 women in the United States. Of those women, 64% were the wives, common-law wives, ex-wives, or girlfriends of the offenders.[10] Geberth[11] suggests the most prevalent sex-related homicides are those that occur between intimate partners. In a recent study by Henry,[1] 44% of sex-related homicides were committed by a current spouse or boyfriend. Of those, 94% had a known history of domestic violence prior to the homicide. Research has repeatedly identified possessiveness and jealously as important risk factors that contribute to men killing their intimate partners,[12-15] and additional studies have determined that sexual assault is another significant risk factor for intimate partner homicide (IPH).[16] Dobash and colleagues'[13] study comparing lethal and nonlethal violence against intimate partners found that IPH was more likely to include sexual violence. Sixty-eight percent of women in one study reported sexual assault at least once by their intimate partner, and of those sexually assaulted, 79% suffered repeated episodes of sexual assault. A second sexual assault by the intimate partner occurred within 1 month of the first in over one-half of the women who reported a sexual assault.[17] Dekeseredy's[18] study found that 74% of women were sexually assaulted by their intimate partner when they expressed a desire to leave the relationship, 49% were sexually assaulted while attempting to leave the relationship, and 33% were sexually assaulted after they left the relationship. The culmination of feelings of jealousy, possessiveness and anger, combined with estrangement or attempted separation (the most dangerous time in a domestic violence relationship), is thought to result in an offender mentality that, if the offender cannot possess his partner, no one will.[11-13,16,19,20] This is an extremely dangerous dynamic that results in the intimate partner engaging in sexual violence during the homicide to punish and demonstrate his ownership of the woman. Because of the high prevalence of sexual assault in IPH, all such homicides should be evaluated for a possible sexual assault[1] and, when identified, should be appropriately coded as a sex-related homicide.

EXAMINING CRIME SCENES FOR EVIDENCE OF SEX-RELATED HOMICIDE

Recognizing signs of sexual behavior that may be present at the crime scene or on the victim's body is necessary to alert investigators that a sex-related homicide may have occurred. According to Meloy:

Sexual behavior might occur before, during, or after the killing, or throughout the event; and the behavior could range from only conscious fantasy, to physiological arousal, to masturbation, or actual penetration (oral, anal, or vaginal) of the victim with a variety of objects, animate or inanimate. Sexual behavior also may be symbolically expressed, often suffused with anger and curiosity, through mutilation of the victim's genitals.[2]

Several indicators of sexual behavior or activity have been identified in sex-related homicides (**Figures 17-1** to **17-17**). See **Table 17-1** for those indicators which have been described by many experts in the law enforcement, psychology, and medical fields.[1-3,5,21-27] For some offenders, the sex-related homicide is part of their deviant sexual fantasy and the killing occurs to fulfill that need; however, most sex-related homicides

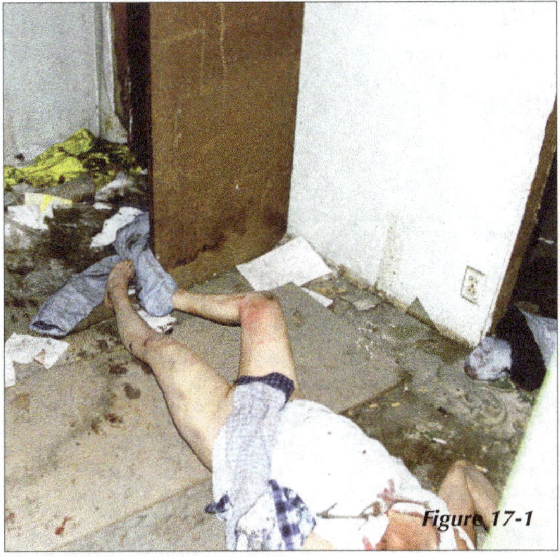

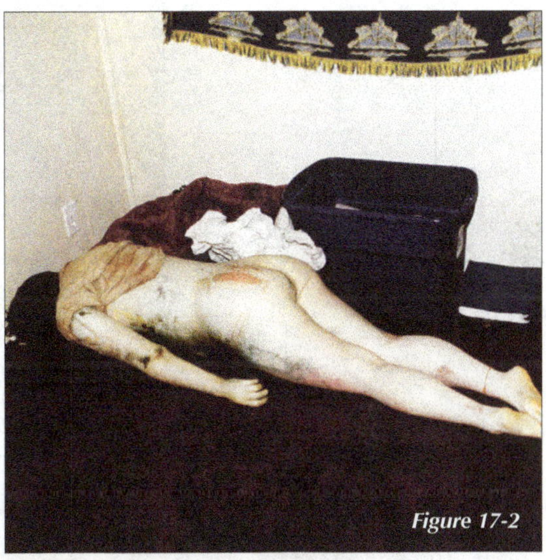

Figure 17-1. *Victim found partially clothed after sex-related homicide. (Contributed by Anchorage Police Department; Anchorage, AK)*

Figure 17-2. *Victim found partially clothed and decomposing after sex-related homicide. (Contributed by Anchorage Police Department; Anchorage, AK)*

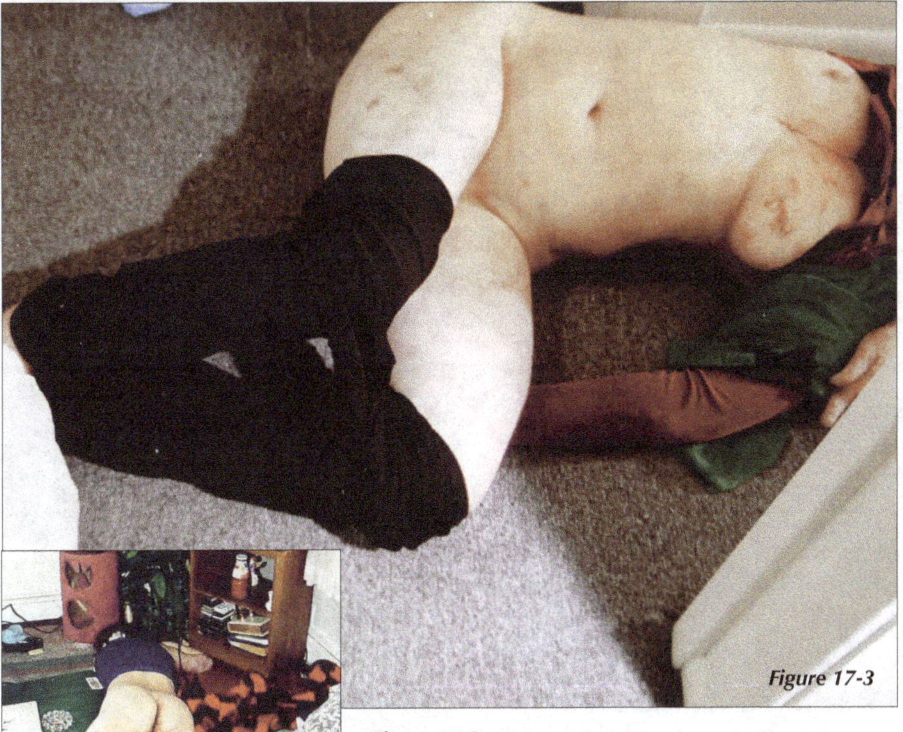

Figure 17-3. *Clothing left positioned exposing breasts and genitalia after sex-related homicide. (Contributed by Anchorage Police Department; Anchorage, AK)*

Figure 17-4. *Body positioned in a sexual manner. (Contributed by Anchorage Police Department; Anchorage, AK)*

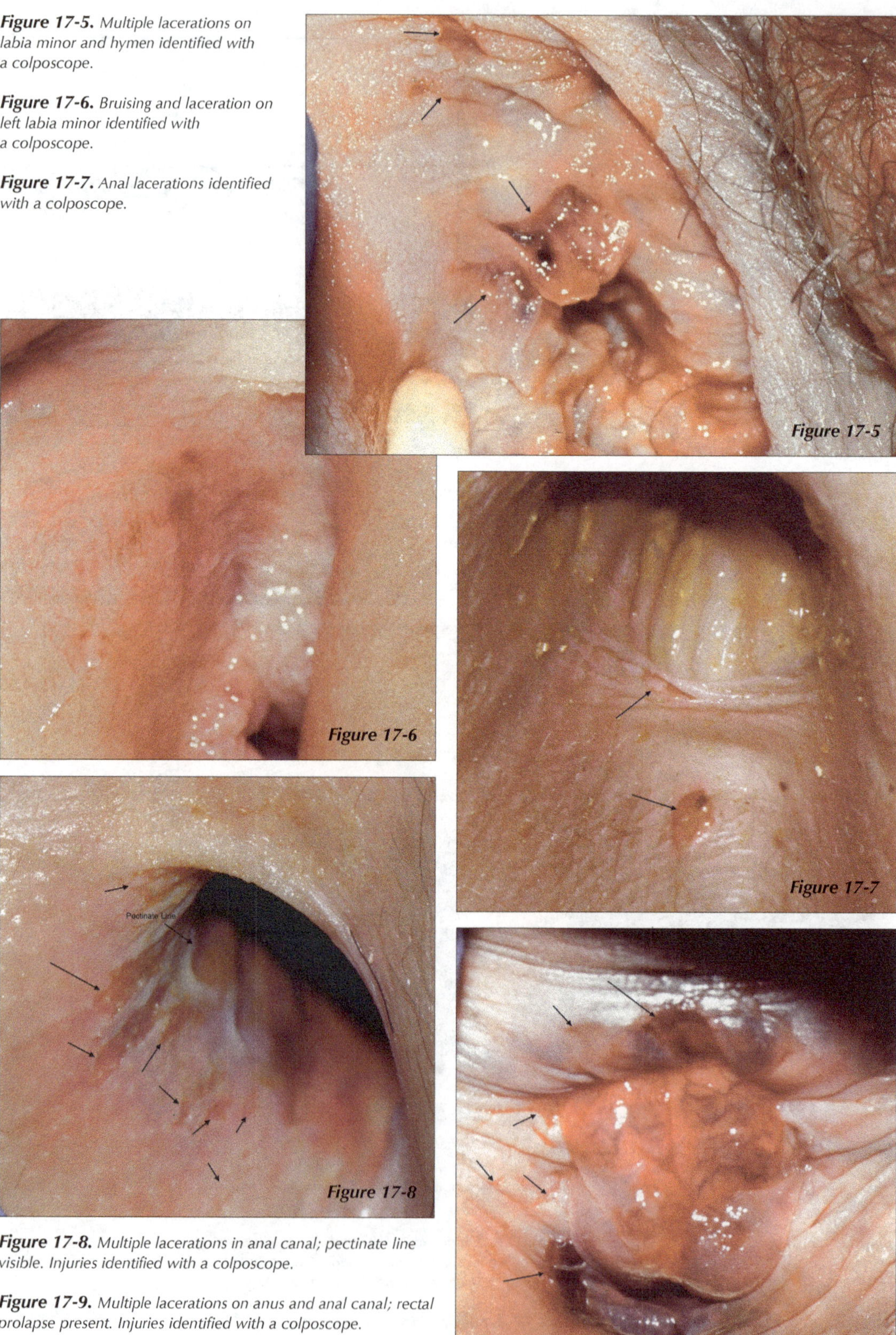

Figure 17-5. *Multiple lacerations on labia minor and hymen identified with a colposcope.*

Figure 17-6. *Bruising and laceration on left labia minor identified with a colposcope.*

Figure 17-7. *Anal lacerations identified with a colposcope.*

Figure 17-8. *Multiple lacerations in anal canal; pectinate line visible. Injuries identified with a colposcope.*

Figure 17-9. *Multiple lacerations on anus and anal canal; rectal prolapse present. Injuries identified with a colposcope.*

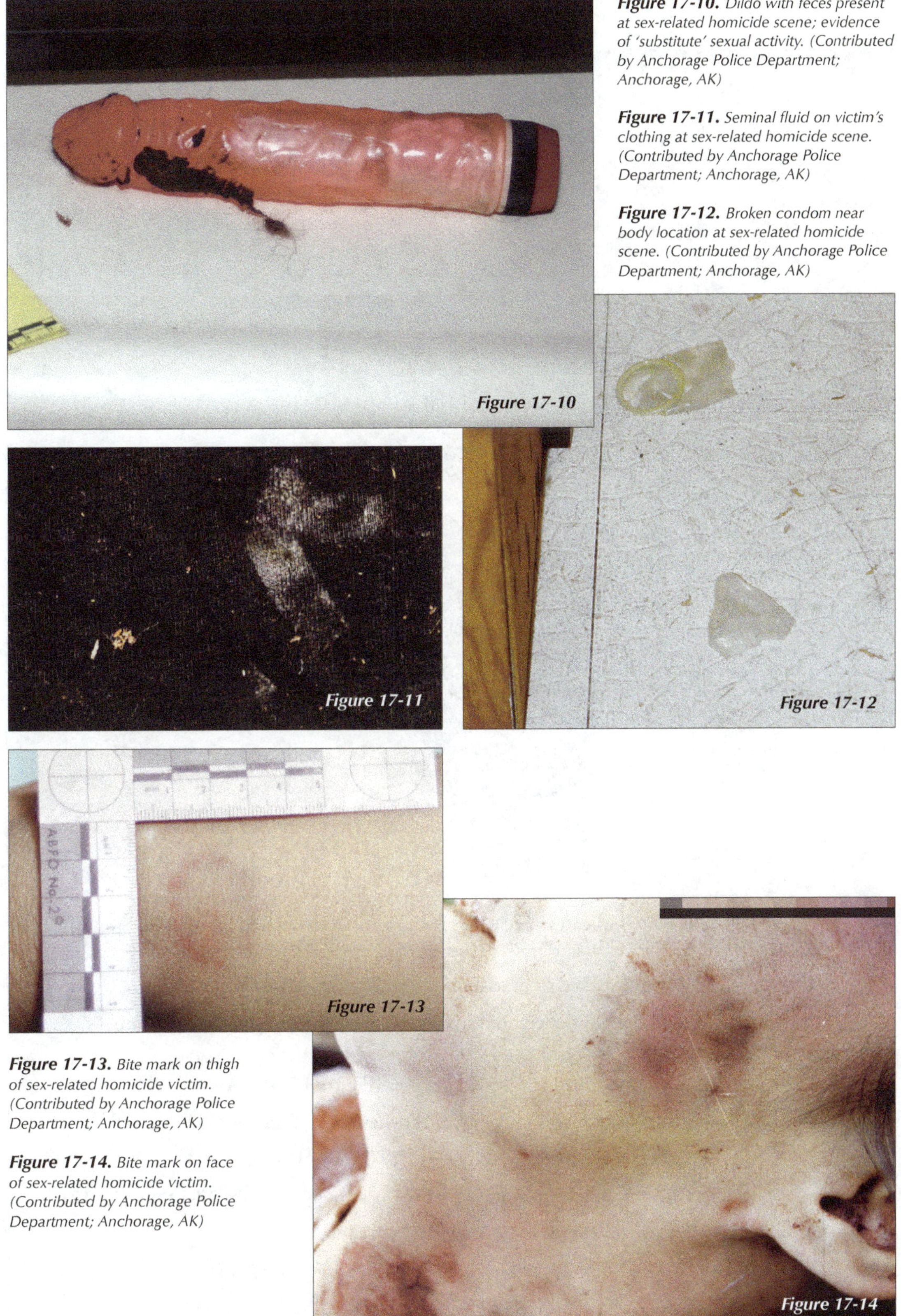

Figure 17-10. Dildo with feces present at sex-related homicide scene; evidence of 'substitute' sexual activity. (Contributed by Anchorage Police Department; Anchorage, AK)

Figure 17-11. Seminal fluid on victim's clothing at sex-related homicide scene. (Contributed by Anchorage Police Department; Anchorage, AK)

Figure 17-12. Broken condom near body location at sex-related homicide scene. (Contributed by Anchorage Police Department; Anchorage, AK)

Figure 17-13. Bite mark on thigh of sex-related homicide victim. (Contributed by Anchorage Police Department; Anchorage, AK)

Figure 17-14. Bite mark on face of sex-related homicide victim. (Contributed by Anchorage Police Department; Anchorage, AK)

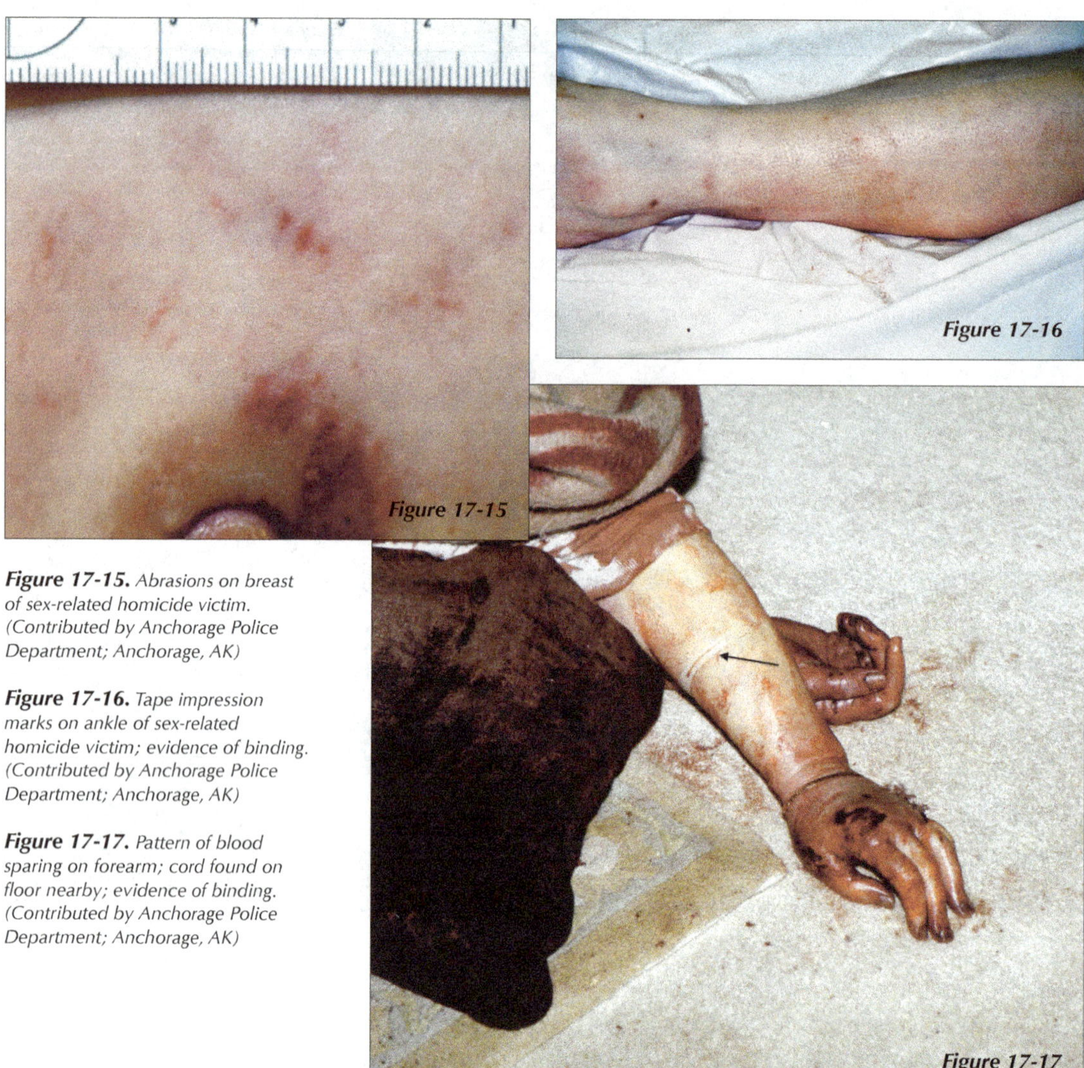

Figure 17-15. *Abrasions on breast of sex-related homicide victim. (Contributed by Anchorage Police Department; Anchorage, AK)*

Figure 17-16. *Tape impression marks on ankle of sex-related homicide victim; evidence of binding. (Contributed by Anchorage Police Department; Anchorage, AK)*

Figure 17-17. *Pattern of blood sparing on forearm; cord found on floor nearby; evidence of binding. (Contributed by Anchorage Police Department; Anchorage, AK)*

Table 17-1. Indicators of Sexual Behavior in Sex-Related Homicides

— Victim is naked or partially clothed (**Figures 17-1** and **17-2**)

— Clothing positioned on the body to expose breasts, genitalia, or buttocks (**Figure 17-3**)

— Body positioned in a sexual manner (**Figure 17-4**)

— Evidence of oral, vaginal, or anal penetration (**Figures 17-5** to **17-9**)

— Evidence of substitute sexual activity (**Figure 17-10**)

— Evidence of seminal fluid in, on, or near body (**Figures 17-11** and **17-12**)

— Bite marks (**Figures 17-13** and **17-14**)

— Breasts, buttocks, or anogenitalia injured (**Figure 17-15**)

— Evidence of bindings or ligatures (**Figures 17-16** and **17-17**) occur as a result of the offender using excessive force during a sexual assault, or to prevent the victim from reporting the sexual assault to law enforcement.[11,26] Cause of death in sex-related homicides is most frequently from strangulation (**Figure 17-18**), stabbing (**Figure 17-19**), or blunt force trauma (**Figure 17-20**). Strangulation is by far the most common cause of death in sex-related homicides.[3,5,9,13,28,29] This is not surprising given the frequency of non-fatal strangulation assaults in living domestic violence and sexual assault victims. In more recent literature, gunshot wounds as a cause of death appear to be more common than previous research has indicated.[1,28] The victim's head, face, neck, and chest suffer the most injury in sex-related homicides, demonstrating the close personal contact and extreme, violent emotion involved. For sex-related homicides committed by an intimate partner, those emotions are often a combination of rage,

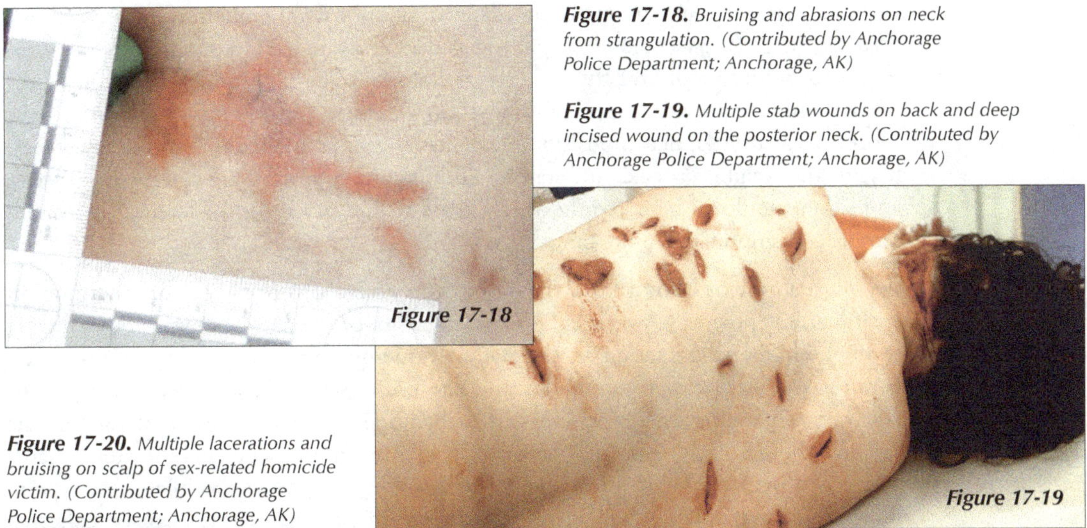

Figure 17-18. Bruising and abrasions on neck from strangulation. (Contributed by Anchorage Police Department; Anchorage, AK)

Figure 17-19. Multiple stab wounds on back and deep incised wound on the posterior neck. (Contributed by Anchorage Police Department; Anchorage, AK)

Figure 17-20. Multiple lacerations and bruising on scalp of sex-related homicide victim. (Contributed by Anchorage Police Department; Anchorage, AK)

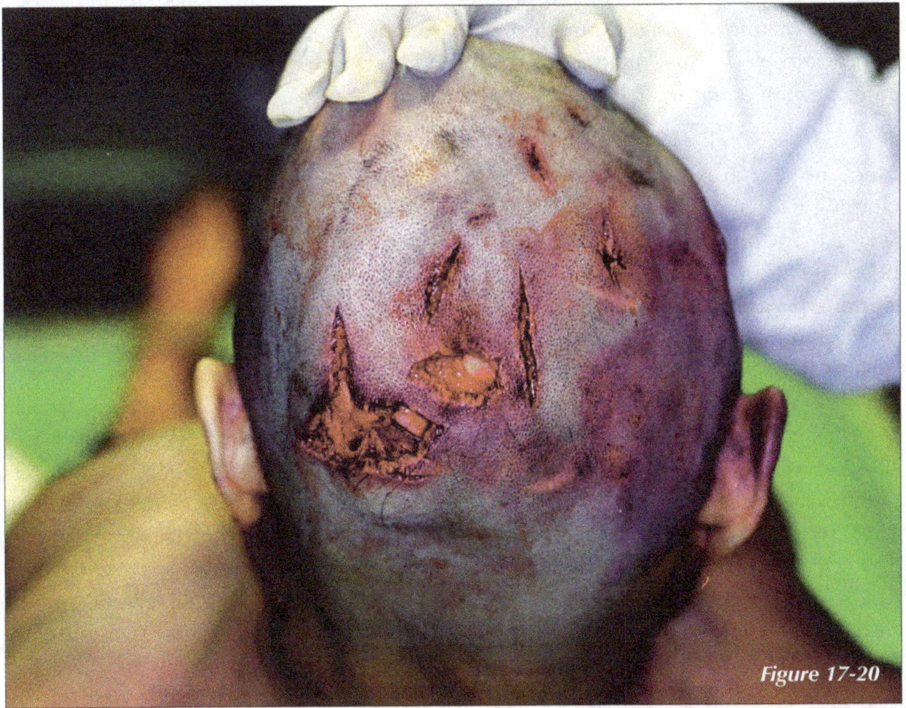

jealously, betrayal, and a perceived loss of control over the victim. That offender chooses to use brutal physical and sexual violence as a way to regain control of, punish, and humiliate the victim. Sex-related homicide in the context of intimate partner violence is the ultimate revenge.

POSTMORTEM EXAMINATION FOR EVIDENCE OF SEX-RELATED HOMICIDE

Forensic nurses or other sexual assault specialists who collaborate with forensic pathologists and law enforcement to examine sex-related homicide victims should follow an examination process similar to that which is performed on living sexual assault victims. First obtain a medical-forensic history. This includes the circumstances surrounding the death, crime scene details, victim's demographics and any known medical, surgical, psychological, and social history available. This is usually obtained from law enforcement and the forensic pathologist. The physical examination of the body should begin with a general evaluation which includes body positioning, rigor mortis, livor mortis, decomposition, evidence of animal predation and insect activity, height, and weight. Presence and state of clothing on the body, bindings, glasses, jewelry, and so on should all be noted; however, items should not be disturbed until pertinent sample collection has been obtained.

Forensic sample collection from the decedent is an important part of the postmortem examination process. Awareness of potential trace evidence should be constant throughout the examination of the body. Numerous types of physical evidence can connect the victim to the offender and the crime scene. Physical evidence present will vary depending on the specifics of each individual case. Assessment for forensic samples should always include examination of the clothing and body for loose hairs, fibers, and debris. This requires a good light source and, when possible, some type of illuminated magnifier. When identified, trace evidence such as this can be collected from the clothing or body by hand-picking or adhesive tape. Hand-picking can be done with the examiner's fingers, but to prevent loss of the item, it is best done with fine tipped forceps. The use of adhesive tape, also known as tape lifting, can be used when hand picking is not feasible, or when a large surface of particles need to be collected. Generally, this is done on a piece of clothing or entire body surface areas.

Once the general examination is complete, physical evidence from the clothing and the clothing itself should be gathered. Clothing should be assessed while still in place on the body for physical evidence, fluid stains, and defects that coincide with wounds or other alterations, such as missing buttons and broken zippers or clasps. In addition, the clothing position on the body should be noted and documented prior to removal. For sex-related homicides, it is common for the body to be naked or the clothing partially missing. When clothing is present on the body, its placement is often altered to expose the breasts, buttocks, or genitalia. Collection of the clothing should be done one article at a time, with the pieces of clothing placed in individual paper bags. Items that are wet should be secured and dried prior to packaging. Examination of any clothing pockets may reveal additional items that assist in identifying the victim (eg, driver's license, social security card, credit cards, photos, cell phone), evidence of lifestyle (eg, cigarettes, lighters, medications, illegal drugs, alcohol), or other clues that may be helpful in determining recent events or contact the victim may have had (eg, receipts, notes, movie tickets). After removal of the clothing, the body should be examined for any jewelry in place. Documentation of the jewelry on the body prior to removal is important. Jewelry and other belongings of the victim are released to the next-of-kin unless there is particular evidentiary value to it (eg, matching earring on body to earring found at scene or with suspect). After removal of the clothing, the body should be systematically and thoroughly assessed for potential forensic evidence and, when identified, collected and packaged appropriately.

In many jurisdictions in the United States, routine collection of pulled head and pubic hairs as reference samples from sexual assault victims is no longer done. Should those known reference samples become relevant in a particular sexual assault case, they can be obtained from the victim at a later date; however, this is not possible if the victim is deceased. Therefore, in postmortem sexual assault examinations, pulled head and pubic hairs must be collected and preserved at the time of initial examination.

Numerous swabs of potential sources of DNA are obtained throughout the postmortem examination. A known blood sample from the victim should be obtained. Any blood stains that appear to be of a source other than the victim should be swabbed and packaged as miscellaneous blood. To identify such stains, it is helpful to have persons with knowledge and expertise in blood spatter patterns present for the external body examination. Swabs of bite marks should be obtained for saliva. The breasts and neck should routinely be swabbed for saliva, regardless of the presence of bite marks, due to the frequent oral contact that occurs at these locations during sexual activity. DNA from skin cells that are transferred onto the surface of an object by simple contact is known as touch DNA.[30] Swabs for touch DNA should be collected from bruises, as skin cells from the offender can transfer to the victim's body when hitting or grabbing. Even without bruises present, swabbing of the victim's neck and extremities may yield touch DNA from the suspect in sex-related homicides. Skin cells or body fluids from the offender may also be found underneath the victim's fingernails if the victim scratched the offender before dying. Fingernail scrapings, clippings, or swabbing of the victim's fingernails should be obtained as a possible source of DNA.

Swabs for seminal fluid should be obtained from the oral cavity, external genitalia, vagina, cervix, anus, and rectum. Other body surface areas that should routinely be assessed for signs of seminal fluid include the face, chest, abdomen, thighs, buttocks, and lower back. A limited number of studies relate to the length of time spermatozoa can be found in body orifices, and the vast majority of those studies have been conducted on live individuals, not decedents. The few publications on deceased individuals identified spermatozoa at a variety of postmortem intervals. Collins and Bennett[31] identified spermatozoa postmortem in the vagina up to 7 days and in the rectum up to 17 hours. Spermatozoan heads were found as far out as 2 ½ months in the vagina (victim was buried) and 2 days in the rectum. Others have reported spermatozoa in the vagina postmortem for 16 days[32] and 34 days.[33] It is likely that the body's state of decomposition and environment significantly contribute to the postmortem preservation of spermatozoa. Further studies should be done to gain a better understanding surrounding this important source of DNA in sex-related homicides.

Samples of blood, urine, and vitreous humor are routinely obtained at autopsy to test for a variety of toxicology and other serology depending on the individual case specifics. These samples are usually obtained by the medical examiner staff once forensic sample collection of physical evidence and DNA sources are complete.

Once the non-genital evidence collection is complete, the anogenital samples and examination should be done. The anogenital examination begins with gross visualization, then ideally should include a detailed inspection and documentation using the colposcope. Like anogenital examinations of living sexual assault victims, each anogenital anatomical site should be assessed for injury (see **Table 17-2**). The speculum can usually be used to assist with sample collection and inspection of the vaginal walls and cervix. Occasionally, if rigor mortis is present, it may be difficult to fully open the speculum. An anoscope may be used to assist with sample collection and inspection of the anal canal and rectum. Oftentimes the anus and anal canal will remain dilated after removal of the anoscope since muscle contractility is no longer possible postmortem.

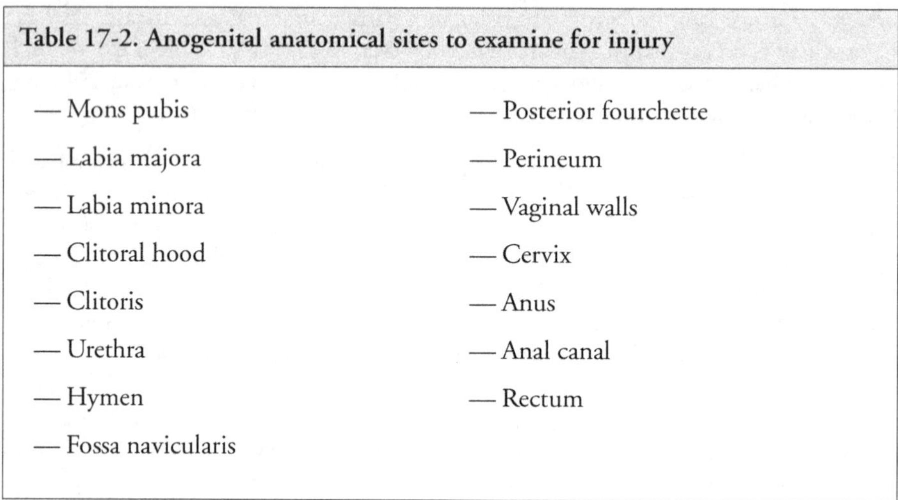

Table 17-2. Anogenital anatomical sites to examine for injury

— Mons pubis	— Posterior fourchette
— Labia majora	— Perineum
— Labia minora	— Vaginal walls
— Clitoral hood	— Cervix
— Clitoris	— Anus
— Urethra	— Anal canal
— Hymen	— Rectum
— Fossa navicularis	

Most of the literature available on sex-related homicide does not focus on the detailed aspects of the anogenital findings identified at autopsy; medical findings in the forensic pathology textbooks, articles, and case reports primarily have demonstrated only the more significant or unusual anogenital findings. This may be due to the fact that anogenital examinations at autopsy have traditionally been performed utilizing gross visualization alone, which can minimize the ability to detect the smaller, more subtle findings present. Over the last decade, however, several forensic pathologists have recognized the benefits of collaborating with forensic nurses who specialize in providing medical-forensic care to living sexual assault victims.[1,34] This collaborative relationship with a sexual assault specialist provides an opportunity for deceased victims of sexual assault to receive a standard of care similar to that currently provided to living victims. The use of a colposcope and toluidine blue dye as tools to enhance visualization of anogenital injury is well documented for living victims of sexual assault.[35-38] Use of similar technology for postmortem sexual assault examinations has not been commonly used. Colposcope (**Figures 17-5** to **17-9**) and toluidine blue dye (**Figures 17-21** and **17-22**) use at autopsy was first described by Bays and Lewman[39] to assist with detection of perineal and anal lacerations in child sexual abuse. Elder[40] also recommended the use of a colposcope postmortem to facilitate visualization of the genitalia for pediatric forensic autopsies. In addition to utilization of a colposcope to assist in the detection of anogenital injuries, Crowley[34] recognized the benefit of its potential for photodocumentation and peer review of postmortem anogenital examinations.

Over the past 25 years, the use of the colposcopes and toluidine blue dye in medical-forensic examinations of sexual assault victims has produced a plethora of literature on the locations and types of anogenital injuries seen post-assault. Other studies have used the same technology to examine women who had engaged in consensual sex. The data published on these populations has significantly contributed to understanding the patterns of anogenital injury sustained in sexual assault and in consensual sex. Such is

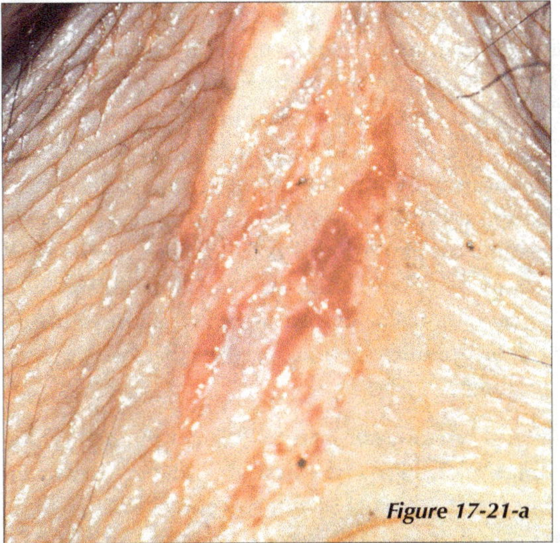

Figure 17-21-a

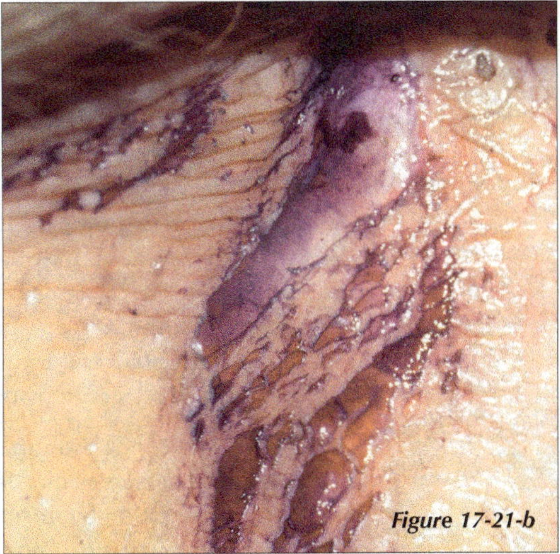

Figure 17-21-b

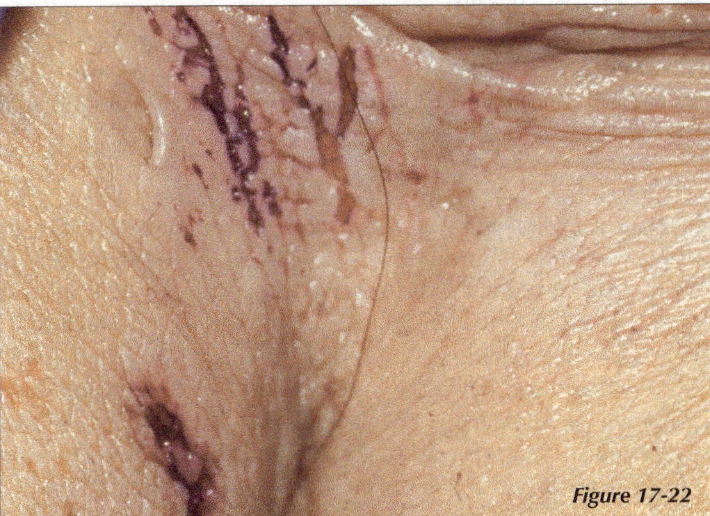

Figure 17-22

Figure 17-21-a. *Multiple lacerations at the 6 o'clock and 8 o'clock positions on the anus of a sex-related homicide victim.*

Figure 17-21-b. *Same lacerations at the 6 o'clock and 8 o'clock positions on the anus of a sex-related homicide victim, stained with toluidine blue dye.*

Figure 17-22. *Lacerations stained with toluidine blue dye on the perineum and buttock of a sex-related homicide victim.*

not the case for anogenital findings in postmortem examinations. To date, only 1 study has been published documenting the characteristics of sex-related homicides in which victims received a comprehensive sexual assault examination using technology and expertise similar to what has been provided to live sexual assault victims for many years.[1] Interestingly, not all of the sex-related homicide victims sustained anogenital injury (58%), which is consistent with research findings from live victims. It is important to keep this in mind when evaluating a possible sex-related homicide victim so as not to assume that lack of anogenital injury means that no sexual activity occurred. The 2 most common sites of anogenital injury in fatal sexual assaults were the labia minora and posterior fourchette, which are also the most common anogenital sites to sustain injury in non-fatal attacks. Significant anogenital trauma in sex-related homicide cases has been documented in the forensic pathology literature.[41-43] Usually, this severe level of trauma is associated with some type of foreign object penetration. According to Henry,[1] fewer than 1% of sexual assault victims sustained anogenital injury significant enough to require emergency care; however, for sex-related homicides, anogenital injury was significant enough to result in death in 22% of the victims.

Upon completion of the anogenital sample collection and colposcope examination, the body can then be washed to allow a thorough evaluation of the nongenital body surface area. The presence and absence of injury and any pertinent marks or anatomical variances should be noted. Injuries should be evaluated in detail for size, color, shape, and characteristics. The nongenital examination should be done simultaneously with the forensic pathologist. The internal autopsy examination is the responsibility of the forensic pathologist; however, the forensic nurse or sexual assault specialist should observe this portion of the examination as part of the collaborative relationship. Observing the internal examination assists the forensic nurse or sexual assault specialist with understanding the scope of violence inflicted, correlating external and internal injuries when possible, and forming their opinions based on the totality of the crime scene and postmortem examination findings.

Documentation of the postmortem sexual assault examination includes photographing the nongenital and anogenital findings, clothing, and physical evidence identified. Written documentation by the forensic nurse or sexual assault specialist should include the medical-forensic history, nongenital and anogenital physical examination findings, and the forensic samples collected. Similar to consults between health care providers who care for living patients, there will be some overlap of documentation between the forensic nurse and the forensic pathologist. It is important for both to have a clear understanding of each other's expertise, professional boundaries, and responsibilities in this collaborative response to sex-related homicides.

CONCLUSION

Sex-related homicides are a combination of the 2 most severe forms of violence against women. As violence against women remains at epidemic levels in the United States, forensic nurses, forensic pathologists, psychologists and law enforcement must form collaborative relationships to improve community responses to sex-related homicides. Sexual violence within the context of intimate partner violence has clearly been demonstrated to be a lethality risk factor for the women in those unfortunate relationships. Henry's[1] study found the most common offender of sex-related homicide was the victim's current spouse or boyfriend. Given the very dangerous connection between intimate partner violence and sexual assault, it is imperative for all suspected intimate partner homicides to be evaluated as sex-related homicides. Recognizing evidence of sexual activity in IPH requires both attention to detail and extensive examination of the crime scene, victim's clothing, and body for trace hairs, fibers, debris, DNA, miscellanous evidence, and non-genital and anogenital injuries. In addition, victims of sex-related homicide deserve to have a community response to their horrific crime that provides comprehensive sexual assault examinations utilizing the most current technology and forensic nurse expertise similar to what is provided to living victims of sexual assault.

REFERENCES

1. Henry T. Characteristics of sex-related homicides in Alaska. *J Forensic Nurs.* 2010;6(2):57-65.

2. Meloy J. The nature and dynamics of sexual homicide: an integrative review. *Aggression Violent Behav.* 2000;5(1):1-22.

3. Abrahams N, Martin L, Jewkes R, Mathews S, Vetten L, Lombard C. The epidemiology and the pathology of suspected rape homicide in South Africa. *Forensic Sci Int.* 2008;178(2-3):132-138.

4. Chan H, Heide K. Sexual homicide: a synthesis of literature. *Trauma Violence Abuse.* 2009;10(1):31-54.

5. Chan H, Heide K. Weapons used by juveniles and adult offenders in sexual homicides: an empirical analysis of 29 years of US data. *J Invest Psychol Offender Profiling.* 2008;5(3):189-208.

6. United States Department of Justice. *Uniform Crime Report.* Washington DC: United States Government Printing Office; 2009.

7. Beauregard E, Stone M, Proulx J, Michaud P. Sexual murders of children: developmental, precrime, crime, and postcrime factors. *Int J Offender Ther Comp Criminology.* 2008;52(3):253-269.

8. Spehr A, Hill A, Habermann N, Briken P, Berner W. Sexual murderes with adult or child victims: are they different? *Sex Abuse J Res Treatment.* 2010;22(3):290-314.

9. Hakkanen-Nyholm H, Repo-Tiihonen E, Lindberg N, Salenius S, Weizmann-Henelius G. Finnish sexual homicides: offence and offender characteristics. *Forensic Sci Int.* 2009;188(1-3):125-130.

10. Violence Policy Center. When men murder women: an analysis of 2008 homicide data. Violence Policy Center Web site. www.vpc.org/studies/wmmw2010.pdf. Published September 2010. Accessed January 4, 2011.

11. Geberth V. *Sex-Related Homicide and Death Investigation: Practical and Clinical Perspectives.* Boca Raton, FL: CRC Press; 2010.

12. Dobash R, Dobash R. What were they thinking? men who murder an intimate partner. *Violence Against Women.* 2011;17(1):111-134.

13. Dobash R, Dobash R, Cavanagh K, Medina-Ariza J. Lethal and nonlethal violence against an intimate female partner. *Violence Against Women.* 2007;13(4);329-353.

14. Leth P. Intimate partner homicide. *Forensic Sci Med Pathol.* 2009;5(3):199-203.

15. Campbell J. *Assessing Dangerousness.* 2nd ed. New York, NY: Springer Publishing Company; 2007.

16. Campbell J, Glass N, Sharps P, Laughon K, Bloom T. Intimate partner homicide: review and implications of research and policy. *Trauma Violence Abuse.* 2007;8(3):246-269.

17. McFarlane J, Malecha A, Watson K, et al. Intimate partner sexual assault against women: frequency, health consequences, and treatment outcomes. *Obstet Gynecol.* 2005:105(1):99-108.

18. DeKeseredy W. Sexual assault during and after separation/divorce: an exploratory study. National Criminal Justice Reference Service Web site. www.ncjrs.gov/pdffiles1/nij/grants/217591.pdf. Published 2007. Accessed July 7, 2008.

19. Aretakis D. Femicide: what were the risk factors. *Nurs Womens Health.* 2008;12(2):146-150.

20. Garcia L, Soria C, Hurwitz E. Homicides and intimate partner violence: a literature review. *Trauma Violence Abuse.* 2007;8(4):370-383.

21. Ressler R, Burgess A, Douglas J. *Sexual Homicide: Patterns and Motives.* New York, NY: Free Press; 1992.

22. Myers W. *Juvenile Sexual Homicide*. San Diego, CA: Academic Press; 2002.

23. Salfati C, Taylor P. Differentiating sexual violence: a comparison of sexual homicide and rape. *Psychol Crime Law*. 2006;12(2):107-125.

24. Schlesinger L. Sexual homicide: differentiating catathymic and compulsive murders. *Aggression Violent Behav*. 2007;12(2):242-256.

25. Stein M, Schlesinger L, Pinizzotto A. Necrophilia and sexual homicide. *J Forensic Sci*. 2010;55(2):443-446.

26. Mieczkowski T, Beauregard E. Lethal outcome in sexual assault events: a conjunctive analysis. *Justice Q*. 2010;27(3):332-361.

27. Schlesinger L, Kassen M, Mesa B, Pinizzotto A. Ritual and signature in serial sexual homicide. *J Am Acad Psychiatry Law*. 2010;38(2):239-246.

28. Van Patten I, Delhauer P. Sexual homicide: a spatial analysis of 25 years of deaths in Los Angeles. *J Forensic Sci*. 2007;52(5):1129-1141.

29. Roberts J, Grossman M. Sexual homicide in Canada: a descriptive analysis. *Ann Sex Res*. 1993;6(1):5-25.

30. Saferstein R. *Criminalistics: An Introduction to Forensic Science*. 10th ed. Upper Saddle River, NJ: Prentice Hall; 2011.

31. Collins K, Bennett A. Persistence of spermatozoa and prostatic acid phosphatase in specimens from deceased individuals during varied postmortem intervals. *Am J For Med Pathol*. 2001;22(3):228-232.

32. Wilson E. Sperm's morphologic survival after sixteen days in the vagina of a dead body. *J Forensic Sci*. 1974;19(3):561-564.

33. Montagna C. The recovery of seminal components and DNA from the vagina of a homcide victim 34 days postmortem. *J Forensic Sci*. 1996;41(4):700-702.

34. Crowley S. Postmortem sexual assault evaluation. In: Lynch V, Duval J, eds. *Forensic Nursing Science*. 2nd ed. St Louis, MO: Elsevier; 2011:234-248.

35. Sommers M, Fargo J, Baker R, Fisher B, Buschur C, Zink T. Health disparities in the forensic sexual assault examination related to color. *J Forensic Nurs*. 2009;5(4):191-200.

36. Anderson S, McClain N, Riviello R. Genital findings of women after consensual and nonconsensual intercourse. *J Forensic Nurs*. 2006;2(2):59-65.

37. Keller P, Lechner M. Injuries to the cervix in sexual assault victims. *J Forensic Nurs*. 2010;6(4):196-202.

38. Jones J, Rossman L, Wynn B, Dunnuck C. Comparative analysis of adult versus adolescent sexual assault: epidemiology and patterns of anogenital injury. *Academic Emerg Med*. 2003;10(8);872-877.

39. Bays J, Lewman L. Toluidine blue in the detection at autopsy of perineal and anal lacerations in victims of sexual abuse. *Arch Pathol Lab Med*. 1992;116(6):620-621.

40. Elder D. Interpretation of anogenital findings in the living child: implications for the paediatric forensic autopsy. *J Forensic Leg Med*. 2007;14(8):482-488.

41. Kovelman I, Vey E, Schober, J. Fatal anorectal trauma in the setting of sexual assault. *Am J Forensic Med Pathol*. 2010;31(3):273-277.

42. Deming J, Mittleman R, Wetli C. Forensic science aspects of fatal sexual assault on women. *J Forensic Sci.*1983;28(3):572-576.

43. Fain D, McCormick G. Vaginal fisting as a cause of death. *Am J Forensic Med Pathol.* 1989;10(1):73-75.

Chapter 18

Intimate Partner Violence and Mental Health Outcomes

Nandrie Steyn, MBChB(Stell), DMH(SA) Diploma in Mental Health
Belinda Bruwer, MBChB(Stell), MMed(Psych), FC Psych(SA)
Soraya Seedat, MBChB, FC Psych (SA), MMed(Psych), PhD

Key Points

1. The mental health outcomes of intimate partner violence (IPV) have been well documented, with posttraumatic stress disorder (PTSD) and deperession being the most commonly identified disorders.

2. Victims of IPV often have additional stressors of poverty, lack of social resources, and parenting stress that stymie recovery from mental health issues.

3. Although research has focused on the mental health outcomes of physical assault, victims have identified psychological abuse as contributing to greater distress. Many victims of IPV are exposed to many types of abuse.

4. Women with severe mental illnesses, including mood and psychotic disorders, have an increased risk of victimization and perpetration of IPV.

5. Clinicians should ensure that patients presenting with mental illnesses are screened for IPV and provided with appropriate and useful information.

Introduction

Long after the physical injuries have healed, victims of intimate partner violence (IPV) struggle with the lasting, often debilitating symptoms of posttraumatic stress disorder (PTSD), depression, suicidality, and substance abuse, among other difficulties. Women exposed to partner violence are at an increased risk of mental disorders and often lack access to and receipt of adequate mental health care. By the same token, women with pre-existing mental illness are more vulnerable to violent behavior at the hands of an intimate partner. In South Africa, for example, IPV is a leading cause of morbidity and mortality among South African women.[1] These women not only have an increased risk of injury and death, but an increased probability of developing short- and long-term morbidity and adopting negative health behaviors, such as alcohol abuse, substance abuse, and smoking, than non-victims.[2,3] Women who are victims of IPV are also at an increased risk of HIV infections.

The Effects of IPV on Mental Health

IPV, specifically physical abuse, negatively affects women's mental and physical health through its impact on psychological well-being.[4-7] The mental health outcomes of IPV have been well documented, with PTSD and depression being the most commonly identified disorders.[8-16] The weighted mean prevalence rate of major depression among battered women is estimated at 48%.[12] In a study conducted in 1999, the rates of PTSD among battered women were found to range from 31%-84%, with a weighted mean prevalence estimate of 64%.[12] This is much higher than rates of PTSD (in the order of 1%-12%) that have been documented among women in general community samples. Depression in battered women is often chronic, with symptoms persisting over a long time for some women, even in the absence of recent revictimization.[8,10,17] To make a bad situation worse, victims of IPV often have additional stressors of poverty, lack of social resources, and parenting stress which makes recovery from PTSD and depression slow and, at times, impossible.[18-20]

STRESS RESPONSE

Stressors cause disruption in a person's equilibrium, resulting in a stress response that aims to restore this equilibrium through an adaptive, physiological response. While much is known about the physiological stress response that follows acute stressors, there is far less empirical data available on response to chronic and repeated stressors. Typically, IPV is a chronic stressor that exerts effects over an extended period of time with long-term repercussions.[21]

Stressors activate the brain's noradrenergic system resulting in catecholamine release from the autonomic nervous system (ANS). In animal models, there is evidence to indicate that tolerance to a specific chronic stressor may develop over time, and decrease the ANS response to that specific stressor but paradoxically result in an enhanced response to a new stressor, thereby leaving the animal more vulnerable to novel stressors. Other neurotransmitters activated by the stress response include serotonin, dopamine, and corticotropin-releasing factor (CRH), amongst others.[21] The hypothalamic-pituitary-adrenal (HPA) axis forms an integral part of the stress response. Stress causes the hypothalamus to secrete CRH which results in adrenocorticotrophic hormone (ACTH) release from the anterior pituitary and in turn stimulates the synthesis and secretion of glucocorticoids, such as cortisol, from the adrenal cortex. Glucocorticoids stimulate the cardiovascular system (flight-or-fight response), promote utilization of energy and inhibit growth, reproduction, and immunity functions in the short term. Under normal conditions, the HPA axis exerts effective negative feedback control at many levels,[21] such as at the level of glucocorticoid receptors in the hippocampus, resulting in a termination of the stress response.[22]

Many other neurochemicals can also influence the HPA axis, such as catecholamines, oxytocin, and vasopressin (secretagogues), and directly cause ACTH release. Interestingly, the stress response can vary depending on the duration and frequency of exposure to the stressor.[21]

Significant neuroendocrine alterations have been found in women with IPV-related PTSD compared to women with no PTSD.[23] However, studies investigating cortisol abnormalities in victims of IPV have produced mixed findings. For example, one study examining cortisol levels in battered women living in shelters found that PTSD severity correlated with a significantly higher cortisol level during the first hour after waking up, while more chronic abuse was associated with lower awakening cortisol levels.[24] In contrast, another study found that women with lifetime IPV-related PTSD had significantly higher cortisol levels across the day compared with IPV-exposed women with no PTSD history, after controlling for age, depression, and severity of abuse.[25] Seedat et al[26] found an inverse relationship between the presence of IPV and morning cortisol levels but no relationship between PTSD and morning cortisol levels, suggesting that lower cortisol levels and HPA alterations might be a consequence of the abuse rather than of PTSD.

PSYCHONEUROIMMUNOLOGY

The concept of *psychoneuroimmunology* implies a network of interactions between the brain, the immune system, and behavior. The immune system plays a vital role in protecting an organism against invading pathogens from the outside and abnormal cells on the inside. Immune cells release cytokines that play an important role in coordinating both innate and specific immune responses.[21] The central nervous system and immune system communicate with each other via the same systems involved in the stress response, namely the HPA and autonomic nervous systems. For example, activation of the sympathetic nervous system can suppress certain immune cell populations while enhancing other aspects of the immune system (humoral immune response), thereby decreasing the ability to destroy viruses that live inside cells but at the same time enhancing the ability to fight bacteria that live outside cells. The HPA axis affects the immune system via suppression of the cellular immune response by cortisol. It is now clear that behaviors and emotions can influence immunity, as psychological responses (expressed in neural activity) are accompanied by neuroendocrine and autonomic function alterations.[21]

There are multiple links between stressors and illnesses, ranging from the physiological effects of stress on the illness to the association of adverse health behaviors, such as overeating, obesity, smoking, and alcohol and drug abuse, that people exposed to stress may resort to.[21,27] Chronic interpersonal stress may worsen tiredness, painful symptoms and limitation in functioning in rheumatoid arthritis patients due to increased IL^6 production.[21] In addition, individuals exposed to psychological stress may have a higher risk of contracting viral infections (eg, Epstein-Barr virus and the common cold), while HIV-infected patients exposed to chronic stress has a more rapid decline in their immune system and higher virus replication.

Stress-related effects of violence (both IPV and childhood maltreatment) can lower immune responses in women, either through direct mechanisms (PTSD→immune status) or through indirect mechanisms (IPV→immune status→PTSD), although, to date, this has been poorly studied.[28,29] Notably, a study in women with IPV found that IPV compromised the immune system, as evidenced by a decrease in immune regulation over herpes simplex virus type 1 (HSV-1), the latent virus that causes cold sores. This suggests an adverse impact of IPV on health through mechanisms of viral reactivation and a diminished ability in abused women to suppress virus proliferation.[30]

RELATIONSHIP BETWEEN TYPES OF IPV AND MENTAL HEALTH OUTCOMES

Intimate partner violence (IPV) has been broadly defined as a pattern of abusive behavior by one or both partners in an intimate relationship, including marriage, homosexual relationships, family, dating, or cohabitation. Much of the existing research has focused on women as victims of IPV, but more recent work has focused on men as victims of IPV, both in heterosexual and homosexual relationships. A study on physical violence among South African men found that 27.5% reported abusing a partner during their current or most recent relationship.

The US National Institute of Mental Health Committee on Family Violence has described a broader definition of IPV as "acts that are physically and emotionally harmful or that carry the potential to cause physical harm....and may also include sexual coercion or assaults, physical intimidation, threats to kill or harm, restraint of normal activities or freedom, and denial of access to resources."[31] This definition includes the 3 primary types of IPV recognized in the literature, namely physical; sexual; and emotional, psychological, or verbal violence.[32,33]

Physical violence is defined as the intentional use of physical force. *Sexual violence* is defined as the use of force to compel a person to engage in a sexual act.[34] *Emotional, psychological,* or *verbal violence* includes threats, humiliation, control of activities, isolation, name calling, and attempts to frighten.[35] Most types of abuse or violence co-occur. To illustrate this, a population-based sample of women in North-Carolina found that 18.4% had experienced at least 1 form of IPV by a recent or current partner, with only 1.9% experiencing physical abuse or assault alone and only 1.1% sexual abuse alone.[36]

In their study among 413 severely battered help-seeking women, Mechanic et al[37] focused on the mental health effects of physical violence, sexual coercion, psychological abuse, and stalking on symptoms of PTSD and depression. The authors specifically tested for the effects of psychological abuse and stalking on mental health outcomes while controlling for physical violence, injuries, and sexual coercion. The study found that psychological abuse and stalking contributed uniquely to the prediction of PTSD and depression. This clearly highlights that IPV is multidimensional and not restricted to physical abuse alone. In other studies, psychological, emotional, and verbal abuse have been found to be clear predictors of depression.[38-40]

Until very recently, much work has focused on mental health outcomes in relation to IPV acts of physical aggression, with psychological abuse and stalking largely neglected.[41] However, in several studies, battered women have identified psychological abuse as contributing to greater distress compared to acts of physical and sexual violence.[40,42] Psychological abuse has also been shown to contribute significantly to PTSD symptoms in battered women and to influence their decisions to end an abusive relationship, even when physical violence is not present.[43] In addition, symptomatic responses to abuse, including PTSD and depression, have been found to be largely predicted by psychological abuse rather than physical violence.[39] Furthermore, emotional abuse in a relationship has been demonstrated to increase the risk of both minor and severe physical injuries.[44]

The role of stalking as a predictor of adverse outcomes among abused women is not clear. There is some evidence to suggest that when stalking is present in an abusive relationship it may be a risk factor for elevated levels of psychopathology and contribute to fears of lethal harm.[45,46] Stalkers pose an unpredictable but omnipresent threat to their victims. This may lead to hypervigilant behavior, and to other symptoms of hyperarousal. Non-physical forms of IPV, like psychological abuse and stalking, are therefore important contributors to PTSD and depression as well as to other adverse emotional outcomes.[38,39,43,47] There is little data available on how sexual violence in relationships impacts on the mental health outcomes of other types of IPV.[48,49] Physical violence, for example, has been found to be more severe if sexual violence is present.[50] However, the effect of sexual coercion in predicting unique variance in PTSD symptomatology has produced mixed findings when other dimensions of IPV are considered in multivariate analyses.[47,49] In contrast, psychological abuse and stalking have been found to contribute uniquely to the prediction of PTSD symptoms.

Many battered women are exposed to multiple, frequent, and sometimes unrelenting traumatic events, even after ending their abusive relationships, with the impact of exposure most likely to be cumulative.[51,52] Exposure to cumulative traumatic events can slowly erode a victim's resources to cope with adversity and lead to chronic stress, distress, and impairment.[51-53] Long-term taunting and degrading behavior has been found to influence depression via its eroding effects on self-esteem and self-worth.[54,55] Dominance and isolation have also been found to significantly predict PTSD in a study of women seeking marital treatment for partner physical violence.[56]

Historically, the focus of treatment programs and research has been on physical violence, with non-physical violence largely neglected; however, it is evident that non-physical forms of IPV not only contribute directly as clear predictors of PTSD and depression, but also hamper recovery from depression in IPV victims.[19,21]

GENDER AND AGE CONSIDERATIONS

In their study describing the epidemiology of IPV in Ukraine, O'Leary et al[57] found that more women than men reported aggression by their spouses (12.7 versus 5.8%). Countries such as Hong Kong[58] and Mexico[59] have reported similar gender patterns while countries such as Canada[60] and the USA[61] have documented no gender differences in IPV. In the aforementioned Ukraine study using data from the World Mental Health (WMH) Survey,[57] the unique risk factors for behaving aggressively in men were being married once, witnessing parental violence, early onset alcohol abuse, and the presence of intermittent explosive disorders (IED). The risk factors for reporting that their wives behaved aggressively were early onset alcohol abuse, IED and marital problems. Among women, the risk factors for behaving aggressively were younger age, unemployment, living in a rural area, early onset alcohol abuse, mood and anxiety disorders, and marital problems. Risk factors for reporting that their husbands' behaved aggressively were younger age, early onset alcohol abuse, and marital problems.

There was an unexpected similarity in risk factors for aggression reported by men and women. The most potent risk factors in both cases were early onset alcohol abuse and IED. Positive assertive mating has been posited as a likely explanation for these findings, given that men and women with a tendency toward externalizing and aggressive behaviors often select spouses with similar behavioral profiles.

One unique factor present in the reports of men who were either engaging in acts of IPV or were victims of IPV, was having witnessed parental aggression during childhood. Violence observed as a child was usually against the mother, or a female figure, rather than the reverse. Further, given the phenomenon of same sex modeling, men may imitate their fathers' behavior more than women may imitate their mothers' behavior. These childhood experiences could, therefore, have stronger effects on later behavior in men compared with women. Men who have witnessed violence against their mothers may develop traditionalist attitudes which favor their dominance over women, played out in violence against female intimate partners. Growing up in a violent home may have a stronger relationship with victimization in female offspring and with perpetration in male offspring. Same-sex modeling provides one possible explanation for this phenomenon.

Studies to date have not convincingly demonstrated an association between age and IPV. For example, population-based studies in the Ukraine and in the US have shown the variance accounted for by age to be relatively small.[57] Violent altercations have been shown to be more common in the age group 30-39 years, with slightly lower rates among older and younger respondents.[62]

An important factor regarding age in women is the age of first menarche.[63] Early menarche has been associated with early first intercourse,[64] which has in turn been associated with early first birth.[65] There is evidence to suggest that early first intercourse is associated with IPV particularly when intercourse is coercive.[66-69] First intercourse at a young age is thus a powerful marker for the experience of early or later partner violence among young women.

IPV AND MENTAL HEALTH IN SAME-SEX COUPLES

Few data are available on IPV in same-sex couples, although it is estimated to affect 15% to 20% of gay and lesbian couples.[70] Men in same-sex relationships experience abuse at similar rates than women in heterosexual relationships.[71,72] Partner abuse has been described as the third most severe health problem among homosexual men, with AIDS and substance abuse being foremost. Men in abusive same-sex relationships have a higher reported rate of depression and also engage in substance abuse or unprotected sex more often than men in non-abusive same-sex relationships.[73] Some researchers have documented reluctance among homosexual men to seek help from agencies that are traditionally used by abused women.[74]

PREGNANCY CONSIDERATIONS AND MENTAL HEALTH

In a comprehensive review of the literature it was found that the prevalence of IPV in pregnancy ranged from 1-20%, depending on the way in which IPV was assessed and the type of population studied.[75] The US Centers for Disease Control and Prevention (CDC) Pregnant Risk Assessment Monitoring Systems (PRAMS) documented a prevalence of 2.9%-5.7%.[76] Similar results were found in a population-based study in New Zealand, where the prevalence of pregnancy-related IPV was found to be 9%.[77,78] Findings have been inconsistent about whether the prevalence of IPV decreases during pregnancy, stays unchanged, or increases during conception and pregnancy. A number of national and international population-based studies have found that pregnant women are no more likely than non-pregnant women to experience IPV and may even be at a lower risk.[79]

Screening for IPV during pregnancy and for associated mental health problems in primary care settings, while of crucial importance, is often not done owing to time constraints and a lack of training. Yet IPV can have significant impacts on reproductive health and pregnancy outcomes.[75,80-84] A number of studies have reported that young age at first pregnancy and subsequent first childbirth are associated with partner abuse.[68,85,86] Numerous reports have identified an association between younger age and pregnancy-related IPV.[87,88] Some national survey reports have suggested near doubling of the risk of pregnancy IPV in women under the age of 20 years.[89] Single women are also at a higher risk for experiencing pregnancy-related IPV than married women.[90]

The clear link that exists between IPV during pregnancy, low birth weight, and prematurity is of great concern, given the numerous adverse outcomes as well as the burden that it places on health care resources. Pregnancy-related IPV is also associated with many mental health consequences, including a 9-fold increase in the risk for mood or anxiety disorders and an increased risk of hospitalizations for mental health–related problems.[91,92] Pregnancy-related IPV has also been associated with negative health behaviors during pregnancy, including poor utilization of prenatal care, smoking, drinking, substance abuse during pregnancy, and inadequate weight gain.[93] The experience of IPV during pregnancy is also associated with multiple adverse newborn outcomes, including decreased infant birth weight, and increased rates of premature births. These are leading causes of neonatal morbidity and mortality and are strong biological predictors of immediate and long-term developmental outcomes.[94] These children will often struggle with cognitive deficits, motor delays, attentional problems, behavioral problems, and other psychological difficulties.[95-97]

CONTRACEPTION AND IPV

With increased recognition of the global impact of IPV, there has been increased interest in understanding the association between violence and coercion within intimate relationships and the use of contraception, unintended pregnancy, and abortion.[98]

Much of this research has been conducted in the USA. In one such study from a 4-state pregnancy monitoring system, it was found that up to 70% of women who experienced violence in relationships had unwanted or mistimed pregnancies.[99] Victims of IPV often report challenges, specifically with regards to male-controlled contraception (eg, condoms). They are less likely to use condoms or to ask a partner to use condoms for fear of verbal, emotional, or physical abuse. They are, therefore, at a significantly higher risk for sexually transmitted diseases.[100,101]

One study in New Zealand found a significantly higher prevalence of family violence among women seeking abortion services compared to the general public.[102] In more traditional cultures, request to use contraception can be seen to affront a male partner's virility thereby inciting violence against women. There is some evidence to show that African women who have been exposed to IPV are more likely to use contraception (65.9%), compared with those who do not report any partner violence (59%).[77,103] This is most likely explained by a desire to avert pregnancy in unfavorable circumstances or as protection against infection with HIV.

Link Between IPV and Severe Mental Illness

The link between IPV and mental health disorders has been clearly shown.[104] IPV may exacerbate pre-existing mental illness while symptoms of mental illness may worsen with the occurrence of victimization.[80] As many as 60% to 90% of battered women have significant mental health problems.[105] For example, in one study, 81% of women treated for psychiatric disorders in the USA reported histories of abuse.[105] In another study, in the Chicago area, between 30% and 90% of abused women had some form of mental illness.[105] Dienemann et al[106] found a 61% lifetime prevalence of physical or emotional IPV among women diagnosed with depression, while Chang et al[107] found the experience of IPV to be more likely if an anxiety disorder, PTSD, bipolar disorder, or problematic substance use were present.

Women with severe mental illness, including mood and psychotic disorders, have an increased risk of being both victims and perpetrators of IPV. As many as half of married female psychiatric inpatients with severe mental illness are victims of IPV, and outpatient rates are similar.[108-110] PTSD in women who have serious mental illness often remains undetected by psychiatrists. Women with mental illness may also exhibit violent behavior toward their partners. In one study, 20% of an inpatient sample had engaged in IPV against their partners.[110] Risk of victimization may be mediated by impairments in judgment, reality testing, and planning.[111] Women who suffer from severe mental illness may also have difficulty in determining whether closeness is assaultive or whether it represents intimacy.[112]

Mental illness is often used as a weapon by abusers against their victims, used to control victims by convincing them that their accounts of the abuse will be ignored as they are known to psychiatric services.[105] As abusers are often involved in the treatment of their victims, they may control or manipulate their medications. Victims often improve and their symptoms will abate once the IPV is addressed.[105]

Interplay Between IPV and Mental Health Related Outcomes

Causal Pathways: Relationship to Childhood and Family Violence

Children and adolescents are often exposed concurrently to various forms of abuse and family violence (eg, witnessing of inter-parental violence), leading to 'poly-victimization'. These youth are at an even greater risk of IPV victimization or perpetration in adult years.[113-117] Multiple studies have examined the relationship between early childhood abuse and later exposure to IPV. A nationally representative study in the USA found that childhood maltreatment victims had a higher likelihood of future violence perpetration and IPV than of victimization.[118] Gender differences were evident: physical abuse and neglect in girls, and sexual abuse in boys, was strongly associated with IPV perpetration. Victimization during adolescence was strongly associated with IPV victimization in men.[118] The cross-sectional, nationally representative South African Stress and Health Study (SASH) found that exposure to parental violence and childhood physical abuse, but not community violence exposure, were 2 significant risk factors for perpetrating intimate partner violence in adult South African men.[119] Another study in the USA found that men having sex with men (MSM) with a history of childhood physical or sexual abuse were at a higher risk of being either a victim or perpetrator of physical or sexual violence against an intimate partner in adulthood.[120]

The family unit represents the foundation where children learn how to behave, to treat others well, and what constitutes acceptable behavior especially within relationships. Children who experience violence directed at them and who witness violence between parents are at an increased risk of being victims or perpetrators of IPV later in life.[121] Thus, maltreatment during childhood can increase antisocial behavior during adolescence and result in perpetration of IPV in adulthood.[122,123] Childhood maltreatment can also result in learned helplessness leaving individuals vulnerable to victimization during adolescence and adulthood.[122,123]

Several confounding factors, including socioeconomic circumstances and education, may influence the association between childhood maltreatment, youth violence, and IPV perpetration.[118] In addition to individual factors, family, and relationships, community and the societal milieu are important[115,124,125] when considering causal relationships between childhood maltreatment and adult IPV.

As previously mentioned, the family unit provides the context where children establish behavioral patterns, to a large extent dependent on how they are treated, and on how their parents treat each other. Children who experience abusive family environments have an increased risk of being involved in violent relationships as perpetrators (this association is more robust for males) or as victims (this association is more robust for females). This may be explained by the interaction between different socialization practices within certain cultures where aggression is reinforced in boys and passivity is reinforced in girls, as well as by imitating and modeling the same-sex parent's behavior.[121] Boys witnessing marital violence may adopt the view that it is acceptable for them to dominate over women,[126] while girls may imitate their mothers' submissive behavior toward marital violence. With regard to victimization, adverse childhood experiences (ie, experiencing childhood abuse and witnessing parental abuse) may increase the risk of experiencing IPV in women and may result in beliefs that partner abuse is an acceptable practice. Women may be left emotionally vulnerable and unable to protect themselves against IPV or unable to engage in healthy adult relationships.[127]

Childhood conduct disorder has shown a strong association with IPV in young adults; however, when conduct disorder is controlled for in analyses, attention-deficit/ hyperactivity disorder (ADHD) has shown a significant association with IPV.[128] Exposure to family violence (witnessing marital abuse and exposure to parent-to-child aggression) has been associated with more depressive symptoms and aggressive behavior in a college student cohort than witnessing inter-parental violence only or not experiencing family violence at all.[129] These findings clearly point towards the importance of directing efforts at preventing childhood maltreatment and at targeted interventions for youth with antisocial behavior, conduct disorder, and ADHD, so as to reduce the incidence of adult IPV.[118,128]

Relationship to Societal Violence and Socio-Economic Factors

Exposure to, and involvement with, community violence has been described as a risk for IPV perpetration.[130,131] In one study in an African American male sample, perpetration of intimate partner abuse was associated with participation in violent neighborhood activities and with living in a community where violence occurred.[132] Involvement with gangsters and exposure to community violence were among the important themes identified in another group of young male IPV perpetrators in the USA.[133] In a young urban female Latina and African American cohort, discrimination was associated with emotional and physical IPV perpetration and victimization, while exposure to community violence was positively associated with emotional IPV victimization.[134]

In a national cross-sectional household survey of 8 southern African countries, the presence of multiple sexual partners among respondents was significantly related to the presence of physical partner abuse. This study did not find a significant association between partner abuse and educational or occupational status, income, size of household, or age.[62] However, a cross-sectional survey in Australia found that separated or divorced women, with low income and educational status, are more likely to be exposed to IPV.[135] Notably, findings from the Demographic and Health Survey conducted in 17 sub-Saharan African countries suggest that uneducated women and unemployed men are more likely to justify IPV against women.[136]

Lower educational levels in a partner and depression have been associated with bidirectional IPV (ie, both partners perpetrating IPV), while illicit drug use has been associated with unidirectional IPV (one partner perpetrating violence) compared with bidirectional IPV and no IPV.[137] In a black, Hispanic, and white United States sample, blacks had higher reported rates of bidirectional IPV than whites, while blacks and Hispanics reported more severe IPV. Findings indicated that women involved in female-to-male unidirectional IPV and bidirectional IPV typically had characteristics indicating a lifetime of severe stressors, while male-to-female unidirectional IPV was associated with men exposed to physical abuse during childhood.[138]

Alcohol use disorders, often in conjunction with other risk factors, such as pre-existing aggressive cognitions and personality disorders, are well-known risk factors for IPV perpetration. Alcohol intoxication may cause disinhibition and impair interpretation of social cues, while long-term heavy alcohol use may cause or contribute to cognitive impairment and dysfunction, leading to violent behavior in the form of IPV.[139] Husbands with an alcohol use disorder were identified as a prominent causative factor of domestic violence in a rural Indian population.[140] Another commonly reported cause was the promotion of wife battering by relatives of the husband.[140]

Intersection with HIV

In certain patriarchal societies where strong emphasis is placed on masculinity, it is often acceptable for men to have multiple sexual partners and to exhibit predatory sexual behaviors. This may lead to power inequity in relationships, resulting in intimate partner violence as well an increased risk of HIV infection. The association between IPV victimization/perpetration and increased HIV infection risk is well-supported by the literature.[141-143] Women in relationships where there is power inequity and IPV are usually unable to influence the circumstances around sexual intercourse, such as insisting on condom usage.[77,144]

Research in India and South Africa has shown that there is a higher incidence of HIV infection in men who are perpetrators of violence, thereby increasing the risk of HIV infection in their partners.[142] A study in Cape Town, South Africa, among promiscuous men found that inadequate condom use, sexually transmitted disease symptoms, transactional sexual activities, alcohol abuse, multiple sexual partners, and a belief that a partner was unfaithful were all associated with IPV perpetration.[145] Therefore, while IPV exposure is associated with an increased HIV infection risk, women with HIV may also be more vulnerable to IPV victimization.[141]

The aforementioned factors contribute to the HIV epidemic in countries such as South Africa[119] and need to be addressed when developing comprehensive prevention and intervention services for people living with HIV as well as those at risk for, or exposed to, intimate partner abuse.[141] For example, women seeking care for intimate partner abuse should be counseled and tested for HIV as well as informed about HIV prevention strategies, while those with HIV or those seeking HIV testing should be screened for IPV victimization or perpetration and counseled about issues such as gender inequity in relationships.[141,146,147]

A study conducted among young people aged 15 to 26 in the Eastern Cape in South Africa found an association between depressive symptoms, risky sexual behavior, and intimate partner abuse. Depressed women were more vulnerable to exposure to IPV, while depressed men had a higher likelihood of perpetrating IPV and were less likely to use condoms correctly or failed to use condoms, thereby increasing HIV risk.[148] HIV infection risk may, therefore, be increased in the context of depressive symptoms and IPV.[148] Post-traumatic stress disorder (PTSD) due to IPV victimization has also been found to be strongly associated with risky sexual behavior in a cohort of low-income women.[149]

Relationship to Physical Health Outcomes

IPV has been associated with injury, mortality (homicide), morbidity (short and long-term), and behaviors that may have adverse effects on physical health.[2] Musculoskeletal, head, and neck injuries were found to be the most common injuries encountered among domestic violence victims seen in a domestic abuse program.[150] Mental illness, such as PTSD, has been shown to be strongly associated with higher levels of pain-related physical health problems in a USA female veteran population.[151]

Some sequelae, such as injury and activity impairment, may be directly related to IPV, while other sequelae, such as fibromyalgia, irritable bowel syndrome, and cardiovascular disease, may be indirectly mediated; for example, stress caused by IPV victimization with consequent effects on the endocrine and immune systems.[152] Another consideration is that while IPV-related stress increases the probability of, and susceptibility to, health problems, the opposite may also be true, ie, health problems may be the cause of stress in relationships leading to an increased risk of IPV.[152]

The association between IPV, health problems, and adverse health behaviors has been documented in both developed as well as developing countries. For example, musculoskeletal illness and injuries, cardiovascular and cerebrovascular disease, asthma, sexually transmitted diseases, functional impairment, and general poor health were more frequently reported among women and men in the USA exposed to IPV than in those not exposed.[152,153] However, in women only was there a significant association between IPV and hypercholesterolemia, cardiovascular disease, and cerebrovascular disease. High rates of behaviors such as alcohol abuse, drug abuse, smoking, and risky behaviors for HIV infection, have also been found in samples exposed to intimate partner violence.[152,154] In a WHO study investigating women's health and domestic violence in 10 developing countries, self-reported poor health as well as health problems such as pain, difficulties with walking and activities of daily living, memory problems, dizziness, and vaginitis were found to be significantly associated with lifetime IPV exposure.[104,155] Similarly, poor self-reported health, cardiovascular problems, ongoing health problems, and numerous somatic complaints were associated with recent IPV in a Mexican American sample.[156]

The SASH study, among South Africans, found that IPV was strongly associated with risky health behaviors, such as cigarette smoking, alcohol, cannabis, sedative and analgesic abuse. There was no significant correlation with chronic medical disease, but illnesses such as hypertension, ischaemic heart disease, and headaches were more frequently reported among abused South African women.[2]

Findings on health-seeking behavior in persons exposed to IPV have been highly variable, and have ranged from increased utilization of health care services,[2] to equivalent use,[154] to decreased frequency of use.[152] Men experiencing IPV are less likely to sustain serious injury and tend to seek health care less frequently than women.[152] Generally, behaviors that may adversely affect health may increase the likelihood of illness. At the same time, increased utilization of health services by abused women may decrease the likelihood of morbidity associated with IPV. Point-of-contact health care services provide an opportunity for health care providers to screen for IPV, associated negative health behaviors, and mental/or physical disease in both men and women so that counseling, intervention, and preventative measures can be instituted in a timely fashion.[2,157]

MANAGEMENT OF MENTAL HEALTH OUTCOMES

SCREENING

Under-detection of IPV is contributed to by the well-known fact that mental health care professionals do not routinely screen for IPV in psychiatric service settings, with studies indicating that less than one-half of patients are asked by their mental health providers about IPV.[106,158,159] Barriers to routine enquiry include concerns about role boundaries (ie, not seen as part of the role of mental health care providers), lack of knowledge and expertise in the area, and a lack of confidence.[160,161] In these settings there is some evidence to suggest that women are more likely than men to be screened.[107] Whether other factors, such as racial or ethnic minority groupings and/or certain mental health diagnoses, result in individuals being more or less likely to be screened is, as yet, unclear and warrants further study. The value of routine screening for IPV remains controversial with several systematic reviews concluding that it would be premature to introduce screening programs for domestic violence routinely into health care settings, given that there is no convincing evidence that routine screening reduces exposure to subsequent violence or impacts on the rates of actual treatment.[162,163] That said, the lack of robust evidence for screening does not mean that inquiry about IPV has no place in a routine mental health assessment. In a review by Ramsay and colleagues,[162] of the 20 studies that were found to be eligible, it is notable that no study included an evaluation of mental health outcomes or other quality of life outcomes in assessment.

MENTAL HEALTH ASSESSMENT

Given the high prevalence and severity of psychiatric sequelae in women and men who experience IPV, mental health professionals require appropriate education and training to recognize, assess for, and address psychopathology. Failure to address IPV can lead to fatal consequences for victims of IPV in the form of homicide and suicide as well as intimate homicide-suicide incidents involving victim, perpetrator, and not uncommonly, other related individuals (family and non-family members).[164,165] Thus, mentally ill women, in particular, with suicidal ideation should be carefully monitored for ongoing IPV, while abused women should be questioned about active suicidal ideation and intent. At a minimum, clinicians need to enquire about the possibility of abuse in presentations with anxiety, depression, substance abuse, unexpected or unexplained stress, physical injuries, and chronic somatic symptoms. Similarly, when women and men report symptoms of depression, PTSD, other anxiety disorder, or a substance use disorder, clinicians should be alert to the possible contributory role of IPV. Clinicians should also distinguish between severity (level) and type of IPV as the mental health effects of IPV can vary according to severity and type. A number of screening tools are available for the detection of commonly occurring symptoms, such as the Symptom Checklist-90-R, Beck Depression Inventory, Hamilton Depression Rating Scale, Beck Anxiety Inventory, Hamilton Anxiety Rating Scale, PTSD Checklist, Alcohol Use Disorders Identification Test, and the Drug Use Disorders Identification Test.

TREATMENTS

As mental health responses to IPV are usually multifaceted, it is important that any approach to intervention be multimodal, so as to address the wide range of psychiatric symptoms, and be tailored to the individual client. This should ideally incorporate referral and access to a wide range of services (eg, social support, legal advocacy, housing, and childcare), offered in the context of a safe, therapeutic relationship.[166,167] In-service training for mental health clinicians should be directed at accurate assessment of domestic violence, understanding the nexus between domestic violence and common mental health outcomes (eg, major depression, PTSD, alcohol, and drug abuse), safety planning, and multidisciplinary collaborative work with other providers whose service systems will be impacted. Training in cognitive-behavioural mental health strategies for those who treat domestic violence victims seem warranted.

Clinicians should also be mindful of ethnic, cultural, gender-related, and socio-economic factors that may impact treatment seeking, treatment acceptability, adherence to treatment, and outcome. Notably, a small qualitative study that sought to evaluate what women with a past or current history of IPV wanted from health care interventions[168] documented that, consistent with other studies, participants most favored counseling on depression, anxiety, and relationship issues, as well as resource-specific information (eg, on legal matters and other services) from their health care providers.

ADVOCACY INTERVENTIONS

In a recent Cochrane review[169] of randomized controlled trials comparing advocacy interventions for women with experience of IPV against usual care, the authors found that while intensive advocacy for women recruited in domestic violence shelters reduced physical abuse 1 to 2 years after the intervention, there was no evidence of a beneficial effect on depression, psychological distress, or quality of life. This is consistent with the findings of a recent assessor-blinded randomized controlled trial[170] of 200 Chinese adult women with IPV, who either received a 12-week advocacy intervention (N=100), comprising empowerment and telephone social support or usual community services (N=100), encompassing health care and promotion, child care, and recreational programs. The advocacy intervention did not result in clinically meaningful improvement in depressive symptoms. This study represents the first to examine the effectiveness of an advocacy intervention for abused Chinese women in a community setting. Notwithstanding, further studies of brief advocacy interventions are needed to more definitively assess their utility for women who choose to leave or who choose to stay with the perpetrating partner.

INTERVENTIONS FOR MENTAL HEALTH OUTCOMES

Few studies have investigated the efficacy of psychological interventions in improving outcomes for patients with psychiatric disorders who have experienced IPV.[161] Similarly, not much is known about the best treatments for IPV among patients entering substance abuse treatment programs.[171] In women with PTSD, individual studies and systematic reviews have shown that a wide range of individual and group psychological interventions, for example cognitive trauma therapy,[172,173] are beneficial in reducing depression, PTSD, and self-esteem. For individual interventions, effect sizes for PTSD ranged from 0.10 to 1.23 and 0.16 to 1.77 for depression, and 0.10 to 2.5 for self-esteem.[163] Findings for efficacy of group interventions have been more equivocal. Johnson and Zlotnick[174] assessed the feasibility and efficacy of an individual cognitive behavioral therapy (CBT) treatment for battered women with PTSD or subthreshold PTSD in shelters using an open trial design. Participants were offered twice-weekly sessions and were followed up at 1-week, 3-months, and 6-months after they left the shelter. While this was a small study (N=18) without a control group, results showed a significant decrease in PTSD symptoms, depressive symptoms, and degree of social impairment, as well as a significant increase in the effective use of community resources, with these gains maintained over time. To date, there have been no published trials of CBT for patients with IPV and severe mental illness.

With regards to interventions among substance-abusing patients, several studies have shown that standard substance abuse treatment decreased both the prevalence and frequency of IPV, moreover among patients who do not relapse posttreatment.[171] Herein lies the main limitation of substance abuse treatments as stand-alone interventions in that reductions in IPV are directly reliant on the ability to remain abstinent from alcohol and drugs.[171] Data from meta-analytic studies examining the effectiveness of referral to domestic violence intervention programs of substance-abusing patients have produced mixed results; however, these studies have been plagued by methodological weaknesses which limit the interpretation of outcomes.[171] Partner-involved conjoint therapy, although controversial, has shown evidence of efficacy in reducing the rates of IPV. For example, behavioral couples therapy (BCT), which is a conjoint treatment used for alcoholism and drug abuse, has demonstrated both clinical and cost effectiveness.[171] It integrates standard substance abuse treatment for the alcoholic or drug-abusing partner, with partner-involved therapy, which comprises elements of positive communication skills, share activities, and negotiation of agreements.[171] BCT has also demonstrated superiority in reducing IPV prevalence compared with standard substance abuse treatment or treatment-as-usual.[175]

Finally, CBT interventions or programs with elements of CBT are frequently used treatments for physically abusive men; however, a recent meta-analysis of CBT trials in men who physically abuse their partners found that evidence for the beneficial effects of CBT is insufficient to draw any conclusions at this point in time.[176] One study examined racial differences in treatment effects among substance-dependent Caucasian and African-American male IPV offenders court mandated to an integrated substance abuse and domestic violence treatment. After treatment (12 weeks) both groups showed a reduction in physical abuse and alcohol abuse; however, Caucasian men showed a reduction in their use of verbal abuse and African American men did not. While these ethnicity differences require further investigation, they do suggest that more targeted and specific interventions may be required in some ethnic groups to maximize treatment outcomes.[177]

CONCLUSION

Assessment for IPV should be included as a routine part of psychiatric evaluation. Published research indicates that women and men exposed to IPV have significantly higher rates of mental health difficulties compared with nonvictimized women and men. Pre-existing mental disorders also render individuals more vulnerable to IPV, which in turn worsens mental health and related outcomes. Effective multi-disciplinary practice and coordination of services are needed with this population. Further research on brief, cost-effective, and culturally transportable interventions that are effective in reducing both psychopathology and abuse are urgently needed.

REFERENCES:

1. Abrahams N, Jewkes R, Martin LJ, et al. Mortality of women from intimate partner violence in South Africa: a national epidemiological study. *Violence Vict.* 2009;24(4):546-556.

2. Gass JD, Stein DJ, Williams DR, et al. Intimate partner violence, health behaviours, and chronic physical illness among South African women. *S Afr Med J.* 2010;100(9):582-585.

3. El-Bassel N, Gilbert L, Witte S, et al. Intimate partner violence and substance abuse among minority women receiving care from an inner-city emergency department. *Womens Health Issues.* 2003;13(1):16-22.

4. Friedman MJ, Schnurr PP. The relationship between trauma, post-traumatic stress disorder, and physical health. In: Friedman MJ, ed. *Neurobiological and Clinical Consequences of Stress: From Normal Adaptation to Post-Traumatic Stress Disorder.* Philadelphia, PA: Lippincott-Raven Publishers; 1995:507-524.

5. Green BL, Kimberling R. Trauma, posttraumatic stress disorder, and health status. In: Schnurr PP, Green BL, eds. *Trauma and Health: Physical Health Consequences of Exposure to Extreme Stress.* Washington, DC: American Psychological Association; 2004:13-42.

6. Schnurr PP, Green BL. A context of understanding the physical health consequences of exposure to extreme stress. In: Schnurr PP, Green BL, eds. *Trauma and Health: Physical Health Consequences of Exposure to Extreme Stress.* Washington, DC: American Psychological Association; 2004:3-10.

7. Schnurr PP, Jankowski MK. Physical health and post-traumatic stress disorder: review and synthesis. *Semin Clin Neuropsychiatry.* 1999;4(4):295-304.

8. Campbell JC, Kub J, Belknap RA, et al. Predictors of depression in battered women. *Violence Against Women.* 1997;3:271-293.

9. Campbell JC, Soeken K. Women's responses to battering: a test of the model. *Res Nurs Health.* 1999;22(1):49-58.

10. Campbell JC, Soeken K. Women's responses to battering over time: an analysis of change. *J Interpers Violence.* 1999;14(1):21-40.

11. Gleason WJ. Mental disorders in battered women: an empirical study. *Violence Vict.* 1993;8(1):53-68.

12. Golding JM. Intimate partner violence as a risk factor for mental disorders: a meta-analysis. *J Fam Violence.* 1999;14(2):99-132.

13. Sutherland C, Bybee D, Sullivan C. The long-term effects of battering on women's health. *Womens Health: Res Gender Behav Policy.* 1998;4(1):41-70.

14. Weaver TL, Clum GA. Psychological distress associated with interpersonal violence: a meta-analysis. *Clin Psychol Rev.* 1995;15(2):115-140.

15. Fauerbach JA, Heinberg LJ, Lawrence JW, et al. Effect of early body image dissatisfaction on subsequent psychological and physical adjustment after disfiguring injury. *Psychosom Med.* 2000;62(4):576-582.

16. Kilpatrick DG, Saunders B, Amick-McMullan A, et al. Victim and crime factors associated with development of crime-related posttraumatic stress disorder. *Behav Ther.* 1989;20(2):199-215.

17. Campbell R, Sullivan CM, Davidson WS. Depression in women who use domestic violence shelters: a longitudinal analysis. *Psychol Women Q.* 1995;19(2):237-255.

18. Anderson DK, Saunders DG, Mieko Y, et al. Long-term trends in depression among women separated from abusive partners. *Violence Against Women.* 2003;9(7): 807-838.

19. Ham-Rowbottom KA, Gordon EE, Jarvis KL, et al. Life constraints and psychological well-being of domestic violence shelter graduates: the "cream of the crop." *J Fam Violence.* 2005;20:109-121.

20. Sutherland C, Bybee D, Sullivan C. Beyond bruises and broken bones: The joint effects of stress and injuries on battered women's health. *Am J Community Psychol.* 2002;30(5):609-636.

21. Sadock BJ, Sadock VA, Ruiz P. *Kaplan & Sadock's Comprehensive Textbook of Psychiatry.* 9th ed. Baltimore, MD: Lippincott Williams & Wilkins; 2009.

22. McEwen BS. Sex, stress, and the hippocampus: allostasis, allostatic load and the aging process. *Neurobiol Aging.* 2002;23:921-939.

23. Scott-Tilley D, Tilton A, Sandel M. Biologic correlates to the development of post-traumatic stress disorder in female victims of intimate partner violence: implications for practice. *Perspect Psychiatr Care.* 2010;46(1):26-36.

24. Johnson DM, Delahanty DL, Pinna K. The cortisol awakening response as a function of PTSD severity and abuse chronicity in sheltered battered women. *J Anxiety Disord.* 2008;22(5):793-800.

25. Inslicht SS, Marmar CR, Neylan TC, et al. Increased cortisol in women with intimate partner violence-related posttraumatic stress disorder. *Ann N Y Acad Sci.* 2006;1071:428-429.

26. Seedat S, Stein MB, Kennedy CM, Hauger RL. Plasma cortisol and neuropeptide Y in female victims of intimate partner violence. *Psychoneuroendocrinology.* 2003;28(6):796-808.

27. Gill JM, Szanton SL, Page GG. Biological underpinnings of health alterations in women with PTSD: a sex disparity. *Biol Res Nurs.* 2005;7(1):44-54.

28. Woods SJ, Wineman NM, Page GG, Hall RJ, Alexander TS, Campbell JC. Predicting immune status in women from PTSD and childhood and adult violence. *ANS Adv Nurs Sci.* 2005;28(4):306-319.

29. Koss MP, Heslet L. Somatic consequences of violence against women. *Arch Fam Med.* 1992;1:53–59.

30. Garcia-Linares MI, Sanchez-Lorente S, Coe CL, Martinez M. Intimate male partner violence impairs immune control over herpes simplex virus type 1 in physically and psychologically abused women. *Psychosom Med.* 2004;66(6):965-972.

31. National Research Council. *Understanding Violence Against Women*. Washington, DC: National Academy Press; 1996.

32. Walton-Moss BJ, Campbell JC. Intimate partner violence: implications for nursing. *Online J Issues Nurs*. 2002;7(1):6.

33. Coggins M, Bullock LFC. The wavering line in the sand: the effects of domestic violence and sexual coercion. *Issues Ment Health Nurs*. 2003;24(6-7):723-738.

34. Petersen R, Saltzman LE, Goodwin MM, et al. *Key Scientific Issues for Research on Violence Occurring Around the Time of Pregnancy*. Atlanta, GA: CDC; 1998.

35. Flitcraft AH, Hadley SM, Hendricks-Matthews MK, et al. American Medical Association diagnostic and treatment guidelines on domestic violence. *Arch Fam Med*. 1992;1(1):39-47.

36. Smith PH, Thornton GE, DeVellis R, et al. A population-based study of the prevalence and distinctiveness of battering, physical assault, and sexual assault in intimate relationships. *Violence Against Women*. 2002;8(10):1208-1232.

37. Mechanic MB, Weaver TL, Resick PA. Mental health consequences of intimate partner abuse. *Violence Against Women*. 2008;14(6):634-654.

38. Sackett LA, Saunders DG. The impact of different forms of psychological abuse on battered women. *Violence Vict*. 1999;14(1):105-117.

39. Dutton MA, Goodman LA, Bennett L. Court-involved battered women's responses to violence: the role of psychological, physical, and sexual abuse. *Violence Vict*. 1999;4(1):89-104.

40. Follingstad DR, Rutledge LL, Berg BJ, et al. The role of emotional abuse in physically abusive relationships. *J Fam Violence*. 1990;5(2):107-120.

41. Arias I. Women's responses to physical and psychological abuse. In: Arriaga XB, Oskamp S, eds. *Violence in Intimate Relationships*. Thousand Oaks, CA: Sage; 1999:139-161.

42. Vitanza S, Vogel LCM, Marshall LL. Distress and symptoms of posttraumatic stress disorder in abused women. *Violence Vict*. 1995;10(1):23-34.

43. Arias I, Pape KT. Psychological abuse: implications for adjustment and commitment to leave violent partners. *Violence Vict*. 1999;14(1):55-67.

44. Thompson MJ, Saltzman LE, Johnson H. Risk factors for physical injury among women assaulted by current or former spouses. *Violence Against Women*. 2001;7:886-899.

45. Harris D, Valdovinos M, Mechanic MB, et al. Mental health effects of stalking among battered women. Poster presented at: Annual Meeting of the Western Psychological Association; 2004; Phoenix, AZ.

46. Mechanic MB, Uhlmansiek MH, Weaver TL, et al. The impact of severe stalking experienced by acutely battered women: an examination of violence, psychological symptoms and strategic responding. *Violence Vict*. 2000;15(4):443-458.

47. Basile KC, Arias I, Desai S, et al. The differential association of intimate partner physical, sexual, psychological, and stalking violence and posttraumatic stress symptoms in a nationally representative sample of women. *J Trauma Stress*. 2004; 17(5):413-421.

48. Bennice JA, Resick PA. Marital rape: history, research, and practice. *Trauma Violence Abuse.* 2003;4(3):228-246.

49. Bennice JA, Resick PA, Mechanic MB, et al. The relative effects of intimate partner physical and sexual violence on posttraumatic stress disorder symptomatology. *Violence Vict.* 2003;18(1):87-94.

50. Frieze IH. Investigating the causes and consequences of marital rape. *Signs.* 1983;8(1):532-553.

51. Dougall AL, Heberman HB, Delahanty DL, et al. Similarity of prior trauma exposure as a determinant of chronic stress responding to an airline disaster. *J Consult Clin Psychol.* 2000;68(2):290-295.

52. Follette VM, Polusny MA, Bechtle AE, et al. Cumulative trauma: the impact of child sexual abuse, adult sexual assault, and spouse abuse. *J Trauma Stress.* 1996;9(1):25-35.

53. Nishith P, Mechanic MB, Resick PA. Prior interpersonal trauma: the contribution to current PTSD symptoms in female rape victims. *J Abnorm Psychol.* 2000;109(1):20-25.

54. Cascardi M, O'Leary KD. Depressive symptomatology, self-esteem, and self-blame in battered women. *J Fam Violence.* 1992;7(4):249-259.

55. Marshall LL. Effects of men's subtle and overt psychological abuse on low-income women. *Violence Vict.* 1999;14(1):69-88.

56. Cascardi M, O'Leary KD, Schlee KA. Co-occurrence and correlates of posttraumatic stress disorder and major depression in physically abused women. *J Fam Violence.* 1999;14(3):227-249.

57. O'Leary KD, Tintle N, Bromet EJ, et al. Descriptive epidemiology of intimate partner aggression in Ukraine. *Soc Psychiatry Psychiatr Epidemiol.* 2008;43(8):619-626.

58. Tang C. Marital power and aggression in a community sample of Hong Kong Chinese families. *J Interpers Violence.* 1999;14(2):586-602.

59. Baker CK, Norris FH, Diaz DMV, et al. Violence and PTSD in Mexico. *Soc Psychiatry Psychiatr Epidemiol.* 2005;40(7):519-528.

60. Kwong MI, Bartholomew K, Dutton DG. Gender differences in patterns of relationship violence in Alberta. *Can J Behav Sci.* 1999;31:150-160.

61. Stets JE, Straus MA. Gender differences in reporting marital violence and its medical and psychological consequences. In: Straus MA, Gelles RJ, eds. *Physical Violence in American Families.* New Brunswick, NJ: Transaction Publishers; 1990:151-165, 227-244.

62. Andersson N, Ho-Foster A, Mitchell S. Risk factors for domestic physical violence: national cross-sectional household surveys in eight southern African countries. *BMC Womens Health.* 2007;7:11.

63. Watson LF, Taft A, Lee C. Associations of self-reported violence with age at menarche, first intercourse, and first birth among a national population sample of young Australian women. *Womens Health Issues.* 2007;17(5):281-289.

64. Edgardh K. Sexual behavior and early coitrache in a national sample of 17 year old Swedish girls. *Sex Transm Infect.* 2000;76(2):98-102.

65. Morgan C, Chapar GN, Fisher M. Psychosocial variables associated with teenage pregnancy. *Adolescence.* 1995;30(118):277-289.

66. Dickson N, Paul C, Herbison P, et al. First sexual intercourse: age, coercion, and later regrets reported by a birth cohort. *Br Med J.* 1998(7124);316:29-33.

67. Dunkle KL, Jewkes RK, Brown HC, et al. Prevalence and patterns of gender-based violence and revictimization among women attending antenatal clinics in Soweto, South Africa. *Am J Epidemiol.* 2004;160(3):230-239.

68. Rickert VI, Wiemann CM, Harrykissoon SD, et al. The relationship among demographics, reproductive characteristics, and intimate partner violence. *Am J Obstet Gynecol.* 2002;187(4):1002-1007.

69. Silverman JG, Raj A, Clements K. Dating violence and associated sexual risk and pregnancy among adolescent girls in the United States. *Paediatrics.* 2004;114 2):e220-e225.

70. Island D, Letellier P. *Men Who Beat the Men Who Love Them: Battered Gay Men and Domestic Violence.* New York, NY: Harrington Park Press; 1991.

71. Greenwood GL, Relf MV, Huang B, et al. Battering victimization among a probability-based sample of men who have sex with men. *Am J Public Health.* 2002;92(12):1964-1969.

72. Seelau EP, Seelau SM, Poorman PB. Gender and role-based perceptions of domestic abuse: does sexual orientation matter? *Behav Sci Law.* 2003;21(2):199-214.

73. Houston E, McKirnan DJ. Intimate partner abuse among gay and bisexual men: risk correlates and health outcomes. *J Urban Health.* 2007;84(5):681-690.

74. Merrill GS, Wolfe VA. Battered gay men: an exploration of abuse, help seeking, and why they stay. *J Homosex.* 2000;39(2):1-30.

75. Gazmararian JA, Lazorick S, Spitz AM, et al. Prevalence of violence against pregnant women. *JAMA.* 1996;275(24):1915-1920.

76. Centers for Disease Control and Prevention. *PRAMS 1996 Surveillance Report.* Atlanta, GA: Division of Reproductive Health, National Center for Chronic Disease Prevention and Health Promotion, Centers for Disease Control and Prevention; 1997.

77. Fanslow J, Whitehead A, Silva M, et al. Contraceptive use and associations with intimate partner violence among a population-based sample of New Zealand women. *Aust N Z J Obstet Gynaecol.* 2008;48(1):83-89.

78. Fanslow JL, Robinson E. Violence against women in New Zealand: prevalence and health consequences. *N Z Med J.* 2004;117(1206).

79. Jasinski JL. Pregnancy and domestic violence: a review of the literature. *Trauma Violence Abuse.* 2004;5(1):47-64.

80. Campbell JC. Health consequences of intimate partner violence. *Lancet.* 2002;359 (9314):1331-1336.

81. Murphy CC, Schei B, Myhr T, et al. Abuse: a risk factor for low birth weight? a systematic review and meta-analysis. *Can Med Assoc J.* 2001;164(11):1567–1572.

82. Gazmararian JA, Peterson R, Spitz AM, et al. Violence and reproductive health: current knowledge and future research directions. *Matern Child Health J.* 2000;4 (2):79-84.

83. Jasinski JL, Kantor GK. Pregnancy, stress and, wife assault: ethnic differences in prevalence, severity, and onset in a national sample. *Violence Vict.* 2003;16(3):219-232.

84. MacMahon PM, Goodwin MM, Stringer G. Sexual violence and reproductive health. *Matern Child Health J.* 2000;4(2):121-124.

85. Saewyc EM, Magee LL, Pettingell SE. Teenage pregnancy and associated risk behavior among sexually abused adolescents. *Perspect Sex Reprod Health.* 2004;36 (3):98-105.

86. Silverman JG, Decker MR, Reed E, et al. Intimate partner violence victimization prior to and during pregnancy among women residing in 26 US states: associations with maternal and neonatal health. *Am J Obstet Gynecol.* 2006;195(1):140-148.

87. Straus MA, Gelles RJ, eds. *Physical Violence in American Families.* New Brusnwick, NJ: Transaction Publishers; 1990.

88. Parker B, McFarlane J, Soeken K, Torres S, Campbell D. Physical and emotional abuse in pregnancy: a comparison of adult and teenage women. *Nurs Res.* 1993;42 (3):173-178.

89. Saltzman LE, Johnson CH, Gilbert BC, et al. Physical abuse around the time of pregnancy: an examination of prevalence and risk factors in 16 states. *Matern Child Health J.* 2003;7(1):31-43.

90. Anderson BA, Marshak HH, Hebbeler DL. Identifying intimate partner violence at entry to prenatal care: clustering routine clinical information. *J Midwifery Womens Health.* 2002;47(5):353-359.

91. Smith MV, Rosenheck RA, Cavaleri MA, et al. Screening for and detection of depression, panic disorder, and PTSD in public obstetric clinics. *Psychiatr Serv.* 2004;55(4):407-414.

92. Lipsky S, Holt VL, Easterling TR, et al. Impact of police-reported intimate partner violence during pregnancy on birth outcomes. *Obstet Gynecol.* 2003;102(3):557-564.

93. Bailey BA. Partner violence during pregnancy: prevalence, effects, screening, and management. *Int J Womens Health.* 2010;2:183-197.

94. Hack M, Klein NK, Taylor G. Long-term developmental outcomes of low birth weight infants. *Future Child.* 1995;5(1):176-196.

95. Kilbride HW, Thorstad K, Daily DK. Preschool outcome of less than 801 gram preterm infants compared with full-term siblings. *Pediatrics.* 2004;113(4):742-747.

96. Marlow N. Neurocognitive outcome after very preterm birth. *Arch Dis Child Fetal Neonatal Ed.* 2004;89:224-228.

97. Taylor HG, Minich NM, Klein N, et al. Longitudinal outcomes of very low birth weight: neuropsychological findings. *J Int Neuropsychol Soc.* 2004;10(3):149-163.

98. Williams CM, Larsen U, McCloskey LA. Intimate partner violence and women's contraceptive use. *Violence Against Women.* 2008;14(12):1382-1396.

99. Gazmararian JA, Adams MA, Saltzman LE, et al. The relationship between pregnancy intendedness and physical violence in mothers of newborns. *Obstet Gynecol.* 1995;85(6):1031-1038.

100. Wingood GM, DiClement RJ. The effects of an abusive primary partner on the condom use and sexual negotiation practices of African-American women. *Am J Public Health.* 1997;87(6):1016-1018.

101. Augenbraun M, Wilson T, Allister L. Domestic violence reported by women attending a sexually transmitted disease clinic. *Sex Transm Dis.* 2001;28(3):143-147.

102. Whitehead A, Fanslow J. Prevalence of family violence amongst women attending an abortion clinic in New Zealand. *Aust N Z J. Obstet Gynaecol.* 2005;45(4):321-324.

103. Alio AP, Daley EM, Nana PN, et al. Intimate partner violence and contraception use among women in Sub-Saharan Africa. *Int J Gynecol Obstet.* 2009;107(1):35-38.

104. Ellsberg M, Jansen HA, Heise L, et al. Intimate partner violence and women's physical and mental health in the WHO multi-country study on women's health and domestic violence: an observational study. *Lancet.* 2008;371(9619):1165-1172.

105. Markham DW. Mental illness and domestic violence: implications for family law litigation. *J Poverty Law and Policy.* 2003;(May-June):23-35.

106. Dienemann J, Boyle E, Baker D, Resnick W, Wiederhorn N, Campbell J. Intimate partner abuse among women diagnosed with depression. *Issues Ment Health Nurs.* 2000;21(5):499-513.

107. Chang JC, Cluss PA, Burke JG, et al. Partner violence screening in mental health. *Gen Hosp Psychiatry.* 2011;33(1):58-65.

108. Friedman SH, Loue S. Incidence and prevalence of intimate partner violence by and against women with severe mental illness. *J Womens Health.* 2007;16(4):471-480.

109. Carlile JB. Spouse assault on mentally disordered wives. *Can J Psychiatry.* 1991;36(4):265-269.

110. Post RD, Willett AB, Franks RD, et al. A preliminary report on the prevalence of domestic violence among psychiatric inpatients. *Am J Psychiatry.* 1980;137(8):974-975.

111. Goodman LA, Rosenberg SD, Mueser KT, et al. Physical and sexual assault history in women with serious mental illness: prevalence, correlates, treatment, and future research directions. *Schizophr Bull.* 1997;23(4):685-696.

112. DeNiro DA. Perceived alienation in individuals with residual-type schizophrenia. *Issues Ment Health Nurs.* 1995;16(3):185-200.

113. Hamby S, Finkelhor D, Turner H. The overlap of witnessing partner violence with child maltreatment and other victimizations in a nationally representative survey of youth. *Child Abuse Negl.* 2010;34(10):734-741.

114. Ehrensaft MK, Cohen P, Brown J, et al. Intergenerational transmission of partner violence: a 20-year prospective study. *J Consult Clin Psychol.* 2003;71(4):741-753.

115. Gil-González D, Vives-Cases C, Ruiz MT, et al. Childhood experiences of violence in perpetrators as a risk factor of intimate partner violence: a systematic review. *J Public Health.* 2007;30(1):14-22.

116. Roberts AL, Gilman SE, Fitzmaurice G, et al. Witness of intimate partner violence in childhood and perpetration of intimate partner violence in adulthood. *Epidemiology.* 2010;21(6):809-818.

117. Jewkes R, Levin J, Penn-Kekana L. Risk factors for domestic violence: findings from a South African cross-sectional study. *Soc Sci Med.* 2002;55(9):1603-1617.

118. Fang X, Corso PS. Child maltreatment, youth violence, and intimate partner violence. *Am J Prev Med.* 2007;33(4):281-290.

119. Gupta J, Silverman JG, Hemenway D, et al. Physical violence against intimate partners and related exposures to violence among South African men. *CMAJ.* 2008;179(6):535-541.

120. Welles SL, Corbin TJ, Rich JA, et al. Intimate partner violence among men having sex with men, women, or both: early-life sexual and physical abuse as antecedents. *J Community Health.* 2011;36(3):477-485.

121. Stith SM, Rosen KH, Middleton KA. The intergenerational transmission of spouse abuse: a meta-analysis. *J Marriage Fam.* 2000;62(3):640-654.

122. Herrenkohl TI, Mason WA, Kosterman R, et al. Pathways from physical childhood abuse to partner violence in young adulthood. *Violence Vict.* 2004;19(2):123-136.

123. Walker L. Battered women and learned helplessness. *Victimology.* 1977;2(3-4):525-534.

124. Heise L. Violence against women. an integrated, ecological framework. *Violence Against Women.* 1998;4(3):262-290.

125. Feldman CM. Childhood precursors of adult inter-partner violence. *Clin Psychol.* 1997;4(4):307-334.

126. Abrahams N, Jewkes R. Effects of South African men's having witnessed abuse of their mothers during childhood on their levels of violence in adulthood. *Am J Public Health.* 2005;95(10):1811-1816.

127. Bensley L, Van Eenwyk J, Simmons KW. Childhood family violence history and women's risk for intimate partner violence and poor health. *Am J Prev Med.* 2003;25(1):38-44.

128. Fang X, Massetti GM, Ouyang L. Attention-deficit/hyperactivity disorder, conduct disorder, and young adult intimate partner violence. *Arch Gen Psychiatry.* 2010;67(11):1179-1186.

129. Howells NL, Rosenbaum A. Examination of sex differences and type of violence exposure in a mediation model of family violence. *J Emotional Abuse.* 2008;8:(1/2) 123-138.

130. Malik S, Sorenson SB, Aneshensel CS. Community and dating violence perpetration among adolescents: perpetration and victimization. *J Adolesc Health.* 1997;21(5):291-302.

131. Abrahams N, Jewkes R, Hoffman M, et al. Sexual violence against intimate partners in Cape Town: prevalence and risk factors reported by men. *Bull World Health Organ.* 2004;82(5):330-337.

132. Reed E, Silverman JG, Welles SL, et al. Associations between perceptions and involvement in neighborhood violence and intimate partner violence perpetration among urban, African American men. *J Community Health.* 2009;34(4):328-335.

133. Reed E, Silverman JG, Raj A, et al. Social and environmental contexts of adolescent and young adult male perpetrators of intimate partner violence: A qualitative study. *Am J Mens Health.* 2008;2(3):260-271.

134. Stueve A, O'Donnell L. Urban young women's experiences of discrimination and community violence and intimate partner violence. *J Urban Health.* 2008;85(3):386-401.

135. Hegarty K, Gunn J, Chondros P, et al. Physical and social predictors of partner abuse in women attending general practice: a cross-sectional study. *Br J Gen Pract.* 2008;58(552):484-487.

136. Uthman OA, Moradi T, Lawoko S. The independent contribution of individual-, neighbourhood-, and country-level socioeconomic position on attitudes towards intimate partner violence against women in sub-Saharan Africa: a multilevel model of direct and moderating effects. *Soc Sci Med.* 2009;68(10):1801-1809.

137. Melander LA, Noel H, Tyler KA. Bidirectional, unidirectional, and nonviolence: a comparison of the predictors among partnered young adults. *Violence Vict.* 2010;25(5):617-630.

138. Caetano R, Ramisetty-Mikler S, Field CA. Unidirectional and bidirectional intimate partner violence among White, Black, and Hispanic couples in the United States. *Violence Vict.* 2005;20:393-406.

139. Clements K, Schumacher JA. Perceptual biases in social cognition as potential moderators of the relationship between alcohol and intimate partner violence: a review. *Aggress Violent Behav.* 2010;15:357-368.

140. Kaur R, Garg S. Domestic violence against women: a qualitative study in a rural community. *Asia-Pac J Public Health.* 2010;22(2):242-251.

141. Tufts KA, Clements PT, Wessell J. When intimate partner violence against women and HIV collide: challenges for healthcare assessment and intervention. *J Forensic Nurs.* 2010;6(2):66-73.

142. Jewkes RK, Dunkle K, Nduna M, et al. Intimate partner violence, relationship power inequity, and incidence of HIV infection in young women in South Africa: a cohort study. *Lancet.* 2010;376(9734):41-48.

143. Decker MR, Seage GR, Hemenway D, et al. Intimate partner violence functions as both a risk marker and risk factor for women's HIV infection: findings from Indian husband-wife dyads. *J Acquir Immune Defic Syndr.* 2009;51(5):593-600.

144. Rountree MA, Mulraney M. HIV/AIDS risk reduction intervention for women who have experienced intimate partner violence. *Clin Soc Work J.* 2010;38(2):207-216.

145. Townsend L, Jewkes R, Mathews C, et al. HIV risk behaviours and their relationship to intimate partner violence (IPV) among men who have multiple female sexual partners in Cape Town, South Africa. *AIDS Behav.* 2011;15:132-141.

146. Christofides N, Jewkes R. Acceptability of universal screening for intimate partner violence in voluntary HIV testing and counseling services in South Africa and service implications. *AIDS Care.* 2010;22(1):279-285.

147. Sikkema KJ, Neufeld SA, Hansen NB, et al. Integrating HIV prevention into services for abused women in South Africa. *AIDS Behav.* 2010;14(2):431-439.

148. Nduna M, Jewkes RK, Dunkle KL, et al. Associations between depressive symptoms, sexual behaviour and relationship characteristics: a prospective cohort study of young women and men in the Eastern Cape, South Africa. *J Int AIDS Soc.* 2010;13:44.

149. Cavanaugh CE, Hansen NB, Sullivan TP. HIV sexual risk behavior among low-income women experiencing intimate partner violence: the role of post-traumatic stress disorder. *AIDS Behav.* 2010;14(2):318-327.

150. Bhandari M, Dosanjh S, Tornetta P III, Matthews D. Musculoskeletal manifestations of physical abuse after intimate partner violence. *J Trauma Injury Infection Critical Care.* 2006;61(6):1473-1479.

151. Campbell R, Greeson MR, Bybee D. The co-occurrence of childhood sexual abuse, adult sexual assault, intimate partner violence, and sexual harassment: a mediational model of posttraumatic stress disorder and physical health outcomes. *J Consult Clin Psychol.* 2008;76:194-207.

152. Breiding MJ, Black MC, Ryan GW. Chronic disease and health risk behaviors associated with intimate partner violence – 18 US states/territories, 2005 *Ann Epidemiol.* 2005;18(7):538-544.

153. Bonomi AE, Anderson ML, Reid RJ, et al. Medical and psychosocial diagnoses in women with a history of intimate partner violence. *Arch Intern Med.* 2009;169(18):1692-1697.

154. Lemon SC, Verhoek-Oftedahl W, Donnelly EF. Preventive health care use, smoking, and alcohol use among Rhode Island women experiencing intimate partner violence. *J Womens Health Gend Based Med.* 2002;11(6):555-562.

155. Garcia-Moreno C, Jansen HAFM, Ellsberg M, et al. Prevalence of intimate partner violence: findings from the WHO multi-country study on women's health and domestic violence. *Lancet.* 2006;368(9543):1260-1269.

156. Lown EA, Vega WA. Intimate partner violence and health: self-assessed health, chronic health, and somatic symptoms among Mexican American women. *Psychosom Med.* 2001;63(3):352-360.

157. Breiding MJ, Black MC, Ryan GW. Prevalence and risk factors of intimate partner violence in eighteen U.S. states/territories, 2005. *Am J Prev Med.* 2008;34(2):112-8.

158. Chang JC, Cluss PA, Burke JG, et al. Partner violence screening in mental health. *Gen Hosp Psychiatry.* 2011;33(1):58-65.

159. Gerber MR, Ganz ML, Lichter E, et al. Adverse health behavior and the detection of partner violence by clinicians. *Arch Intern Med.* 2005;165(9):1016-1021.

160. Rose D, Trevillion K, Woodall A, Morgan C, Feder G, Howard L. Barriers and facilitators of disclosures of domestic violence by mental health service users: qualitative study. *Br J Psychiatry.* 2011;198(3):189-194.

161. Howard LM, Trevillion K, Agnew-Davies R. Domestic violence and mental health. *Int Rev Psychiatry.* 2010;22(5):525-534.

162. Ramsay J, Richardson J, Carter YH, Davidson LL, Feder G. Should health professionals screen women for domestic violence? systematic review. *BMJ.* 2002;325(7359):314.

163. Feder G, Ramsay J, Dunne D et al. How far does screening women for domestic (partner) violence in different health-care settings meet criteria for a screening programme? systematic reviews of nine UK National Screening Committee criteria. *Health Technol Assess.* 2009;13(16):iii-iv,xi-xiii,1-113,137-347.

164. Campbell JC, Glass N, Sharps PW, Laughon K, Bloom T. Intimate partner homicide: review and implications of research and policy. *Trauma Violence Abuse.* 2007;8(3):246-269.

165. Daniels K. Intimate partner violence & depression: a deadly comorbidity. *J Psychosoc Nurs Ment Health Serv.* 2005;43(1):44-51.

166. Hien D, Ruglass L. Interpersonal partner violence and women in the United States: an overview of prevalence rates, psychiatric correlates and consequences and barriers to help seeking. *Int J Law Psychiatry.* 2009;32(1):48-55.

167. Briere J, Jordan CE. Violence against women: outcome complexity and implications for assessment and treatment. *J Interpers Violence.* 2004;19(11):1252-1276.

168. Chang JC, Cluss PA, Ranieri L, et al. Health care interventions for intimate partner violence: what women want. *Women's Health Issues.* 2005;15(1):21-30.

169. Ramsay J, Carter Y, Davidson L, et al. Advocacy interventions to reduce or eliminate violence and promote the physical and psychosocial well-being of women who experience intimate partner abuse. *Cochrane Database Syst Rev.* 2009;(3):CD005043.

170. Tiwari A, Fong DY, Yuen KH, et al. Effect of an advocacy intervention on mental health in Chinese women survivors of intimate partner violence: a randomized controlled trial. *JAMA.* 2010;304(5):536-43.

171. Klostermann K, Kelley ML, Mignone T, Pusateri L, Fals-Stewart W. Partner violence and substance abuse: treatment interventions. *Aggress Violent Behav.* 2010;15(3):162-166.

172. Kubany ES, Hill EE, Owens JA. Cognitive trauma therapy for battered women with PTSD: preliminary findings. *J Trauma Stress.* 2003;16(1):81-91.

173. Kubany ES, Hill EE, Owens JA, et al. Cognitive trauma therapy for battered women with PTSD (CTT-BW). *J Consult Clin Psychol.* 2004;72(1):3-18.

174. Johnson DM, Zlotnick C. A cognitive-behavioral treatment for battered women with PTSD in shelters: findings from a pilot study. *J Trauma Stress.* 2006;19(4):559-564.

175. Fals-Stewart W, Kashdan TB, O'Farrell TJ, Birchler GR. Behavioral couples therapy for drug-abusing patients: effects on partner violence. *J Subst Abuse Treat.* 2002;22(2):87-96.

176. Smedslund G, Dalsbø TK, Steiro AK, Winsvold A, Clench-Aas J. Cognitive behavioural therapy for men who physically abuse their female partner. *Cochrane Database Syst Rev.* 2007;(3):CD006048.

177. Scott MC, Easton CJ. Racial differences in treatment effect among men in a substance abuse and domestic violence program. *Am J Drug Alcohol Abuse.* 2010;6(6):357-362.

Chapter 19

SUICIDE AND INTIMATE PARTNER VIOLENCE

Pamela Marcus, RN APRN/PMH-BC

KEY POINTS

1. Identify individuals who would be at risk for suicidal thoughts and behavior after sustaining intimate partner violence (IPV).

2. List four assessment questions that are helpful to determine the level of risk of suicide in an individual who has experienced IPV.

3. Identify three interventions that are clinically proven to prevent suicide for people who have has IPV.

INTRODUCTION

Understanding the link between intimate partner violence (IPV) and suicidal intent, including death by suicide, is important to prevent further loss of life. One aspect of providing comprehensive care for individuals who have experienced IPV is to assess the individual for potential suicidal thoughts and behaviors. It is estimated that 50 000 people die as a result of violence, according to the Surveillance for Violent Deaths – National Violent Death Reporting System. In 2006, the National Violent Death Reporting System received data from 16 states that participate in this CDC sponsored reporting system. The data showed that 15 007 fatalities occurred in these states. Of the reported deaths, 55.9% were individuals who died by suicide. The National Violent Death Reporting System listed suicide as a consequence of intimate partner violence.[1,2]

Washington State collected data on the correlation of childhood abuse, adult interpersonal violence, and suicidal ideation. Data collected by the Behavioral Risk Factor Surveillance System yielded a large sample size of 4081 individuals. The results of this research demonstrated the most significant risk factor for suicidal ideation was physical abuse that occurred in adulthood. In this population, individuals had suicidal ideation over 27 times higher than individuals who had not experienced interpersonal violence. Adults who had been abused sexually were 5 times more likely to have suicidal ideation than individuals who had experienced sexual abuse as an adult. Individuals who were sexually abused as children were 3 times more likely to experience suicidal ideation in adulthood than those who did not experience childhood sexual abuse. Individuals who had experienced childhood physical abuse had 2.31 times likely to experience suicidal ideation than the rest of the population.[3] People who have PTSD due to experiencing a psychological trauma have a significantly higher rate of suicide attempts and deaths.[4] Krysinska et al[4] state that individuals who have sustained repeated and prolonged psychological trauma due to IPV had a higher rate of suicide attempts. The possibility of suicidal thoughts and attempts increases if the individual had physical or sexual abuse during childhood.[4]

INDIVIDUALS AT RISK FOR
SUICIDAL THOUGHTS AND BEHAVIOR AFTER IPV

Most of the literature and research on IPV focuses on women. It is important to study the possibility of suicidal behavior in men who are involved in IPV. An important predictor of adult behavior is to consider male adolescent behavior. In a study by Kerr and Capaldi,[5] adolescent aggression and suicidal behavior increased the probability of romantic partner dissatisfaction, with jealousy and low relationship satisfaction as well as IPV and suicidal behavior. Key stressors that are important to monitor to prevent IPV and suicidal behavior in men are: financial stressors, substance abuse, depression, and low self-esteem.[6]

Leiner et al studied IPV and suicidal behavior in African American women.[7] This study concluded that African American women who have experienced IPV have a higher risk of suicidal ideation and suicidal attempts than those African American women who have not experienced IPV. Women who demonstrated symptoms of depression and IPV had an increased rate of suicidal ideation. This study also found that African American women who had experienced IPV and developed PTSD had increased symptoms of depression. This study encourages clinicians to assess individuals who have had IPV to evaluate for depression and PTSD as well as suicidal ideation.

IPV and suicidal behavior is not limited to any one culture or country. In a 2010 WHO World Mental Health Survey researchers studied the relationship between suicidal behavior in response to psychological trauma exposure. This study had 102 245 participants from 21 countries. The countries represented nations all over the world, such as Africa (Nigeria; South Africa), the Americas (Brazil; Colombia; Mexico; United States), Asia and the Pacific (India; Japan; New Zealand; Beijing; and Shanghai in the People's Republic of China), Europe (Belgium; Bulgaria; France; Germany; Italy; the Netherlands; Romania; Spain; Ukraine), and the Middle East (Israel and Lebanon). One important finding of this study was that suicidal ideation and attempts are significantly associated with psychological trauma. Interpersonal violence and sexual violence are highly associated with unplanned suicide attempts.[8]

In a study of university students internationally, Chan et al studied 16 000 students in 22 universities from 21 different countries.[9] There were large differences between countries; however, the prevalence of violence between partners was similar throughout the research sample. Both men and women were reported to be physically abusive towards their partners. Sexual coercion as well as physical abuse was reported by both sexes in this study. Suicidal ideation was reported by students who have symptoms of depression as well as a history of dating violence.

China's suicide rate accounts for one third of the global suicide statistics. Wong and Phillips[10] conducted a study of 353 women who were admitted to the emergency department of 9 rural general hospitals in China for a suicidal attempt,[11] spousal conflict was the most frequent precipitating factor for this incidence of crisis. One third of the study participants reported physical abuse by their spouses. The women in this study who had sustained physical abuse were younger, with more chaotic relationship patterns in their family systems and a higher rate of divorce. These women expressed sadness at not having completed the suicidal act. This placed them at a high risk for a future suicide.[10]

A study was conducted in Hong Kong, China to determine the implications of childhood sexual abuse on IPV in later adult dating relationships. A total of 1154 individuals participated in this study. Of this study sample, 1.7% reported childhood sexual abuse, mostly women. There was no gender differences reported for individuals who had experienced either adult sexual victimization or IPV. The subjects reported an increase incidence of IPV when the couple engaged in substance abuse, sexual activity, sex with a partner, and/or experienced low self-esteem. Suicidal ideation increased with substance abuse, childhood trauma (such as witnessing parental IPV), childhood sexual abuse, and low self-esteem.[12]

Haarr studied 400 women in 3 districts of Tajikistan who had experienced intimate partner abuse.[13] The findings of this study appear to suggest that when an abused partner reveals the sexual or physical abuse to a friend, the likelihood of a suicidal attempt increases. The family relationship is a closed system; seeking help may be seen as going against this principle. This is important to consider when providing care for an individual who discloses intimate partner abuse.

A study conducted in West Delhi, India explored the rate of domestic violence against women between the ages of 15 and 49 year old (15-49). Of the 350 women who were interviewed, 34.9 % reported physical or sexual abuse, with 29.1% reporting either physical or sexual abuse within the year prior to the study. Twelve percent (12%) of the women in this research study stated that they had mental health issues, which included suicidal thoughts or behaviors. This study concluded that women who have reported IPV have a higher probability of mental health concerns, including a risk for suicide.[14]

There are 2 studies involving Latino populations in the United States that are helpful to understand the link between IPV and the risk for a suicidal attempt. One study was done using a self reporting survey given to individuals 11 to 13 years old. This survey was administered to 322 participants who reported 14.4 % physical dating violence within the year prior to the study for girls and 12.9 % for boys. The statistics demonstrated that girls became at risk for physical dating violence when they engaged in binge drinking. The boys had the following variables associated with and elevated risk for dating violence: carrying a gun, drinking alcohol, and having suicidal thoughts. This study has implications for IPV in adulthood.[15]

The second study described 146 adult Latino women who were receiving care at an urban family medical practice. Twenty one percent (21%) of this group stated that they had experienced IPV in their current relationship. Of these individuals, 64.5% reported depression. This high percentage of women who experience depression along with IPV indicates a high risk for suicide.[16]

ASSESSMENT OF SUICIDAL RISK

It is important to assess an individual for the risk of suicide after determining that he or she has sustained IPV. The person may feel embarrassed by the violence within their relationship and therefore may be reluctant to disclose their feelings of hopelessness, and possible suicidal thoughts and/or behaviors. It is not unusual for people who have suicidal thoughts and/or a plan for completion to withhold this information from a clinician. This may be due to several factors such as: embarrassment of these thoughts, a value system that identifies talking about suicide with another person as a taboo, a belief that contemplating suicide is a sin, concern that the clinician may label the individual as mentally ill and in need of hospitalization. The individual feels death would be a relief and does not identify any other options for living. Shea points out that individuals who have suicidal ideation may withhold information until they determine how safe it is to share their true suicidal intent with the interviewing professional.[17,18] Shea's equation for suicidal intent is:

Real Suicidal Intent = Stated Intent + Reflected Intent + Withheld Intent

CASE APPROACH

Assessing an individual for their true suicidal intent is more than asking the standard questions of: *"are you thinking of committing suicide and if so, do you have a plan?"* A comprehensive assessment takes into consideration the individual's potential reluctance to discuss their level of hopelessness and intent to die by suicide. Shea's interviewing strategy; the CASE Approach (Chronological Assessment of Suicide Events) assists the clinician to utilize well formulated questions to elicit the individual's deep thoughts on suicide. This method takes into consideration the person's possible feelings of shame or embarrassment by the manner that the questions are asked. CASE relies on the clinician asking questions using 4 principles: (1) Behavioral Incident; (2) Gentle Assumption; (3) Symptom Amplification; and (4) Denial of the Specific.

The principle of **Behavioral Incident** is based on getting beyond the patient's unconscious defense mechanisms or conscious withholding of information. Using the principle of Behavioral Incident, the clinician asks a series of questions that encourage the individual to describe their suicidal intent step by step. Using questions such as "what happened next," and "then what did you do?" the clinician can obtain a step by step picture of the individual's suicide attempt or thought pattern. The second principle of **Gentle Assumption** uses a series of questions that the clinician asks as though the behavior is occurring. This method is useful when the clinician is sensing that the individual is withholding information. It is important to keep in mind that the method of Gentle Assumption can be considered leading questions, and therefore is not advisable to use for children who have been sexually or physically abused and individuals who are involved in legal proceedings. An example of Gentle Assumption is the following: "I understand that you are in a lot of emotional pain with all of the losses you have had after leaving your husband and going to a Safe House. I wonder if you have ever had plans to complete suicide that you have never said aloud." **Symptom Amplification**, the third principle in CASE, asks the individual to estimate the exact quantity of the symptom. An example of the types of questions the clinician asks in this principle is the following: "How many times have you thought about suicide in the past 48 hours? All the time, 75% of the time or 50% of the time?" "How many times did you pick up your gun and unlock the safety?" "Ten times? Five times? Or Two times?" This quantity helps the clinician determine the level of risk for the individual to act on their lethal thoughts. **Denial of the Specific** is a principle used to illicit information that the person may be withholding, either because of embarrassment or not wanting to share the level of lethality of their thought pattern. Examples of these types of questions are the following: "Have you thought about using your medications in an overdose attempt?" "Have you ever thought of jumping into a subway track or jumping from a bridge?" The clinician should ask each method of suicide separately and give the individual the opportunity to respond before asking the next question. This method of questioning assists the person to become more specific with their answers and determine a more accurate risk of suicide.

Using the 4 principles of the CASE Approach, the clinician asks the individual information about his or her presenting suicidal events:

1. Within the last 48 hours

2. Recent suicide attempts, within the last 2 months

3. Past suicide thoughts and behaviors, from the last 2 months to the full past history of the person's suicidal thoughts and behaviors

4. Current, immediate suicidal intent.

These questions will explore the individual's suicidal risk in depth while using the 4 principles of interviewing described above. This comprehensive interview system gives

Table 19-1. The CASE Approach (Chronological Assessment of Suicide Events)

1. Behavioral Incident	Encourages the client to describe his/her suicidal intent step by step through asking a series of questions.
2. Gentle Assumption	The clinician asks a series of questions to the client as though the behavior is occurring. Caution, the questions may be considered leading and cannot be used for children or individuals who are involved in an active legal case.
3. Symptom Amplification	Is used to illicit information that the person may be withholding, either because of embarrassment or not wanting to share the level of lethality of their thought pattern.
4. Denial of the Specific	The clinician asks the individual to estimate the exact quantity of the symptom.

EACH STEP TAKES INTO CONSIDERATION QUESTIONS ABOUT THE FOLLOWING:

1. Thoughts and behavior that occurred within the last 48 hours

2. Recent suicide attempts, within the last 2 months

3. Past suicide thoughts and behaviors, from the last 2 months to the full past history of the person's suicidal thoughts and behaviors

4. Current, immediate suicidal intent.

the clinician and the individual a clear picture, which Shea calls a "verbal videotape" in order to determine the suicidal risk and treatment to decrease the level of risk of dangerousness of this crisis (see **Table 19-1**).[17,18]

SUICIDE ASSESSMENT FIVE-STEP EVALUATION AND TRIAGE (SAFE-T)

After a thorough assessment of suicidal intent, understanding the overall threat is the next step. The Suicide Prevention Resource Center (www.sprc.org) suggests a 5 step program, called SAFE-T (Suicide Assessment Five-step Evaluation and Triage). This is useful for clinicians to determine the level of probability for a risk for suicide and implement the most appropriate intervention for the individual. The first step in this program is to determine the risk factors. This includes the information the clinician has obtained using the CASE Approach for assessment of the individual's current suicidal risk and the history of the person's past suicidal attempts. Augment the CASE interview with the following information:

1. Current and past psychiatric disorders

2. Current key symptoms

3. Family history of suicide and psychiatric disorders

4. Current stressors and interpersonal problems that can cause humiliation or shame, such as IPV

5. Any change in psychiatric treatment

6. Any access to firearms

The second step in SAFE-T is to Identify Protective Factors. These are categorized as internal or external protective factors. Internal factors are the ability to problem solve, cope with stress and frustration and spiritual beliefs that assist the person during challenging emotional periods. External protective factors are relationships, support systems and individuals or animals that the person values and is responsible for meeting their basic needs. The third step in the SAFE-T is the suicide inquiry which was accomplished in depth using the CASE Approach. The fourth step is to determine the risk level and intervention. The risk level is categorized in 3 stages, high, moderate, and low. An individual with a high risk factor has several serious risk factors, such as a history of severe psychiatric disorders or an acute precipitating event, such as IPV. This person has possibly one or more plans for a lethal suicide attempt or persistent suicidal ideation. The CASE Approach helps the clinician to know how strong this ideation is, the duration and the plan or plans the person is contemplating. The person with a moderate level of risk, according to SAFE-T has several risk factors, such as a current or past psychiatric disorder, a family history of suicide, or a serious crisis, such as IPV. An individual with a moderate risk has a few protective factors, such as a spiritual belief system or the love of a child that needs parenting. This person has suicidal ideation and has a plan, but no intent to utilize this plan. A person with a low risk of suicide, according to SAFE-T, has a few risk factors, such as an interpersonal stressor, and both internal and external protective factors.[19]

The American Association of Suicidology has a mnemonic to outline the warning signs of impending suicide (**Box 19-1**).

Box 19-1. IS PATH WARM

I Ideation expressed or communication of suicide ideation

S Substance abuse

P Purposelessness

A Anxiety

T Trapped

H Hopelessness

W Withdrawal from friends, family and work/school peers

A Anger

R Recklessness

M Mood Change

Adapted from the American Association of Suicidology.[20]

INTERVENTIONS TO PREVENT SUICIDE

Individuals, who have a high risk level as defined by SAFE-T, are in need of acute psychiatric hospitalization. These individuals may be admitted to the hospital either on a voluntary or an involuntary basis. If the individual is at a high risk for suicidal behavior, the emergency number 911 can be called and the police will take the person to an Emergency Department for assessment for possible hospitalization. While a person is hospitalized, he or she is in a safe, structured milieu with constant monitoring to prevent a suicidal attempt and professional staff to talk to and determine new strategies to use when thinking about the precipitating problems. Hospitalization is an intervention used to prevent eminent suicidal behavior. If the individual is able to safely stay at home overnight, a partial hospitalization program may assist in reducing the suicide drive. Individuals with a moderate level of risk, according to the SAFE-T should develop a list of potential actions to take to prevent a suicide. This list of potential actions to prevent a suicide assists the person with a blueprint of actions to take if the suicidal drive increases. An example of a protective action is teaching the client how to use the Suicide Prevention Hotline at 1-800-273-TALK (8255) if he or she experiences an increase in suicidal thoughts. Another action the person can take is to go to the local Emergency Department for safety and an evaluation if the suicidal drive increases. It is helpful for the individual to attend regular psychotherapy sessions to address the issues that caused the suicidal ideation. Individuals with a low risk level, identified by SAFE-T, generally receive a referral for outpatient psychotherapy and emergency numbers to use if the suicidal ideation increases. All of the assessment data, risk level, and treatment plan need to be documented as the fifth stage of the SAFE-T intervention (See **Table 19-2**).[19]

Table 19-2. SAFE-T Suicide Assessment Five-step Evaluation and Triage

I. Assessment of risks:
   a. Current and past psychiatric disorders
   b. Current key symptoms
   c. Family history of suicide and psychiatric disorders
   d. Current stressors and interpersonal problems that can cause humiliation or shame, such as IPV
   e. Any change in psychiatric treatment
   f. Any access to firearms.

II. Protective factors:
   a. Internal factors:
     1. The ability to problem solve and cope with stress and frustration.
     2. Spiritual beliefs that assist the person during challenging emotional periods.
   b. External factors
     1. Relationships
     2. Support systems
     3. Individuals or animals that the person values and is responsible for meeting their basic needs.

III. Suicide inquiry
   a. The CASE Approach
   b. An in-depth evaluation for suicidal intent
   c. Objective tests, such as the Beck Suicidal Inventory or Suicide Intent Questionaire (SIQ)

(continued)

Table 19-2. SAFE-T Suicide Assessment Five-step Evaluation and Triage *(continued)*	
IV. Determine the suicidal risk level and intervention	a. High: Hospitalization or PHP b. Medium: Develop a list of things to do to prevent an escalation of suicidal drive, including psychotherapy c. Low: Outpatient psychotherapy and emergency numbers

V. Documentation	a. Assessment
	   1. Potentiating risk factors
	   2. Warning signs
	   3. Protective factors
	b. History of suicide attempts
	c. Formulation of risk
	   1. Data from clinical interview
	   2. Use of clinical evaluation tool
	d. Interventions
	e. Client teaching and education

THE GRADY NIA PROJECT

Specific culturally congruent interventions are a powerful means of suicide prevention and safety for an individual experiencing IPV. Researchers at Grady Hospital developed the Grady Nia Project for African American women who have suicidal thoughts and/or attempts and IPV. This intervention has been tested in research and has been demonstrated as being efficacious. The Grady Nia Project consists of ten 90 minute group meetings that are designed with the evidence based interventions guiding the therapy. The first group meeting is an introduction meeting which includes an agreement of safety with the goal of beginning a positive relationship between the participants and the group facilitators. The second group meeting provides information about IPV and suicide. This group discusses the correlation of IPV and suicide in the African American family. Group meetings 4 and 5 explore intrapersonal risk factors for an increase in IPV as well as suicidal ideation and/or behavior. This includes providing education about psychiatric disorders and racial identity issues that co-occur with suicide attempts and IPV. The groups emphasize protective factors, such as coping strategies, problem solving tools, and positive identification with African American women who have overcome adversity and are viewed as role models. The participants are encouraged to develop a philosophy for living and coping. Group meeting 6 works on reducing stress between partners in order to stop the cycle of violence. The women learn their patterns within their own relationship and ways to reduce their risk of injury. The focus of this group is to learn to listen and communicate while setting limits and boundaries to prevent future abuse. If a woman desires to leave their relationship, this session discusses safe ways to do so. Group meeting 7 concentrates on defining social support systems, what to expect from them, and how to ask for help. Meeting 8 assists the women to learn how to secure resources in the community. Community leaders who provide services for women who have been abused and/or suicidal take an active part in teaching the women how to utilize their organizations. Group meeting 9 focuses on obtaining employment and the reduction of depression and suicidal drive. Assistance is given to the women from the community and the participants are encouraged to use role playing to plan ways to call community agencies that can help to secure employment. Meeting 10 is a review of the information from prior meetings and a termination session. This group meeting ends with a party, a certificate of completion and cards with the positive statements from meeting 4 that the women are encouraged to use in the future (see **Table 19-3**).[21]

Table 19-3. The Standard Skeletal Survey

Meeting I	Introduction and commitment to safety
Meeting II	Education about IPV and suicide
Meeting III	Safety planning for IPV and suicidal behavior
Meetings IV and V	Reduce intrapersonal risk factors and enhance intrapersonal protective factors
Meetings VI and VII	Reduce social and situational risk factors, such as relationship problems and interpersonal problem areas
Meetings VIII and IX	Reduce cultural and environmental risk factors and enhance associated protective factors
Meeting X	Review and develop aftercare plans, graduation and feedback

The Grady Nia Project points out important factors to include in interventions with all individuals who have experienced IPV. It is essential to assist the person to develop a sense of empowerment to problem solve the complex situations that may result in suicidal behaviors. It is also necessary to help the individual to identify steps to take to promote personal safety and prevent a suicidal attempt and encourage and assist the individual to identify and enhance protective factors that strengthen the person's positive abilities and hope.

CONCLUSION

Community resources that provide assistance for an individual who has experienced IPV and is suicidal are becoming more readily available. One important program is mental health services that are provided in conjunction with the local Police Department. This has been done in a number of ways. Some Police Departments have a relationship with the local Suicide Hotline, others have teams of Mental Health professionals who either ride with the police or are on call to the department when there is a mental health emergency. Having a relationship between the Police Department and the local crisis response system assists the community in 2 ways. This partnership allows the police to concentrate on crime reduction while the mental health needs are met by professional counselors. The individual receives a thorough mental health evaluation, and the level of care provided matches the person's need. This partnership can reduce unnecessary trips to the emergency department and can offer the individual the appropriate level of care necessary to prevent a suicidal attempt.[22]

The care of the individual who has sustained IPV must include an assessment for suicidal risk. This assessment should be done in a comprehensive manner, sensitive to the person's cultural background and the level of negative self-feelings that occur after an incident of IPV. Interventions ought to be based on the level of risk of death by suicide and the community resources available to facilitate a balanced crisis plan, keeping in mind the individual's family structure as well as the risk for future IPV. Individuals should be encouraged to use the Suicide Hotline 1-800-273-TALK (8255). Reaching out for care should be encouraged in the community's safe houses or shelters as well as the local emergency department.

REFERENCES

1. Centers for Disease Control and Prevention. Intimate partner violence: consequences. Centers for Disease Control and Prevention Web site. http://www.cdc.gov/Violence Prevention/intimatepartnerviolence/consequences.html. Accessed May 10, 2011.

2. Center for Disease Control and Prevention. National violent death reporting system. Centers for Disease Control and Prevention Web site. http://www.cdc.gov/violence prevention/NVDRS/index.html. Retrieved May 10, 2011.

3. Calder J, McVean A, Yang W. History of abuse and current suicidal ideation: results from a population based survey. *J Fam Viol.* 2010;25:205-214.

4. Krysinska K, Lester D, Martin G. Suicidal behavior after a traumatic event. *J Trauma Nurs.* 2009;16:103-111.

5. Kerr DCR, Capaldi DM. Young men's intimate partner violence and relationship functioning: long-term outcomes associated with suicide attempt and aggression in adolescence. *Psychol Med.* 2011;41:759-770.

6. Tilley DS, Rugari SM, Walker CA. Development of violence in men who batter intimate partners: a case study. *J Theory Constr Test.* 2008;12:28-34.

7. Leiner AS, Compton MT, Houry D, Kaslow NJ. Intimate partner violence, psychological distress, and suicidality: a path model using data from African American women seeking care in an urban emergency department. *J Fam Viol.* 2008;23:473-481.

8. Stein DJ, Chiu WT, Hwang I, et al. Cross-national analysis of the associations between traumatic events and suicidal behavior: findings from the WHP World Mental Health Surveys. PlosOne Web site. http://plosone.org/article/info:doi/10.1371/journal.pone.0010574. Published May 13, 2010. Accessed September 23, 2011.

9. Chan KL, Straus MA, Brownridge DA, Tiwari A, Leung WC. Prevalence of dating partner violence and suicidal ideation among male and female university students worlkwide. *J Midwifery Women's Health.* 2008;53(6):529-535.

10. Wong SP, Phillips MP. Nonfatal suicidal behavior among Chinese women who have been physically abused by their male intimate partners. *Suicide Life Threat Behav.* 2009;39:648-659.

11. Crosby AE, Ortega L, Melanson C. *Self-directed Violence Surveillance: Uniform Definitions and Recommended Data Elements.* Atlanta, GA: Centers for Disease Control and Prevention, National Center for Injury Prevention and Control, Division of Violence Prevention; 2011.

12. Chan KL, Yan E, Brownridge DA, Tiwari A, Fong DYT. Childhood sexual abuse associated with dating partner violence and suicidal ideation in a representative household sample in Hong Kong. *J Interpers Violence.* 2011;26:1763-1772.

13. Haarr RN. Suicidality among battered women in Tajikistan. *Violence Against Women.* 2010;16:764-768.

14. Vachher A, Sharma A. Domestic violence against women and their mental health status in a colony in Delhi. *Indian J Community Med.* 2010;35:403-405.

15. Yan FA, Howard DE, Beck KH, Shattuck T, Hallmark-Kerr M. Psychosocial correlates of physical dating violence victimization among Latino early adolescents. *J Interpers Violence.* 2010;25(5):808-831.

16. Chen PH, Rovi S, Vega M, Jacobs A, Johnson MS. Relation of domestic violence to health status among Hispanic women. *J Health Care Poor Underserved.* 2009;20:569-583.

17. Shea SC. Suicide Assessment: Part 1: Uncovering suicidal intent a sophisticated art. *Psychiatric Times.* Psychiatric Times Web site. http://www.psychiatrictimes.com/display/article/10168/1491291. Published December 3, 2009. Accessed May 12, 2011.

18. Shea SC. Suicide Assessment Part 2: Uncovering suicidal intent using the Chronological Assessment of Suicide Events (CASE Approach). *Psychiatric Times.* Psychiatric Times Web site. http://www.psychiatrictimes.com/display/article/10168/1501845.Published December 21, 2009. Accessed May 12, 2011.

19. Suicide Prevention Resource Center. Suicide Assessment Five-step Evaluation and Triage for Mental Health Professionals SAFE-T. Suicide Prevention Resource Center Web site. www.sprc.org/library/safe_t_pcktcrd_edc.pdf. Accessed July 25, 2013.

20. American Association of Suicidology. IS PATH WARM: know the warning signs. American Association of Suicidology Web site. http://www.suicidology.org/stats-and-tools/suicide-warning-signs. Accessed May 5, 2011.

21. Davis SP, Arnette NC, Bethea KS, et al. The Grady Nia Project: a culturally competent intervention for low-income, abused, and suicidal African American women. *Prof Psychol Res Pr.* 2009;40:141-150.

22. Young AT, Fuller J, Riley B. On-scene mental health counseling provided through police departments. *J Ment Health Couns.* 2008;30:345-362.

Chapter 20

Intimate Partner Violence During Pregnancy

Theresa Fay-Hillier, MSN, PMHCNS-BC
Susan Solecki, MSN, FNP-BC, PNP-BC
Paul Thomas Clements, PhD, RN

Key Points

1. It has been estimated that between 9% and 25% of pregnant women experience intimate partner violence (IPV). One in 8 pregnant teenagers reports being physically abused by the father of her baby.

2. Pregnancy itself can be a stressor that can trigger an initial act of violence or heighten pre-existing aggression against a women and her unborn child.

3. There are many characteristics that are common in those who abuse their intimate partners. These include jealousy, controlling behaviors, poor communications skills, and substance abuse.

4. Pregnant women who reported IPV were more likely to report their pregnancies were unintended, had weak support systems and resources, less education, less likely to be married, less likely to be employed, more likely to receive Medicaid, and more likely to use tobacco, drugs, and alcohol.

5. IPV during pregnancy can have a negative impact on the outcome of the pregnancy, including a higher risk of preterm birth and placental abruption. There are often also psychological side effects for the victim of IPV during pregnancy.

6. Health care providers should assess pregnant women for IPV, using the relevant screening tools, and should provide victims of IPV with the necessary support, information, and links to community services.

Introduction

Intimate partner violence (IPV), especially when experienced by pregnant women, is a global public health issue.[1] IPV encompasses actual or threatened physical, psychological, sexual, or economic abuse including emotional degradation, intimidation, and threats from an intimate partner. Additionally, IPV can happen to anyone regardless of race, age, sexual orientation, religion, or gender and affects people of all socioeconomic backgrounds and education levels. IPV occurs in both opposite-sex and same-sex relationships and can happen to intimate partners who are married, living together, or dating.[2] Whether in an emotionally stable partnership or a precarious tenuous relationship, the state of pregnancy itself can be a stressor that can trigger an initial act of violence or heighten pre-existing aggression against a woman and her unborn child.[3,4] Health care providers are uniquely situated to assess, provide advocacy, treatment, and safety for the abused pregnant client and her unborn child or newborn.

INCIDENCE AND PREVALENCE

Women's reproductive health has been identified to have inherent risks for intimate partner violence [IPV].[3-7] Specifically, IPV-related homicide has been determined to be a leading cause of death for women during pregnancy and 1 year postpartum.[5-10] It has been estimated that 9-25% of pregnant women are abused and are at greater risk for the initiation or escalation of violence during pregnancy.[11,12] Further, in a study conducted by Wiemann et al that focused on teen pregnancy, they found that 1 out of every 8 pregnant adolescents stated having been physically assaulted by the father of her baby.[13] In addition to homicide, pregnant women who are abused have been found to be at greater risk for other health related problems including anemia, infections, HIV, first and second trimester bleeding, low birth weight infants, maternal depression, suicide attempts, and substance abuse.[4,14,15]

The impact that IPV has on both the victim and the family also reflects the financial burden placed on the community. It is estimated that 5.3 million victimizations occur each year among women in the US. The result of the abuse is that nearly 2 million are injured and 1300 are murdered. According to the CDC the overall cost of IPV in 1995 exceeded $5.8 billion. The overall cost of IPV was updated to 2003 dollars which resulted in the adjusted figures: the overall cost of IPV exceeded $ 8.3 billion, which included $460 million for rape, $6.2 billion for physical assault, $461 million for stalking, and $1.2 billion in value of lost lives.[16,17]

It has also been noted that children who live in a home where there is IPV are at greater risk of being victims of child abuse.[18-20] IPV is an identified public health issue because of its high incidence and prevalence, which, of course is actually higher than realized due to the ongoing issues related to lack of screening, lack of reporting, and under-reporting.[21] Additionally, children who live in such a chaotic environment, particularly when the mother is once again pregnant, are also at risk for direct abuse from the battering partner. Subsequently, it is imperative that health care providers address the need for enhanced screening and subsequent intervention and referral for pregnant mothers, and any children, relative to IPV.[22]

Health care providers have the opportunity (and responsibility) to provide information about available options (ie, providing abuse support agency numbers, offering social services, legal information) to women they encounter, who are found to be victims of abuse. Health care providers who work with women during their reproductive years are often the only provider who a woman might encounter and it is essential that screening for IPV and appropriate interventions be provided. In direct response to the pandemic levels of IPV, both the American College of Obstetricians and Gynecologists (ACOG) and Women's Health and Education Center (WHEC) recommend routine screening throughout the reproductive years regardless of the health care setting.[23, 24]

Historically, studies that investigated screening for IPV in health care settings found that most health care providers believed that the training needed to confidently screen for IPV was not provided in their education. It was found that such education should include a comprehensive framework that focuses on both theory and practice in addressing the complexity of IPV. Without the appropriate training in the undergraduate and graduate health professions curricula or medical programs, many providers might not screen for IPV, even if provided with universal tools in their practice, due to the lack of foundational educational training to provide support in the development of their screening skills. This includes incorporating specific information on screening in all women's health curricula across disciplines particularly for nurse midwives, obstetricians, and gynecologists.[4,22,25-30]

As noted by Miller and colleagues concerning practices of health care providers in addressing IPV, "less than a third of female adolescent patients were ever screened by a health care provider for experiences of IPV."[31] Studies that interview women about their feedback related to health care provider practices of screening all their patients for abuse identified a majority of the women who participated in the surveys expected to be screened for intimate partner violence. Many women further identified that they would not disclose abuse unless they were asked directly.[32-34] In a survey by Stewart and Cerutti on physical abuse during pregnancy, it was noted that although 24 pregnant women (66.7%) received medical treatment for abuse, only one (2.8%) told the prenatal care provider of her abuse.[35]

Although pregnancy has not been identified as a protective factor against abuse and is a time where health care providers can develop a relationship with their patients, there is a lack of consistent research that has identified either an increase or decrease in disclosure of that abuse during pregnancy.[36,37] Research has consistently presented that women are more likely to disclose abuse to health care providers who have taken the time to develop a trusting relationship as well as the women being in a position to actually disclose the abuse and perhaps make a change.[37-39] An ideal opportunity is provided for the development of a trusting relationship while a woman is pregnant due to the frequent health care appointments throughout the maternity process.

CHARACTERISTICS OF AN ABUSER

Women can be most vulnerable for violence when they are pregnant. The abuser is often known to the pregnant woman and usually is a current partner or one in the past with whom she had an intimate relationship.[40] Stress and frustration over a pregnancy, especially if it is unintended or unwanted, may direct acts of violence by a jealous, insecure partner as a demonstration of power over them.[41,42] Many women who are victims of abuse have identified common characteristics of possessiveness, insecurity, and jealousy in their abusive male partners.[40] The new baby may be perceived as a threat to a man's sense of being the primary person in a family that could monopolize his partner's time and attention.[41,42] Battering is not an isolated incident of a male partner "blowing up," but rather an established set of control skills and coercive behaviors used by a man who abuses his partner and children.[43] The reality is that the perpetrator is not an individual who is out of control, but one who is very much in control.[44] Findings from a large survey by Tjaden and Thoennes also supports this theory that violence perpetrated against women by intimate partners is often part of a systematic pattern of dominance and control.[45] Controlling for socioeconomic characteristics, having a verbally abusive partner was the variable most likely to predict that a woman would be victimized by an intimate partner.

Pregnant victims of violence are more likely to report that their partners engage in patriarchal domineering behavior and engage in attempts to socially isolate them as opposed to those women who do not experience violence during pregnancy.[46] Most abusers were abused themselves or witnessed the abuse of a loved one during their own childhood.[47] Other traits of abusers include substance abuse, aggressive behavior, low self-esteem, difficulty expressing oneself, and a belief in rigid sex role stereotypes with many abusers presenting as extremely seductive, possessive, and manipulative.[47]

The following behaviors have been described as red flag characteristics for abusive partners which can become more pronounced when a women is pregnant (adapted from AARDVARC[44]) (see **Table 20-1**).

Table 20-1. Red Flag Characteristics for Abusive Partners

Low self esteem	— Batterers may appear to be tough, strong, and confident, but more often than not they really suffer from low self-esteem.
	— If emotionally needy, may become dependent on their partner; may feel threatened by potential loss of partner becoming controlling and jealous.
	— Batterer may become jealous of the fetus that the woman is carrying viewing the pregnancy as an added distraction in the dysfunctional relationship (true in heterosexual relationships as well as in gay and lesbian relationships).
	— Male abusers may overcompensate with hyper-masculinity if insecure in the area of their own sex stereotype.
Rushing into relationships	— Many victims date or know their abuser for less than 6 months before they are engaged or living together.
	— Abusers can come on like a whirl-wind claiming "love at first sight," and using flattery such as "you are the only person I could ever talk to" or "I have never felt loved like this by anyone."
	— There is often a progression to an all or nothing approach to the relationship.
	— Abusers often pressure the other partner to commit to a relationship before the victim is truly ready. This information might be helpful for the health care provider to learn during the screening process.
Excessive jealousy	— Abusers often say that jealousy is a sign of love when on the contrary it's a sign of possessiveness and lack of trust.
	— In a healthy relationship, the partners trust each other unless one of them has legitimately done something to break that trust.
	— Jealousy is not always a sign of potential abuse, but when it becomes a disruptive force in a relationship, the jealousy can progress toward increased attempts at controlling and isolating the partner.
	— The batterer may accuse their partner of being unfaithful and question the paternity of the fetus, which can lead toward escalation of anger and violence.
Controlling behavior	— Often at the beginning of a relationship, a batterer will say that controlling behavior is out of concern for the partner's safety.
	— Abusers will be angry if the partner is late coming back from the store or an appointment and might be questioned closely about where she went and who she talked to.
	— As controlling behavior worsens, the abuser may not let the partner make personal decisions about the house, clothing, or even going to church.
	— Abusers may keep all the money or may make the partner ask permission to leave the house.
	— These types of behaviors mimic the parent/child relationship and thus by definition cannot be part of an equal and healthy relationship.

(continued)

Table 20-1. Red Flag Characteristics for Abusive Partners *(continued)*	
Unrealistic expectations or demands	— Abusers often expect their partner to meet all of their needs: the perfect partner, lover, and friend. They say things like "if you love me, I'm all you need and you're all I need." — Abusers may have unnatural or unhealthy expectations of their partner to fulfill all of their emotional, physical, and sometimes economic needs.
Isolate their partner	— Frequently, an abuser tries to cut the partner off from all resources. — If the partner has friends, terms such as "whore," "slut," or "cheater" may be used. — If the partner is close to family, they may be told that they are "tied to the apron strings." — Abusers will accuse supportive people of the victim as causing trouble and may restrict phone use. — Abusers may gradually isolate the partner from all friends and family. — Abusers may not let the partner use a car (or have one that is reliable), and may refrain them from working or going to school. — Sometimes this process can take years and then suddenly a victim looks up and realizes that they've been moved across the country, away from family, friends, and a support system and without a job or resources of their own making them completely isolated and totally dependent on the abuser.
Believe in male supremacy and the stereotyped masculine role in the family	— Abusers are often obsessive about appearing to be the man [or head] of the house and they tend to hold very high and rigid rules about how they get to act because they are the man - often leading them to feel the need to dominate and control and to expect their word and their needs to be catered to at all times, including in the bedroom. — These abusers see the partner as unintelligent, inferior, responsible for menial tasks, and less than whole without the relationship. — They will often tell the partner that no one else would want them or that they are nothing without them. — They will remind the partner of their provider role - everything they have done, thus using guilt and convoluted logic to pressure them to into servile behaviors.
Use force during sex	— Abusers may show little concern about whether the partner wants to have sex and use sulking or anger to manipulate her into giving in to sex. — Abusers may initiate sex while the partner is sleeping with no regards to consent or may demand sex even when the partner is ill or tired. — This behavior reflects that the abuser is just in it for himself and/or is enjoying the power of coercing sex knowing that the partner is less than willing. — The abuser may want to make up after having sex even though it was done with physical or verbal abuse to the partner. Sex under these conditions is just an extension of the power and control exerted by the prior abuse.

(continued)

Table 20-1. Red Flag Characteristics for Abusive Partners *(continued)*

Poor communication skills	— Abusers not only talk with their words, but also with their actions (fists, weapons, punishment, etc).
	— Abusers typically have trouble with discussing emotions, especially very strong ones like anger or frustration.
	— Some male abusers may feel that having feelings and talking out problems goes against the stereotypical role expected of men.
	— Without the skills or self-permission to express himself in constructive ways (ways that feel uncomfortable or a sense of inadequacy) can lead to lashing out with violence.
Use of negative behaviors as coping mechanisms for stress (drugs, alcohol, battering)	— Studies suggest that abusers, in general, have a higher incidence of drug and alcohol abuse than non-abusers.
	— This does not mean that drugs or alcohol cause the abuse, rather it lowers inhibitions making an already frustrated and violence-prone person more likely to fall back on violence as a crutch, especially when confronted with a lack of communication skills and feelings of inadequacy.
Blame others for their actions	— Commonly, abusers use the actions of others as excuses for their own behavior.
	— Abusers often blame the person who made them angry.
	— Statements to the victim may include, for example, "why did you make me do that?"
	— If the abuser is chronically unemployed, he may claim that someone is always doing him wrong or is out to get him.
	— He may make mistakes and then blame the partner for upsetting him.
	— Abusers may make statements to the partner such as "it's your fault" for almost anything that goes wrong.
	— Abusers often see themselves as the victim in the relationship, and do not take responsibility for their own feelings or behaviors.
Hypersensitive	— Abusers are easily insulted taking the slightest setback as a personal attack.
	— Abusers will rant and rave about the injustice of things that are really just a part of living, such as having to get up for work, getting a traffic ticket, or being asked to help with chores.

(continued)

Table 20-1. Red Flag Characteristics for Abusive Partners *(continued)*

Manipulative, deceitful	— Many abusers are also excellent at manipulation causing the most frustration for the victim.
	— Abusers may appear to function well at work, with friends and family, etc.
	— Sometimes only the victim is aware of the true personality of the abuser.
	— This behavior often makes it difficult for a victim to reach out for support from friends and family because those persons may try to talk the victim out of thinking that their partner is abusive.
	— Often friends and family of the victim will go on and on about "what a great partner you've got there"—because the abuser has successfully hidden their violence at home.
	— Frustrating ensues for the victim when members of their support system try to turn the tables and say things like "well, just don't make him/her mad," thereby inappropriately putting the blame on the victim and not on the offender.
	— When this occurs, the violent partner unwittingly gets re-enforcement from the very people the victim needs for support.
Cruelty to animals or children	— Some abusers may punish animals brutally or be insensitive to their pain.
	— Abusers may also expect children to be capable of doing things beyond their ability.
	— Abusers may tease children until they cry.
	— Abusers may be very critical of other people's children, especially any children from a previous relationship.
	— It has been estimated that 60% of people who beat their partner also beat their children.
	— Abuse also models the role of violence to the children as they grow and develop toward forming relationships of their own.

CHARACTERISTICS OF VICTIMIZATION

No matter how positive a woman's situation may be, any woman can potentially be at risk for abuse.[40] Characteristics of IPV victims vary, but research has indicated some consistent common elements of women that may put them at greater risk for experiencing IPV. Increased awareness and enhanced assessment of these facets can promote early identification of the problem and subsequent implementation of proactive measures. The results of a study by Reichenheim et al indicate that knowledge of certain characteristics of pregnant women who seek health care services can alert professionals to those who are potentially at high risk for IPV.[48] For example, variations by maternal age suggest that special attention is required in the pregnant teen population as the highest rate of abuse is found among adolescents.[40] In their study, Leone et al found that pregnant women who reported IPV were more likely to report their pregnancies were unintended, had weak support systems and resources, less education, less likely to be married, less likely to be employed, more likely to receive Medicaid, and more likely to use tobacco, drugs, and alcohol.[49] In a contrasting study, Taylor and Nabors found females who are more highly educated than their male partners are at an increased risk for femicide compared to those women who are not killed.[50] One possible theory for this incompatibility in educational attainment is that men may feel the need to exert dominance over a partner who has achieved greater academic success to compensate for the perceived power differential.

While obtaining a health history and performing a physical exam on the pregnant victim, some characteristic red flags of abuse may be evident including:

— Bruises, abrasions, burns, lacerations often most commonly to the head, abdomen, breasts, neck, genitals, and forearms

— An explanation of the injury that is inconsistent with the type of injury

— A prior history of trauma

— A delay between onset of injury and seeking treatment

— Psychological distress manifested as depression, anxiety, sleep disorders, or suicidal ideation.[40,51]

In one seminal study, abused women were twice as likely to delay access to prenatal care until the third trimester of their pregnancy as women who did not report being in an abusive relationship.[52] Subsequent studies have continued to demonstrate that reluctance to disclose abuse may include shame, embarrassment, fear, and issues related to emotional and economic dependence to their perpetrators.[40,53,54] Health care providers should also be alert for signs of abuse that could be attributed to other physiologic or psychosocial factors such as poor weight gain, malnutrition, preterm labor, low birth weight, anxiety, or depression.[40]

EFFECTS OF INTIMATE PARTNER ABUSE DURING PREGNANCY

Violence affecting pregnant women is a major factor associated with complications in pregnancy.[55] The occurrence of battering in pregnant women occurs more frequently than hypertension, gestational diabetes, or any other antepartum complication.[40] IPV remains one of the leading causes of injury and death in women, with victims of IPV being more likely to report negative physical health effects including poor health status, poor quality of life, and increased use of health care services.[56] Abused pregnant victims recount calamitous acts against them including being choked, kicked, punched, scalded, thrown down stairs, threatened with knives, pushed out of moving cars, and having objects thrown at them.[57] Other injuries experienced as a result of brutality include cuts, bruises, fractures, concussions, persistent head¬aches, dental injuries, stab wounds, and vaginal bleeding.[57] Brownridge et al concur that women who experience violence during pregnancy are twice as likely to be sexually assaulted, 2.9 times more likely to be physically assaulted, 3.5 times more likely to have been hit with something that could cause injury, and 3.7 times more likely to be kicked, bit, or hit with a fist.[46] Research has demonstrated a significant prevalence of sexual assaults with physical IPV culminating in higher associations of morbidities including increased rates of urinary tract infections (UTIs), sexually transmitted infection (STIs), and Human Immunodeficiency Virus (HIV) that can affect maternal and neonatal outcomes.[4,58,59]

Shah and Shaw identified, in a systematic review of 30 studies, significantly increased unadjusted and adjusted odds of low birth weight (LBW), preterm births (PTB), and small for gestational age (SGA) births among infants born to women exposed to IPV compared with those not exposed to IPV.[60] Findings by Leone et al indicate that women who report experiencing IPV during prenatal care have more than 30 times the odds of a clinical diagnosis of pregnancy trauma and approximately 5 times the odds of experiencing placental abruption.[49] Chambliss notes that an estimated 10% of hospitalizations due to injury in pregnancy are a result of intentional injuries inflicted upon the pregnant woman.[61] Campbell identifies a report from the United Kingdom in which 70 out of 295 women who died during pregnancy or within 6 weeks of giving birth had a history of IPV and 19 of those women were murdered.[62]

Women's mental health status has also been demonstrated to be adversely affected by IPV. The Centers for Disease Control and Prevention report that the emotional harm caused from IPV may result in victims experiencing trauma symptoms including flashbacks, panic attacks, and trouble sleeping.[5] In a study by Rose et al on the impact of abuse, many women who had experienced abuse reported higher scores for depression and post-traumatic stress disorder (PTSD).[63] IPV is also linked to unhealthy coping behaviors including smoking, drinking, taking drugs (illicit and/or prescription), or having risky sex.[5] Edin et al state that other than sexual abuse, emotional violence often encompasses and appears to be the worst aspect in abusive relationships.[36] They additionally noted that severe forms of intimidation include threats to shoot the woman, to kill her, or to kidnap the baby. Jaffe notes that 5% of abusive fathers threaten to kill the mother during visitation.[64] Liss and Stahly report that 34% of abusive fathers threaten to kidnap their children with 11% actually abducting them.[65] One study found that 25% of abusive male partners of battered women living in shelters had kidnapped their children, 35% threatened to take the children in a custody action, and used visitation to verbally abuse (25%) or physically abuse (10%) the children's mothers.[65]

At the expense of their mental health, women experiencing IPV during pregnancy and after birth may experience changes in their self-perception with the internalization of repeated negative messages by their abuser, reportedly seeing themselves as nothing.[63]

CYCLE OF VIOLENCE

Not all women who are victims of abuse disclose that there was a specific pattern that they experienced from their abuser, but many women who have been victims of abuse have been able to identify a pattern and process of violent encounters (refer to **Figure 20-1**). The actual violent episodes for many victims are followed by periods of remorse by the abuser. The remorsefulness period is then followed by a slow build-up of tension by the abuser that ultimately leads to another violent episode. As noted by Varcarolis, the abuse is a process that increases in intensity and risk for potentially lethal results over time.[66] The actual abusive cycle was foundationally described by Walker as a Cycle of Violence.[67] The cycle was described as primarily consisting of 3 stages. The first stage in the process is known as the *tension building stage* where there is no actual violence, there is an increase in criticism and annoyance by the abuser toward the victim. As this stage escalates, the victim becomes increasingly aware that with each day, there is an increased risk for a violence episode towards them by their abuser. The next stage in the cycle is the *acute explosive phase.* During the acute explosive phase there is actual violence toward the victim. Usually the length of the violent phase increases over time along with potential life threatening injuries. The *honeymoon phase* is identified to occur between the other stages of abuse and is described as the abuser displaying outward signs of remorse. The abuser might make promises to change and provide gifts to the victim. As

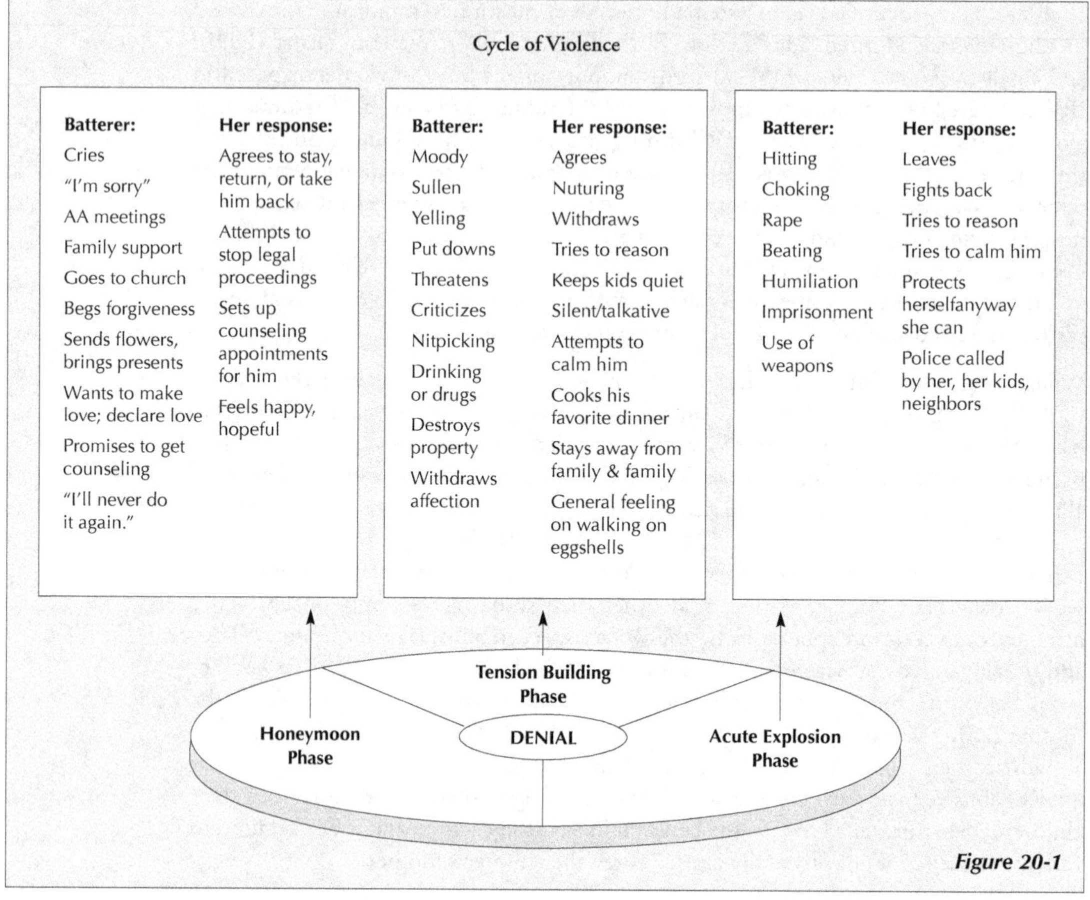

Figure 20-1. *The recurrent behaviors associated in the Cycle of Violence (from Arkansas Coalition Against Domestic Violence).*[68]

the abuse continues, this stage often decreases in length and intensity only to re-enter the cycle with tension building eventually followed by explosive episodes.

A qualitative study examining advanced practice nurses experiences with intimate partner violence by Brykczynski et al identified that a discussion of the cycle of abuse should also include the cycle that many victims encounter as they attempt to leave an abusive relationship.[69] It is not uncommon for victims to return to the abuser for many reasons such as financial or perceived safety issues during the process of ending the abusive relationship. They can also return due to being homeless and due to limited resources not being able to access a shelter.[70,71] As the length of time away from the abusive relationship increases over time, there are victims who can develop a feeling of empowerment that provides them with the needed strength to terminate the abusive relationship.

A woman who is pregnant may be more likely to leave the abusive relationship to protect her unborn child or newborn.[20] Asking if the woman feels safe, and discussing the use of an emergency kit (money, checkbook, important documents, keys, change of clothes, and medications) are foundationally important. At a minimum, all agencies should have referral sources available. The health care provider should also have the contact numbers for the local police department, social services (if available at the site where the woman was screened), and printed material for the patient to read in private.[72]

Johnson discusses 4 different types of intimate partner violence rather than 1 specific pattern to describe abuse.[73] The types of patterns are: *intimate terrorism* (when the abuser includes some or all of physical, economic, or psychological abuse to gain control and power over the victim); ***violent resistant*** (the victim uses violence against abuser to resist the intimate terrorism); ***situational couple violence*** (the violence is usually in response to a specific incident that is not associated with power and control and can be initiated by either partner); ***mutually violent*** (both partners use violence in attempts to intimidate and control). Johnson describes the need to distinguish the types of abuse encountered during the IPV relationship: "With respect to the general importance of distinguishing among types of violence, I [Johnson] believe that they have different causes, different patterns of development, different consequences, and that they require different forms of intervention."[73] Johnson's model could be dovetailed into the assessment process which should necessarily include a systematic process of continually assessing and modifying interventions based on the individual responses of the patient.[73] Clinician inquiry appears to be one of the strongest determinants of communication with patients about partner abuse and it can take up to at least 6 interactions with a health care provider for a woman who is abused to disclose the violence.[74,75] Asking the questions on each visit during pregnancy and for the first year postpartum is based on the fact that pregnancy may be a time for increase violence or when the violence starts.[20] The concept of obtaining the specific experience of the IPV encounter of the victim in describing the violent encounters would support the foundational premise of this, which is individualizing and adapting interventions based on the patient's feedback and response to care.

THE ROLE OF HEALTH CARE

The process of assessment, diagnosis, planning, interventions, and evaluation can be used to structure the health care role in addressing IPV. It is imperative that health care providers address primary, secondary, and tertiary interventions. Assessment of family dynamics is essential to identify risk factors that may promote violence during the adaptation to pregnancy and the addition of a new child.[76] During the prenatal period, health care providers must use opportunities to screen women and their partners for certain physical, psychological, social, and environmental risk factors that could promote IPV.

On a federal level, in 1994, Congress passed the Violence Against Women Act (VAWA) which provided federal dollars to state and local programs to address IPV.[77] In addition, the Joint Commission of Accreditation of Health Care Organizations established the requirement that hospital personnel consistently assess for abuse.[78] Over 1 in 10 women who are victims of violent crimes is a victim of IPV; as such there is a need for health care providers to screen and provide interventions that address the safety of both the victim and other family members.

Based on the fact that IPV during pregnancy increases mortality and health complications, health care practitioners who work directly with pregnant women are obligated to screen for abuse. For example, since women's health care providers are in a position to screen for IPV on a routine basis, having a tool that is interactive and designed to be administered on each visit will assist in consistent screening that denotes continuous caring and works synchronously with the developing relationship between the pregnant woman and the health care provider.

Since pregnant women have the opportunity to be seen by their practitioner at routine visits throughout their pregnancy and postpartum, a screening tool designed to promote interaction between the health care provider and the woman at each visit would be an attribute. Some victims of IPV might be reluctant to share the information about abuse on an initial health visit not because they do not want to share, but rather they might need to witness the consistent professional caring behavior of the practitioner prior to actually sharing information about abuse. Some other barriers to reporting abuse may be shame, embarrassment, or reluctance due to the emotional or economic dependency the victim has with her abuser. Abused women may feel anxious reporting an abusive partner by thinking it may escalate the violence and put themselves or others in their family in further danger.[40]

The trusting relationship can be developed through the engagement during routine visits, a consistent display by the health care professional of being concerned with the woman's health, and using a consistent screening tool that would be repeated at each prenatal visit to promote interactions between the woman and their health care provider.[79,80] The repetition of the assessment may also alert the woman to the importance of reporting IPV and assist her to reflect on her situation. The American College of Obstetricians and Gynecologists[81] and the American Nurses Association[82] have established position papers recommending that women be screened routinely at preconception, family planning, and gynecology visits as well as the first prenatal visit, once per trimester, and at the postpartum checkup.

SCREENING TOOLS FOR IPV

A review of literature of major screening tools for IPV that were used in practice was sponsored by the Centers for Disease Control and completed by Basilel and Hertz.[83] Each tool was evaluated for several key factors which included: the characteristic of the scale, the population that it was developed, and the psychometric properties. The tools were divided into Intimate Partner Violence and Sexual Violence. Thirty-four IPV screening tools were identified and 14 for Sexual Violence (SV). The process of examining the screening tools by the authors of this study was based on the following criteria:

— The tool will be used with pregnant women and, should screen for both Intimate Partner Violence (IPV) and Sexual Violence (SV) Abuse.

— It should be administered by a clinician to encourage interaction between the clinician and the patient,

— Contain guidelines for the clinician in reference to the process of screening and interventions that could be offered to the woman if she is identified as being a victim of abuse.[83]

Of the 48 screening tools evaluated, only 1, the Abuse Assessment Screen (AAS) was specifically designed to be used with pregnant women, screening for both IPV and SV, and provides some guidelines that can be used for clinicians.

The Abuse Assessment Screen (AAS) was developed by McFarlane et al to screen for physical, emotional, and sexual abuse of women by their intimate partners.[52] The definition of abuse by the developers of the AAS "as having been hit, slapped, kicked, or otherwise physically hurt by someone."[84] The objective of the AAS model is that the screening process should be collaborative between the woman being screened and the health care provider. Health care practitioners who use the AAS are encouraged to use the tool on each visit. The AAS consists of 5 questions or items. The first 3 questions focus on the frequency and severity of the abuse as well as on the identification of the perpetrator. The woman being screened is asked to provide a number from 1 to 6 to rate the frequency and severity of the abuse. The fourth question focuses on the extent of sexual abuse, and the fifth question focuses on emotional abuse. The health care provider interviewing the patient uses the questions to screen for abuse. If the woman shares that she is a victim of physical abuse, the woman is given a body map of a pregnant woman to document the location of areas on the body that were targets of the assaults.[84-86] The AAS includes a protocol that consist of seven specific guidelines to be followed throughout the screening process. The steps start with the actual setting that should be used to administer the tool (private without children or spouse) and ends with possible interventions based on the results of the screening.

There are 3 general IPV screening tools that have been noted to be sound in both reliability and validity. They are also frequently used by researchers to establish the validity of new or revised tools. The tools are the Conflict Tactics Scale (CTS), the Index of Spouse Abuse Scale (ISA), and the Danger Assessment Screen (DAS). All 3 of these tools were used for validity analysis of the Abuse Assessment Tool (AAS).[52,84]

The CTS was developed by Murray Straus in 1972 who stated the following:

It measures both the extent to which partners in an intimate relationship engage in psychological and physical attacks on each other and also their reasoning and negotiation to deal with conflicts....Conflict theory was used as the framework to develop the tool. The theory assumes that conflict is an inevitable part of all human associations, whereas violence as a tactic to deal with conflict is not.... The CTS measures the extent to which specific tactics, including acts of physical violence, have been used.[87]

The tool was also designed to be given to both partners to evaluate each of their behaviors in the relationship.[87,88] As noted by McFarlane et al:

The CTS is a 19 item scale that measures the use of 'reasoning, verbal aggression and violence' tactics to settle differences between spouses and partners within the past year. Items are weighted in accord with the frequencies indicated by the response categories presented to the respondent, and 4 frequencies weighted subcale scores are computed: Reasoning, Verbal Aggression, Minor Violence, and Severe Violence.[52(p198)]

The validity and reliability of the CTS have been supported and tested through hundreds of studies that have used the CTS when performing both research and for clinical practice. Content validity was obtained through qualitative interviews and reviews by expert clinicians. Construct validity has been consistently supported through hundreds of studies that have found that there is a positive correlation between the CTS scores and independent studies that examine related to IPV violence. The theoretical findings in research support the scores measured by the CTS. Some of the risk factors that have been consistently identified as risk factors such as inequality between partners, poverty, unemployment, stress, and isolation from either community or family support are measured by the CTS. The reliability for the CTS has been measured through both internal consistency and test-retest correlations. Based on 41 studies that measured internal consistency reliability of the CTS, the alpha coefficient mean was found to be 0.77. The results from the few studies that actually completed a test-retest reliability measure were, the overall mean of the coefficients for the studies to be 0.72.[84] The tool can be helpful for a therapist for on-going therapy, research as the gold standard when developing another tool, or perhaps in mental health facilities as an initial screening tool in the development of the treatment process. It appears to be very useful for health care professionals whose primary focus is not on the treatment of mental health issues. However, CTS can be complicated to score and does not provide the clear documentation needed by victims of abuse who are seeking legal options in reference to the objective signs of physical abuse that were reported and observed during the interview.

The next tool which was evaluated was the ISA. The ISA is a 30-item summated scale designed for use in clinical settings that is written at a high school reading level. The 30-items on the ISA are organized into 2 subscales that assess 2 forms of abuse: physical (11 items) and nonphysical violence (19 items).[84,89,90] The tool is completed by answering all of the items using a scale from 1 (never) to 5 (very frequently). Each item on the scale represents varying degrees of abuse. After all answers are completed, there are 2 scores that are computed: 1 score is known as the ISA-P score that measures the severity of physical abuse and the other is known as the ISA-NP score which measures the severity of non-physical abuse. The scores on both scales range from 0-100.[92]

The internal reliability of the ISA was noted to be measured in 2 studies with both results having a coefficient alpha reliability of over 0.90.[84,90] Several studies were completed in the initial development of the tool to test validity. "A principal component factor analysis procedure with a varimax rotation was used to confirm the two dimensions of the ISA that were designed to measure physical and nonphysical abuse. Factors with eigenvalues of 1 or higher were selected for the tool".[91] Construct validity was measured by testing the ISA against clinical interviews in 2 studies.[52,90] The ISA is not designed to be interactive and does not provide guidelines to the health care provider in reference to interventions for victims identified as being abused. The tool does not provide the clear documentation needed by victims of abuse when seeking legal options in reference to the objective signs of physical abuse that were reported and observed during the interview. Based on the noted deficits of the tool, this author would not recommend that this tool be used as a routine screening tool.

Another tool that has been used by health care providers is the Danger Assessment (DA) Screen. The DA was developed by Campbell in 1981 and was designed to be self-administered and assist women who have been identified as being abused determine their potential danger of homicide.[50] The DA is divided into 2 parts. In the first part of the scale the woman is provided with a calendar that is used to assess the severity and frequency of the battering over the past year. The woman is asked to mark the days when physical abuse occurred and then rank the severity of the abuse using a scale of 1 (a slap or pushing where there was no visible physical injury) to 5 (use of a weapon). The calendar was used as a tool to provide concrete documentation for the abused woman about the severity of the abuse and hopefully decrease the minimization of the abuse that is often seen when attempting to provide interventions to the woman.[92,93] The second part of the scale is a 15-item yes/no response that is associated with intimate partner homicide. It takes approximately 20 minutes to complete the entire form. The DA is scored by counting up the "yes" responses with no noted cut score. After counting up the positive items or "risk factors" the health care provider reviews them with the respondent. The goal is that the respondent will use the information in making choices that would decrease her risk of homicide.[94]

Content validity of the original tool was supported through consultation with women who were abused, shelter workers, law enforcement officials, and clinical experts in working with intimate partner violence.[92,95] Several studies have measured and reported internal consistency reliability that ranged from 0.60 to 0.86.[96-98] The initial study to measure the test-retest reliability on 9 participants out of the original 30 in the study one week after the first test was found to have a Pearson's r was determined to be 0.97.[94] This scale is best used by health providers who work in mental health or in clinical areas where an on-going patient-provider relationship exists. Health care providers who work with pregnant women might find this tool useful after a woman admits to being in an abusive relationship and she is reluctant to discuss any available options. This tool takes at least 20 minutes to complete and therefore might not be practical in all health care settings.

Another foundational process that has been used in health care settings but was not specifically designed for pregnant women is a tool identified as RADAR. The name of the screening tool is an acronym that stands for the following: (1) Routinely inquire about present and past violence; (2) Ask direct questions about the abuse; (3) Document the findings using direct quotes and specific descriptions of any physical injuries; (4) Assess the victim for current safety; and (5) Review available options to the victim as well as provide appropriate resources and referrals. This screening tool has been found to support health care providers in screening and for abuse and structuring interventions that support the safety and autonomy of the patient.[27,99,100]

As noted by Rodríguez et al in reference to the active involvement and skill of the clinician in screening for IPV, clinician inquiry appears to be one of the strongest determinants of communication with patients about partner abuse.[75] Other factors that need to be addressed include patient perceptions regarding clinicians' time and interest in discussing abuse, fear of police or court involvement, and patient concerns about confidentiality. Screening is only the first step; having appropriate interventions directly attached to the screening tool is imperative in order to promote the health of the pregnant woman and her fetus. As noted by Moracco and Cole, health care providers who screen for abuse should also provide interventions that provide for social and community support in order to prevent further abuse.[101]

Health care providers are also in a position to support any legal action that a victim elects to seek by carefully documenting any identified physical and psychological findings. In one observational study by Kendall and colleagues, patients who were screened and provided with referrals found that "legal assistance and/or law enforcement were considered the most beneficial resource referral."[102] An example of the impact documentation can have on supporting the victim of IPV is noted by Laughon et al, by revising the Abuse Assessment Screening Tool (which screens for IPV) to include documentation of episodes of non-lethal strangulation.[85] One of the reasons for the modification was so that it can be used by women who elect to pursue criminal charges. The impact of the documentation of health care providers in reference to nonlethal strangulation has been noted to change charges against abusers who have attempted to strangle their partner during an abusive episode from a misdemeanor to a felony charge.[103]

Providing victims who report abuse with empathetic and supportive responses is the first step in the development of a trusting and effective relationship. After abuse is disclosed, health care providers should assess for safety and current danger. Interventions should include information about safety which includes informing the women, particularly when she elects to return home, that when violence is imminent to avoid the kitchen and bathrooms, packing a bag, and disclosing the abuse to a trusted relative or friend who can assist with supporting an escape if necessary.[100]

Health care providers should be aware of local, statewide, and national victim assistance numbers that they can provide during the encounter with the victim. As noted in the seminal work by Fishwick in the development of interventions for women who disclose abuse:

It is essential to understand that an 'effective response' is not synonymous with 'fixing the problem.' Women who disclose abuse are not expecting or wanting their problem to be solved for them...The most important interventions include the provision of emotional support, safety assessment, accurate information, and links to community services that focus on the myriad needs of women in abusive relationships.[104]

Additionally, health care educators are encouraged to incorporate assessing for IPV during child-bearing years into undergraduate and graduate curricula in order to improve implementation of early interventions to increase the safety of victims.[4,27] Brykczynski et al in their qualitative study further supported the need for health care education to include more consistent training in both the assessment and interventions of victims of violence.[69] The reluctance of health care professionals to ask directly about IPV and the hesitation of abused women to disclose spontaneously that they are in a harmful relationship or "keeping up a front" during antenatal care visits may result in the lack of identification of those pregnant women who are at risk for negative consequences to themselves and their children.[36,105-107]

CONCLUSION

Multiple challenges present themselves in the ongoing efforts to thwart IPV in pregnant women. Ongoing research for effective strategies to prevent, identify, and intervene for pregnant victims of IPV is warranted to expand knowledge and resources against this devastating social abhorrence. Pregnant women experiencing abuse necessitate the care of health care providers whose mission is to advocate for a health care system that will detect, protect, and treat those individuals most vulnerable to this harmful threat to maternal and infant health.

RESOURCES

— **Rape, Abuse and Incest National Network. The Online Hotline.**
http://www.rainn.org/get-help/national-sexual-assault-online-hotline

— **Rape, Abuse and Incest National Network. Search for a Local Crisis Center.**
http://centers.rainn.org/

— **US Department of Justice. Violence against women: Local resources by state.**
http://www.ovw.usdoj.gov/statedomestic.htm

— **US Department of Health and Human Services. Tips for Domestic Violence A-Z**
http://healthfinder.gov/scripts/SearchContext.asp?topic=253

— **The Danger Assessment. The Institute for Johns Hopkins Nursing.**
http://www.dangerassessment.org

REFERENCES

1. World Health Organization. Violence against women. World Health Organization Web site. http://www.who.int/mediacentre/factsheets/fs239/en/. Pubished 2011.

2. Unites States Department of Justice. Domestic Violence. The United States Department of Justice Web site. http://www.ovw.usdoj.gov/domviolence.htm. Published 2011.

3. Centers for Disease Control and Prevention. Intimate partner violence during pregnancy: a guide for clinicians. Centers for Disease Control and Prevention Web site. http://www.cdc.gov/reproductivehealth/violence/IntimatePartnerViolence/. Published 2009.

4. Tufts KA, Clements PT, Wessell J. When intimate partner violence against women and HIV collide: challenges for health care assessment and intervention. *J Forensic Nurs.* 2010;6(2):66-73.

5. Centers for Disease Control and Prevention. Understanding intimate partner violence fact sheet. Centers for Disease Control and Prevention Web site. http://www.cdc.gov/violenceprevention/pdf/IPV_factsheet-a.pdf. Published 2009. Accessed July 17, 2013.

6. Martin SL, Harris-Britt A, Li Y, Moracco KE, Kupper LL, Campbell JC. Changes in intimate partner violence during pregnancy. *J Fam Violence.* 2004;19(4):201-210.

7. National Association of County and City Health Officials. Intimate partner violence among pregnant and parenting women: local health department strategies for assessment, intervention and prevention. National Association of County and City Health Officials Web site. www.naccho.org/topics/HPDP/mch/upload/IPV-Issue-Brief-6-11-08.pdf. Published 2008.

8. Chang J, Berg CJ, Saltzman LE, Herndon J. Homicide: a leading cause of injury deaths among pregnant and postpartum women in the United States, 1991–1999. *Am J Public Health.* 2005;95(3):471–7.

9. McFarlane J, Parker B, Moran B. *Abuse During Pregnancy: A Protocol for Prevention and Intervention.* 3rd ed. White Plains, NY: March of Dimes; 2007.

10. Campbell J, Webster D, Koziol-McLain J, et al. Risk factors for femicide in abusive relationships: results from a multisite case control study. *Am J Public Health.* 2003;93(7):1089-1097.

11. Martin S, Mackie L, Kupper L, Buescher P, Moracco K. Physical abuse of women before, during, and after pregnancy. *JAMA.* 2001;285:1581-1584.

12. Schoening AM, Greenwood JL, McNichols JA, Heermann JA, Agrawal S. Effect of an intimate partner violence educational program on the attitudes of nurses. *J Obstet Gynecol Neonatal Nurs.* 2004;33(5):572-579.

13. Wiemann CM, Agurcia CA, Berenson AB, Volk RJ, Rickert VI. Pregnant adolescents: experiences and behaviors associated with physical assault by an intimate partner. *Matern Child Health J.* 2000;4(2):93-101.

14. Dunn LL, Oths KS. Prenatal predictors of intimate partner abuse. *J Obstet Gynecol Neonatal Nurs.* 2004;33(1):54-63.

15. Family Violence Prevention Fund. *National Consensus Guidelines: On Identifying and Responding to Domestic Violence Victimization in Health Care Settings.* 2nd ed. San Francisco, CA: Family Violence Prevention Fund; 2004.

16. Centers for Disease Control and Prevention. Intimate partner violence: consequences/cost to society. Centers for Disease Control and Prevention Web site. http://www.cdc.gov/violenceprevention/intimatepartnerviolence/consequences.html. Published 2012.

17. Max W, Rice D, Finkelstein E, Bardwell BA, Leadbetter S. The economic toll of intimate partner violence against women in the United States. *Violence Vict.* 2004;19(3):259-272.

18. Children's Defense Fund. Children who witness domestic violence. Children's Defense Fund Web site. http://cdf.childrensdefense.org/site/DocServer/children-who-witness-domestic-violence-ohio.pdf?docID=9961. Published 2009.

19. Lemmey D, McFarlane J, Wilson P, Malecha A. Intimate partner violence: mothers' perspectives of effects on their children. *Matern Child Nurs.* 2001;26(2):98-103.

20. Watts N. Screening for domestic violence: a team approach for maternal/newborn nurse. *AWHONN Lifelines.* 2004;8(3):210-219.

21. Goodman PE. Intimate partner violence and pregnancy. In: Mitchell C, Anglin D, eds. *Intimate Partner Violence: A Health-Based Perspective.* New York, NY: Oxford University Press; 2009:253-264.

22. Tufts KA, Clements PT, Karlowicz KA. Integrating intimate partner violence content across curricula: developing a new generation of nurse educators. *Nurse Educ Today.* 2009;29(1):40-7.

23. American College of Obstetricians and Gynecologist (ACOG). IPV screening encouraged in OB/Gyn clinical settings. Family Violence Preventio Program Web site. http://xnet.kp.org/domesticviolence/news/ipv_screening.html. Published, 2013.

24. Women's Health and Education Center (WHEC). Domestic violence: screening and interventions. Women's Health and Education Center Web site. http://www.womenshealthsection.com/content/vaw/vaw012.php3. Published June 2010. Accessed July 17, 2013.

25. American College of Obstetricians and Gynecologists (ACOG). Special issues in women's health: intimate partner violence and domestic violence. Washington, DC: American College of Obstetricians and Gynecologists: 2005.

26. Bailey B. Partner violence during pregnancy: prevalence, effects, screening, and management. *Int J Women's Health.* 2010;2,183-197.

27. Clements PT, Holt KE, Hasson CM, Fay-Hillier T. Enhancing assessment of interpersonal violence (IPV) pregnancy-related homicide risk within nursing curricula. *J Forensic Nurs.* 2011;7(4):195-202.

28. Hinderliter D, Dougherty AS, Delaney K, Pitula C, Campbell J. The effect of intimate partner violence education on nurse practitioners' feelings of competence and ability to screen patients. *J Nurs Educ.* 2003;42(10):449-454.

29. Lapidus G, Cooke MB, Gelven E, Sherman K, Duncan M, Banco L. A statewide survey of domestic violence screening behaviors among pediatricians and family physicians. *Arch Pediatr Adolesc Med.* 2002;156:332-336.

30. Women's Health and Education Center (WHEC). Domestic violence during pregnancy. Women's Health and Education Center Web site. http://www.womenshealthsection.com/content/vaw/vaw011.php3. Published 2011.

31. Miller E, Decker MR, Raj A, Reed E, Marable D, Silverman JG. Intimate partner violence and health care-seeking patterns among female users of urban adolescent clinics. *Matern Child Health J.* 2010;14:901-917.

32. Caralis PV, Musialowski R. Women's experiences with domestic violence and their attitudes and expectations regarding medical care of abuse victims. *South Med J.* 1997;90(11):1075-1080.

33. Duncan MM, McIntosh PA, Stayton CD, Hall CB. Individualized performance feedback to increase prenatal domestic violence screening. *Matern Child Health J.* 2006;10:443-449.

34. Messinger AM, Davidson LL, Rickert VI. IPV among adolescent reproductive health patients: the role of relationship communication. *J Interpers Violence.* 2011;26(9):1851-1867.

35. Stewart DE, Cerutti A. Physical abuse in pregnancy. *CMA.* 1993;19(9):1257-1263.

36. Edin KE, Dahlgren L, Lalos A, Högberg U. Pregnancy, and antenatal care, "Keeping Up a Front:" narratives about intimate partner violence. *Violence Against Women.* 2010;16: 189.

37. Feder GS, Hutson M, Ramsay J, Taket AR. Women exposed to intimate partner violence: expectations and experiences when they encounter health care professionals: a meta-analysis of qualitative studies. *Arch Intern Med.* 2006;166:22-37.

38. Ramsay J, Richardson J, Carter YH, Davidson LL, Feder G. Should health professionals screen women for domestic violence? Systemic review. *BMJ.* 2002;325:314-318.

39. Wathen CN, MacMillian. Interventions for violence against women: scientific review. *JAMA*. 2003;289:589-600.

40. Giardino ER, Aggeles TB. Uncovering abuse in the pregnant woman. Nurse. com Web site. http://ce.nurse.com/ce205-60/uncovering-abuse-in-the-pregnant-woman-2/coursepage/. Published 2013. Accessed July 13, 2013.

41. Bacchus L, Mezey G, Bewley S. A qualitative exploration of the nature of domestic violence in pregnancy. *Violence Against Women*. 2006;12(6):588-604.

42. Campbell JC, Oliver C, Bullock L. Why battering during pregnancy? *AWHONN'S Clin Issues Perinat Womens Health Nurs*. 1993;4:343-349.

43. Stark E. *Coercive control: How Men Entrap Women in Personal Life*. New York, NY: Oxford University Press; 2007.

44. Abuse, Rape and Domestic Violence Aid and Resource Collection. Abusers, Batterers, Domestic Violence Offenders. An Abuse, Rape, Domestic Violence Aid and Resource Collection Web site. http://www.aardvarc.org/dv/batterer.shtml. Published 2011.

45. Tjaden P, Thoennes N. Extent, nature, and consequences of intimate partner violence: findings from the National Violence Against Women Survey. National Institute of Justice and The Centers for Disease Control and Prevention. Nations Institute of Justice Web site. http://www.ojp.usdoj.gov/nij/pubs-sum/181867.htm. Published July 2000. Accessed July 12, 2011.

46. Brownridge DA, Taillieu TL, Tyler KA, Tiwari A, Chan KL, Santos SC. Pregnancy and intimate partner violence: risk factors, severity, and health effects. *Violence Against Women*. 2011;17:858.

47. Schwartz MR. When closeness breeds cruelty: helping victims of intimate partner violence. *American Nurse Today*. 2007;2(6). American Nurse Today Web site. http://www.americannursetoday.com/article.aspx?id=4676&fid=4662.

48. Reichenheim ME, Patricio TF, Moraes CL. Detecting intimate partner violence during pregnancy: awareness-raising indicators for use by primary health care professionals. *Public Health*. 2008;122:716–724.

49. Leone JM, Lane SD, Koumans EH, et al. Effects of intimate partner violence on pregnancy trauma and placental abruption. *J Women's Health*. 2010;19(8): 1501-1509. Doi: 10.1089/jwh.2009.1716.

50. Taylor R, Nabors EL. Pink or blue…black and blue? examining pregnancy as a predictor of intimate partner violence and femicide. *Violence Against Women*. 2009;15(11):1273-1293.

51. King MC, Ryan J. Woman abuse: the role of nurse-midwives in assessment. *J Nurse Midwifery*. 1996;41(6):436-441.

52. McFarlane J, Parker B, Soeken K, Bullock L. Assessing for abuse during pregnancy: severity and frequency of injuries and associated entry into prenatal care. *JAMA*. 1992;267(23):3176-3178.

53. Brookoff D, O'Brien KK, Cook CS et al. Characteristics of participants in domestic violence: assessment at the scene of domestic assault. *JAMA*. 1997;277(17):1369-1373.

54. Wright RJ, Wright RO, Isaac NE. Response to battered mothers in the pediatric emergency department: a call for an interdisciplinary approach to family violence. *Pediatrics*. 1997;99(2):186-192.

55. Hockenberry M, Wilson D. *Wong's Nursing Care of Infants and Children*. 9th ed. St. Louis, MO: Elsevier; 2011.

56. Campbell JC. Health consequences of intimate partner violence. *Lancet*. 2002;359:1331-1336.

57. Bacchus L, Mezey G, Bewley S. A qualitative exploration of the nature of domes¬tic violence in pregnancy. *Violence Against Women*. 2006;12:588-604.

58. McFarlane J, Malecha A, Watson K, et al. Intimate partner sexual assault against women: frequency, health consequences, and treatment outcomes. *Obstet Gynecol*. 2005;105:99-108.

59. Silverman JG, Decker MR, Reed E, Raj A. Intimate partner violence victimization prior to and during pregnancy among women residing in 26 U.S. states: associations with maternal and neonatal health. *Am J Obstet Gynecol*. 2006;195:140–8.

60. Shah P, Shah J. Maternal exposure to domestic violence and pregnancy and birth outcomes: a systematic review and meta-analyses. *J Women's Health*. 2010;19(11):2017-2031.

61. Chambliss LR. Intimate partner violence and its implication for pregnancy. *Clin Obstet Gynecol*. 2008;51:385-397.

62. Campbell D. A question of maternal health. *World of Ir Nurs Midwifery*. 2010;18(9):53-55.

63. Rose L, Alhusen J, Bhandari S, et al. Impact of intimate partner violence on pregnant women's mental health: mental distress and mental strength. *Issues in Ment Health Nurs*. 2010;31:103-111.

64. Jaffe PG. Children of domestic violence: special challenges in custody and visitation dispute resolution. In: Carter J, Hart B, Hostler C, eds. *Domestic Violence and Children: Resolving Custody and Visitation Disputes, A National Judicial Curriculum*. San Francisco, CA: The Family Violence Prevention Fund; 1995:19-30.

65. Liss MB, Stahly GB. Domestic violence and child custody. In: Hensen M, Hawaway N, eds. *Battering and Family Therapy: A Feminist Perspective*. Newbury Park, CA: Sage Publications; 1993:181-183.

66. Varcarolis EM. *Essentials of Psychiatric Mental Health Nursing: A Communication Approach to Evidence-Based Care*. 2nd Edition. St. Louis, MO; Elsevier; 2013:409.

67. Walker L. *The Battered Women*. New York, NY: Harper & Row; 1979.

68. Power and control wheel. Arkansas Coalition Against Domestic Violence Web site. http://www.domesticpeace.com/ed_wheel.html. Published 2011. Accessed July 17, 2013.

69. Brykczynski KA, Crane P, Medina CK, Pedraza D. Intimate partner violence: advanced practice nurses clinical stories of success and challenge. *J American Acad Nurse Pract*. 2011;23:143-152.

70. National Coalition for the Homeless. Domestic violence and homelessness. National Coalition for the Homeless Web site. http://www.nationalhomeless.org/factsheets/domestic.html. Published 2009. Accessed July 17, 2013.

71. National Network to End Domestic Violence (NNEDV). Domestic Violence Counts 12: A 24-Hour Census of Domestic Violence Shelters and Services Across the United States. Washington, DC: National Network to End Domestic Violence; 2012. National Network to End Domestic Violence Web site. http://www.nnedv. org/downloads/Census/DVCounts2012/DVCounts12_NatlReport_Color.pdf.

72. Pennsylvania Coalition Against Domestic Violence. Report of the Pennsylvania domestic violence task force. Pennsylvania Coalition Against Domestic Violence Web site. http://www.pcadv.org/Resources/s_00273.pdf. Published 2010.

73. Johnson MP. Conflict and control: gender symmetry and asymmetry in domestic violence. *Violence Against Women.* 2006;12:1003-1018.

74. Mayer B. Female domestic violence victims: perspectives on emergency care. *Nurs Sci Q.* 2000;13:340-346.

75. Rodríguez MA, Sheldon WR, Bauer HM, Pérez-Stable EJ. The factors associated with disclosure of intimate partner abuse to clinicians. *J Fam Pract.* 2001;50(4):338-44.

76. Hagan JF, Shaw JS, Duncan PM, eds. *Bright Futures: Guidelines for Health Supervision of Infants, Children, and Adolescents.* 3rd ed. Elk Grove Village, IL: American Academy of Pediatrics; 2008.

77. United States Department of Justice: Office on Violence Against Women. About the Office on Violence against Women. United States Department of Justice Web site. http://www.ovw.usdoj.gov/docs/about-ovw-factsheet.pdf. Accessed July 17, 2013.

78. Joint Commission on Accreditation of Health Care Organizations. *Accreditation manual for hospitals. Volume -Standards.* Oakbrook Terrace, IL; 1992.

79. Anderson BA, Marshak HH, Hebbeler DL. Identifying intimate partner violence at entry to prenatal care: clustering routine clinical information. *J Midwifery Women's Health.* 2002:47(5):353-359.

80. McFarlane J, Soeken K, Wiist W. An evaluation of interventions to decrease intimate partner violence to pregnant women. *Public Health Nurs.* 2000;17(6):443-451.

81. American College of Obstetricians and Gynecologist (ACOG). *Domestic violence (ACOG Technical Bulletin).* Washington, DC: ACOG; 1995.

82. American Nurses Association. *Position statement on physical violence against women.* Washington, DC: ANA; 1991.

83. Basilel KC, Hertz MF. Intimate partner violence and sexual violence victimization assessment instruments for use in health care settings. Centers for Disease Control and Prevention. Centers for Disease Control Web site. http://www.cdc.gov/ncipc/ pub-res/images/ipvandsvscreening.pdf. Published 2007.

84. Soeken KL, McFarlane J, Parker B, Lominack MC. The abuse assessment screen: a clinical instrument to measure frequency, severity, and perpetrator of abuse against women. In: Campbell JC, ed. *Empowering Survivors of Abuse: Health Care for Battered Women and Their Children.* Thousand Oaks, CA: Sage; 1998:195-203.

85. Laughon K, Renker P, Glass N, Parker B. Revision of the abuse assessment screen to address nonlethal strangulation. *J Obstet Gynecol Neonatal Nurs.* 2008;37(4):502-507.

86. Renker P. Physical abuse, social support, self-care, and pregnancy outcomes of older adolescents. *J Obstet Gynecol Neonatal Nurs.* 1999;28(4):377-388.

87. Straus MA, Hamby SL, Boney-McCoy S, Sugarman DB. The revised conflict tactics scales (CTS2): development and preliminary psychometric data. *J Fam Issues.* 1996;17(3):283-316

88. Straus MA. Conflict tactics scales. In: Jackson NA, ed. *Encyclopedia of domestic violence.* New York, NY: Routledge; 2007:190-197.

89. Cook SL, Conrad L, Bender M, Kaslow NJ. The internal validity of the index of spouse abuse in African American women. *Violence and Victims.* 2003;18(6):641-657.

90. Hudson W, McIntosh S. The index of spouse abuse: two quantifiable dimensions. *J Marriage Fam.* 1981;43:873-888.

91. Campbell D, Campbell J, King C, Parker B, Ryan J. The reliability and factor structure of the index of spouse abuse with African American women. *Violence and Victims.* 1994;9(30):259-274.

92. Campbell JC. Misogyny and homicide of women. *Adv Nurs Sci.* 1981;3:67-85.

93. Ferraro KJ, Johnson JM. How women experience battering: the process of victimization. *Soc Probl.* 1983;30:325-339.

94. Stuart EP, Campbell JC. Assessment of patterns of dangerousness with battered women. *Issues in Ment Health Nurs.* 1989;10(3-4):245-260.

95. Browne A. *Battered Women Who Kill.* New York, NY: Free Press; 1987.

96. Campbell JC. Nursing assessment for risk of homicide with battered women. *Adv Nurs Sci.* 1986;8:36-51.

97. McFarlane J, Parker B, Soeken K. Abuse during pregnancy: associations with maternal health and infant birth weight. *Nurs Res.* 1996;45(1):37-42.

98. McFarlane J, Parker B, Soeken K, Silva C, Reed, S. Research exchange: severity of abuse before and during pregnancy for African American, Hispanic, and Anglo women. *J Nurse-Midwifery.* 1999;44(2):139-144.

99. Alpert EJ, Fred KM, Park CC, Patel JC, Sovak MA. Partner violence: how to recognize and treat victims of abuse. Waltham, MA: Massachusetts Medical Society; 1992.

100. Griffin M, Koss M. Clinical screening and intervention in cases of partner violence. *Online J Issues in Nurs.* 2002;7(1).

101. Moracco KE, Cole TB. Preventing intimate partner violence: screening is not enough. *JAMA.* 2009;302(5):568-70.

102. Kendall J, Pelucio M, Casaletto J, et al. Impact of emergency department intimate partner violence intervention. *J Interpers Violence.* 2009;24(2):280-306.

103. Strack GB, McClane GE, Hawley D. A review of 300 attempted strangulation cases part 1: criminal legal issues. *J Emerg Med.* 2001;21(3):303-309.

104. Fishwick NJ. Assessment of women for partner abuse. *J Obstet Gynecol Neonatal Nurs.* 1998;27:661-670.

105. Edin KE, Hogberg U. Violence against pregnant women will remain hidden as long as no direct questions are asked. *Midwifery.* 2002;18:268-278.

106. Peterson R, Moracco KE, Goldstein KM, Clark KA. Moving beyond disclosure: women's perspectives on barriers and motivators to seeking assistance for intimate partner violence. *Women's Health.* 2004;40:63-76.

107. Plichta SB. Interactions between victims of intimate partner violence against women and the health care system: policy and practice implications. *Trauma Violence Abuse.* 2007;8:226-239.

Chapter 21

The Continuum of Intimate Partner Violence and Child Maltreatment: Definitions, Epidemiology, and Health Consequences

Megan H. Bair-Merritt, MD, MSCE
Jonathan D. Thackeray, MD

Key Points

1. It has been estimated that, in 2009, 9.3 per 1000 children in the US were victims of maltreatment. Over three quarters of this maltreatment took the form of neglect, while 18% of these children were victims of physical abuse.

2. 15 million children a year in the US witness intimate partner violence (IPV), with half of these witnessing severe IPV, such as beatings or violence involving a weapon.

3. Co-occurrence rates of IPV and child maltreatment have been estimated at about 30% to 60%.

4. Both IPV and child maltreatment are risk factors for poor physical and emotional health.

5. Pediatric professionals should seek to identify children who are exposed to IPV or who are abused, and must report any suspected cases of child maltreatment to Child Protective Services. Requirements for reporting childhood exposure to IPV vary by State, such that providers should learn that particular State's laws.

Introduction

In response to the World Health Assembly's 1996 declaration that violence is a leading public health problem, the World Health Organization developed a 'typology' of violence to characterize the various forms of violence and the connections between them.[1] The proposed typology divides violence into 3 broad categories according to characteristics of those committing the violent act: self-directed violence, collective violence, and interpersonal violence. These 3 categories are further subdivided to reflect more specific types of violence. Self-directed violence is subdivided into suicidal behaviors and actions and self-abuse, such as self-mutilation. Collective violence is divided into social, political, and economic violence. Interpersonal violence is subdivided into community violence and family and intimate partner violence (IPV). Community violence includes violence between individuals who are unrelated and generally takes place outside of the home, while family violence and IPV are defined as violence that occurs "largely between family members and intimate partners, usually, though not exclusively, taking place in the home" and includes child and elder maltreatment.[1] This classification of family violence takes into account the nature of the violent act, the relevance of the setting, and the relationship between the perpetrator and the victim. It is also in accordance with how most would see family violence in its broadest sense—an umbrella term that incorporates child maltreatment, IPV, sibling violence, and elder maltreatment.[2]

Despite the World Health Organization's conceptualization of family violence,[1] researchers have long disagreed about standard definitions. This lack of consensus on how to define family violence, IPV, and child maltreatment limits uniform collection and analysis of data and likely accounts for the wide range of published estimates of violence incidence and prevalence. Is a violent act, for example, only an act that includes the use of physical force? For an act to be considered violent, must it result in injury or death?

Research in the field of IPV demonstrates inconsistencies with respect to what constitutes violence and who represents an intimate partner. Specifically, early IPV research focused only on physical acts of aggression against women with no mention of emotional abuse, sexual abuse, or consideration for male victims.[2] In an effort to promote consistency in the use of terminology and data collection related to IPV, the National Center for Injury Prevention and Control and the Centers for Disease Control and Prevention (CDC) produced recommendations in 1999.[3] In this recommendation, IPV is defined as "a pattern of coercive behaviors that may include repeated battering and injury, psychological abuse, sexual assault, progressive social isolation, deprivation, and intimidation. These behaviors are perpetrated by someone who is or was involved in an intimate relationship with the victim," a category defined by the CDC as current, divorced, or separated spouses (including common-law), and current or former dating or non-marital partners, irrespective of gender, history of sexual involvement, or cohabitation status.[3]

Likewise, consistent definitions of child maltreatment are lacking, and legal definitions may differ from those used in medical care and research. Child maltreatment is broadly defined by the World Health Organization as "all forms of physical or emotional ill-treatment, sexual abuse, neglect or negligent treatment or commercial or other exploitation, resulting in actual or potential harm to the child's health, survival, development or dignity in the context of a relationship of responsibility, trust, or power."[4] While it is generally accepted that child maltreatment is comprised of physical abuse, sexual abuse, neglect, and emotional abuse, universally accepted definitions for each of these subtypes do not exist.[5]

EPIDEMIOLOGY OF CHILD MALTREATMENT AND CHILDHOOD EXPOSURE TO IPV

CHILD MALTREATMENT

The Child Abuse Prevention and Treatment Act (CAPTA), enacted in 1974, was the first piece of federal legislation to focus specifically on child abuse and neglect. Although each state currently has its own definition of child maltreatment, CAPTA sets a minimum federal definition; states must meet this minimum definition to receive CAPTA-related funding. CAPTA has been amended numerous times with 1988 and 1996 amendments specifying that the Department of Health and Human Services (DHHS) should establish a national database of Child Protective Services (CPS) reports. States receiving federal CAPTA dollars must provide information about CPS reports to this database, known as the National Child Abuse and Neglect Data System (NCANDS).

Based on 2009 data from national CPS reports, the Administration of Children and Families estimated that 9.3 per 1000 children in the United States were victims of maltreatment.[6] The majority of reports were for neglect (78%), with physical abuse (~18%) the second most common form of maltreatment. Boys and girls were almost equally affected; children less than 1 year had the highest rates of victimization at 20.6 per 1000 children.[6]

The federal government also tracks statistics about child maltreatment through the National Incidence Study (NIS) of Child Abuse and Neglect. The goal of NIS is to conduct a needs assessment for child maltreatment. Therefore, in contrast to NCANDS, NIS gathers information not only from CPS reports but also from community professionals who encounter children and families and who are mandated reporters of child abuse.[7] Using data from 2005-2006, NIS-4 found that overall rates of child maltreatment were lower than in NIS from prior years. NIS-4 estimated that 17 in 1000 (or 1 in 58) children were abused or neglected, as defined by an act instigated by a caregiver leading to demonstrable harm.[7] A higher rate of children (1 in 25) was endangered, meaning that they were either directly harmed or put into danger as a result of child maltreatment.[7]

CHILDHOOD IPV EXPOSURE

Textbooks and research publications frequently cite that "between 3.3 and 10 million children are exposed to IPV each year."[8] These numbers are likely inaccurate, however, because they are extrapolated from 1970s and 1980s surveys of families that were designed to measure the frequency of IPV and not child exposure to IPV.[8] Likely more precise prevalence estimates can be gleaned from a study that sought specifically to determine national prevalence of childhood IPV exposure through a random-digit dialing telephone survey.[8] This study estimated that 15 million children in the United States are exposed to IPV each year, with almost half of these 15 million children being exposed to severe IPV such as parents beating each other, or violence involving a knife or gun.[8] The 2008 National Children's Exposure to Violence Survey (NCEVS) sponsored by the Department of Justice and Center for Disease Control and Prevention is a second rigorous study that likely better reflects prevalence of childhood IPV exposure.[9] The NCEVS estimated that 1 in 10 children witness family assault each year.

Rates of IPV are disproportionately high in families with a child less than 5 years of age.[10] Higher rates in these families may relate to younger women, who have higher risk of IPV than older women, having younger children, or to the stressors of caring for an infant or toddler. Children less than 5 years are more likely than older children to directly witness IPV; though, when IPV is occurring, children of all ages often are in the same room or overhear the violence from an adjacent room.[11] Although studies looking at the relationship between race/ethnicity and childhood IPV exposure are limited, one study using statewide Department of Health surveillance data found that Latino and African American children were more likely than White children to be present at a police-reported IPV incident.[12]

CHILD MALTREATMENT AND IPV

IPV and child maltreatment commonly co-occur in the same families. Systematic reviews and meta-analyses have suggested a range of frequencies of overlap between the 2 forms of family violence.[13,14] Edleson reviewed over 30 studies and reported that co-occurrence rates of IPV and child physical abuse were between 30 and 60%.[13] A similar review by Appel reported co-occurrence ranging from 10% to 100%, with a median overlap of 40% for clinical samples including families involved with CPS and families living in IPV shelters.[14] Rates of overlap in community-based samples were lower, though still notable. Studies included in these 2 reviews had a wide range of percentages for co-occurrence; differences in percentages were likely related to differences in study methodologies including who was included in the sample population and how each form of violence was defined.

Men who use IPV are more likely than men who do not use IPV to threaten and perpetrate child physical and sexual abuse.[15,16] However, emerging research suggests that, when there is co-occurrence between IPV and child physical abuse, most often there is not a single perpetrator of both the IPV and the child maltreatment. More commonly, both parents are using physical aggression in their relationship, and one or both are abusive to the child.[17,18] Further study would be helpful to confirm the most common patterns of perpetration in families with multiple types of violence.

Early studies of overlap, including the ones in Edleson and Appel's reviews, focused predominantly on the co-occurrence of physical aggression between partners and physical child abuse.[13,14] Increasingly, however, evidence supports that psychological abuse between partners also increases risk for child maltreatment. For example, a study conducted by Chang and colleagues emphasized that risk of physical and emotional child maltreatment is higher not only in families in which there is physical abuse between adult partners, but also in families in which there is inter-parental emotional abuse; rates of neglect increased when there was male-perpetrated psychological IPV.[19]

Additionally, IPV increases risk for multiple types of aggression directed toward the child. Analysis of telephone survey data from a two-state population-based sample found that in homes where the mother reported IPV, there was increased risk for all forms (ie, physical, sexual, and emotional abuse as well as neglect) of child maltreatment.[20] In a random sampling of state CPS data, IPV was present in 1 out of every 5 cases of all cases referred for investigation and almost half of all cases assigned a high level of investigation.[21] Finally, when parents engage in mutual IPV, the odds of using corporal punishment almost double.[22]

When IPV and child maltreatment co-occur, some research suggests that IPV commonly precedes the child maltreatment. Because of this research, the American Academy of Pediatrics has stated that "intervening on behalf of an abused mother may be one of the most effective means by which to prevent child abuse."[23] One study, for example, found that the risk of child maltreatment significantly increased if there was IPV within the first 6 months of the child's life; when IPV occurred within this time period, children had over 3 times the risk of physical child abuse and 2 times the risk of emotional abuse by their fifth year.[24] When IPV is occurring, certain risk factors, including young maternal age, poverty, lower parental education, and lack of religious beliefs may increase risk of future child maltreatment.[25] The risk of child maltreatment also increases significantly as the number of acts of past year IPV increases.[18] Maternal separation from her partner and high levels of maternal support, in contrast, may buffer the increased risk of child maltreatment in families with IPV.[25]

In families with both IPV and child maltreatment, IPV increases the risk of continued, serious child maltreatment. Specifically, in families reported to CPS for possible child maltreatment, risk of re-report and child placement into foster care doubles within an 18-month period if there is co-occurring IPV.[26,27] IPV also increases the risk of child abuse-related fatalities,[26] and rates of child sexual abuse are higher in homes in which IPV is occurring.

When IPV is occurring within a family, children also may be injured during incidents of IPV. Younger children, in particular, can be injured if they are in a parent's arms when the violence begins. Older children commonly try to "get in the middle" of a fight to stop the violence, and may therefore be injured.[28] Anonymous interviews with 111 abused women in 4 US cities found that over a third of women stated that their child was unintentionally injured during an IPV episode, while one quarter reported that their partner had intentionally hurt their child when their child had tried to intervene.[29] Latino children were at greatest risk for both unintentional and intentional injuries.[29] Additionally, Latina women in this study were the most likely, and African American women least likely, to be injured by their partner when they were trying to protect their child from injury.[29]

THEORIES EXPLAINING CO-OCCURRENCE OF CHILD MALTREATMENT AND IPV

Explanations of co-occurrence generally focus on characteristics of individuals or of families. Within the field of IPV, researchers have examined individual profiles of men who batter and have established typologies based on the severity and frequency of violence, the degree to which the violence is familial only versus extra-familial and the presence of psychopathology or personality disorders.[30] If a violent family member has a personality disorder, or general problem handling anger with a tendency to use violence, the person may use violence both with his partner and with his child. Individuals who tend to use violence across relationships also often engage in substance abuse or have mental health issues. A second explanation, focusing on the family, posits that when families experience significant stress, risk of IPV and child maltreatment both increase. This explanation is supported by the fact that rates of IPV and child maltreatment may be disproportionately high in socioeconomically disadvantaged families and in families experiencing multiple stressors.[31] A final theory, entitled the *spillover hypothesis*, states that one form of family violence sets the stage, or "spills over" to the other. For example, the anger experienced by a parent during an IPV episode gets directed toward the child.[17] Alternatively, women experiencing abuse are dealing with significant stress; this stress may translate into a limited capacity to handle the challenges of parenting, and increase risk for child maltreatment.

TOXIC STRESS AND IMPACT ON CHILDREN'S ANATOMY AND PHYSIOLOGY

The interplay between stressful stimuli, such as child maltreatment or exposure to IPV, and a person's subsequent physical and emotional health is complex. An expanding body of evidence indicates that IPV exposure, child maltreatment, and other adverse experiences, individually and collectively, are independent risk factors for poor physical and emotional health. Some studies suggest the ramifications of early childhood trauma are "dose-dependent,"[32,33] and children who experience chronic maltreatment or multiple forms of victimization have poorer outcomes.[34-37]

The effects of stress are evident in brain development early in life. Emphasizing this relationship, Shonkoff established the term *toxic stress* to refer to significant childhood stressors that impact neurophysiology.[38] By definition, toxic stress is chronic, uncontrollable to the child, and occurs without the support of a primary caregiver.[38] Child maltreatment and exposure to IPV are both toxic stressors; abused and IPV-exposed children commonly live with significant fear and anxiety. Chronic fear and anxiety affect health by dysregulating neuroendocrine function and altering brain architecture.

Explaining the developmental neurobiology of childhood stress and trauma, Teicher and colleagues describe the brain as a dynamic organ frequently in a state of flux during childhood.[39] The developing neonatal brain contains 2 to 3 times the amount of neurons seen in adulthood, and in a process largely influenced by corticosteroid levels, approximately half of these undergo cell death before birth. Production of new neurons ceases at this time in most areas of the brain, with the exception of the hippocampal dentate gyrus. During the first several years of childhood, there is myelination of fiber tracts and a resultant rapid increase in brain mass. Similar to the neonatal overproduction of neurons, at this time a marked overproduction and rapid growth of dendrites, axons, and synapses is seen.

These elements are then "pruned back" to varying degrees based on the age of the child, gender of the child, location within the brain, and additional genetic factors. It has been proposed that this happens because the brain overproduces the necessary elements during childhood to allow for maximization of information intake and skill acquisition. As the child develops, redundancies in the system are removed to improve efficiency and reduce metabolic demands – what Jacobson terms "neuronal modification by selective depletion."[40] As Teicher describes the process: "Genes dictate the basic architecture, but there is insufficient genetic information to detail the specific wiring. The final form and connection patterns are sculpted by experience."[39] In other words, the brain remodels itself in response to what it has experienced.

This process of remodeling has been studied extensively in the context of child response to toxic stress. An illustrative example is the "fight or flight" response mounted repeatedly in children exposed to maltreatment or IPV. This response is adaptive in urgent situations - the proverbial running away from the bear. However, repeatedly activating this stress response leads to pathologic changes, including alterations in the hypothalamic-pituitary-adrenal (HPA) axis, an area known to be strongly regulated by social environment.

Cortisol secretion typically exhibits a diurnal rhythm, with levels high at awakening, a peak shortly after awakening, and a drop throughout the course of the afternoon; cortisol also is secreted during times of stress (reactivity). Maltreated children demonstrate alterations in diurnal cortisol and cortisol reactivity. Patterns of disruption of cortisol vary based on factors such as the type and timing of the abuse. Maltreated children often demonstrate exaggerated cortisol responses, which are particularly notable early in the day, although blunted reactivity and diurnal patterns have also been noted.[41]

A small number of studies have measured cortisol in IPV-exposed children. Saltzmann and colleagues obtained random cortisol samples on IPV-exposed children and on non-IPV exposed children seeking care in a mental health center and found that IPV-exposed children had higher levels of cortisol.[42] Linares was interested in how different types of maltreatment differentially affected diurnal cortisol. In a population of children in foster care, the authors found that 80% of children with abnormal diurnal cortisol patterns had been IPV-exposed as compared to ~15% with normal cortisol patterns.[43] Finally, in a longitudinal study of children from infancy to 24 months, Hibel, et al., determined that IPV exposure was related to increased cortisol reactivity at 24 months. Interestingly, interaction with a sensitive mother buffered children from this reactivity.[44]

Altered cortisol levels then impact brain development and architecture. Animal studies demonstrate that developing rats subjected to stressors (prolonged maternal separation, for example) experience overproduction of ACTH and cortisol.[45] Exposure to varying levels of these stress hormones has direct impact on the development of specific areas of the brain, including those areas which house functions related to memory (hippocampus); behavior (amygdala); and attention, cognition, and affect (cerebellar vermis).

Child Maltreatment, Intimate Partner Violence, and Health

Felitti and colleagues were among the first to report the association between adverse childhood experiences and adult disease outcomes. The Adverse Childhood Experience (ACE) studies enrolled over 15 000 adults participating in a health maintenance organization.[46] The participants were surveyed about their health and questioned specifically about adverse childhood experiences, including childhood psychological, physical or sexual abuse, violence against the mother, or living with household members who were substance abusers, mentally ill or suicidal, or had been imprisoned. Felitti, et al., demonstrated that a graded relationship exists between the number of adverse childhood experiences and the risk of having multiple diseases as an adult, including hypertension, obesity, and depression.[46] Additional sub-analyses have identified associations between adverse childhood experiences with onset of smoking at an earlier age and heavier smoking,[22] risk of attempted suicide, sexually-transmitted infection, and high-risk sexual behaviors.[47-49] Additionally, exposure to an abused mother independently increased odds of alcoholism, drug use, and depression.[50,51]

Much of the work of Felitti, et al., evaluates the cumulative effect of multiple adverse experiences on adult physical health. Additional research, which is summarized below, has further attempted to isolate the specific associations between child maltreatment or exposure to IPV on child and adult physical, social, and emotional health.

Physical Health

IPV Exposure

Four population-based empirical studies have linked IPV exposure to higher incidence and prevalence of asthma.[52-55] Interestingly, one study of asthma incidence reported that while odds of developing asthma increased for IPV-exposed children, this increase in developing asthma was buffered when there was an engaged, positive mother-child relationship.[52] Additionally, when children are exposed to chronic IPV during infancy and preschool, they have 80% increased odds of becoming obese by 5 years of age.[56] International studies report that IPV exposure is associated with excessive child morbidity and mortality.[57] A study of families in India found increased child mortality in homes with IPV; in Bangladesh, children of mothers experiencing IPV had higher rates of acute respiratory infections and diarrhea than children of mothers not experiencing IPV.[58]

Child Maltreatment

Recent studies have begun to examine the link between child abuse and physical health consequences for children throughout their lives (see **Table 21-1**). Analysis of data from a longitudinal study of over 6000 children demonstrated that children with a history of reported maltreatment had a 74 to 100% higher risk of hospital treatment for asthma, cardio-respiratory and non-sexually transmitted infection than children without reported maltreatment.[35] The authors also documented that multiple reports for maltreatment predicted a higher number of admissions for hospital care.[35] These deleterious effects on physical health persist into adulthood. Springer and colleagues, for example, found that adults who self-reported physical abuse as a child had higher odds ratios of asthma, high blood pressure, liver disease and ulcers as compared to adults who did not experience childhood physical abuse.[59] Those who were physically abused as children also reported a significantly higher frequency of cardiopulmonary symptoms, constitutional symptoms, and musculoskeletal symptoms than the cohort who had not experienced physical abuse. Additional research suggests a strong correlation between child maltreatment and chronic pain syndromes, such as fibromyalgia.[60] Two recent meta-analyses explored the relationship between child maltreatment and adult health and reinforce the strong influence of childhood abuse on poor physical health as an adult.[61,62]

SOCIAL-EMOTIONAL HEALTH

IPV Exposure

Infants exposed to IPV are more likely than non-exposed infants to demonstrate signs of trauma. For example, IPV-exposed infants have more frequent crying, dysregulated sleep and feeding patterns, and difficulties responding to adults. Infants form attachment relationships with primary caregivers. When IPV is occurring, there is increased risk of insecure attachments and exposed infants can be irritable and difficult to soothe. Infant symptoms are particularly pronounced when their mothers are experiencing

Table 21-1. Effects of Childhood IPV Exposure and Child Maltreatment

Infants and toddlers	— Difficulty with caregiver attachment relationships
	— Excessive crying
	— Poor sleep hygiene
	— Dysregulated feeding patterns
	— Irritable and difficult to soothe
	— Separation anxiety
	— Developmental delay, particularly language
	— Aggression with peers
	— Tantrums
	— Lower rates of well-child visits
	— Higher likelihood of under-immunization
	— Higher rates of emergency department visits
	— Increased risk of developing asthma
	— Increased risk of obesity
	— Post-traumatic stress disorder (PTSD)
School age	— Aggression with peers (externalizing problems)
	— Anxiety and depression (internalizing problems)
	— Learning difficulties including truancy and suspension from school
	— Higher rates of emergency department visits
	— Higher rates of hospitalization
	— PTSD
Adolescence	— Need to assume "parental" roles
	— Higher rates of entering into intimate relationship with dating violence
	— Higher rates of substance use
	— Increased sexually risky behavior
	— PTSD

post-traumatic stress symptoms as a result of the abuse.[63] IPV exposure during infancy may impact the child's social and emotional health through compromising attachment or through inconsistent parenting.

Toddlers must learn self-regulation and achieve social competence. Achieving these developmental milestones, however, may be difficult in the face of IPV. Compared to peers, toddlers who are exposed to IPV are more likely to have nightmares and have excessive separation anxiety. IPV-exposed children learn that it is acceptable to use violence and intimidation to resolve conflict and control others, and that it is acceptable to blame the victim; children may model this behavior with their peers. Children in homes with male-perpetrated IPV also may internalize gendered stereotypes including the message that women are inferior to men.[64] Some literature also suggests that IPV exposure is associated with delayed language and social development. For example, Graham-Bermann studied the verbal abilities of 87 pre-school-age children compared to national norms using the Wechsler Preschool and Primary Scale of Intelligence. She found that IPV-exposed children had significantly lower verbal sub-scale scores.[11] In a twin study, Koenen found that IPV-exposed 5 year old children had average IQs that were 8 points lower than non-exposed children.[65]

When IPV is occurring, school-aged children commonly worry about their own and their families' safety. School-age children who have been exposed to IPV display both internalizing (depression and anxiety) and externalizing (aggression and inattention) disorders at higher rates than non-IPV exposed children.[66] Some research suggests that the magnitude of IPV effect on social-emotional health differs by race, with White children more likely to exhibit externalizing symptoms than African American children.[67] School age children exposed to IPV are twice as likely as their peers to be suspended from school and 1.5 times as likely to be truant.[68] They also have higher rates of school nurse visits for injuries, social and emotional concerns, and alcohol or drug assessments.[68]

Adolescents who live in homes with IPV may be inappropriately required to take on a "parental" role, offering support and care-giving to the parent experiencing the abuse or to younger children. Batterers may also inappropriately use adolescents as confidants, sometimes in an attempt to manipulate or bias the child. This early requirement of heightened familial responsibility may have an adverse impact on emotional health. IPV-exposed adolescents also often enter into their own dating relationships with violence; in particular, boys exposed to IPV are more likely than those not exposed to perpetrate IPV while IPV-exposed girls are more likely to be abused.[69] They engage in risk-taking behaviors, including risky sexual practices and substance abuse at higher rates than their peers.[70]

Child Maltreatment

Children who have experienced personal maltreatment are more likely to exhibit internalizing behaviors, including depression and anxiety, as well as externalizing behaviors, such as rule-breaking behaviors and attention disorders.[71,72] These children are more likely to be aggressive and have difficulty establishing and maintaining peer relationships.[73,74] Post-traumatic stress disorder (PTSD) is another common mental health outcome for children who have experienced maltreatment.[75] In one retrospective cohort study, odds were five times more likely that a child who had experienced abuse would carry the diagnosis of PTSD one year out from the event.[76]

Adults who have experienced childhood maltreatment are more likely to manifest antisocial behaviors.[77] Additionally, self-reported histories of childhood sexual abuse are associated with significant mental health problems seen in adults. In fact, both sexual and physical abuse, independently and collectively, have been associated with common mental health disorders, such as depression,[33,59] suicidal ideation,[51] anxiety,[59,77] and eating disorders.[33] In 2001, Molnar and colleagues published analysis of data from the National Comorbidity Survey, a nationally representative study of nearly 6000 participants.[78] Female adults who had experienced childhood sexual abuse were more likely to have depression (odds ratio 1.8), dysthymia (odds ratio 1.9) or mania (odds ratio 9.1) as compared to controls. Women in this study were also more likely to manifest anxiety disorders, including panic attacks and social phobias. The authors concluded that a history of childhood sexual abuse was significantly associated with 14 various mood, substance use, and anxiety disorders in women and 5 such disorders in men.[78]

HEALTH CARE UTILIZATION

IPV Exposure

Patterns of health care use are altered in children exposed to IPV. Specifically, compared to children not exposed to IPV, children exposed to IPV are less likely to have the recommended 5 well-child visits during the first year of life.[79] Mothers experiencing abuse trust their child's doctor less, and tend to give him or her less favorable overall ratings.[79] IPV-exposed children are, however, more likely to have visits to the emergency department and to mental health providers, and they cost health plans ~17% more than non-exposed children.[80,81]

Child Maltreatment

Given the link between childhood maltreatment and adult health adversity, it should not be surprising that health care utilization and costs are significantly greater among those who have experienced abuse as a child.[82] In an attempt to quantify health care use and costs among abused children, Tang and colleagues examined the relationship between childhood maltreatment and health care utilization.[83] Analyzing self-reported health care utilization and self-reported histories of childhood maltreatment, the authors concluded that having a history of sexual and physical abuse nearly doubled the mean annual ambulatory health care costs as compared to women without history of these abuses.[83] In an effort to quantify actual health care expenditures in relation to specific types of maltreatment, Bonomi and colleagues randomly sampled and interviewed over 3000 women participating in a group insurance and health services plan.[36] Health care utilization, including visits to primary, specialty, urgent, and behavioral health care, the emergency department and the hospital, and use of pharmacy, laboratory, and radiology services were analyzed. Women were asked to self-report a history of childhood physical abuse, sexual abuse, combined abuse, or no abuse. The authors report significantly higher annual health care utilization for women with a history of child abuse. Adjusted annual health care costs were found to be 36% higher for women with both abuse types as compared to women without any history of abuse. Work by Lanier, et al., suggests that these and other previous reports of health care utilization may represent significant underestimates as they do not take into account the burden of child health care issues.[35]

"DOUBLE WHAMMY": HEALTH IMPACT OF
CO-OCCURRING IPV & CHILD MALTREATMENT ON HEALTH

In 1988, Hughes referred to child maltreatment and IPV-exposure as a "double whammy" for children's health.[84] In this study, Hughes reported that rates of behavioral problems were higher for abused children who were also IPV-exposed as compared to children who were only IPV exposed.[84] Literature on the health effects of concurrent IPV and child maltreatment subsequent to Hughes's study is limited, but suggests that experiencing both forms of family violence is more detrimental to children than experiencing only one. There is not enough empirical data, however, to know whether the risk of adverse outcomes when both forms of violence are occurring is additive or multiplicative.[85]

Similar to Hughes, O'Keefe found among a population of children in IPV shelters that children who were abused themselves had higher rates of behavioral problems than non-abused children.[86] Kernic examined internalizing and externalizing behaviors for IPV-exposed children and for IPV-exposed and maltreated children.[66] Children with both forms of family violence had higher risk of both internalizing and externalizing behaviors. In a meta-analysis, Wolfe examined 4 studies that compared outcomes for children exposed to IPV as compared to children who were exposed and who were victims themselves.[87] These 4 studies indicated that children experiencing both forms of violence had worse outcomes than children who were only maltreated.[87]

Increasing rates of health problems for children who are personally maltreated and are exposed to IPV may be related to higher accumulated levels of toxic stress. Additionally, children living in homes with both types of violence learn from multiple dyadic relationships within the family that violence is an acceptable means by which to resolve conflict, and this message may be more powerfully reinforced than in families with only one form of violence.[86] Finally, families with both forms of violence generally display more maladaptive functioning, and this maladaptive functioning may be responsible for higher rates of poor child outcomes.[26]

RESPONSE TO CO-OCCURRING IPV AND CHILD MALTREATMENT WITHIN PEDIATRICS

As described above, childhood exposure to IPV has potentially devastating effects on a child's development and health that may last the entirety of the child's life. In much the same way that pediatric providers advocate for children by discussing appropriate sleep positioning, car seat safety, and benefits of vaccination, providers who provide care for children are obligated to identify and address issues of IPV whenever possible. Physicians often cite inadequate time, discomfort in discussing sensitive issues with the family, or inadequate knowledge of the dynamics of IPV as barriers to addressing IPV with the family.[88] These barriers, while real, should not dissuade the pediatric provider from identifying violence and subsequently intervening on behalf of the child and the caregiver.

Ideally, the pediatric provider should develop an action plan or protocol to guide response when IPV is identified in a child's life. Knowledge of and coordination with local resources such as victim advocacy groups, shelters, and social services is critical. Free resources are available through Futures Without Violence.[89] The American Medical Association and The American Academy of Pediatrics have each published a clinical report to provide health care providers with specific guidance in rendering this type of care.[23,90] Pediatric providers should maintain an awareness of personal, systemic and cultural barriers that may prevent a caregiver from wanting to discuss IPV. Women experiencing abuse also may be reluctant to discuss IPV, given that American society remains largely patriarchal – women who disclose IPV may encounter providers who usurp their decision-making power, and systems (eg, police, courts, etc.) that do not provide adequate support and protection. An appreciation for the unique dangers related to IPV disclosure is necessary, and provision of educational information and recommendations for ongoing care should be tailored accordingly. A supportive and protective atmosphere should be provided to both the child and the caregiver at all times.

Above all else, the pediatric provider must determine if the child is at risk for harm from living in an environment in which he or she is exposed to IPV or child maltreatment. This determination should involve inquiry about direct injury to the child, an assessment of potential for danger, questioning regarding presence of drugs or weapons in the home, an assessment of the caregiver's strengths and supports and the ability to provide adequately for the child's safety, and a careful, unclothed physical exam. Additionally, family courts may not understand the increased risk for abuse so careful examination and documentation is essential. If the pediatric provider is concerned that the child is being abused or is at risk due to IPV exposure, then a report to CPS is legally mandated. Of note, in some states all childhood IPV exposure requires a CPS report regardless of the pediatrician's risk assessment; providers therefore need to know their states' reporting requirements. Providers should stay actively involved after making a CPS referral to help advocate for the non-abusing parent and child throughout the process. While the experience of CPS involvement is difficult for all families, some research suggests that women of color may face particular biases and challenges.[91]

CPS agencies vary in their response to a report of child exposure to IPV or to a report of co-occurring IPV and child maltreatment. Some CPS agencies have well-developed protocols for responding to childhood IPV exposure or co-occurring IPV and child maltreatment, while other agencies face continual budgetary and staffing constraints that may limit their ability to respond to these cases. In 1999, for example, the state of Minnesota redefined exposure to IPV as a reportable form of child maltreatment.[92] This legislative change obligated mandated reporters to report children suspected of having witnessed IPV to child protective services or local law enforcement. Almost immediately, many counties experienced a 50 to 100% increase in reports to CPS agencies and an estimated $30 million expansion of services to accommodate the increased volume of reports. The Minnesota legislature repealed the change the following year.

If the pediatric provider is not practicing in a state with mandated reporting of childhood IPV exposure and determines that the exposure does not rise to a level of reportable harm and there is no immediate concern for the child's well-being, he or she should continue to provide support and avoid judgment of the caregiver. The impact of exposure to IPV should be discussed and referrals to voluntary care, including mental health referrals for the child, should be offered. The attitude and behaviors of the caregiver experiencing IPV have been described using a transtheoretical ("Stages of Change") model and knowledge of this may help health care providers appropriately re-address the issue at subsequent visits.[93]

CONCLUSION

The study of the frequency, co-occurrence, and outcomes of both child maltreatment and IPV represents an evolving field of research. Although establishment and use of standardized definitions will allow for more precise measurement of incidence and prevalence of each, it is clear that the 2 share many risk factors and are often intertwined. The interplay between each of these stressful stimuli and a person's subsequent physical, emotional, and mental health is complex. A growing body of literature demonstrates that child abuse and IPV, both individually and collectively, have adverse effects on the well-being of the child. These adversities carry forward into adulthood and are associated with increased utilization of health care resources and many of the leading causes of human morbidity and mortality. Although the child protective system response may vary from location to location, the health care provider should consistently address these issues of maltreatment proactively, honestly, and supportively.

REFERENCES

1. Krug EG, Dahlberg LL, Mercy JA, Zwi AB, Lozano R. World report on violence and health. World Health Organization Web site. http://www.who.int/violence_injury_prevention/violence/world_report/en/introduction.pdf. Published 2002. Accessed March 26, 2013.

2. Straus M, Gelles R, Steinmetz S. *Behind Closed Doors: Violence in the American Family.* Newbury Park, CA: Sage Publications; 1980.

3. Saltzman LE, Fanslow JL, McMahon PM, Shelley GA. Intimate partner violence surveillance: uniform definitions and recommended data elements. Centers for Disease Control and Prevention, National Center for Injury Prevention and Control Web site. http://www.cdc.gov/ncipc/pub-res/ipv_surveillance/Intimate%20Partner%20Violence.pdf. Published 1999. Accessed March 26, 2013.

4. World Health Organization, International Society for Prevention of Child Abuse and Neglect. Preventing child maltreatment: a guide to taking action and generating evidence. France, UK: World Health Organization; 2006.

5. Manly J. Advances in research definitions of child maltreatment. *Child Abuse Negl.* 2005;29:425-439.

6. US Department of Health and Human Services, Adminstration for Children and Families, Aministration on Children, Youth, and Families, Children's Bureau. Child Maltreatment 2009. Administration for Children and Families Web site. http://archive.acf.hhs.gov/programs/cb/pubs/cm09/cm09.pdf. Published 2010. Accessed March 26, 2013.

7. Sedlak A, Mettenburg J, Basena M, et al. Fourth National Incidence Study of Child Abuse and Neglect (NIS-4): Report to Congress. Administration for Children and Families Web site. http://www.acf.hhs.gov/programs/opre/research/project/national-incidence-study-of-child-abuse-and-neglect-nis-4-2004-2009. Published 2010. Accessed March 26, 2013.

8. McDonald R, Jouriles E, Ramisetty-Mikler S, Caetano R, Green C. Estimating the number of American children living in partner-violent families. *J Fam Psychol.* 2006;20:137-142.

9. Finkelhor D, Turner H, Ormrod R, Hamby S, Kracke K. Children's exposure to violence: a comprehensive national survey. Juvenile Justice Bulletin, US Department Of Justice Web site. https://www.ncjrs.gov/pdffiles1/ojjdp/227744.pdf. Published 2009. Accessed March 26, 2013.

10. Fantuzzo J, Boruch R, Beriama A, Atkins M, Marcus S. Domestic violence and children: prevalence and risk in five major US cities. *J Am Acad Child Adolesc Psychiatry.* 1997;36:116-122.

11. Graham-Bermann S, Perkins S. Effects of early exposure and lifetime exposure to intimate partner violence on child adjustment. *Violence Victim.* 2010;25:427-439.

12. Gjelsvick A, Verhoek-Oftedahl W, Pearlman D. Domestic violence incidents with children witnesses: findings from Rhode Island surveillance data. *Womens Health Issues.* 2003;13:68-73.

13. Edleson J. The overlap between child maltreatment and woman battering. *Violence Against Women.* 1999;5:134-154.

14. Appel A, Holden G. The co-occurrence of spouse and physical child abuse: a review and appraisal. *J Fam Psych.* 1998;12:578-599.

15. McCloskey L, Figueredo A, Koss M. The effect of systemic family violence on children's mental health. *Child Dev.* 1995;66:1239-1261.

16. Bowker L, Arbitell M, McFerron R. On the relationship between wife beating and child abuse. In: Yllo K, Bograd M, eds. *Feminist Perspectives on Wife Abuse.* Newbury Park, CA: Sage; 1988:159-174.

17. Jouriles E, McDonald R, Slep A, Heyman R, Garrido E. Child abuse in the context of domestic violence: prevalence, explanations, and practice implications. *Violence Victim.* 2008;23:221-235.

18. Smith Slep A, O'Leary S. Parent and partner violence in families with young children: rates, patterns, and connections. *J Consult Clin Psych.* 2005;73:435-444.

19. Chang J, Theodore A, Martin S, Runyan D. Psychological abuse between parents: associations with child maltreatment from a population-based sample. *Child Abuse Negl.* 2008;32:819-829.

20. Zolotor A, Adrea D, Coyne-Beasley T, Runyan D. Intimate Partner Violence and Child Maltreatment: Overlapping Risk. *Brief Treatment and Crisis Intervention.* 2007;7:305-321.

21. English D. Domestic violence in one state's child protective caseload: a study of differential case dispositions and outcomes. *Child Youth Serv Rev.* 2005;27:1183-1201.

22. Taylor C, Lee S, Guterman N, Rice J. Use of spanking for 3-year-old children and associated intimate partner aggression or violence. *Pediatrics.* 2010;126:415-424.

23. Thackeray J, Hibbard R, Dowd M, Neglect CoCAa, Committee on Injury V, and Poison Prevention. Intimate partner violence: the role of the pediatrician. *Pediatrics.* 2010;125:1094-1100.

24. McGuigan W, Pratt C. The predictive impact of domestic violence on three types of child maltreatment. *Child Abuse Negl.* 2001;25:869-883.

25. Cox C, Kotch J, Everson M. A longitudinal study of modifying influences in the relationship between domestic violence and child maltreatment. *J Fam Viol.* 2003;18:5-17.

26. English D, Marshall D, Stewart A. Effects of family violence on child behavior and health during early childhood. *J Fam Viol.* 2003;18:43-57.

27. Casanueva C, Martin S, Runyan D. Repeated reports for child maltreatment among intimate partner violence victims: findings from the National Survey of Child and Adolescent Well-Being. *Child Abuse Negl.* 2009;33:84-93.

28. Christian C, Scribano P, Seidl T, Pinto-Martin J. Pediatric injury resulting from family violence. *Pediatrics.* 1997;99:e8.

29. Mbilinyi L, Edleson J, Hagemeister A, Beeman S. What happens to children when their mothers are battered? Results from a four city anonymous telephone survey. *J Fam Viol.* 2007;22:309-317.

30. Holtzworth-Munroe A, Meehan J. Typologies of men who are maritally violent: scientific and clinical implications. *J Interpers Viol.* 2004;19:1369-1389.

31. Hartley C. The co-occurrence of child maltreatment and domestic violence: examining both neglect and child physical abuse. *Child Maltreatment.* 2002;7:349-358.

32. Wise L, Zierler S, Krieger N, BL H. Adult onset of major depressive disorder in relation to early life violent victimization: a case-control study. *Lancet.* 2001;358:881-887.

33. Kendler K, Bulik C, Silberg J, Hettema J, Myers J, Prescott C. Childhood sexual abuse and adult psychiatric and substance use disorders in women: an epidemiological and cotwin control analysis. *Arch Gen Psychiatry.* 2000;57:953-959.

34. English D, Graham J, Litrownik A, Everson M, Bangdiwala S. Defining maltreatment chronicity: are there differences in child outcomes? *Child Abuse Negl.* 2005;29:575-595.

35. Lanier P, Jonson-Reid M, Stahlschmidt M, Drake B, Constantino J. Child maltreatment and pediatric health outcomes: a longitudinal study of low-income children. *J Pediatr Psychol.* 2010;35:511-522.

36. Bonomi A, Cannon E, Anderson M, Rivara F, Thompson R. Association between self-reported health and physical and/or sexual abuse experienced before age 18. *Child Abuse Negl.* 2008;32:693-701.

37. Turner H, Finkelhor D, Ormrod R. Poly-victimization in a national sample of children and youth. *Am J Prev Med.* 2010;38:323-330.

38. Shonkoff J, Boyce W, McEwen B. Neuroscience, molecular biology, and the childhood roots of health disparities: building a new framework for health promotion and disease prevention. *JAMA.* 2009;301:2252-2259.

39. Teicher M, Andersen S, Polcari A, Anderson C, Navalta C. Developmental neurobiology of childhood stress and trauma. *Psychiatr Clin North Am.* 2002;25:397-426.

40. Jacobson M. Genesis of neuronal specificity. In: Rockstein M, ed. *Development and Aging in the Nervous System.* New York, NY: Academic Press; 1973:105.

41. Tarullo A, Gunnar M. Child maltreatment and the developing HPA axis. *Horm Behav.* 2006;50:632-639.

42. Saltzman K, Holden G, Holahan C. The psychobiology of children exposed to marital violence. *J Clin Child Adol Psych.* 2005;34:129-139.

43. Linares L, Stovall-McClough K, Li M, et al. Salivary cortisol in foster children: a pilot study. *Child Abuse Negl.* 2008;32:665-670.

44. Hibel LC, Granger DA, Blair C, Cox MJ, The Family Life Project Key Investigators. Maternal sensitivity buffers the adrenocortical implications of intimate partner violence exposure during early childhood. *Dev Psychopath.* 2011;23(2):689-701.

45. Liu D, Diorio J, Tannenbaum B, et al. Maternal care, hippocampal glucocorticoid receptors, and hypothalamic-pituitary-adrenal responses to stress. *Science.* 1997;277:1659-1662.

46. Felitti V, Anda R, Nordenberg D, et al. Relationship of childhood abuse and household dysfunction to many of the leading causes of death in adults: the Adverse Childhood Experiences (ACE) study. *Am J Prev Med.* 1998;14:245-258.

47. Hillis S, Anda R, Felitti V, Marchbanks P. Adverse childhood experiences and sexual risk behaviors in women: a retrospective cohort study. *Fam Plann Perspect.* 2001;33:206-211.

48. Hillis S, Anda R, Felitti V, Nordenberg D, Marchbanks P. Adverse childhood experiences and sexually transmitted diseases in men and women: a retrospective study. *Pediatrics.* 2000(106):E11.

49. Dietz P, Spitz A, Anda R, et al. Unintended pregnancy among adult women exposed to abuse or household dysfunction during their childhood. *JAMA.* 1999;282:1359-1364.

50. Dube S, Anda R, Felitti V, Edwards V, Williamson D. Exposure to abuse, neglect, and household dysfunction among adults who witnessed intimate partner violence as children: implications for health and social services. *Violence Vict.* 2002;17:3-17.

51. Dube S, Anda R, Felitti V, Chapman D, Williamson D, Giles W. Child abuse, household dysfunction, and the risk of attempted suicide throughout the lifespan: findings from the Adverse Childhood Experiences Study. *JAMA.* 2001;286:3089-3096.

52. Suglia S, Enlow M, Kullowatz A, Wright R. Maternal intimate partner violence and increased asthma incidence in children: buffering effects of supportive caregiving. *Arch Pediatr Adolesc Med.* 2009;163:244-250.

53. Subramanian S, Ackerson L, Subramanyam M, Wright R. Domestic violence is associated with adult and childhood asthma prevalence in India. *Int J Epid.* 2007;36:569-579.

54. Breiding M, Ziembroski J. The relationship between intimate partner violence and children's asthma in 10 US states/territories. *Pediatr Allergy Immunol.* 2010.

55. Suglia S, Duarte C, Sandel M, Wright R. Social and environmental stressors in the home and childhood asthma. *J Epidemiol Community Health.* 2010;64:636-642.

56. Boynton-Jarrett R, Fargnoli J, Suglia S, Zuckerman B, Wright R. Association between maternal intimate partner violence and incident obesity in preschool-aged children: results from the Fragile Families and Child Well-being Study. *Arch Pediatr Adolesc Med.* 2010;164:540-546.

57. Ackerson L, Subramanian S. Domestic violence and chronic malnutrition among women and children in India. *Am J Epidemiol.* 2009;167:1188-1196.

58. Silverman J, Decker M, Gupta J, Kapur N, Raj A, Naved R. Maternal experiences of intimate partner violence and child morbidity in Bangladesh: evidence from a national Bangladesh sample. *Arch Pediatr Adolesc Med.* 2009;163:700-705.

59. Springer K, Sheridan J, Kuo D, Carnes M. Long-term physical and mental health consequences of childhood physical abuse: results from a large population-based sample of men and women. *Child Abuse Negl.* 2007;31:517-530.

60. Katon W, Sullivan M, Walker E. Medical symptoms without identified pathology: relationship to psychiatric disorders, childhood and adult trauma, and personality traits. *Ann Intern Med.* 2001;134:917-925.

61. Wegman H, Stetler C. A meta-analytic review of the effects of childhood abuse on medical outcomes in adulthood. *Psychosom Med.* 2009;71:805-812.

62. Irish L, Kobayashi I, Delahanty D. Long-term physical health consequences of childhood sexual abuse: a meta-analytic review. *J Pediatr Psychol.* 2010;35:450-461.

63. Bogat G, DeJonghe E, Levendosky A, Davidson W, Von Eye A. Trauma symptoms among infants exposed to intimate partner violence. Child Abuse Negl. 2006;30:109-125.

64. Graham-Bermann S, Brescoll V. Gender, power, and violence: assessing the family stereotypes of the children of batterers. *J Fam Psych.* 2000;14:600-612.

65. Koenen K, Moffitt T, Caspi A, Taylor A, Purcell S. Domestic violence is associated with environmental suppression of IQ in young children. *Dev Psychopathol.* 2003;2003:297-311.

66. Kernic M, Wolf M, Holt V, McNight B, Huebner C, Rivara F. Behavioral problems among children whose mothers are abused by an intimate partner. *Child Abuse Negl.* 2003;27:1231-1246.

67. Spilsbury J, Belliston L, Drotar D, et al. Clinically significant trauma symptoms and behavioral problems in a community-based sample of children exposed to domestic violence. *J Fam Viol.* 2007;22:487-499.

68. Kernic M, Holt V, Wolf M, McNight B, Huebner C, Rivara F. Academic and school health issues among children exposed to maternal intimate partner abuse. *Arch Pediatr Adolesc Med.* 2002;156:549-555.

69. Delsol C, Margolin G. The role of family-of-origin violence in men's marital violence perpetration. *Clin Psychol Rev.* 2004;24:99-122.

70. Polillo L. The effects of domestic violence on children. *Clin Fam Pract.* 2003;5:177-193.

71. Grogan-Kaylor A. Relationship of corporal punishment and antisocial behavior by neighborhood. *Arch Pediatr Adolesc Med.* 2005;159:938-942.

72. Gershoff E. Corporal punishment by parents and associated child behaviors and experiences: a meta-analytic and theoretical review. *Psychol Bull.* 2002;128:539-579.

73. Finzi R, Cohen O, Sapir Y, Weizman A. Attachment styles in maltreated children: a comparative study. *Child Psychiatry Hum Dev.* 2000;31:113-128.

74. Flores E, Cicchetti D, Rogosch F. Predictors of resilience in maltreated and nonmaltreated Latino children. *Dev Psychol.* 2005;41:338-351.

75. Ruggiero K, Smith D, Hanson R, et al. Is disclosure of childhood rape associated with mental health outcome? Results from the National Women's Study. *Child Maltreatment.* 2004;9:62-77.

76. Scott K, Smith D, Ellis P. Prospectively ascertained child maltreatment and its association with DSM-IV mental disorders in young adults. *Arch Gen Psychiatry.* 2010;67:712-719.

77. MacMillan H, Fleming J, Streiner D, et al. Childhood abuse and lifetime psychopathology in a community sample. *Am J Psychiatry.* 2001;158:1878-1883.

78. Molnar B, Buka S, Kessler R. Child sexual abuse and subsequent psychopathology: results from the National Comorbidity Survey. *Am J Public Health.* 2001;91:753-760.

79. Bair-Merritt M, Crowne S, Burrell L, Caldera D, Cheng T, Duggan A. Impact of intimate partner violence on children's well-child care and medical home. *Pediatrics.* 2008;121:e473-480.

80. Bair-Merritt M, Feudtner C, Localio A, Feinstein J, Rubin D, Holmes W. Health care use of children whose female caregivers have intimate partner violence histories. *Arch Pediatr Adolesc Med.* 2008;16(2):134-139.

81. Rivara F, Anderson M, Fischman P, et al. Intimate partner violence and health care costs and utilization for children living in the home. *Pediatrics.* 2007;120:1270-1277.

82. Walker E, Unutzer J, Rutter C, et al. Costs of health care use by women HMO members with a history of childhood abuse and neglect. *Arch Gen Psychiatry.* 1999;56:609-613.

83. Tang B, Jamieson E, Boyle M, Libby A, Gafni A, MacMillan H. The influence of child abuse on the pattern of expenditures in women's adult health service utilization in Ontario, Canada. *Soc Sci Med.* 2006;63:1711-1719.

84. Hughes H. Psychological and behavioral correlates of family violence in child witnesses and victims. *Am J Orthopsychiatry.* 1988;58:77-90.

85. Litrownik A, Newton R, Hunter R, English D, Everson M. Exposure to family violence in young at-risk children: a longitudinal look at the effects of victimization and witnessed physical and psychological aggression. *J Fam Viol.* 2003;18:59-73.

86. O'Keefe M. Predictors of child abuse in maritally violent families. *J Interpers Viol.* 1995;10:3-25.

87. Wolfe D, Crooks C, Lee V, McIntyre-Smith A, Jaffe P. The effects of children's exposure to domestic violence: a meta-analysis and critique. *Clin Child Fam Psych Rev.* 2003;6:171-187.

88. Waalen J, Goodwin M, Spitz A, Petersen R, Saltzman L. Screening for intimate partner violence by health care providers. Barriers and interventions. *Am J Prev Med.* 2000;19:230-237.

89. Groves B, Augustyn M, Lee D, Sawires P. *Identifying and Responding to Domestic Violence: Consensus Recommendations for Child and Adolescent Health.* San Francisco, CA: Family Violence Prevention Fund; 2004.

90. American Medical Association diagnostic and treatment guidelines on domestic violence. *Arch Fam Med.* 1992;1(1):39-47.

91. Johnson S, Sullivan C. How child protection workers support or further victimize battered mothers. Affilia: *J Women Soc Work.* 2008;23(3):242-258.

92. Zink T, Kamine D, Musk L, Sill M, Field V, Putnam F. What are providers' reporting requirements for children who witness domestic violence? *Clin Pediatr (Phila).* 2004;43:449-460.

Chapter 22

Intergenerational Transmission of Intimate Partner Violence

Jill Malik, MS*
Richard E. Heyman, PhD‡

Key Points

1. One study has found that 94.5% of homes reporting interparental intimate partner violence (IPV) also reported some parent-child physical abuse. In 22.4% of the homes with severe interparental IPV, there were also reports of severe parent-child physical violence.

2. Child exposure to parental IPV could at least double the risk for IPV perpetration in adulthood. However, isolating the effect of exposure to IPV is difficult, as so many families experiencing IPV also experience other types of violence.

3. Some evidence suggests that exposure to IPV in childhood puts the child at a greater risk of IPV victimization in adulthood.

4. Many theories have been put forward to explain the way the intergenerational transmission of violence works. These models can suggest possible interventions or preventative measures that could be taken.

Introduction

Intimate partner violence (IPV) is a problem of substantial magnitude worldwide, affecting the mental and physical health of both adult partners and their children.[1,2] One of the most longstanding "common sense" hypotheses regarding the causes of IPV is that violence is transmitted from generation to generation.[3] Given the vast body of work demonstrating the powerful effects of modeling, observation, and imitation in learning behaviors,[4] this was more than a product of armchair psychology. As evidence accumulated about the effects of noxious environments on children's psychological and neurological development[5,6] and of gene x environment interactions on violence,[7] this assumption seemed obviously true on its face. But what does scientific study say?

This chapter will examine the evidence for this assumption. We will begin by defining IPV (a more contentious endeavor than those outside the field would presume), providing information on IPV prevalence and measurement, and sketching the overlap of IPV and parent-child violence. To provide context for the intergenerational transmission hypothesis, we review literature on risk and protective factors at varying ecological levels. Finally, we present the evidence and theory regarding intergenerational transmission of family violence via IPV.

Jill Malik's preparation of this chapter was supported by the National Institute on Aging, National Institute of Health, Grant F31/AG037529-01.
‡*Richard Heyman's preparation of this chapter was supported by the National Institute for Dental and Craniofacial Research, Grant R21DE01953701A1.*

DEFINING INTIMATE PARTNER VIOLENCE

IPV refers to physical, psychological, or sexual violence that is perpetrated by a current or former romantic partner. Definitions of IPV range widely, from any physical act during conflicts (eg, throwing objects or using weapons) to physical acts that inflict injury (eg, beating) and further to any physical, psychological, or sexual act with the intent or perceived intent to cause harm. IPV can therefore vary widely in type and severity as well as in the nature of the intimate relationship of the parties. This wide range of definitions has been an impediment to the field, and, as will be discussed later, is one of the primary difficulties in evaluating whether intergenerational transmission of IPV exists.

As noted first by Straus and Johnson, there has been controversy about what constitutes partner maltreatment largely because of the existence of 2 distinct subfields.[8,9] One subfield studies individuals or couples from the general population and typically operationalizes IPV as a single act of physical aggression; the other studies women who have been highly victimized (eg, women in shelters) and men who have faced legal adjudication (eg, men in court-mandated abuse treatment programs).

PROBLEMS WITH DEFINING PHYSICAL AND EMOTIONAL IPV WITH SINGLE BEHAVIORAL ACT

The most commonly used measures of physical and emotional IPV are the Conflicts Tactics Scale (CTS) and the Revised Conflict Tactics Scale (CTS2).[10,11] The CTS is an 18-item list of non-aggressive constructive conflict behaviors, putatively emotionally aggressive tactics, and physically aggressive tactics arranged in order of severity. Respondents indicate the frequency of each behavior, ranging from "never" to "more than 20 times." The most typical time span in the instructions is 1 year, although the CTS is often modified to include other periods (eg, lifetime or since pre-test). The CTS2 is a 39-item measure, updated by ordering items randomly (ie, not in increasing severity and not grouped by type of IPV), expanding emotional and physical aggression items, and adding sexual coercion, sexual assault, and physical impact questions.

Most general population studies solely report or emphasize prevalence of a single act of physical assault or purported emotionally aggressive behavior (even when impact was measured) on the CTS or CTS-like measure.[8,12,13] Defining either physical or emotional IPV as a "single aggressive act in the last year" (with or without impact) is of questionable validity for 2 reasons. First, despite near universal expert belief that "true" abuse — that which significantly harms the victim or evokes fear substantial enough to control the victim or to constrict her culturally-expected freedoms — is largely a male-perpetrated phenomenon, women are equally or more physically and emotionally aggressive toward their partners than men in all age groups.[14] The high prevalence of female-to-male IPV cannot be due to self-defense, as women attribute their actions to self-defense less than 25% of the time and a substantial proportion of reported female-to-male IPV occurs in the absence of male-to-female IPV.[15,16] Second, again running counter to expert beliefs about "true abuse," reported instances of IPV typically are not severe,[17] are infrequent,[8] and often desist spontaneously;[18] victims typically are uninjured and report minimal psychological impact.[8,19]

EMERGING CONSENSUS FOR DEFINING IPV

Because most prevention, intervention, and public policy efforts are targeted at IPV that either directly harms victims or prevents victims from living freely without fear of harm, several recent conceptualizations have gone beyond using only reported acts of physical or emotional aggression to define intimate partner maltreatment. Research definitions by the World Health Organization,[1] United States Centers for Disease Control and Prevention,[20] and a growing number of researchers[21-25] have made clearer distinctions between impactful assaults (ie, those that cause or have a high potential to cause injury, harm, or death) and non-impactful assaults.

RESEARCH TESTED CRITERIA FOR IPV

Heyman and Slep have developed and field tested a set of reliable and valid definitions for all forms of IPV (and child maltreatment) via a rigorous program of research.[26-30] The criteria, which demonstrated over 90% agreement in everyday usage between clinical field raters and those of master raters, can be summarized as follows:

— Intimate partner maltreatment comprises physical, verbal/symbolic, or sexual acts (or, in the case of neglect, omissions) that cause—or have reasonable potential to cause—harm to an intimate partner.

  — Physical Abuse—Non-accidental acts of physical force that result, or have reasonable potential to result, in physical harm to an intimate partner or which evoke significant fear in the partner.

  — Emotional Abuse—Non-accidental verbal or symbolic acts that result in significant psychological harm to an intimate partner.

  — Sexual Abuse—Forced or coerced sexual acts with an intimate partner or sexual acts with an intimate partner who is unable to consent.

  — Neglect—Acts or omissions that result, or have reasonable potential to result, in physical harm to an intimate partner who is incapable of self-care.

Full operationalizations of the criteria can be found at http://dx.doi.org/10.1037/a0017011.supp.

PREVALENCE OF IPV

Physical IPV, when defined as any physical assault from pushes to punches, has a yearly prevalence of approximately 16% in nationally representative studies from the United States[8,31] and 12-20% in similar studies in England, Greece, Germany, Portugal, and Spain.[32-35] More severe forms of violence, such as battering, are reported to be far less common (eg, hitting reported by approximately 1% and need of medical attention reported by 2%).[8] Hostile couple interactions have dramatic and widespread effects, including increases in blood pressure,[36] lower immunological functioning,[37] elevated endocrine activity, especially affecting stress hormone levels,[38] and slower wound healing.[39] Moreover, IPV often causes lasting physical (eg, chronic disease)[21] and psychological difficulties, such as depressive symptoms[40,41] and Posttraumatic Stress Disorder (PTSD).[42]

Further, the 1985 National Family Violence Survey data indicates that 17.9% of respondents with children at home reported IPV in the last year.[43] A study of a generalizable sample of parents with a 3-7 year-old found the rate of IPV to be 48%; if emotional IPV (ie, severe psychological aggression on the CTS2) is included, the rate rose to 63%.[44] Exposure to IPV also impacts children in affected households, 75% of whom see or hear it.[45,46] Nearly all children in such homes are exposed when indirect effects (eg, witnessing sequelae or exposure to maternal depression) are considered.[5] A meta-analysis of 118 studies about children exposed to parental IPV found that on a host of outcomes (internalizing problems, externalizing problems, social problems, academic problems, negative affect or distress, negative cognitions), children exposed to IPV fared significantly worse than non-exposed children (d = -0.34).[5]

Overlap with Parent-Child Violence

In the best study of co-occurrence yet conducted, Slep and O'Leary, using anonymous self-reports from 453 families including a 4-8 year old child that were recruited through random digit dialing, found that 94.5% of the homes with any interparental IPV also had some parent-child physical violence.[44] Further, 22.4% of the homes with severe interparental IPV also had severe parent-child physical violence.

Risk and Protective Factors

In the following review of the current research, studies on individual risk and protective factors (for both perpetrators and victims) are presented first, followed by interpersonal, environmental, and, lastly, cultural factors. Because physical IPV is the most highly studied, for the purposes of this chapter we will focus on physical forms of IPV and will limit our discussion to research focused on that form (although families with both emotional or sexual and physical IPV would still be included in these studies). For more detailed reviews of perpetrator risk factors for physical IPV, see Schumacher et al;[47] Slep and O'Leary;[48] and Stith et al.[49] For reviews of risk factors for emotional IPV, see Schumacher et al[50]; for sexual IPV, see Black et al.[51]

Individual Risk Factors

Perpetrator Variables

The relationship between demographic variables and IPV has been examined across several studies. The 2 variables showing a consistent link with perpetrating IPV are age and income. However, although youth and lower incomes have consistently been found to be linked with IPV perpetration,[49] averaged across studies the effect sizes are weak for men (age r = -.13; income r = -.08). Slep et al found that youth was a unique predictor for both men's and women's perpetration of IPV and clinically significant IPV (CS-IPV; defined as violence that leads to injury or fear).[52] Stith et al also noted a weak negative association between education and male perpetrated IPV (r = -.13).[49] Last, although several studies have found that Black or Hispanic men may be at a slightly higher risk for perpetrating IPV than White, non-Hispanic, men[8,53] this has not been supported by all studies. For example, after controlling other factors (eg, age and socioeconomic status), Kantor et al did not find a link between Hispanic descent and IPV.[54] Field and Caetano also did not find any differences between Hispanic and White perpetrators after controlling for other demographics;[55] however, black couples remained 2 times more likely than white couples to engage in female-to-male partner violence. Career and life stress is moderately associated with male partner violence (r =.24).[49]

In clinical samples of mostly court-mandated IPV perpetrators, men who commit IPV tend to have higher degrees of psychopathology and poorer psychological functioning than their non-violent counterparts.[49] Perpetrators, compared with controls or norms, report more anger and hostility[56-58] and have lower self-esteem.[59,60] In addition, men who commit IPV have higher rates of depressive symptoms,[52] PTSD,[61-64] and drug problems (overall effect size =.31 across 6 studies) than men who do not.[49] Furthermore, Slep et al found that alcohol problems were a unique risk factor for both men's and women's IPV and CS-IPV;[52] moreover, Stith et al calculated a moderate effect size (r =.24 across 22 studies) for male perpetrators.[49] Similarly, on measures assessing for Axis II psychopathology, men who perpetrate IPV score higher on narcissistic, avoidant, borderline personality, antisocial, and schizotypal subscales.[56,65] Finally, attitudes condoning violence were also a strong positive predictor of IPV perpetration (r =.30).[49] However, a separate study by Dibble and Straus reported that, even if a man condoned male-to-female IPV, he was unlikely to perpetrate IPV unless his partner also used IPV.[66]

These differences were striking (9% vs. 76%, respectively), indicating that attitudes may interact with behavioral patterns within the home to result in IPV.

Taken together, results of studies on characteristics of men who perpetrate IPV suggest that these individuals tend to be younger and from lower SES, have more alcohol and drug problems, have directly experienced or witnessed violence during childhood (see below), and have more psychopathology than non-violent men. However, future research needs to enhance our understanding of the complex causal relationships that result in IPV and to disentangle population-level risk for clinically significant IPV from factors that might result in court-mandated involvement.

Victim Characteristics

Several researchers have also investigated victim characteristics that may serve as risk factors for IPV victimization, but this area of research is more controversial because of the concern that such research may imply that the victim is to blame. However, to succeed in preventing IPV, we must know who is at greatest risk for victimization. Moreover, as with other social problems, risk factors are not synonymous with causal factors.

Victim risk factors investigated have included demographic variables, childhood victimization experiences, and psychological variables. Overall, there are not as many links between victim characteristics and IPV as there are between perpetrator characteristics and IPV. Similar to examinations of perpetrator factors, results have been inconsistent and effect sizes weak (ie, below r =.10) for employment, age, and education; Stith et al concluded that these variables were not useful in further understanding and identifying risk of female victimization.[49] Similarly, childhood emotional or verbal abuse is the only form of violence that has shown a consistent link with being a victim of IPV;[67] witnessing interparental IPV, experiencing child physical abuse, and experiencing child sexual abuse do not appear to be risk factors.[49] Victims' social support or isolation has produced inconsistent findings.[68-71] Stress has also been implicated as a moderate risk factor (r =.26) for IPV victimization.[49] Across studies, the strongest risk factor for women's IPV victimization was perpetrating IPV toward men (r = -.41).[49]

Studies assessing psychological variables cannot definitively show whether the psychological difficulties are precursors or consequences of IPV. Some studies have attempted to deal with this confound by assessing past history of Axis I disorders,[52,72,74] studying disorders that rarely have an adult onset, or assessing the presence of Axis II disorders[72,73,75,76]—traits and symptoms of which almost emerge in childhood and adolescence and are therefore unlikely to be the result of violence that occurs in adulthood. In general, the results of studies assessing psychopathology of IPV victims are not as robust as results from studies assessing the psychopathology of IPV perpetrators. Women experiencing IPV have been found to be slightly more likely to have histories of depression (r =.28 across 6 studies),[71] current symptoms of psychosis,[72,73] eating disorders,[72] and PTSD.[74] Furthermore, they are more likely than women who have not experienced IPV to have symptoms of antisocial personality disorder.[72,73] In addition, the Psychopathic Deviant Subscale of the MMPI (eg, disregard for societal norms, marital and family conflicts, conflicts with authority, poor judgment) has been linked to IPV victimization.[75,76] Specifically, this study found that battered women endorsed elevated levels of family discord and self-alienation.[76]

Victim's own alcohol and drug use have been inconsistently linked to IPV victimization. Overall, Stith et al found a weak effect size for alcohol use (r =.13).[49] Inconsistent assessment of substance use may be accountable for these discrepancies, as non-standardized measures are often used to assess alcohol and drug use or dependence.

Regarding other psychological variables, Star found that IPV victims had higher ego strength, were more emotionally sensitive or less emotionally mature, and were more irritable and negative than non-victims.[77] Replication of this study is necessary, however, before any conclusive statements can be made about the potential of these personality styles as risk factors for IPV. Walker also found that college-aged battered women reported their self-esteem as higher than that of other women, and interprets this finding by suggesting that battered women have an inaccurate perception of themselves.[78] Stith et al also indicated that fear of partner violence was moderately correlated with female victims of IPV (r =.27).[49] However, it is also noted that it is less likely that fear precipitates partner violence that that it is a consequence of it.

Taken together, the research on victim risk factors suggests that experiencing childhood verbal or emotional victimization (see below), fear of IPV, depressive symptoms, and having anti-social personality traits or disorders are related to IPV victimization. On the other hand, evidence suggesting a relationship between IPV victimization and age, race, religion, unemployment, education, or drug use is inconsistent or weak. Longitudinal studies conducted on the link between psychological functioning need to be conducted to help tease apart the relationship between Axis I psychopathology, other personality factors, and subsequent IPV.

Relationship Factors

In general, relationships in which IPV occurs differ from those in which IPV does not occur. The strongest relationship predictors of physical IPV are emotional IPV and forced sex (r =.49 and r =.45, respectively).[49] Men's and women's relationship discord and conflict have consistently been found to be linked to IPV[52] (for review, see Stith et al),[79] a finding that is not surprising given that most IPV occurs during a conflict or argument.[80,81] IPV perpetration is related to relationship dissatisfaction for both men and women (r =.30 and r =.25, respectively),[79] although male perpetrators are significantly less satisfied in their relationships than are female perpetrators.[79] Men in relationships characterized by IPV also report higher levels of jealousy,[58,68,82] though the effect size is small.[49] Moreover, male IPV perpetrators consistently reported moderately higher levels of anger and hostility, compared with nonviolent men in discordant relationships (d = 0.60).[83] Norlander and Eckhardt found that males who perpetrated IPV, compared with males that did not, reported higher anger and hostility (d =51).[83] A man's actual or perceived power in the intimate relationship may also play an important role in the occurrence of IPV. Men engaging in IPV appear to have higher power needs than do non-IPV men.[84] At the same time, men who enact IPV also perceive themselves as low in decision making power and that they have more concerns than men not engaging in IPV that their partners will engage in unpleasant or unpredictable behaviors.[85-87]

Overall, the communication style and affective responses of IPV couples are more negative and hostile than those of couples without IPV. Laboratory studies coding communication patterns of couples asked to discuss a relationship problem have revealed that men who perpetrate IPV engage in fewer positive and facilitative behaviors,[88,89] and more negative and aversive behaviors than non-IPV men.[89-91] Moreover, IPV men report less mutually constructive communication and more mutual blame.[92] Male IPV perpetrators have also been found to act with significantly more belligerence and contempt toward their partners than men not engaging in IPV, whereas women from IPV couples have been found to exhibit significantly more anger and tension or fear than women from couples without IPV.[93] Similarly, in a study of couples' interactions in their homes, Margolin et al found that IPV-men exhibited more overt hostility than non-IPV men.[94] The results of this study also revealed that men who engaged in IPV reported more anxiety, anger, feelings of being attacked, and overall negative emotion post-discussion than non-IPV men. Stith et al concluded that, for male IPV perpetration, anger and hostility had an overall effect size of r =.26.[49]

Several studies have demonstrated differences in attachment styles, with IPV-perpetrating, compared with non-perpetrating, men found to have less secure, less trusting, and more fearful attachments to their partners and higher levels of anxiety over abandonment, more avoidance of dependency, and more discomfort with closeness.[82]

In sum, it appears that several couple variables may be important risk factors for IPV, including low relationship satisfaction, negative communication styles, insecure attachment, and power differences. Again, due to the nature of the majority of the above studies, care must be taken when interpreting these findings, since chronology cannot be determined and some of the patterns may have emerged after IPV had been initiated and become established.

Environmental and Cultural Factors

Environmental risk factors, such as the geographic area of residence (eg, urban versus rural) and perpetrator social support, have not received adequate empirical attention. Recently, Slep et al found that community (eg, social support) and workplace variables (eg, support from leadership) were indirect predictors of both men's and women's IPV and CS-IPV.[52] With regard to geographic regions, differences were found in the relationship between workplace support from leadership and male perpetrated CS-IPV, in that associations were strongest for men in the Midwestern United States whereas associations were weaker for men living in the South, West, and no association was found for men living in the Northeast.[52]

Similarly, cultural factors are thought to impact IPV but have received little empirical attention. One of the broadest cultural factors is a culture's attitude towards family violence. In the United States, there is broad rejection of the acceptability of male-to-female IPV.[95] For example, in a 1994 national survey conducted by the U.S. Centers for Disease Control and Prevention (N = 5238), 1.35% of women and 2.05% of men thought it was "OK for a man to hit his wife or girlfriend to discipline her or keep her in line" and 7.2% of women and 9.75% of men thought it was "OK for a man to hit his wife or girlfriend if she hits him first."[95] Approval for female-to-male violence was considerably higher: positive responses to the questions were 4.4% for women and 4.95% for men regarding a woman hitting to discipline or keep her male partner in line and 26.65% for women and 33.75% for men regarding women hitting after being hit first.[95] Of note, non-Hispanic Blacks were nearly 3 times as likely and Hispanics over 5 times as likely as Whites to endorse men hitting women to keep them in line (even after adjusting for gender, age, marital status, income, education, and urbanicity). Those who did not graduate from high school were more than twice as likely to endorse hitting women to keep them in line as those who did graduate (controlling all other variables), as were those making less than $20 000 annually compared with those earning more.

Intergenerational Transmission of Violence

The intergenerational transmission of violence is one of the most widely studied phenomena in family violence. The global question of "Does IPV exposure as a child lead to adult family violence?" becomes much more complicated when one has to specify the type of adulthood family violence, not to mention the gender of the child and parental IPV victim(s) and perpetrator(s), the severity of both IPV and later violence, and the child's developmental stage - to name only a few factors. When one considers the number of permutations possible, it is no wonder that the answer to "Does IPV exposure as a child lead to adult family violence?" has often been obscured by a tangle of inconsistent findings and methodological pitfalls.[3,79,96]

To be as clear as possible about the variables studied in the research summarized below, we have adopted the following conventions:

— IPV: any act of physical force used against a romantic partner, typically measured by self-report measures such as the CTS.

— Parent-Child Physical Violence (PCPV): any act of physical force used by a parent or parental figure against a child, typically measured by self-report measures such as the Parent Child CTS.[97]

— Exposure to Parental IPV: reports that a child witnessed parental IPV or "[saw] the results (eg, bruises), or experienced its aftermath when interacting with parents."[98]

Note that most studies combine types of maltreatment (eg, physical, emotional, and sexual abuse and neglect) together, making it nearly impossible to isolate the differential effects for the type of maltreatment.

Additionally, one of the most common and difficult issues in exploring the intergenerational transmission of IPV is its interaction with other adverse individual, couple, and family dynamics. Many times IPV exposure is just one adverse environmental factor in a host of noxious family elements. Unfortunately, most literature to date has not been able to split apart the impact of IPV as a specific environmental risk verses other factors that occur within maltreating families.

Compared with other types of negative environmental factors, IPV is relatively infrequent. Therefore, at this point in time, it is nearly impossible to specifically study exposure to IPV alone. In our review of the literature below, we will focus on studies related to IPV and transmission of IPV from one generation to the next; however, the reader should not infer that these findings are due to exposure to IPV alone without exposure to other noxious family environmental forces. Additional methodological caveats are discussed after the presentations of the research on intergenerational transmission.

Different Forms of Intergenerational Transmission of Violence
Does Child Exposure to Parental IPV Lead to IPV Perpetration in Adulthood?
Ehrensaft et al found in a 20-year prospective study of 543 randomly selected children from upstate New York that exposure to parental IPV tripled the risk for IPV perpetration in adulthood.[99] Even when controlling for numerous other significant factors, exposure still more than doubled the risk for adulthood perpetration.

Stith et al conducted a meta-analysis that found weak effect sizes for the link between childhood exposure to parental IPV and IPV perpetration (r =.18, n = 29 studies).[96] Increased risk related to exposure to parental IPV was stronger for men (r =.21, n = 20 studies) than for women (r =.13, n = 9 studies) and in clinical samples of IPV victims (r =.35, n = 17 studies) than in representative samples of community members (r =.11, n = 12 studies). Here the strongest relation accounted for less than 13% of the variance in adult IPV. Additional studies located by Schumacher et al found similar effect sizes.[47]

Schumacher, Feldbau-Kohn et al noted the difficulty of interpreting the effect sizes because most families with parental IPV also use PCPV.[47] Doumas et al attempted to isolate the unique effects of family violence in the family of origin.[100] They studied a convenience sample of 181 families. Parents reported on the frequency of:

— being "physically or verbally abused" as a child,

— being exposed to "physical or verbal abuse" between parents as a child, and

— the occurrence of IPV ever in the relationship.

For men, but not for women, frequency of parental IPV exposure was significantly related to use of IPV at some point in the relationship, whereas frequency of child abuse victimization was not. The effect size was weak, accounting for less than 5% of the variance in risk for IPV.

A longitudinal study of 213 adolescents found a moderate correlation between interparental IPV and adolescent/young adult perpetration of IPV (r =.39, p <01).[101] Effects were similar for both physical and verbal IPV with no significant gender differences. The relation between interparental IPV and later adult IPV was partially mediated through parents' aggression toward the participant as an adolescent. Black et al also found significant but weak positive associations linking interparental psychological IPV to early adulthood IPV and interparental physical IPV to early adult physical IPV in a sample of 233 college students (rs =21, p <001).[102]

Does Child Exposure to Parental IPV lead to IPV Victimization in Adulthood?

Stith et al conducted a meta-analysis that found weaker effect sizes for the link between childhood exposure to parental IPV and IPV perpetration (r =.14, n =17 studies).[96] Risk for IPV victimization related to exposure to parental IPV was stronger in clinical samples of IPV victims (r =.24, n = 5 studies) than in representative samples of community members (r =.13, n = 12 studies); there was no differential effect for gender (men: r =.14, n = 14; women: r =.10, n = 3). Additional studies located by Schumacher and colleagues found similar effect sizes.[47]

Similarly, the 20-year prospective study conducted by Ehrensaft et al found that exposure to parental IPV increased the risk for adulthood IPV victimization by 17%;[99] however, the association was not significant when other risk factors were controlled for. Similarly, Cui et al found that exposure to parental IPV was moderately positively correlated with adult IPV victimization (r =.35, p <01);[101] however, this relationship was fully mediated by exposure to parental aggression in adolescence.

Does Child Exposure to Parental IPV lead to Child Maltreatment Perpetration in Adulthood?

Using data from the 1985 National Family Violence Survey, a nationally representative telephone survey, Straus found a weak relation (r =.20; effect size calculated by Black et al)[102] between exposure to parental IPV as a child and using severe (but likely non-substantiated, or unverified by formal agencies) PCPV as an adult.[103] Straus and Smith further broke down the data.[104] Both men and women who were exposed to their mothers hitting their fathers had higher rates of severe PCPV than did those who did not report such exposure. Similar results for exposure to father-to-mother IPV were found, but for females only. Given the paucity of studies investigating this relation (and the gender of the perpetrator), it is unclear whether this is a spurious result or whether women's parenting is more affected by exposure to father-to-mother IPV than is men's.

PROBLEMS WITH INTERGENERATIONAL TRANSMISSION OF VIOLENCE RESEARCH

Widom summarized methodological problems with intergenerational transmission of violence research, most of which are still applicable to much research published to date (see **Table 22-1**).[3]

<table>
<tr><td>

Table 22-1. Methodological Problems with Research on Intergenerational Transmission of Violence

1. Questionable criteria for abuse and neglect, including non-substantiated cases

2. Designs weakened by questionable accuracy of information due to retrospective nature of data or reliance on second-hand information

3. Weak sampling techniques, involving convenience or opportunity samples

4. Reliance on correlational studies

5. Failure to distinguish between abused and neglected children, treating them as one group

6. Lack of appropriate comparison or control groups and failure to consider statistical base rates

7. Tendency to examine generalized delinquent behavior, with less focusing on violent criminal behavior

8. Lack of knowledge of long-term consequences of abuse and neglect into adulthood.

See Widom for a more detailed discussion of each problem.[3]

</td></tr>
</table>

Besides the problem with definitions that we have discussed above, the studies that we reviewed were either drawn from representative samples or had a control group. The strongest threat to validity not thoroughly discussed, then, is that of retrospective reporting. However, Widom and Shepard found that retrospective CTS reports of childhood PCPV related fairly well with child maltreatment substantiation records.[104] Their participants were substantiated victims of child maltreatment in 1967-71 who were interviewed 2 decades later. Because the participants were not a clinical group of family violence perpetrators, they had no incentive to overreport childhood victimization and, in fact, were more likely to underreport it. Widom and Shepard's findings imply that, at least in nonclinical samples, retrospective reports of maltreatment are likely valid (yet conservative).[104]

Additionally, more research is needed that focuses on female IPV perpetrators and male victims. According to a review by Stith et al, only 1 study at that time was examined that exclusively focused on female perpetrators.[79] Additionally, more research needs to be conducted on diverse samples (eg, lower SES and different ethnic backgrounds) in relation to martial satisfaction and IPV, as most studies examine violence among white, middle-class couples.[79]

A significant optimistic development, however, is the publication of longitudinal studies of IPV.[40,99,101,105,106] Although not always narrowly focusing on the intergenerational transmission of violence (as defined here), these studies portend that prospective data may soon allow for more definitive conclusions regarding the various intergenerational transmission of violence hypotheses.

Finally, moderating factors need to be considered. Although no comparable meta-analysis exists for intergenerational transmission, a meta-analysis by Stith et al looked at several moderators in a parallel phenomenon—the association between relationship satisfaction and IPV.[79] Stith et al found that use of standardized instruments yielded stronger effect sizes than non-standardized instruments, that effect sizes was stronger for male than for female perpetrators, and that they were stronger for female than male IPV victims.[79] Further, IPV victims reported lower levels of relationship satisfaction and higher levels of discord than did IPV perpetrators and clinical samples of IPV yielded larger effect sizes for satisfaction versus discord than did community samples.

SUMMARY

Despite the problems with the literature, across the permutations of the intergenerational transmission of violence reviewed above there was support for the hypothesis that violence begets violence. The effect, however, is weak, and the majority of children exposed to parental IPV do not seem to grow up to either perpetrate or be victimized by IPV.

HOW DOES THE INTERGENERATIONAL TRANSMISSION OF VIOLENCE OPERATE?

OBSERVATIONAL LEARNING

Most researchers interested in the intergenerational transmission of violence point to observational learning (also known as modeling) as a prime source of such transmission.[4,107] Through observational learning, one sees the success of strategies performed by others and imitates them. When the imitated behavior is performed, the rewards increase the likelihood of future performance of the behavior (ie, operant conditioning). Thus, children see that coercion and violence against loved ones works in getting something desired. When violence is imitated later, it is typically rewarded by the environment (eg, violence succeeds in wresting a toy from a peer); thus, the victimized child learns to victimize others. Simons et al in a study of the intergenerational transmission of harsh (but not necessarily abusive) parenting, found that punitive beliefs about discipline or hostile personality organizations were not required mediators; rather, "repeated exposure to aggressive parenting provides individuals with a model of the parent role that they use with their own children in a reflexive way, with little awareness of alternatives or concern with rationalization."[108] Thus, modeled violence may be performed later by the child and reinforced by the environment. Through frequent performance and success, the link between aversive environmental cues (especially those emitted by loved ones) and violence may become fast and without cognitive mediation (ie, automated), just as complex behaviors such as driving become automated.[109]

COERCION THEORY

Perhaps the most developed and influential operant behavioral model of dyadic conflict is Patterson and colleagues' *Coercion Theory*, which explains how, via negative reinforcement, negative escalation sequences can be reinforcing for both members of a dyad, despite their unpleasant and destructive qualities.[110] Thus, Coercion Theory addresses the processes that sometimes lead to IPV (which are being modeled for the child) and the dysfunctional operant learning that often occurs in such families between parents and children (which may cement coercive strategies in the child's repertoire).[80]

Coercion Theory posits that people learn coercive behavior through the ways in which conflicts are resolved. Over time, if Person A responds to Person B's escalating aversive behavior by giving in (thus ceasing his or her own aversive behavior), Person B learns to escalate to get his or her way. Importantly, both partners' behaviors are maintained through reinforcement. Person B is negatively reinforced for escalating (via Person A shutting up) and may be positively reinforced as well (via Person A doing what Person B was asking for in the argument). Person A is negatively reinforced for giving in (via the termination of Person B's aversive behavior). Over time, these conflicts serve as learning trials. Of course, Person B doesn't always win. Sometimes, Person A's aversive escalation leads to Person B giving in. Thus, once a coercive process takes hold, both members of the dyad are faced with an unfortunate choice: (a) give in and lose the battle, or (b) win via out-escalating the other. This process leads to ever darker, bitterer battles. In Patterson's exquisite phrasing, each person is both the "victim and architect of a coercive system."[111]

BIOLOGICAL AND GENETIC FACTORS

Inherited biological and genetic factors that predispose one generation toward violence may be passed on to the offspring, especially if assortative mating provides higher genetic loadings for violence from both parents.[112] Given gene-environment interactions, biological predispositions may be exacerbated by hormonal responses to the environmental factors discussed above. For further review on the biological contribution to the intergenerational transmission of violence, see Hines and Saudino[112]; DiLalla and Gottesman[113]; and Widom.[114]

NEUROBIOLOGICAL THEORIES OF TRAUMA

Evolutionarily functional, innate, organized behavioral patterns exist to respond to danger (eg, fight/flight response) and can be shaped through environmental interaction, especially childhood exposure to noxious environments, including IPV.[7] Although humans, like all animals, are born with perceptual and behavioral systems to scan for and respond to danger, these systems are plastic and responsive to environmental influences. LeDeux posited 2 information pathways, a danger related pathway from the thalamus to the amygdala and a slower, non-threat-based pathway from the cortex to the amygdala.[115] The former, although adaptive in the face of real environmental dangers, can become primed to such an extent via traumatic experience that hyperarousal and hypervigilance result. The latter, although more accurate, is not evolutionarily advantageous in danger-rich environments. Thus, through exposure to a dangerous, traumatic environment, neural connections can be formed and strengthened that favor attention to danger-cues in social information processing.

ATTACHMENT THEORIES

Attachment Theory focuses on the primacy of the caregiver-caretaker relationship in establishing people's representations of the interpersonal world.[116,117] These representations are first formed via interactions with the primary caregiver (typically the mother) but are updated in later development via relationships with important others (eg, romantic partners). Cummings and Davies' ***Emotional Security Hypothesis*** (ESH) is perhaps the most extensively studied and best validated example of an attachment-informed approach relevant to how childhood exposure to IPV may be involved in intergenerational transmission.[118] The ESH suggests that emotional security is a goal that motivates and directs children's reactions to events, such as exposure to IPV, in their environment.[119] Under the ESH, exposure to IPV does not have a direct impact on child outcomes. Rather, it is the extent to which elements of the exposure to IPV threaten or disrupt the child's sense of security that drives their responses, which, over time, can evolve into patterns that are generally maladaptive but serve in the moment to help the child regain security.[120] Research suggests that elements of couple conflict that may threaten security (eg, how it was resolved or how heated the conflict became) are more tightly related to child outcomes than children's exposure to IPV per se.[121]

CONCLUSION

Childhood exposure to IPV appears to have a reproducible but weak relation to later IPV perpetration, victimization, and violence toward one's own children. Considering the multi-determined nature of IPV,[122] it is not surprising that a distal variable such as childhood exposure would not be an overpowering factor in the occurrence of adulthood family violence, considering the number of proximal influences operating. However, reduction of IPV in the homes of children would have an important impact in reducing children's risk for later violence and should not be dismissed. Thus, intergenerational transmission of family violence neither seals a child's fate in adulthood nor should it be ignored as a screening factor for prevention.

REFERENCES

1. Krug EG, Dahlberg LL, Mercy JA, Zwi AB, Lozano R, eds. *World Report on Violence and Health.* Geneva: World Health Organization; 2002.

2. Carbone-López K, Kruttschnitt C, Macmillan R. Patterns of intimate partner violence and their associations with physical health, psychological distress, and substance use. *Public Health Rep.* 2006;121(4):382–392.

3. Widom C. Does violence beget violence? a critical examination of the literature. *Psychol Bull.* 1989;106(1):3-28.

4. Bandura A. *Social Foundations of Thought and Action: A Social Cognitive Theory.* Englewood Cliffs, NJ US: Prentice-Hall, Inc; 1986.

5. Kitzmann K, Gaylord N, Holt A, Kenny E. Child witnesses to domestic violence: a meta-analytic review. *J Consult Clin Psychol.* 2003;71(2):339-352.1

6. Repetti R, Taylor S, Seeman T. Risky families: family social environments and the mental and physical health of offspring. *Psychol Bull.* 2002;128(2):330-366.

7. Jonson-Reid M, Presnall N, Constantino J, et al. Effects of child maltreatment and inherited liability on antisocial development: an official records study. *J Am Acad Child Adolesc Psychiatry.* 2010;49(4):321-332.

8. Straus MA, Gelles RJ. *Physical Violence in American Families: Risk Factors and Adaptation to Violence in 8,145 Families.* New Brunswick, NJ: Transaction Publishing; 1990.

9. Johnson H. *Dangerous Domains: Violence Against Women in Canada.* Scarborough, Ontario: International Thomas Publishing; 1996.

10. Straus M. Measuring intrafamily conflict and violence: the Conflict Tactics (CT) Scales. *J Marriage Fam.* 1979;41(1):75-88.

11. Straus M, Hamby S, Boney-McCoy S, Sugarman D. The revised Conflict Tactics Scales (CTS2): Development and preliminary psychometric data. *J Fam Issues.* 1996;17(3):283-316.

12. Ellsberg M, Heise, L. *Researching Violence Against Women: A Practical Guide For Researchers And Activists.* Washington, DC: World Health Organization and Program for Appropriate Technology in Health; 2005.

13. Tjaden P, Thoennes N. *Full Report of the Prevalence, Incidence and Consequences of Violence Against Women: Research Report.* Washington, DC; National Institute of Justice; 2000. NCJ 183781.

14. Archer J. Sex differences in aggression between heterosexual partners: a meta-analytic review. *Psychol Bull.* 2000;126:651-680.

15. Cascardi M, Vivian D. Context for specific episodes of marital violence: gender and severity of violence differences. *J Fam Violence.* 1995;10(3):265-293.

16. Straus MA. Women's violence toward men is a serious social problem. In: Gelles RJ, Loseke DR, eds. *Current Controversies on Family Violence.* 2nd ed. Newbury Park, CA: Sage Publications; 2004:55-77.

17. Caetano R, Cunradi C, Schafer J, Clark C. Intimate partner violence and drinking patterns among white, black, and Hispanic couples in the US. *J Subst Abuse.* 2000;11(2):123-138.

18. Quigley B, Leonard K. Desistance of husband aggression in the early years of marriage. *Violence Vict.* 1996;11(4):355-370.

19. Ehrensaft M, Vivian D. Spouses' reasons for not reporting existing marital aggression as a marital problem. *J Fam Psychol.* 1996;10(4):443-453.

20. Saltzman LE, Fanslow JL, McMahon PM, Shelley GA. Intimate partner violence surveillance: uniform definitions and recommended data elements. http://www.cdc.gov/ncipc/pub-res/ipv_surveillance/intimate.htm. Published 1999. Accessed April 1, 2013.

21. Coker A, Davis K, Smith P, et al. Physical and mental health effects of intimate partner violence for men and women. *Am J Prev Med.* 2002;23(4):260-268.

22. Graham-Kevan N, Archer J. Physical aggression and control in heterosexual relationships: the effect of sampling. *Violence and Victims.* 2003;18(2):181-196.

23. Heyman RE, Feldbau-Kohn S, Ehrensaft M, Langhinrichsen-Rohling J, O'Leary K. Can questionnaire reports correctly classify relationship distress and partner physical abuse? *J Fam Psychol.* June 2001;15(2):334-346.

24. The differential effects of intimate terrorism and situational couple violence: findings from the national violence against women survey. *J Fam Issues.* 2005;26(3):322-349.

25. Smith P, Thornton G, DeVellis R, Earp J, Coker A. A population-based study of the prevalence and distinctiveness of battering, physical assault, and sexual assault in intimate relationships. *Violence Against Women.* October 2002;8(10):1208-1232.

26. Heyman RE, Slep AMS. Creating and field-testing diagnostic criteria for partner and child maltreatment. *J Fam Psychol.* 2006a;20(3):397-408.

27. Heyman RE, Slep AMS. Relational diagnoses: from reliable, rationally derived criteria to testable taxonic hypotheses. In: Beach SRH, Wamboldt M, Kaslow N, Heyman RE, First M, Underwood LG, Reiss D, eds. *Relational Processes and DSM-V: Neuroscience, Assessment, Prevention, and Treatment.* Washington, DC: American Psychiatric Association; 2006b:139-155.

28. Heyman RE, Slep AMS. Reliability of family maltreatment diagnostic criteria: 41 site dissemination field trial. *J Fam Psychol.* 2009;23(6):905-910.

29. Heyman RE, Collins PS, Slep AMS, Knickerbocker L. Evidence-based substantiation criteria: improving the reliability of field decisions of child maltreatment and partner abuse. *Protecting Child.* 2010;25:35-46.

30. Slep AMS, Heyman RE. Creating and field-testing child maltreatment definitions: improving the reliability of substantiation determinations. *Child Maltreat.* 2006;11(3):217-236.

31. Schafer J, Caetano R, Clark CL. Rates of intimate partner violence in the United States. *Am J Public Health.* 1998;88:1702-1704.

32. Machado C, Gonçalves M, Matos M, Dias A. Child and partner abuse: self-reported prevalence and attitudes in the north of Portugal. *Child Abuse Negl.* 2007;31(6):657-670.

33. Medina-Ariza J, Barberet R. Intimate partner violence in Spain: findings from a national survey. *Violence Against Women.* 2003;9(3):302-322.

34. Ruiz Pérez I, Plazaola Castaño J. Intimate partner violence and mental health consequences in women attending family practice in Spain. *Psychosom Med.* 2005:67:791–797.

32. Stathopoulou G. Greece. *International Perspectives on Family Violence and Abuse: A Cognitive Ecological Approach.* Mahwah, NJ: Lawrence Erlbaum Associates Publishers; 2004:131-149.

36. Ewart C, Taylor C, Kraemer H, Agras W. High blood pressure and marital discord: not being nasty matters more than being nice. *Health Psychol.* 1991;10(3):155-163.

37. Kiecolt-Glaser J, Malarkey W, Chee M, Newton T. Negative behavior during marital conflict is associated with immunological down-regulation. *Psychosom Med.* 1993;55(5):395-409.

38. Malarkey W, Kiecolt-Glaser J, Pearl D, Glaser R. Hostile behavior during marital conflict alters pituitary and adrenal hormones. *Psychosom Med.* January 1994;56(1):41-51.

39. Kiecolt-Glaser J, Loving T, Glaser R, et al. Hostile marital interactions, proinflammatory cytokine production, and wound healing. *Arch Gen Psychiatry.* 2005;62(12):1377-1384.

40. Magdol L, Moffitt T, Caspi A, Silva P. Hitting without a license: testing explanations for differences in partner abuse between young adult dates and cohabitors. *J Marriage Fam.* February 1998;60(1):41-55.

41. Reid R, Bonomi A, Thompson R, et al. Intimate partner violence among men: prevalence, chronicity, and health effects. *Am J Prev Med.* 2008;34(6):478-485.

42. Jones L, Hughes M, Unterstaller U. Post-traumatic stress disorder (PTSD) in victims of domestic violence: a review of the research. *Trauma Violence Abuse.* 2001;2(2):99-119.

43. Gelles RJ, Straus MA; University of New Hampshire Family Research Laboratory. Physical Violence in American Families, 1985. Ann Arbor, MI: Inter-University Consortium for Political and Social Research; 1994.

44. Slep AMS, O'Leary S. Parent and partner violence in families with young children: rates, patterns, and connections. *J Consult Clin Psychol.* June 2005;73(3):435-444.

45. Mahoney A, Donnelly W, Boxer P, Lewis T. Marital and severe parent-to-adolescent physical aggression in clinic-referred families: mother and adolescent reports on co-occurrence and links to child behavior problems. *J Fam Psychol.* March 2003;17(1):3-19.

46. O'Brien M, John R, Margolin G, Erel O. Reliability and diagnostic efficacy of parents' reports regarding children's exposure to marital aggression. *Violence Vict.* 1994;9(1):45-62.

47. Schumacher J, Feldbau-Kohn S, Slep AMS, Heyman RE. Risk factors for male-to-female partner physical abuse. *Aggression Violent Behav.* 2001;6(2-3):281-352.

48. Slep AMS, O'Leary S. Distinguishing risk profiles among parent-only, partner-only, and dually perpetrating physical aggressors. *J Fam Psychol.* 2009;23(5):705-716.

49. Stith S, Smith D, Penn C, Ward D, Tritt D. Intimate partner physical abuse perpetration and victimization risk factors: a meta-analytic review. *Aggression Violent Behav.* 2004;10(1):65-98.

50. Schumacher J, Slep AMS, Heyman RE. Risk factors for male-to-female partner psychological abuse. *Aggression Violent Behav.* March 2001;6(2-3):255-268.

51. Black D, Heyman RE, Slep AMS. Risk factors for child physical abuse. *Aggression Violent Behav.* 2001;6(2-3):121-188.

52. Slep AMS, Foran H, Heyman RE, Snarr J. Ecological risk factors for intimate partner violence and clinically significant intimate partner violence. 2011.

53. Leonard K, Blane H. Alcohol and marital aggression in a national sample of young men. *J Interpers Violence.* March 1992;7(1):19-30.

54. Kantor G, Jasinski J, Aldarondo E. Sociocultural status and incidence of marital violence in Hispanic families. *Violence Vict.* 1994;9(3):207-222.

55. Field C, Caetano R. Intimate partner violence in the US general population: progress and future directions. *J Interpers Violence.* 2005;20(4):463-469.

56. Beasley R, Stoltenberg C. Personality characteristics of male spouse abusers. *Professional Psychol Res Pract.* 1992;23(4):310-317.

57. Dutton D, Saunders K, Starzomski A, Bartholomew K. Intimacy-anger and insecure attachment as precursors of abuse in intimate relationships. *J Appl Soc Psychol.* 1994;24(15):1367-1386.

58. Dutton D, van Ginkel C, Landolt M. Jealousy, intimate abusiveness, and intrusiveness. *J Fam Violence.* 1996;11(4):411-423.

59. Lawson D, Brossart D, Shefferman L. Assessing gender role of partner-violent men using the Minnesota Multiphasic Personality Inventory-2 (MMPI-2): comparing abuser types. *Professional Psychol Res Pract.* 2010;41(3):260-266.

60. Murphy C, Meyer S, O'Leary K. Dependency characteristics of partner assaultive men. *J Abnorm Psychol.* 1994;103(4):729-735.

61. Campbell J, Lewandowski L. Mental and physical health effects of intimate partner violence on women and children. *Psychiatric Clin North Am.* 1997;20(2):353-374.

62. Cascardi M, O'Leary K, Schlee K. Co-occurrence and correlates of posttraumatic stress disorder and major depression in physically abused women. *J Fam Violence.* 1999;14(3):227-249.

63. Fergusson D, Horwood L, Ridder E. Partner violence and mental health outcomes in a New Zealand birth cohort. *J Marriage Fam.* 2005;67(5):1103-1119.

64. Sherman M, Sautter F, Jackson M, Lyons J, Han X. Domestic violence in veterans with posttraumatic stress disorder who seek couples therapy. *J Marital Fam Ther.* 2006;32(4):479-490.

65. Thornton A, Graham-Kevan N, Archer J. Adaptive and maladaptive personality traits as predictors of violent and nonviolent offending behavior in men and women. *Aggressive Behav.* 2010;36(3):177-186.

66. Dibble U, Straus M. Some social structure determinants of inconsistency between attitudes and behavior: the case of family violence. *J Marriage Fam.* 1980;42(1):71-80.

67. Cascardi M, O'Leary K, Lawrence E, Schlee K. Characteristics of women physically abused by their spouses and who seek treatment regarding marital conflict. *J Consult Clin Psychol.* 1995;63(4):616-623.

68. Barnett O, Martinez T, Bluestein B. Jealousy and romantic attachment in maritally violent and nonviolent men. *J Interpers Violence.* 1995;10(4):473-486.

69. Carlson B, McNutt L, Choi D, Rose I. Intimate partner abuse and mental health: the role of social support and other protective factors. *Violence Against Women.* 2002;8(6):720-745.

70. Zlotnick C, Kohn R, Peterson J, Pearlstein T. Partner physical victimization in a national sample of American families: relationship to psychological functioning, psychosocial factors, and gender. *J Interpers Violence.* 1998;13(1):156-166.

71. Zlotnick C, Johnson D, Kohn R. Intimate partner violence and long-term psychosocial functioning in a national sample of American women. *J Interpers Violence.* 2006;21(2):262-275.

72. Danielson KK, Moffitt TE, Caspi A, Silva PA. Comorbidity between abuse of an adult and DSM-III-R mental disorders: evidence from an epidemiological study. *Am J Psychiatry.* 1998;155:131-133.

73. Magdol L, Moffitt T, Caspi A, Silva P. Developmental antecedents of partner abuse: a prospective-longitudinal study. *J Abnorm Psychol.* 1998;107(3):375-389.

74. Becker K, Stuewig J, McCloskey L. Traumatic stress symptoms of women exposed to different forms of childhood victimization and intimate partner violence. *J Interpers Violence.* September 2010;25(9):1699-1715.

75. Harris R, Lingoes J. Subscales for the Minnesota Multiphasic Personality Inventory [mimeographed materials]. Department of Psychiatry, University of California, San Francisco; 1968.

76. Rhodes N. Comparison of MMPI Psychopathic Deviate scores of battered and nonbattered women. *J Fam Violence.* 1992;7(4):297-307.

77. Star B. Comparing battered and non-battered women. *Victimology.* 1978;3(1-2):32-44.

78. Walker LE. The battered woman syndrome study. In: Finkelhor D, Gelles RJ, Hotaling GT, Straus MA, eds. *The Dark Side of Families.* Beverly Hills, CA: Sage; 1983:31-48.

79. Stith SM, Green NM, Smith DB, Ward DB. Marital satisfaction and marital discord as risk markers for intimate partner violence: a meta-analytic review. *J Fam Violence.* 2008;23(3):149-160.

80. Babcock J, Costa D, Green C, Eckhardt C. What situations induce intimate partner violence? a reliability and validity study of the Proximal Antecedents to Violent Episodes (PAVE) Scale. *J Fam Psychol.* 2004;18(3):433-442.

81. Flynn A, Graham K. "Why did it happen?" a review and conceptual framework for research on perpetrators' and victims' explanations for intimate partner violence. *Aggression Violent Behav.* 2010;15(3):239-251.

82. Holtzworth-Munroe A, Stuart G, Hutchinson G. Violent versus nonviolent husbands: differences in attachment patterns, dependency, and jealousy. *J Fam Psychol.* 1997;11(3):314-331.

83. Norlander B, Eckhardt C. Anger, hostility, and male perpetrators of intimate partner violence: a meta-analytic review. *Clin Psychol Rev.* 2005;25(2):119-152.

84. Dutton D, Strachan C. Motivational needs for power and spouse-specific assertiveness in assaultive and nonassaultive men. *Violence Vict.* 1987;2(3):145-156.

85. Rehman U, Holtzworth-Munroe A, Herron K, Clements K. 'My way or no way': anarchic power, relationship satisfaction, and male violence. *Pers Relationships.* 2009;16(4):475-488.

86. Sagrestano L, Heavey C, Christensen A. Perceived power and physical violence in marital conflict. *J Soc Issues.* 1999;55(1):65-79.

87. O'Leary KD, Curley, A.D. Assertion and family violence: correlates of spouse abuse. *J Marital Fam Ther.* 1986;12:281-289.

88. Berns S, Jacobson N, Gottman J. Demand–withdraw interaction in couples with a violent husband. *J Consult Clin Psychol.* 1999;67(5):666-674.

89. Cordova J, Jacobson N, Gottman J, Rushe R, Cox G. Negative reciprocity and communication in couples with a violent husband. *J Abnorm Psychol.* 1993;102(4):559-564.

90. Burman B, John R, Margolin G. Observed patterns of conflict in violent, nonviolent, and nondistressed couples. *Behav Assess.* 1992;14(1):15-37.

91. Margolin G, John RS, Gleberman L. Affective responses to conflictual discussion in violent and nonviolent couples. *J Consult Clin Psychol.* 1988;56:24 33.

92. Holtzworth-Munroe A, Smutzler N, Stuart G. Demand and withdraw communication among couples experiencing husband violence. *J Consult Clin Psychol.* 1998;66(5):731-743.

93. Jacobson N, Gottman J, Waltz J, Rushe R, Babcock J, Holtzworth-Munroe A. Affect, verbal content, and psychophysiology in the arguments of couples with a violent husband. *Prev Treatment.* 2000;3(1):982-988.

94. Margolin G, Burman B, John R. Home observations of married couples reenacting naturalistic conflicts. *Behav Assess.* 1989;11(1):101-118.

95. Simon T, Anderson M, Thompson M, Crosby A, Shelley G, Sacks J. Attitudinal acceptance of intimate partner violence among US adults. *Violence Vict.* 2001;16(2):115-126.

96. Stith S, Rosen K, Middleton K, Busch A, Lundeberg K, Carlton R. The intergenerational transmission of spouse abuse: a meta-analysis. *J Marriage Fam.* 2000;62(3):640-654.

97. Straus M, Hamby S, Finkelhor D, Moore D, Runyan D. Identification of child maltreatment with the Parent–Child Conflict Tactics Scales: development and psychometric data for a national sample of American parents. *Child Abuse Negl.* 1998;22(4):249-270.

98. Holden G. Introduction: the development of research into another consequence of family violence. In: Holden G, Geffner R, Jouriles E,eds. *Children Exposed to Marital Violence: Theory, Research, and Applied Issues.* Washington, DC: American Psychological Association; 1998:1-18.

99. Ehrensaft MK, Cohen P, Brown J, et al. Intergenerational transmission of partner violence: A 20-year prospective study. *J Consult Clin Psychol.* 2003;71(4):741-753.

100. Doumas D, Margolin G, John R. The intergenerational transmission of aggression across three generations. *J Fam Violence.* 1994;9(2):157-175.

101. Cui M, Durtschi JA, Donnellan MB, Lorenz FO, Conger RD. Intergenerational transmission of relationship aggression: a prospective longitudinal study. *J Fam Psychol.* 2010;24(6):688-697.

102. Black DS, Sussman S, Unger JB. A further look at the intergenerational transmission of violence: witnessing interparental violence in emerging adulthood. *J Interpers Violence.* 2010;25(6):1022-1042.

103. Straus M. *Beating the Devil Out of Them.* New York, NY: Lexington Books; 1994.

104. Widom C, Shepard R. Accuracy of adult recollections of childhood victimization: Part 1. childhood physical abuse. *Psychol Assess.* 1996;8(4):412-421.

105. Capaldi D, Clark S. Prospective family predictors of aggression toward female partners for at-risk young men. *Dev Psychol.* 34(6):1175-1188.

106. Halpern C, Spriggs A, Martin S, Kupper L. Patterns of intimate partner violence victimization from adolescence to young adulthood in a nationally representative sample. *J Adolesc Health.* 2009;45(5):508-516.

107. Bandura A. *Social Learning Theory.* Oxford, UK: Prentice-Hall; 1977.

108. Simons R, Whitbeck L, Conger R, Wu C. Intergenerational transmission of harsh parenting. *Dev Psychol.* 1991;27(1):159-171.

109. Bargh J, Williams E. The automaticity of social life. *Curr Dir Psychol Sci.* 2006;15(1):1-4.

110. Patterson G. *Coercive Family Process.* Eugene, OR: Castalia; 1982.

111. Patterson G. The aggressive child: victim and architect of a coercive system. In: Hamerlynck LA, Mash EJ, Handy LC, eds. *Behavior Modification and Families: I. Theory and Research.* New York, NY: Brunner & Mazel; 1976:1-30.

112. Hines DA, Saudino KJ. Intergenerational transmission of intimate partner violence: a behavioral genetic perspective. *Trauma Violence Abuse.* 2002;3(3):210-255.

113. DiLalla L, Gottesman I. Biological and genetic contributors to violence: Widom's untold tale. *Psychol Bull.* 1991;109(1):125-129.

114. Widom C. A tail on an untold tale: response to 'biological and genetic contributors to violence: Widom's untold tale'. *Psychol Bull.* 1991;109(1):130-132.

115. LeDeux J. *Synaptic Self: How Our Brains Become Who We Are.* New York, NY: Viking; 2002.

116. Ainsworth M, Blehar M, Waters E, Wall S. *Patterns of Attachment: A Psychological Study of the Strange Situation.* Oxford, UK: Lawrence Erlbaum; 1978.

117. Bowlby J. *Attachment and Loss.* New York, NY: Basic Books; 1969.

118. Davies PT, Cummings EM. Marital conflict and child adjustment: an emotional security hypothesis. *Psychol Bull.* 1994;116:387-411.

119. Cummings EM, Davies PT. *Marital Conflict and Children: An Emotional Security Perspective.* New York, NY. The Guilford Press; 2010.

120. Cummings E, Davies PT. Emotional security as a regulatory process in normal development and the development of psychopathology. *Dev Psychopathol.* 1996;8:123-139.

121. Cummings EM, Goeke-Morey MC, Papp LM, Dukewich TL. Children's responses to mothers' and fathers' emotional and tactics in marital conflicts in the home. *J Fam Psychol.* 2002;16:478-492.

122. O'Leary KD, Slep, AMS, O'Leary SG. Multivariate models of men's and women's partner aggression. *J Consult Clin Psychol.* 2007;75:752-764.

Chapter 23

Intimate Partner Violence and the Mother Who Kills

Marie E. Mugavin, PhD, FNP-BC, SAFE-A

Key Points

1. Each year women experience about 4.8 million intimate partner related physical assaults and rapes. IPV resulted in 2340 deaths in 2007, 70% of which were female.[1]

2. Factors that increase the risk an individual will hurt an intimate partner include, but are not limited to, a history of violence or aggression, childhood victimization, drug and alcohol abuse, and unemployment.

3. Partner abuse is a significant risk factor for all forms of violence against children with women being more than twice as likely to abuse their children if they are in a violent intimate partner relationship.

4. Those women who feel they have no power to influence their own experiences are not likely to take immediate action to control stressful events in their lives.

5. Research is less typically focused on women abused during pregnancy, although the violence during that period can be more severe than that which occurs when women are not pregnant.

6. An external locus of control was diathetic to the development of emotional and psychological difficulties that ultimately lead to the death of their children.

Introduction

Intimate partner violence (IPV), which is also referred to as domestic violence, occurs between 2 people in a close relationship including current and former spouses and dating partners.[1] IPV exists along a continuum from a single episode of violence to ongoing battering and includes physical, sexual, and emotional abuse. It generally starts with emotional abuse and then progresses to physical or sexual assault. Poverty and a low level of education are stronger risk factors for IPV than other sociodemographic features such as ethnicity and marital status perhaps because such constraints provide women with fewer choices to end a violent situation and may influence her selection of a partner. Each year women experience about 4.8 million intimate partner related physical assaults and rapes. IPV resulted in 2340 deaths in 2007, 70% of which were female.[1]

An unfortunate byproduct of this phenomenon is that children are more likely to be victims of fatal and nonfatal child abuse if there is intimate partner violence in their family.[2] Some women abuse and kill in conjunction with the male partner or fail to intervene, both of which demonstrate the serious, intersecting issues of IPV and child maltreatment. In 2008, there were 905 000 confirmed cases of child abuse and 1740 child fatalities. Both parents were involved in more than 75% of the filicides, and the mother acted alone (maternal filicide) in more than 1/4 (26.6%) of these cases.[3]

Filicide lies on the extreme end of the IPV continuum and refers to the murder of a child up to the age of 18 years. The perpetrator may be the natural parent or other caregivers such as stepparents or legal guardians.[4] The most dangerous time for children is the first 3 years of life. According to NCAND Child Maltreatment Report,[3] 32.6% of children abused and 79.8% of children who were killed were between the ages of birth to 3 years with the first year of life being the most perilous for the child.

There is a robust relationship between victimization history and locus of control.[5] *Locus of control* is a concept that concerns the attitudes of people about the control they have over their life circumstances.[6] Those who believe they can make choices to affect their life circumstances have an *internal locus of control,* while those who believe their circumstances are controlled by external forces are said to have *external locus of control.*[6] This manner of thinking about and responding to the world can become a relatively stable characteristic of an individual.

Victimization and an external locus of control predict problems such as depression, anxiety, dissociation, and hostility.[7] The focus of this chapter is the relationship between intimate partner violence and maternal filicide as suggested by women incarcerated for said crime. Their narratives resonated feelings of victimization, oppression, and regret. An external locus of control was diathetic to the development of emotional and psychological difficulties that ultimately lead to the death of their children. The data was gathered during interviews with 43 women incarcerated for killing their children across 3 states in 3 different prison systems. A university and 3 prison Internal Review Boards approved the study.

The women interviewed were largely part of the general prison population. Two were in solitary confinement. None of the women were deemed incompetent due to reason of insanity, although more than half of the participants had one or more Axis I diagnoses (prior to their incarceration) including but not limited to, clinical depression, anxiety disorder, bipolar disorder, posttraumatic stress disorder, and attention deficit hyperactivity disorder. Common Axis II disorders included borderline personality disorder, antisocial personality disorder, histrionic personality disorder, dependent personality disorder and intellectual disabilities.

FILICIDE: A SNAPSHOT

How are women who kill their children broadly evaluated by criminal justice and health service personnel after the crime? They have been categorized according to the perpetrator's psychopathology, social and psychiatric stress factors, the source of impulse to kill, and the suspect's alleged motive for the crime.[8-11] Patterns seen among women incarcerated for filicide or abuse include the presence of multiple, severe stressors such as persistent poverty, mental illness, history of substance abuse, limited social support and education, unemployment, serving as the primary caregiver for at least one young child, and being victims of childhood abuse.[9,11,12]

Maternal mental illness plays a varying role in these crimes.[13] Filicidal mothers drawn from psychiatric populations have shown high rates of depression, suicidality, psychosis, prior use of psychiatric services, and, in some cases, decreased intelligence.[9] Smithey[14] asserted filicide was the result of a culmination of predisposing factors evolving from the mothers' socialization experiences and precipitating factors, such as economic deprivation and a lack of interpersonal support.

Korbin[15] concentrated on the role of a mother's social network in the facilitation of a filicide. She underscored the repetitive nature of abuse preceding some child fatalities with an emphasis on the fact that it is extremely difficult to predict whether child abuse will result in a fatality. Korbin identified a positive feedback process whereby maternal denial of the seriousness of previous abuse and minimization of the maltreatment by members of her support networks augmented each other and undermined the urgency with which the cases might otherwise have been viewed. The deceased children in her study were perceived by mothers as having had a range of health problems and behavioral difficulties that made them difficult to care for.

What is being addressed in this chapter is the proclivity for some women with a trauma history to become involved with a man who is equally unhealthy and who exploits her vulnerabilities. Intrapsychic responses are viewed from the standpoint of women who may never have felt a sense of empowerment or control in their lives. Based on the narratives, it seems external forces have shaped their thinking and as an extension, responses to abusive partners and their children. To this end, there is an emphasis on external locus of control in the women. Although broad categorization is important to understanding patterns in a given population and to advancing knowledge, what is most pertinent in the context of this chapter is the more nuanced exploration of perpetrator narratives. In these narratives we learn how the women perceive the role of IPV in the demise of her child(ren).

The Male Perpetrator of IPV

Factors that increase the risk an individual will hurt his partner include but are not limited to a history of violence or aggression, childhood victimization, drug and alcohol abuse, and unemployment. Men who batter often select partners they perceive will be dependent, meet their emotional needs, or physically attractive.[16] They make an effort to create emotional vulnerability and dependency as the relationship progresses. Frequent attempts are made to isolate their partners by disrupting support networks and interfering with job-related or school-related activities. Partner selection may be influenced by needs arising from their varied personality disorders and styles. Interestingly, rapists and sex offenders demonstrate this tendency during victim selection in that they look for children and adolescents with low self-esteem who appear lonely and emotionally needy.[16] Male perpetrators are often demanding in a relationship and use varied approaches to maintain control.

AB, a 42-year-old Hispanic woman, high school dropout, responsible for the death of 3 children reported:

"My husband turned me on to drugs when we first got together. I was weakened and confused allowing the drug to take me over and allowing my husband to abuse me and my children. I was a very sick person."

The men are inclined to intimidate naïve or unsuspecting women with the goal of breaking their will. This is not difficult given the victims they choose. JT, a 30-year-old paralegal incarcerated for killing her 2-year-old son:

"The physical abuse greatly changed my life. I married my first husband at 18 and I changed as a result of the abuse. I feel that it took away my positive attitude and innocence. My outlook on life and relationships changed."

AZ, a 26-year-old clerk in insurance company incarcerated for killing her 8-month-old child:

"I didn't have very much love for myself back then. I let myself down and had no confidence in myself from all the abuse - it helped break me down to nothing as a person and made me very depressed."

RG, a 24-year-old sales representative incarcerated for killing her 4-month-old:

"He kept me trapped from venturing out and being productive in raising my children. I didn't want to fail in his eyes so we went without — we always stayed home. I became addicted to drugs to deal with the fear, anger and pain. The most drastic affect my drug addiction had and continues to have on my kids is that I was physically but not mentally there for them. Now I am physically absent cause of my crime which continues to impact our lives and my daughter is dead."

One woman reported being weakened by childhood abuse and her regret of inviting those dynamics back into her home with a new husband. AZ, a 26-year-old exotic dancer incarcerated for killing her 26-month-old child:

"My father was an alcoholic. I was afraid of authority, rejection, and always felt like I was not good enough, not doing enough. I was a single mom - the best mom I knew to be. My children that are alive are very close to me – the problems began when I married a very controlling and abusive man. Those experiences he put us through produced a confused and desperate and terrified person (me). I could not be myself and feared speaking and what my actions might provoke. What affected me with my children was that I never left the abuse therefore I didn't give my children enough attention and they suffered badly."

NM, a data entry clerk whose child died at 5 years of age, shared:

"I was always filled with fear - not knowing the reason for things he did to me. I was desperate because he would beat me and I knew it would affect the kids - I had maternal instinct - but I always felt rejected, not worthy, not good enough – too scared to go. He told me I would never make it without him."

WOMEN AND VIOLENCE

Partner abuse is a significant risk factor for all forms of violence against children[17] with women being more than twice as likely to abuse their children if they are in a violent intimate partner relationship.[18-22] Battered women are more likely to have suffered child sexual or physical abuse than women who are not battered.[16] They are susceptible to selection by male perpetrators largely due to high rates of depression, anxiety, posttraumatic stress disorder, and having an external locus of control. Intimate partner violence has also been linked to a women's use of harsh parental discipline such as screaming, hitting and, threatening behaviors. For example, the Second National Family Violence Survey[23] showed that mothers abused by their partners more often employ corporal punishment as a means of disciplining them than those women who were not abused.[16]

JT: "I used drugs because I was so desperate for love from their father, and feared being alone with the kids. I neglected the kids and hit them a lot especially when I was high, but I loved them. It was really my husband who took all my energy and time. That was the way he wanted it. I think my kids were affected by witnessing the mental and physical abuse of their father because my son would try to protect me and my daughter would scream and cry."

The pain and humiliation of long-term abuse flared in one woman who claimed that experiences of physical and sexual abuse and feelings of revenge still have a profound affect on her thinking. MM, a 26-year-old teen advocate for the State whose daughter died at 5 months of age shared:

"I was beaten as a child and then as a wife. I hate my husband for sexually abusing me for so many years. I want to hurt people that hurt me in the past. The abuse happening said I meant nothing to nobody in this world not even God. Now I see them as experiences that eventually got me in prison. My husband isolated me, family members were not allowed in my life, I was alone and scared to death. My baby was too young to know that, I didn't mean to hurt him; I wanted to hurt my husband. I just kept hitting and hitting him and then he stopped moving. Now my son is dead, I am in prison and my husband is on the outside living his life like nothing happened."

Research is less typically focused on women abused during pregnancy, although the violence during that period can be more severe than that which occurs when women are not pregnant.[24] Careful consideration of IPV directed against women during pregnancy and the women's later abuse of their infants is important. Newborns are more vulnerable and frail than older children making the physical abuse of infants more deleterious on the development and functioning of the child's brain. Infants exposed to maternal abuse may develop attachment and various types of psychiatric disorders.[2]

GA, a 26-year-old college student incarcerated for killing her 5-month-old child:

"The abuse began during my pregnancy. Until then I never even thought of him hurting me. He didn't have a job, was always angry with me like it was my fault. He used to punch me in the stomach and curse at the baby. One time he beat me so bad I had to have the orbit of my eye fixed. He took the phones and locked me in during the day. I couldn't see my family. They didn't know where we lived. When the baby was five months old my husband threatened to take him away by saying I wasn't a good mother. Being close to my baby was very meaningful to me. I never wanted to be separated from him and I wanted for him to feel no matter what, he could rely on me, so I stayed in the abuse. One day I was so hurt and angry after a beating from my husband and the baby kept crying. I shook and hit him until he stopped and went back to sleep – I kept seeing my husband's face while I was doing it—all I felt was pain and extreme anger. A few hours later when I went to check on the baby he was dead— I wish it was my husband who died. I'll never forgive myself for killing my child."

THE TRIFECTA OF POWER, OPPRESSION, AND CONTROL IN THE MOTHER WHO KILLS HER CHILDREN

Popular media in the United States reinforces a feminine stereotype lacking in self-efficacy and personal control. Women are socialized to hold a more external locus of control view than men. Lefcourt[25] postulated that those women who feel they have no power to influence their own experiences are not likely to take immediate action to control stressful events in their lives. They begin to believe after multiple negative experiences that their behavior will have little if any effect on outcomes.

Some investigators have questioned whether there is a primary gain for the woman in having her children removed from an abusive household by an authority rather than making the decision to leave the violent situation with her children. While that perspective is worthy of consideration by health care providers and scholars, the women interviewed and discussed in this chapter reported across the board, that they were afraid to report issues of domestic violence or child abuse for fear of the child being removed from their custody.

Many women stay in relationships where they are victimized because they are acclimated to violence and do not perceive their partner to be very dangerous. Part of the confusion may be because abuse occurs over minor disagreements followed by expressions of remorse, affection, and gift giving.[24] Women incarcerated for killing their children often have severe child abuse histories in which their experiences and pain were never validated. Although the spouse was violent, the remorse can be a temporary salve to a woman unaccustomed to kindness and generosity in the context of abuse. In this group, perpetrators cycle from generosity to withholding affection and economic resources. Emotional abuse has a profound, long-term affect on the women long after their physical wounds have healed. It is common for harmless interactions to transform into violent struggles to satisfy the perpetrators need for control and power.

A rather provocative explanation for ongoing intimate partner violence was proposed by Freud[26] which asserted masochist tendencies in abused women. The main premise is that maintenance of suffering is all that matters to abused women. The suffering is required in an effort to ameliorate underlying guilt related to competing with her mother for her father's attention. The woman unconsciously provokes paternal aggression with her partner thereby reducing deep feelings of guilt associated with her desire for her father.

Other theorists suggest that feelings of helplessness and long periods of dependency in infancy predispose women to the masochistic process. In this context, women are viewed as afraid to resist, refuse, offend, or insist on limits. These coping mechanisms (or lack thereof) are seeded in early childhood. As an adult they maintain an obedient and cooperative manner complying with the partner's demands usually in an effort to survive. Diminished social support and isolation lead to feelings of hopelessness.

Anger directed against the self or others is always a central problem in the lives of people who have been violated. Van der Kolk[27] considers this cycle re-enactment of real events from the trauma. Disruptions or distortions of attachment bonds lead to post-traumatic stress syndromes. Strong emotional ties with abusers can lead to confusion between feelings of pain and love. When experiencing stress and anxiety, previously traumatized people tend to return to familiar patterns, even if they cause pain and feelings of powerlessness.

For some women, children can represent both a significant source of power and oppression. They have relatively little power both outside and inside the home yet considerable responsibility for and control over their children.[28] The juxtaposition may underlie perpetuation of maternal violence toward her children: that is, aggression toward those who have even less power than she does.[29] When the perpetrator externalizes blame for his attacks, it is common to berate the victim for being a poor wife and mother. Accusations related to role as spouse and mother are of particular sensitivity to the population of mothers discussed in this text.

NT, 24-year-old high school drop-out incarcerated for killing 3 of her 4 children:

"My father's alcohol use and the way he treated my mom colored the way I looked at all men. I thought I made a good decision with my boyfriend, I never believed he would lay a hand on me, but I was so wrong. My children witnessed the abuse and I think our relationship was strained because of it. My abuse from him numbed me to recognizing how I caused serious injuries in my kids. The drug use also did this to me. I believe that after being physically abused as a child and the fear I suffered then froze me to where I couldn't fight back like I wanted to. Being a good mom was all I ever wanted to do up until I took my children's lives. I really believed I was being a good mom. I was so naïve, he had all the control."

Many mothers are afraid to reach out and ask for help, but there is evidence that women who have been abused or killed by their partner used the health care system with some regularity. They sought care for injuries from domestic violence, but more often for physical or mental health issues including depression, anxiety, and substance abuse. Children were brought in for well-child and acute health care needs.[24] TJ, 17-year-old high school dropout, convenience store cashier before incarcerated for filicide of 3-month-old child, reported:

"I remember bringing my child into the ED about two weeks before he died. I shared my concerns about not being able to manage him, not understanding his behavior and that we had some problems at home. I tried to cover my own substance abuse and the fact that I was a runaway minor. I was intimidated by people in general and scared of the doctors and nurses at the hospital. I covered my bruises with long sleeves and make up. I was raised in the manner of "what went on inside the house stayed inside the house" but really wished someone could have helped me – that I had been more open. I was so scared and confused."

LOCUS OF CONTROL AND THE PRISON SETTING

The women interviewed were all incarcerated for the crime of filicide. The external locus of control view was proliferated in the prison setting with mothers being highly stigmatized victims of abuse and relentlessly reminded of their stations at the bottom of the prison pecking order. Many were afraid to self-identify, avoiding grief and group therapy meetings, thereby further diminishing their opportunities for evaluation.[15,30,31] Prisons tend to maintain stringent control over inmates with activities continually observed and regulated by members of the prison staff. Unpredictable, random behaviors of prison staff toward inmates are encouraged including personal and room searches, mail censorship, and telephone conversation monitoring.

Behavioral and psychological adjustment is also influenced by the prisoner subculture. Strong controls on inmate behavior are imposed and one must define her standing within the social hierarchy and manufacture acceptable responses to other inmates and the prison staff.[32] The inmate code requires experimentation on the part of new arrivals to test limits of acceptable behavior including that of sexual orientation. There were reports by a few study participants of intimate partner violence within the prison, but those individuals experienced shame related to taking female lovers and would not provide details of the maltreatment.

Fellow inmates bestow rewards or sanctions in an effort to induce normative prisoner behavior.[32] The transition was confusing and the women felt little control over how people responded to them. There was a significant shift toward externality. The longer they were incarcerated, the more developed their external locus of control. Interestingly, classes offered regarding self-reflection, parenting, religious study, and addiction counseling helped the women begin to build on fragments of an internal locus of control that became more cohesive with time spent in prison. They learned to survive with a shift toward externality, yet also began to grow internally. At the time of the interviews not one victim of intimate partner violence was still associated with her male partner/perpetrator. It seemed the profundity of the loss of their child(ren) coupled with the opportunity to develop self-knowledge through prison programs and counseling sobered them and inspired belief that they can make choices to effect positive change in their lives and to contribute in a meaningful way.

CLINICAL IMPLICATIONS

In the clinical setting, questions pertaining to whether a woman feels threatened by her partner or has an inclination to hurt her child do not always inform one's risk assessment. There may not be a perception of danger on the woman's part and her commitment to portraying the role of "good mother" can obscure identification of those at risk for being hurt or for hurting their children. The most effective way to communicate with a vulnerable woman who feels easily threatened and in denial of the danger she experiences day-to-day is to maintain a nonjudgmental manner during interviews and to reassure her she is safe to share concerns.

The idea that she may have an external locus of control can serve the clinician. We must be sentient that simple measures including a reassuring manner and tone of voice will help build a foundation of trust in a woman who may not have been able to trust anyone else in her life. If the woman believes her circumstances are controlled by external forces the clinician may influence a situation by focusing on the need to protect the child as an important element of being a good mother. A focus on the maternal role and the child's safety may be an important catalyst to moving women away from dangerous environments and preventing further intimate partner abuse and the unfortunate death of a child.

CONCLUSION

Partner abuse is a significant risk factor for all forms of violence against children. Women are more than twice as likely to abuse their children if they are in a violent intimate partner relationship. Those with a significant history of childhood abuse may experience anxiety, depression, dissociation, hostility, and have a largely external locus of control. This predisposition makes them easy targets for male perpetrators. Narratives of this sample resonated feelings of oppression, fear, and regret around events that lead to the unfortunate demise of their children. Inherent in each scenario was the use of illicit substances and need for validation from the male perpetrator at the expense of tending to the needs of their children.

It can be difficult to identify women in the clinical setting who are at risk for being hurt or hurting their children. They may feel easily threatened and in denial of the danger experienced day-to-day. It is appropriate to maintain a nonjudgmental manner during interviews and to reassure the mother she is safe to share concerns.

The external locus of control perspective can serve the clinician. Simple measures including a reassuring manner and tone of voice will help build a foundation of trust. A focus on maternal role and the child's safety can be important catalysts to moving women away from dangerous environments and preventing further intimate partner abuse and the unfortunate death of a child.

REFERENCES

1. Centers for Disease Control and Prevention. Intimate Partner Violence. Centers for Disease Control and Prevention Web site. http://www.cdc.gov/violenceprevention/ intimatepartnerviolence/index.html. Published 2011. Updated April 2013. Accessed July 17, 2013.

2. Casanueva CE, Martin SL. Intimate partner violence during pregnancy and mothers' child abuse potential. *J Interpers Violence.* 2007;22:603-620.

3. National Child Abuse and Neglect Data system (NCANDS). Office of the Assistant Secretary for Planning and Evaluation Web site. aspe.hhs.gov/hsp/06/catalog-ai-an-na/NCANDS.htm. Published 2008. Accessed March 4, 2011.

4. West SG, Friedman SH, Resnick PJ. Fathers who kill their children: an analysis of the literature. *J Forensic Sci.* 2009;54(2):463-468.

5. Porter C, Long P. Locus of control and adjustment in female adult survivors of childhood sexual abuse. *J Child Sex Abuse.* 1999;8(1):3-25.

6. Rotter JB. Generalized expectancies for internal versus external control of reinforcement. *Psychol Monogr.* 1966;80:1-28.

7. Lefcourt HM. *Locus of Control: Current Trends in Theory and Research.* Hillsdale, NJ: Lawrence Erlbaum Associates; 1976.

8. Baker J. *You Can't Let Your Children Cry: Filicide in Victoria 1978-1988* [master's thesis]. Victoria, Australia: University of Melbourne; 1991.

9. Hatters SF, Horwitz S, Resnick PJ. Child murder by mothers: a critical analysis of the current state of knowledge and a research agenda. *Am J Psychiatry.* 2005;162(9):1578-1587.

10. McKee GR. *Why Mothers Kill: A Forensic Psychologist's Casebook.* New York, NY: Oxford University Press; 2007.

11. Resnick PJ. Child murder by parents: a psychiatric review of filicide. *Am J Psychiatry.* 1969;126(3):325-334.

12. Lewis CF, Bunce SC. Filicidal mothers and the impact of psychosis on maternal filicide. *J Am Acad Psychiatry Law.* 2003;31:459-470.

13. Spinelli MG. Maternal infanticide associated with mental illness: prevention and the promise of saved lives. *Am J Psychiatry.* 2004;161(9):1548-1557.

14. Smithey M. Infant homicide at the hands of mothers: toward a sociological perspective. *Deviant Behav.* 1997;18:255-272.

15. Korbin JE. Fatal maltreatment by mothers: a proposed framework. *Child Abuse Negl.* 1989;13:481-489.

16. Saunders D, Fennel J, Diechert K, Kenna C. What attracts men who batter to their partners? an exploratory study. *J Interpers Violence.* 2011;26(14).

17. Tajima EA. The relative importance of wife abuse as a risk factor for violence against children. *Child Abuse Negl.* 2000;24(11):1383-1398.

18. Straus M, Gelles R. *Physical Violence in American Families.* New Brusnwick, NJ: Transaction Publishing; 1990.

19. Holden G, Ritchie K. Linking extreme marital discord, child rearing, and child behavior problems: evidence from battered women. *Child Dev.* 1991;62:311-327.

20. Holden G, Stein J, Ritchie KL, Harris SD, Jouriles E. Parenting behaviors and beliefs of battered women. In: Holden G, Geffner R, Jouriles E, eds. *Children Exposed to Marital Violence: Theory, Research, and Applied Issues.* Washington, DC: American Psychological Association; 1998:289-334.

21. Levendosky A, Graham-Bermann S. Parenting in battered women: the effects of domestic violence on women and their children. *J Fam Violence.* 2001;16(2):171-192.

22. Osofsky J. The impact of violence on children. Future of Children. 1999;9(3):33-49.

23. Straus M. *Breathing the Devil out of them: Corporal Punishment in American Families.* San Francisco, CA: Jossey-Bass/Lexington Books; 1994.

24. Campbell J. Helping women understand their risk in situations of intimate partner violence. *J Interpers Violence.* 2004;19(12):1464-1477.

25. Lefcourt HM. Internal versus external control of reinforcement: a review. *Psychol Bull.* 1966;65(4):206–20.

26. Rieff P. *Freud: The Mind of the Moralist.* New York, NY: Anchor Books; 1959.

27. Van der Kolk BA, Perry JC, Herman JL. Childhood origins of self-destructive behavior. *Am J Psychiatry.* 1991;148(12):1665-1671.

28. Meyer CL, Oberman M. *Mothers Who Kill Their Children: Understanding the Acts of Moms from Susan Smith to the "Prom Mom."* New York, NY: New York University Press; 2001.

29. Cole SG. Child battery. In: Guberman C, Wolf M, eds. *No Safe Place: Violence Against Women and Children.* Toronto, Ontario: Women's Press; 1985.

30. Banks C. *Women in prison.* Santa Barbara, CA: ABC-CLIO, Inc; 2003.

31. Enos S. *Mothering from the Inside: Parenting in a Women's Prison.* New York, NY: State University of New York Press; 2001.

32. Griffith J, Pennington-Averett A, Bryan I. Women prisoners' multidimensional locus of control. *Crim Justice Behav.* 1981;8(3):375-389.

Chapter 24

THE FEMINIST PERSPECTIVE: INTIMATE PARTNER VIOLENCE AND THE INTERSECTION WITH HEALTH CARE

Grace Mattern*
Carol Post[‡]

KEY POINTS

1. The feminist perspective of intimate partner violence recognizes that violence against women is connected to women's unequal access to power and autonomy both in and out of the family.

2. Feminist, victim-centered advocacy recognizes that every victim of intimate partner violence is the best judge of her own experiences and can best determine what next steps are best for her.

3. The battered women's movement has focused on shifting power imbalances between men and women in the public sphere, including the civil and criminal justice systems, in order to support women's empowerment in the private sphere.

4. The feminist model asserts that women should be considered as independent, empowered agents of change in their own lives and should have access to state systems of justice and protection.

5. Feminist advocacy has promoted a model of collaboration with other systems, including police, prosecutors, judges, welfare officials, health care professionals, faith leaders, and child protection workers, in order to establish empowering responses to victims so they could access the services and support needed to remain free of the control of batterers.

6. Framing intimate partner violence as a health care issue of paramount importance creates an opportunity to identify victims and offer them support and assistance that could prevent future violence.

Research has consistently found since the 1980s that intimate partner violence (IPV) and sexual violence are common experiences for women, with over half of all women experiencing some form of abuse in their lifetimes. The National Violence Against Women Survey (NVAWS) conducted by the Centers for Disease Control and the National Institute of Justice,[1] the largest published prevalence survey to date, found that 33% of women have experienced an assault by an intimate partner and that 17.6%

*Executive Director, NH Coalition Against Domestic and Sexual Violence
[‡]Executive Director, Delaware Coalition Against Domestic Violence

of women have been sexually assaulted, with 14.8% including penetration. Questions from the NVAWS have been replicated in several states, including New Hampshire. State replication surveys have found similar or higher rates of violence against women. In 2006, the New Hampshire Violence Against Women Survey[2] found that 33.4% of women have experienced intimate partner violence and 22.7% have been sexually assaulted, with 19.5% of women having been sexually assaulted with penetration.

INTRODUCTION

Current recognition of the pervasive and destructive reality of intimate partner violence in the lives of women first arose out of women's advocacy groups in the late 1960s. Women who were involved in various movements, such as the civil rights and anti-war movements, began to share experiences across the multiple arenas in which they were organizing. As women came together to talk about their struggles for leadership and autonomy within mostly male-led social action movements, they articulated a variety of common struggles, including a lack of economic, political, and personal power in all spheres of their lives. Women's centers and activist groups were organized to address these common concerns, and it soon became evident that many participants had been victims of sexual assault and/or physical and emotional abuse at the hands of their intimate partners.

Out of these early gatherings in women-centered spaces emerged the beginnings of the battered women's movement. As women recognized their own stories of abuse in what other women recounted, a growing awareness developed of the commonality of violence in women's lives. These nascent advocates soon realized that criminal laws against wife abuse were rarely enforced, divorce was difficult to obtain, and services for victims of abuse were essentially nonexistent.[3] In response, women began to organize hotlines and emergency shelters for victims, using volunteer resources, private homes, and telephones to provide a safety net for women fleeing abusive partners.[4]

THEORETICAL ADVANCES

The first research documenting the level of violence in American families was published soon after the emergence of supportive services for victims, providing concrete evidence of violence against women by intimate partners. Early studies, such as the landmark 1980 study conducted by Straus, Gelles, and Steinmetz,[5] found high rates of violence in families and described a number of structural and situational factors that contribute to violence among family members. Authors such as Del Martin in Battered Wives[6] and Lenore Walker in The Battered Woman[7] offered descriptive accounts of what living with abuse was like for women abused by their male partners. With early research confirming what advocates and activists knew from their own experiences and what they heard from the other women in their lives, a theoretical feminist framework that could help explain the origins of violence against women, including intimate partner violence and sexual assault, began to take shape.

As scholarly work on intimate partner violence began to emerge, 3 main theoretical perspectives were developed to provide an analysis of violence in families and intimate relationships. The first, rooted in psychology, attempts to explain domestic abuse at the individual behavior level. The second, a sociological perspective, hypothesizes that socioeconomic factors, family systems, and cultural norms, lie at the root of intimate partner violence. The third framework, the feminist perspective, offers a gender-based analysis of violence in intimate relationships. Although these 3 theoretical frameworks originate from fundamentally different standpoints, they are not mutually exclusive and there can be considerable overlap among them. Individual behavior influences the function of social institutions, such as the family and the legal system, and social institutions affect how individuals operate within particular social contexts.

Of these 3 models, the feminist perspective has gained the most acceptance among those providing services to victims of domestic violence since the 1980s, because it places violence against women in the context of women's unequal access to power and autonomy both in and outside of the family. In 1983, researchers Dobash and Dobash[8] defined marriage as the social institution upon which the patriarchal structure of society is organized and within which the ideology of male supremacy is reproduced. They considered violence against wives to be primarily an expression of the gender relations of a society in which men were entitled to control women through the use of force if necessary. Thus, as Dobash and Dobash stated, "it is within marriage that a woman is most likely to be slapped or shoved about, severely assaulted, killed, or raped."[8] According to this perspective, as long as women were primarily responsible for domestic labor, child care, and the emotional sustenance of the family and men were primarily defined in terms of work outside the home, wife abuse would continue.

Early feminist research on intimate partner violence attempted to describe the broader circumstances that defined the lives of battered women. Numerous studies documented the experiences of abused women within the family,[9,10] in medical institutions,[11,12] in shelters,[13] and within the criminal justice system.[14,15] Feminist approaches also sought to link various forms of female oppression and male domination by examining the connections between domestic violence, sexual assault, and pornography.[16-18]

Bograd[19] described this feminist perspective as an approach which emphasized relations of gender and power to explain wife abuse and provided an analysis of the family as an historically situated social institution, which validated the experiences of women, and helped develop research models and theories that more accurately reflected those experiences. Consequently, while a feminist analysis of domestic violence does not deny the existence of psychological and social factors which may contribute to the incidence of violence in intimate relationships; it does require that those factors be placed within the context of institutionalized male domination. Whether the subject of study is the behavior of individuals or the structure of institutions, the gender relations of power must be at the root of any meaningful feminist analysis.

The strategies of the battered women's movement have thus been designed to provide services to victims, while challenging the societal, legal, and structural basis of men's power and abuse of women. For advocates, a major part of this challenge has been to expand and legitimize the feminist analysis and model of empowerment-based services commonly practiced within programs for battered women to any system or institution with which a victim might interact, including the health care system.

Empowerment Model

From the beginning, services for women who were experiencing intimate partner violence were structured within a peer-led empowerment model.[20] Volunteers offering safe shelter and crisis intervention for battered women helped victims of domestic violence identify choices for addressing the violence in their lives and then supported them in enacting those choices. Instead of telling victims what to do, early battered women's advocates encouraged women to make their own choices, thus helping reclaim some of the power they had been denied by their abusive partners. Rather than developing a professional or clinical network of supportive services for victims, the foundation of the battered women's movement created a model of peer support that recognized the centrality of violence in the lives of many women. This model helped victims of domestic violence understand that they were not alone in their experience of abuse, and promoted the view that anyone could be abused. Further, early advocates believed that battered women were the real experts on their own lives and capable of making decisions about their best course of action.[20] This fundamental peer empowerment model of services for victims of intimate partner violence still underlies most domestic violence programs operating in the country today.

EARLY FEMINIST IPV ACTIVISM

Shelters and Support

By first addressing the physical integrity and safety of victims of intimate partner violence, feminist organizers provided a foundation for the development of services to victims. As shelters and hotlines for battered women organized across the country, the experiences of women who were fleeing abusive relationships shaped the expansion of services provided by domestic violence programs. Beyond physical violence, victims described ongoing patterns of control and power manipulation that affected their lives as much, if not more, than the physical violence.[20] The coercive control of batterers defined victims' lives in ways that were often replicated by the legal and social service systems that victims turned to for safety and support. Police who were called to homes during violent incidents did little more than try to calm down abusers, often leaving the scene and the victim vulnerable to even worse abuse.[21] Prosecutors did not proceed with criminal prosecutions even when batterers were charged with crimes, or if prosecutors brought charges, judges rarely imposed significant sentences.

As advocates addressed the detrimental effects of exposing children to battering, child welfare systems responded by blaming mothers for allowing their children to be subjected to abuse and charged them with "failure to protect." When victims turned to social service agencies, faith communities, and other systems of public assistance seeking support and safety, they were often confronted with questions about what they had done to enrage their abuser, or why they had put up with past abuse.[22] Victims who did manage to get away from abusers and engage with local domestic violence service programs described ongoing control on the part of intimate partners and social systems that reinforced the disempowering messages of batterers: that the abuse was the victim's own fault, that no one would support or believe her, and that she would never get away. Thus, in turning to the justice and social services systems for relief, advocates and the battered women they were trying to assist often encountered systems built on a patriarchal model that represented the very power structure feminist advocates were challenging.

In response to the spoken experiences of victims trying to access legal and social services support, domestic violence programs expanded beyond advocacy with individual women to systems level advocacy. Working with local police departments, prosecutors, judges, welfare officials, health care professionals, faith leaders, and child protection workers, domestic violence advocates provided training and education about the dynamics of intimate partner violence. Advocates formed collaborations with local service providers and developed protocols that outlined empowering responses to victims so they could access the services and support needed to remain free of the control of batterers. Since the 1980s, the feminist perspective of intimate partner violence has continued to inform and influence domestic violence services, systems advocacy initiatives, and research efforts all across the country and around the world. Advocate and volunteer training at local service programs routinely includes a component on the feminist roots of the movement to end violence against women and stresses the centrality of a victim-centered, empowerment approach to advocacy. Within a few years of the development of the first volunteer programs to assist battered women, advocates for victims began to secure government and private funding for direct service programs on the local, state, and national level. As domestic violence programs became more established, they continued to provide services for victims that were based on the experiences of victims themselves. Built on a feminist model of social change and empowerment, domestic violence service programs organized around the needs of victims. Rather than tell victims how to resolve the difficult choices they faced in fleeing abusers, domestic violence programs provided information to victims on their legal and social services options, then supported victims in the choices they made. By allowing victims to control their own process of disengaging from violent partners, advocates empowered women to realize their own capacities and strengths. Advocates also affirmed the resilience of victims, recognizing that no one knows better than the victim what choices will be safest and most effective for her.

Legal Reforms

In the 1970s, as programs assisting victims organized across the country, the societal structures that upheld men's ownership of women and children were still firmly in place. Historically, the behavior of men towards their wives and children was regulated only marginally, usually when abuse of children came to the attention of authorities. Rarely was men's violence against their female partners considered a crime, and even violence as severe as murder was often portrayed as an uncontrollable response by a man to the threat of "losing" his woman. Most recently, so called "honor killings" among Middle Eastern traditional cultures have placed an additional focus on this view that men control women and can be "shamed" by women acting independently of the wishes of the dominant men in their lives.[23,24]

Feminist perspectives brought to light important dimensions to the issue of intimate violence by considering gender relations of power and dominance and how those relations are reflected and reinforced in the public sphere. Early on, advocates recognized the need for fundamental change in how civil and criminal justice systems responded to domestic violence cases. Until the early 1980s, the criminal justice system largely ignored the problem of intimate partner violence. Law enforcement and the courts took a laissez-faire approach to the plight of battered women, responding only in the most egregious cases and, even then, arrests and prosecutions were rare. For example, a 1971 report from Kansas City, MO noted that 40% of all homicides were spouse killings and 50% of these murders were cases in which the police had been called to the house 5 times or more in preceding 2 years.[25] The law also vigorously regulated the private domain of the family including marriage and property rights, divorce settlements, and the custody of children, in a way which upheld male privilege.[26] Thus, while women were still largely excluded from the public sphere, they were also denied legal redress for wrongs committed against them in the private domestic sphere. Implicitly and explicitly, the message was conveyed to both men and women that injustices which occur within the realm of the family are not matters for legal intervention.[15] The movement to help battered women called into question the legitimacy of a legal system that ignored the rights of women who were victims of violence in their own homes. Activists began to advocate for changes in laws and policies that would toughen arrest laws and hold perpetrators of violence and abuse accountable.

The historical belief in men's entitlement to ownership of women and children, and access to sexual gratification whenever men chose, was still largely supported by existing statutes during the 1970s. In 1979, New Hampshire passed its first statute providing protection for victims of intimate partner violence, RSA 173-B. Like statutes that were being drafted and passed in many states, RSA 173-B provided emergency legal relief to victims in civil court, restraining batterers from abusing, contacting, or in any way further harassing or harming victims and members of their families. For the first time across the country, laws were enacted that framed violence against an intimate partner as a crime, rather than a private family dysfunction. Domestic violence statutes were written to provide civil court relief from abuse, and mechanisms for charging violence against an intimate partner as a crime. Other states sought to toughen existing laws as a means to improve protections for battered women. For example, in 1984 Delaware passed a warrantless arrest statute in direct response to the activism of domestic violence advocates. Reforms such as these made it easier for law enforcement to make an arrest if there was evidence that a crime had been committed, and, as a result, placed responsibility for the arrest in the hands of the police rather than the victim of the assault.

A significant number of battered women were also victimized by marital rape,[17] yet in every state up until 1975, there was still a spousal exception to sexual assault statutes. Until that time, by getting married, women relinquished their right to refuse to have sex with their husbands. In New Hampshire the statute read, "[a] person is guilty of sexual assault except as between legally married spouses." In 1981, New Hampshire became one of the first states to delete the spousal exception, adding language that states, "[a]n actor commits a crime under this chapter even though the victim is the actor's legal spouse." Even after the elimination of a marital exception in Delaware, rape laws included a provision that resulted in lesser charges if the victim was the voluntary social companion of the accused up until 1998. It wasn't until 1993 that every state made rape within marriage illegal, and still in many states forced sexual activity within marriage is not codified as the same crime as raping a stranger or acquaintance.

The emergence of statutory responses to intimate partner violence and sexual assault was a concrete illustration of the fundamental social change that early pioneers of the movement to end violence against women believed was necessary to prevent future violence. By creating new civil and criminal legal responses to violence against women, early organizers were creating a new social and statutory framework in which intimate partner violence, including sexual assault, would not be tolerated. Further, domestic violence statutes creating civil protection orders were intentionally written to provide legal relief that would be available to anyone, without legal representation or any cost to the victim, thus putting the power to address intimate partner violence directly into the hands of the victims. These efforts had a basic feminist intention at their core – that women should be considered as independent, empowered agents of change in their own lives, and should have access to state systems of justice and protection that did not rely on a man as a gateway to power.

CRITIQUES ON THE FEMINIST PERSPECTIVE OF IPV

However, the feminist perspective has not been universally accepted. Early on, sharp disagreements arose between family violence researchers and those espousing a gender analysis over how to measure the incidence of violence in families. For example, the National Family Violence Survey results seemed to at first demonstrate that women and men were equally likely to use violence in relationships. Feminist researchers and advocates argued that simply counting self-reported acts of abuse as defined by the Conflict Tactics Scale, a tool frequently used by family violence researchers,[5,27] failed to account for the context in which such acts occurred and that women's use of violence was often in self-defense or self-protection. Moreover, in contrast to the Straus et al findings, official crime statistics, as well as hospital and police reports, demonstrated that the victims of domestic violence incidents were overwhelmingly women.[11]

Feminism has faced criticism for being too narrowly focused on the experiences of white middle class women, and the battered women's movement has faced a similar critique. The early founders of the movement were largely white, heterosexual, middle class, educated women whose focus on understanding domestic violence and sexual assault using a gender analysis of violence and oppression has been viewed by many as insensitive to or ignoring the experiences of women of color, poor women, and lesbians. Scholars, activists, and new generations of feminists have called for a more complex understanding of the intersections of race, ethnicity, class, and gender and how these intersections play out for women and men in marginalized communities.[28,29] While the earliest research and activism focused almost exclusively on male inflicted female violence, feminists now recognize that intimate partner violence between same sex partners has similar prevalence, consequences, and dynamics as male inflicted female battering.[30,31] Finneran and colleagues examined the reporting of IPV among a sample of 2368 men who had sex with men in an internet recruited sample drawn from the US, Canada, Australia, the United Kingdom, South Africa and Brazil. Reporting of physical IPV ranged from 5.75% in the US to 11.75% in South Africa where as experiencing sexual violence was less commonly reported ranging from 2.54% in Australia to 4.52% in the US. Homophobic discrimination, internalized homophobia and seeing heterosexuality as superior and the only normal behavior were all found to increase odds of reporting IPV in all countries.[32]

Feminists have also been criticized for looking to reform the justice system as the centerpiece of activism and social change efforts rather than taking a broader view of women's needs from a more holistic or human rights perspective. Others have questioned whether successes that led to legal reform, government funding of programs, and a push toward professionalism have left the battered women's movement and its feminist roots co-opted by the very systems it once sought to reform.[21]

Despite these critiques, the feminist perspective has proven to be an invaluable tool when examining the relationship between gender and intimate partner violence. Feminism and the battered women's movement continue to be enriched as a deeper, more complex understanding of women's lives and diverse experiences evolving over time. The feminist perspective provides the theoretical and philosophical basis for a movement that has, at its core, a belief in the power of dedicated advocates to create fundamental social change through individual empowerment and system transformation.

FEMINIST ADVOCACY, INTIMATE PARTNER VIOLENCE, AND HEALTH CARE PROFESSIONALS

Since 2000, many local and state domestic violence programs and coalitions have engaged with the health care community as a primary means of addressing intimate partner violence. The health impact of domestic violence has been established by numerous studies which document poor health outcomes for victims compared to those who have not been abused. The New Hampshire Violence Against Women Survey found that women who report having a chronic disease or medical condition were more likely to report sexual and physical violence than women who do not report having a chronic disease or medical condition.

Framing intimate partner violence as a health care issue of paramount importance creates an opportunity to identify victims and offer them support and assistance that could help prevent future violence or abuse. A knowledgeable and well-trained health care provider should not only provide acute medical treatment but should also assess a patient to determine if they have experienced domestic or sexual violence and make appropriate referrals. In some health care settings, advocacy services are available on-site. When that is not possible, referral protocols can be developed with local service providers to ensure that victims who disclose abuse in a medical setting have confidential, supportive services available. In many jurisdictions comprehensive protocols have been developed, such as the Domestic Violence Protocol for Health Care Professionals developed by the New Hampshire Governor's Commission on Domestic and Sexual Violence. The Family Violence Prevention Fund has developed National Consensus Guidelines on Identifying and Responding to Domestic Violence Victimization in Health care Settings.[33] The American Medical Association Advisory Council on Violence and Abuse[34] has also issued policy guidelines for responding to intimate partner violence and "recommends that questions to assess risk for family violence should be included within the context of taking a routine social history, past medical history, history of present illness, and review of systems as part of emergency, diagnostic, preventive, and chronic care management."

All of these protocols, guidelines, and collaborative efforts have a common theme of delineating the complimentary roles of health care providers and advocates. Unlike other health conditions providers would seek to cure, intimate partner violence is a long-term problem that cannot be solved by a health care provider alone. In fact, developing plans for safety, support, and on-going assistance should be done by an advocate who is specifically trained to provide services to victims within the empowerment model. Proper screening, support, and referral procedures for health care providers, once the acute medical needs of the patient are addressed, are outlined in the numerous publications available that address the health care response to intimate partner violence.[35]

Along with the information available to health care providers on responding to intimate partner violence, there is also a wealth of information on successful collaborations between domestic violence advocacy services and health care systems. In all successful collaborations, the roles of each provider are clearly understood by all, and victims are supported within a feminist, empowerment model. This model is not complicated, it simply recognizes that every victim of intimate partner violence is the best judge of her own experiences and has the ability to determine the next steps that are best for her if she is given honest and accurate information about the support services and legal remedies available in her community. In using a feminist empowerment model, advocates acknowledge that the options available to women will vary due to the intersections of race, ethnicity, economics, gender orientation, and a host of other issues that affect each woman differently. The feminist model calls for working with individual victims where they are and with the resources they have, recognizing that those who are victimized by an intimate partner do not need to be saved or cured but rather need choices, support, and freedom to make those choices.

By screening patients for intimate partner violence as an essential component of addressing medical needs and following established protocols for documentation and referrals for services, health care providers can contribute to the safety and health of victims. The feminist perspective supports providing all victims with the information and support they need in order to most effectively plan for their own safety as they move beyond their victimization into more fully realized lives.

REFERENCES

1.   Tjaden P, Thoennes N. *Full Report of the Prevalence, Incidence, and Consequences of Violence Against Women: Findings From the National Violence Against Women Survey.* Washington, DC: DOJ CDC; 2000. NCJ 183781.

2.   University of New Hampshire, the New Hampshire Division of Public Health Services, and the New Hampshire Coalition Against Domestic and Sexual Violence. *Violence Against Women in New Hampshire.* Concord, NH: 2006.

3. Mandel M, Hindin MJ. Men's controlling behaviors and women's experiences of physical violence in Malawi. *Matern Child Health J.* 2013;17(7):1332-1338.

4. Schechter S. *Women and Male Violence: The Visions and Struggles of the Battered Women's Movement.* Boston, MA: South End Press; 1982.

5. Straus MA, Gelles RJ, Steinmetz SK. *Behind Closed Doors: Violence in the American Family.* Garden City, NY: Anchor Books; 1980.

6. Martin D. *Battered Wives.* San Francisco, CA: Volcano Press; 1981.

7. Walker LE. *The Battered Woman.* New York, NY: Harper and Row; 1980.

8. Dobash RE, Dobash R. *Violence Against Wives: A Case Against the Patriarchy.* New York, NY: Free Press; 1983.

9. Stanko EA. *Intimate Intrusions: Women's Experience of Male Violence.* London; Boston: Routledge & Kegan Paul; 1985.

10. Kelly L. How women define their experience of male violence. In: Bograd M, Yllo K, eds. Feminist Perspectives on Wife Abuse. Newberry Park, CA: Sage Publications; 1988:114-132.

11. Kurz D, Stark E. Not so benign neglect: the medical response to battering. In: Bograd M, Yllo K, eds. *Feminist Perspective on Wife Abuse.* Newberry Park, CA: Sage Publications; 1988:249-266.

12. Warshaw C. Limitation of the medical model in the care of the battered women. *Gender and Society.* 1989;3:506-517.

13. Gondolf EW, Fisher ER. *Battered Women As Survivors: An Alternative to Treating Learned Helplessness.* Lexington, MA: Lexington Books; 1988.

14. Ferraro KJ. The legal response to woman battering in the United States. In: Hammer J, ed. *Women, Policing, and Male Violence.* London: Routledge; 1989.

15. Taub N. Adult domestic violence: the law's response. *Victomology.* 1983;8(1-2):152-171.

16. Klein D. Violence against women: some considerations regarding its causes and its elimination. *Crime and Delinquency.* Jan 1981;27(1):64-80.

17. Russell DEH. *Rape in Marriage.* New York, NY: Macmillan; 1982.

18. Sommers EK, Check JVP. An empirical investigation of the role of pornography in the verbal and physical abuse of women. *Violence and Victims.* 1987;2(3):189-209.

19. Bograd M. Feminist perspectives on wife abuse: an introduction. In: Bograd M, Yllo K, eds. *Feminist Perspectives on Wife Abuse.* Newberry Park, CA: Sage Publications; 1988:11-26.

20. Cerulli C, Poleschuck E, Raimondi C, Veale S, Chin N. "What fresh hell is this?" victim of intimate partner violence describe their experiences of abuse, pain, and depression. *J Fam Violence.* 2012;27(8):773-781

21. Pence E. Advocacy on Behalf of Battered Women. In: Renzetti CM, Edleson JL, Bergen RK, eds. *Sourcebook on Violence Against Women.* Thousand Oaks, CA: Sage Publications; 2001:329-343.

22. Uthman OA, Moradi T, Lawoko S. Are individual and community acceptance and witnessing of intimate partner violence related to its occurrence? multilevel structural equation model. PLoS ONE 6(12) e27738. Doi: 10.1371/journal.pone.0027738. December 14, 2011.

23. Bibi S, Ashfaq S, Shaikh F, Qureshi PMA. Prevalence, instigating factors and help seeking behavior of physical domestic violence among married women of Hyderabad, Sindh. *Pak J Med Sci.* 2014;30(1):122-125.

24. Ghanim D. Internalizing Middle Eastern Violence. In: Ghanim A, ed. *Gender and Violence in Middle East.* Westport, CT: Praeger. 2009:1-11.

25. History of battered women's movement. Indiana Coalition Against Domestic Violence. Indiana Coalition Against Domestic Violence Web site. http://www.icadvinc.org/what-is-domestic-violence/history-of-battered-womens-movement/. Published 1999. Accessed June 9, 2014.

26. Okin SM. *Justice, Gender, and the Family.* New York, NY: Basic Books; 1989.

27. Straus MA, Gelles RJ. *Physical Violence in American Families: Risk Factors and Adaptations to Violence in 8,145 Families.* New Brunswick, NJ: Transaction Publishers; 1990.

28. Renzetti CM. Violence and abuse in lesbian relationships: theoretical and empirical issues. In: Bergen RK, ed. *Issues in Intimate Violence.* Thousand Oaks, CA: Sage; 1998:117-127.

29. Volpp L. A black feminist reflection on the antiviolence movement. In: Sokoloff NJ, Pratt C, eds. *Domestic Violence: Readings on Race, Gender, and Culture.* New Brunswick, NJ: Rutgers University Press; 2005.

30. Hirth J, Berenson A. Racial/ethnic differences in depressive symptoms among young women: the role of intimate partner violence, trauma, and posttraumatic stress disorder. *J Womens Health.* 2012:21(9):966-974.

31. Arnold G, Ake J. Reframing the narrative of the battered women's movement. *Violence Against Women.* 2013;19(5):557-578.

32. Finneran C, Chard A, Sineath C, Sullivan P, Stepheneon R. Intimate partner violence and social pressure among gay men in six countries. *West J Emerg Med.* 2012;13(3):260-271.

33. *National Consensus Guidelines On Identifying and Responding To Domestic Violence Victimization in Health Care Settings.* San Francisco, CA: Family Violence Prevention Fund; 2004

34. *Policy Compendium.* Chicago, IL: American Medical Association National Advisory Council on Violence and Abuse; 2008.

35. Giardino AP, Datner EM, Asher JB. Sexual Assault Victimization Acrsos the Life Span a Clinical Guide. St. Louis, MO; STM Learning, Inc.; 2003.

Chapter 25

LGBTQ Culture: Considerations

Kassia Wosick PhD
Diana Faugno MSN, RN, CPN, SANE-A, SANE-P, FAAFS, DF-IAFN

Key Points

1. Same-gender relationships can experience domestic violence, but face unique barriers in terms of reporting, support, and advocacy.

2. Communities like LGBTQ are an important way to maintain social identities and offer specific resources to individuals who share similarities.

3. LGBTQ violence and sexual victimization continues to be under-reported due to social stigma and assumptions that same-sex victimization does not occur.

4. Homophobia continues to be a major social problem, and victimization is a major consequence of homophobia in school settings for LGBTQ youth.

5. Transgender and intersexual individuals often distinguish between their gender identity and their sexual orientation.

6. Health care providers should have a positive attitude that demonstrates particular understanding and sensitivity to LGBTQ patients.

Introduction

While domestic violence has become a major concern for health care professionals over the past several decades, examining intimate partner violence, domestic violence, and spousal abuse within same-gender relationships has remained relatively nonexistent.[1] This is due, in part, to the limited visibility of homosexuality and bisexuality in general, but is also the result of misconceptions about prevalence and lack of information and resources for same-gender partner violence.[2]

Recently, researchers and practitioners have begun to identify, assess, and treat partner abuse within same-gender relationships.[3] The purpose of this chapter is to contextualize intimate partner violence by focusing on the gay, lesbian, bisexual, queer, and transgender population. The chapter begins by defining sexualities, and provides a brief history of sexual diversity in the United States before detailing the role of community in the lives of LGBTQ individuals. Next, the chapter examines the impact of homophobia and heterosexism, and then moves to articulating cultural considerations for LGBTQ populations. The remainder of the chapter is devoted to sexual assault and violence within a same-gender relational context, and briefly articulates suicide in LGBTQ youth. The chapter concludes with considerations and resources for both intervention and prevention for intimate partner violence, domestic violence, and abuse.

DEFINING SEXUALITIES

Sexual orientation is an enduring emotional, romantic, sexual, or affectional attraction to another person (APA). Gender is the basis for sexual orientation, in that one's attraction may be to someone of the opposite gender (heterosexual), same gender (homosexual), both genders (bisexual), or neither gender (asexual). In recent years, the term queer has also been invoked, whether in reference to one's sexual orientation as "different" from heterosexual, or to resist standard identity labels such as gay/lesbian/bisexual. Regardless of the term or label used, sexual orientation can best be described as a spectrum of possibilities.

Sexuality refers to the combination of one's sexual orientation, sexual desire, sexual behavior, identity, and gender. Sexuality is best thought of in the plural; there is such diversity with regard to orientations, desires, behaviors, identities, and genders that researchers must confront the changing landscape of sexualities in contemporary society.

In thinking about sexuality and sexual orientation, a common mistake is to refer only to the sexual practices of sexual minorities. Being gay, lesbian, bisexual, queer, and even heterosexual involves a wide array of sexual and nonsexual interactions that facilitate everyday life. Nevertheless, the purpose of this chapter is to illuminate relationship violence within the context of LGBTQ lives, which has been systematically overlooked until recently.

Historically, sexualities have been socially controlled through various institutions in an effort to "protect" individuals and society from the perils of sexual diversity and expression. Religion has characterized some forms of sexuality as sinful, the legal system has criminalized certain sexual behaviors, and the medical community has medicalized certain forms of sexuality as a disease or an illness, namely homosexuality. However, social attitudes have changed to encompass a wider range of sexual normalcy as well as acceptance of sexual diversity. For example, the American Psychiatric Association removed homosexuality from the mental health manual as a diagnosis of mental disorders in 1973.[4]

Sexual identity politics have attempted to expose the social and political inequalities of a heterosexist society through focusing on gay, lesbian, bisexual, and transgender equality rights. The American Gay Rights Movement has been successful over the past 70 years in mobilizing efforts to outlaw discrimination on the basis of sexual orientation and gender diversity, deem sodomy laws unconstitutional, ensure domestic partner benefits, and obtain civil unions and same-sex marriage rights. Such political and social success has been achieved, in part, through the community-wide efforts of the LGBTQ population.

LGBTQ COMMUNITIES

As social beings, humans have a tendency to congregate in groups like communities for solidarity, support, and life resources. Research acknowledges the role of community in establishing and supporting social identities.[5-7] However, the definition of what is actually considered a community has remained complex due to geographical changes in population as well as an increase in technologically-based social networks.

Communities serve to bring people together socially, provide a foundation for generating and maintaining shared social identities, and offer resources specific to the needs of both individuals and the community as a whole.[7,8] Gay, lesbian, bisexual, transgender, and queer communities provide a supportive atmosphere that accepts same-gender orientations and behaviors as valid, and allows for a range of romantic and sexual expression.[8] A majority of cities in the United States and throughout the world have some sort of LGBTQ resource center, and there are numerous on-line resources for individuals in need of information, support, and community involvement specific to LGBTQ issues.

While communities have the power to include those with shared identities and experiences, they also have the power to exclude those who deviate from shared identities.[7] During the initial phases of the gay and lesbian movement, gay men often excluded lesbians from their political and social efforts, while some lesbians later distinguished themselves as a separate political entity in the 1970s.[9] More recently, gays and lesbians have worked together in efforts to legalize same-sex marriage, ensure equal rights, and challenge widely-held misconceptions about homosexuality in general. Bisexuals are often included in reference to the "gay and lesbian" community, although such inclusion has been tenuous throughout political and social efforts for equal rights and social acceptance.[10,11] Because bisexuality is often mistakenly regarded as a transition to homosexuality, or an experimental phase rather than a distinct sexual orientation, bisexuals have experienced biphobia in both heterosexual and homosexual contexts. Some bisexuals align with the gay and lesbian community because they do not conform to a heterosexist culture and may be involved in same-gender relationships. Others have formed their own communities that provide specific support for bisexuals in ways that the gay and lesbian community cannot.[7,12,13] Bisexual communities tend to support individuals who have "dual gender" attractions, and provide resources for specific bisexual issues and concerns.

Similar to bisexuals, transgender individuals have experienced both inclusion and exclusion from the gay and lesbian community. *Transgender* is an inclusive term used to describe individuals who cannot (or choose not) to conform to society's gender norms.[14] Transgender individuals transgress traditional gender boundaries through a variety of means; some physiologically augment their bodies through hormonal supplements and/ or surgeries (transsexuals), present themselves as another gender (drag queens/kings, cross dressers), or remain decidedly androgynous as part of a personal or political agenda to challenge gender binaries (gender queer, androgyne).

Regardless of self-identification, transgender individuals often distinguish between their gender identity and their sexual orientation. For example, studies on transgendered sexual practices find that significant portions of postsurgical transsexuals identify as homosexual, while many identify as heterosexual.[15,16] In other words, individuals who have transitioned to another gender can be gay, lesbian, heterosexual, queer, or bisexual in terms of identifying their sexual orientation. The gay and lesbian community has played an increasingly integral role in combating transphobia and providing resources for transgender persons, regardless of sexual orientation. As noted later in this chapter, transgender persons have unique struggles and concerns in terms of both gender and sexuality that may not be met by inclusion in the gay and lesbian community.

Like transgender individuals, intersexuals have also become increasingly active within the LGBTQ community. *Intersexuality* is a newer term that refers to "a variety of conditions in which a person is born with a reproductive or sexual anatomy that does not seem to fit the typical definitions of female or male."[17] What is considered intersexual depends on certain chromosomal, external genitalia, and internal reproductive combinations or ambiguities that are usually diagnosed at birth but may present at a later age. Therefore, results vary in terms of how common intersexuality actually is, but range between 1 in 1500 to 1200 births.[17,18] Most children born intersexual undergo a series of surgeries to alter their genitalia in order to conform to typical male/female anatomy. However, recent activism by the Intersex Society of North America (ISNA), adult intersexual survivors of sex reassignment surgery, and various vocal members of the medical community has been successful in reducing the number of genital alterations through advocacy, information, and research.

Intersexuals have recently been incorporated into the LGBTQ community because intersexual bodies also transgress typical sexual and gender norms. Intersexuals, like transgender individuals, range in terms of sexual orientation, and also may struggle with healthy sexual expression and sexual behavior because of atypical physical constraints. Further, intersexuals encounter a range of prejudice and phobia that parallels gender and sexual minorities. They also have unique concerns when dealing with sexual or intimate partner violence. Health care personnel should always remember that sensitivity and understanding is necessary when working with the transgender or intersexual patient in any capacity.

Historically, the LGBTQ community has been reluctant to provide resources and advocacy for intimate partner violence and spousal abuse, for several reasons. First, the LGBTQ community has focused their efforts primarily on HIV and AIDS research, prevention, and resources. Secondly, intimate partner violence is often perceived as an issue within heterosexual relationships, due to the gendered pattern of violence. However, intimate partner violence and sexual assault do occur among the LGBTQ population. The lack of research, resources, and support for victims of intimate partner violence within the LGBTQ community can be considered a result of heterosexism on a larger scale.

HETEROSEXISM, HOMOPHOBIA, AND DISCRIMINATION

The most damaging effects of heterosexism and homophobia have resulted in inadequate prevention efforts, insufficient legal protection, and sparse social resources for same-gender relationships experiencing intimate partner violence. *Heterosexism* refers to an ideological system that denies, denigrates, and stigmatizes any nonheterosexual form of behavior, identity, relationship, or community.[19] Heterosexism occurs at both the institutional and individual level, much like sexism or racism. At the institutional level, heterosexism pervades the legal system through, for example, a lack of protection against anti-gay discrimination, and scattered gay marriage rights. At the individual level, heterosexism impacts how heterosexuals regard sexual minorities and sexual diversity. Heterosexism is the foundation for animosity, disgust, hostility, and hatred of gay, lesbian, bisexual, transgender, and queer persons and practices. Researchers note a strong correlation between accepting negative stereotypes about the LGBTQ population and incidences of heterosexual expressions of hostility.[20] Another pervasive effect of heterosexism is that people are usually assumed to be heterosexual, and assume others to be heterosexual. Such assumptions remain problematic, especially for health professionals who are responsible for intimate partner violence, victim response, and care. And although attitudes about sexual minorities have, in fact, shifted in recent years due to increased visibility, availability of LGBTQ information and resources, and personal contact with gay and bisexual people, heterosexism continues to pervade both institutional and psychological arenas. Part of this continuation has to do with homophobia.

Homophobia is often defined as an "irrational fear and avoidance of homosexuals,"[21] although some have used the term more generally to describe any negative attitude, belief, or action toward homosexuals.[22,23] While homophobia remains the attitudinal basis for acts of discrimination, heterosexism is a more useful way to characterize widespread institutional ideology and personal prejudice against sexual minorities.

Heterosexism and homophobia both contribute to the experiences of victims (and perpetrators) of same-sex intimate partner violence, as well as how rates of same-sex relationship violence are reported and subsequently handled. Heterosexism certainly influences our perceptions of whether intimate partner violence occurs within a same-sex relationship context, and affects how victims are assessed and treated, and how perpetrators are arrested and prosecuted.

Case Study 25-1.

Scott is a 35 year old gay man who has been living with Jimmy, his 41 year old boyfriend of 10 years in a small Oregon community. Jimmy is a local artist who financially supports Scott and their adopted 3 year old daughter, Eliza. In the past several months, Jimmy and Scott had been arguing more frequently about bills, parenting, and a possible career switch for Jimmy. During one particular disagreement, Jimmy pinned Scott up against a wall and began punching him. Although the fight quickly ended, Jimmy was horrified and immediately began apologizing for what he had done. Another argument ensued a few weeks later. This time, Jimmy gave Scott 2 black eyes and fractured his left cheekbone. Scott decided he wanted to file a police report, but changed his mind while in the parking lot of the local police station. He was worried about being taken seriously by the male police officers he saw entering and exiting the station doors, even though he had visible physical injuries. Scott and Jimmy continued their relationship, which continued to be plagued by spouts of domestic violence.

SAME-SEX INTIMATE PARTNER VIOLENCE: AN OVERVIEW

A vast majority of research on intimate partner violence and domestic violence focuses on heterosexual couples. Johnson and Ferraro[24] articulate 2 broad themes in the literature on partner violence. First, there is a distinction between different types of violence, motives of perpetrators, and cultural context in which violence occurs.[24] Second, there is a theme in the feminist literature that argues that partner violence is primarily a problem of men using violence to maintain control over women.[24] Johnson and Ferraro do note that domestic violence occurs within gay male and lesbian couples, although their family literature review of the 1990s is decidedly focused on heterosexual couples.

What research exists on intimate partner violence among gay, lesbian, and bisexual relationships is limited, and has emerged only within the past 30 years.[3] According to Burke and Follingstad,[25] several factors have contributed to the slow evolution of research on same-sex partner violence. First, there is a general reluctance to acknowledge the existence of same-sex intimate relationships, although this has changed in recent years. Second, most assume that domestic violence occurs between male perpetrators and female victims. It is worth noting that the feminist discourse on intimate partner violence has often perpetuated this assumption through emphasizing that patriarchy and sexism are the root causes of domestic violence and women as victims.[26,27]

Several studies suggest that rates of intimate partner violence are similar between heterosexual couples and nonheterosexual couples.[27,28] Further, same-sex domestic violence is likely to follow the "cycle of violence" seen in opposite-sex domestic violence situations.[29-31] In reviewing both classical and contemporary literature on same-sex intimate partner violence and spousal abuse, there are several main themes: social stigma, LGBTQ-specific resources, gay/bisexual men, lesbian/bisexual women, and transgender and intersexual individuals.

SOCIAL STIGMA

Rachel Baum, national program coordinator for NCAVP, characterizes domestic violence as the "hidden secret of the LGBTQ community."[31] Baum suggests that since LGBTQ relationships are already stigmatized, shame and denial prevent many from disclosing experiences with domestic violence in an attempt to avoid airing one's dirty laundry. Other researchers similarly find that investigating or acknowledging intimate partner violence among gay male and lesbian relationships may further negative stereotypes of the LGBTQ community and risk what advancements have been made in combating homophobia.[29,33]

Research indicates that because gay and lesbian relationships are seen as less serious than heterosexual relationships, same-sex domestic violence is therefore perceived as less serious than opposite-sex domestic violence,[27,34] and that gay and lesbian victims are treated differently than heterosexual victims of domestic violence.[35]

COMMUNITY RESOURCES TO OVERCOMING BARRIERS

Baum, along with other researchers, suggests several problems with resources for victims of intimate partner violence within the LGBTQ community. First, a majority of shelters and agencies that offer LGBTQ services tend to focus on homosexual and bisexual women, often neglecting transgender individuals, and rarely assist men of any sexual orientation or gender identity.[36] Second, staff is often insufficiently trained to handle LGBTQ-specific concerns, and many mental health professionals continue to harbor homophobic attitudes that can influence treatment and services.[35,37-39]

LGBTQ individuals must also navigate legal barriers in accessing assistance and protecting victims of same-sex intimate partner violence. Because homophobia remains an issue in the judicial system, many LGBTQ individuals are reluctant to report domestic violence to authorities.

While rates of intimate partner violence are fairly similar between heterosexual and LGBTQ relationships, the National Coalition of Anti-Violence Programs has identified 5 ways in which perpetrators of IPV in the LGBTQ community can psychologically or emotionally abuse their victim (see **Table 25-1**).

In addition to these 5 issues, several researchers have examined specific sexual minority groups in exploring same-gender intimate partner violence. Since most data on bisexual men and women originates from studies that combine bisexual and homosexual respondents, both orientations are discussed together.

Table 25-1. Types of Psychological and Emotional Abuse within the LGBTQ Community

1. "Outing" or threatening to out a partner to friends, family, employers, police, or others.

2. Reinforcing fears that no one will help a partner because s/he is lesbian, gay, bisexual or transgender, or for this reason, the partner "deserves" the abuse.

3. Alternatively, justifying abuse with the notion that a partner is not "really" lesbian, gay, bisexual or transgender; ie, s/he may once have had or may still have relationships with other people, or express a gender identity inconsistent with the abuser's definitions of these terms.

4. Telling the partner that abusive behavior is a normal part of LGBTQ relationships, or that it cannot be domestic violence because it is occurring between LGBTQ individuals.

5. Portraying the violence as mutual and even consensual, especially if the partner attempts to defend against it, or has an expression of masculinity or some other "desirable" trait.

GAY AND BISEXUAL MEN

According to Cruz and Firestone,[30] domestic violence is the third largest health issue facing gay men, after HIV and substance abuse. Rates of domestic violence range from 11-39% among gay male relationships.[25] Merrill and Wolfe,[29] find that gay men experience different types of abuse; 87% reported severe physical abuse, 85% reported emotional abuse, and 73% reported some type of sexual abuse.

While researchers suggest similarities in the prevalence and cycle of violence between gay male and heterosexual relationships,[30,32,40] some have suggested noticeable differences in how gay and bisexual men experience intimate partner violence. Letellier[40] finds that gay and bisexual males have more difficulty conceptualizing themselves as victims, are more likely to fight back against abusive partners, and are less likely to seek treatment or assistance due to internalized homophobia and institutional heterosexism.[30,41]

LESBIAN AND BISEXUAL WOMEN

According to Kulkin et al,[2] most studies pertaining to same-gender partner abuse examine lesbian relationships more often than gay male relationships,[2] although few have studied correlates of such violence.[28]

Since women have traditionally been reported as the victims of intimate partner violence, same-gender relationships introduce a different dynamic. McLaughlin and Rozee[42] suggest that the "lesbian community may not be conceptualizing violence in lesbian relationships as domestic violence"[42] and what violence takes place may be minimized and concealed in an attempt to normalize lesbian relationships.

Mental health providers have been reported to perceive lesbian battering as less violent, and therefore less significant, than a comparable heterosexual battering.[34] Still, 47.5% of lesbians reported being victimized by a same-sex partner.[43]

TRANSGENDER AND INTERSEXUAL INDIVIDUALS

As previously mentioned, transgender individuals have both similar and unique concerns when dealing with intimate partner violence and victimization. There is a massive need for published research on intimate partner violence within the transgender community, in part because most researchers incorporate transgender data into a catch-all LGBTQ population impacted by sexual assault and domestic violence. According to the FORGE (For Ourselves: Reworking Gender Expression) organization, transgender people have fears and concerns similar to those of the gay, lesbian, bisexual, and queer population in terms of reporting, resources, and experiences.

Like LGBTQ victims, transgender and intersexual persons are hesitant to address intimate partner violence for fear that it will taint the community's myth of non-violence. Further, many transgender and intersexual individuals hesitate to use shelters, since they are typically female (and sometimes male) oriented, and may not even be allowed entrance due to their gender/genital/legal status. Many victims fear losing their privacy by being "outed" to utilize resources, or may fear revictimization (like many lesbian, gay, bisexual, and queer victims) due to transphobia, hostility, or prejudices from service provides and legal representatives.

SEXUAL ASSAULT AND VIOLENCE IN A LGBTQ CONTEXT

An overwhelming amount of sexual assault research focuses on heterosexual (usually female) victims and perpetrators (usually male).[44] Yet studies indicate that LGBTQ individuals report significantly higher lifetime rates of sexual victimization than their heterosexual peers.[45,46] There are 2 main issues to address in terms of sexual assault and violence within an LGBTQ context. First, rates of reporting, regardless of the victim's sex, continues to be the most underreported of all violent crimes.[44,47] This is even more true for LGBTQ victims involved in both opposite-sex and same-sex victimization situations, due in part to assumptions that same-sex victimization does not occur, or is a problem within the gendered "heterosexual world" rather than the LGBTQ community. Secondly, a particular form of sexual assault (and hate crime), anti-gay rape, is a direct result of heterosexism and homophobia.[48]

Perpetrators of anti-gay rape are usually heterosexual men who are asserting their heterosexist masculinity over an LGBTQ individual; if the victim is a male, the perpetrator is still "straight." If the victim is a female, the perpetrator is still "straight," but indicates through the rape that the victim is "not really a lesbian," or needs "a good dick" to set her straight. Regardless of reasoning, anti-gay rape is a hate crime, punishable as such in a majority of states.

According to the New Mexico Coalition of Sexual Assault Programs, LGBTQ sexual assault survivors are, in most ways, no different from their heterosexual counterparts. However, they may have unique issues and needs that warrant special attention. While perpetrators of sexual assault can literally be anyone; a friend, a date, a family member, a partner, or a stranger, if the victim is raped specifically because he or she is a sexual minority, the rape can also be considered a hate crime (depending on state law).

Victims of same-sex sexual assault may feel anger due not only to the assault, but also from the cultural oppression of LGBTQ persons in general. Further, if the perpetrator is a lover, he or she may feel doubly victimized by someone similar who shares in being a victim of cultural heterosexism.

While heterosexual victims of sexual assault are often fearful about reporting the assault, LGBTQ victims face additional fears. For example, the LGBTQ victim may fear judgment about his/her sexual orientation in addition to the assault, or may be fearful of being "outed" due to the assault. She or he may consider that the LGBTQ community is relatively small, and worry about disclosing the assault to others. Further, he or she may worry about being discriminated against by the criminal justice system, which is still plagued by heterosexism and individuals who may be unsympathetic to LGBTQ victims.

Transgender individuals are often sexually targeted specifically because of their gender status, and intimate partners who discover one's gender transgression can verbally, psychologically, physically, and sexually abuse the victim.[49] According to Courvant and Cook-Daniels,[50] 50% of transgender respondents from the Gender, Violence, and Resource Assess Survey had been raped or assaulted by a romantic partner. Like LGBTQ sexual assault victims, many transgender persons are reluctant to report the attack for reasons similar to those within LBGTQ communities, such as retraumatization within the criminal justice and legal systems, as well as transphobia and trans-prejudice among service providers and health care professionals.

Intersexuals face similar consequences when reporting sexual violence, in that the criminal justice and legal system, as well as the medical community, is largely unaware of intersexual bodies and issues. Further, social exposure and further trauma are specific concerns that intersexual survivors of sexual violence may face. According to Jordan,[51] "when seeking help [there is] the possibility that their intersex status, if previously hidden, might become known and expose them to more violence." Of particular concern for the health care provider is that, "often an intersex survivor has a unique body and/ or a unique vulnerability to the emotional aftermath of sexual violence," which Jordan argues can make it difficult to discuss the abuse or sexual violence with an unfamiliar victims' advocate.[51]

Case Study 25-2.

Tanish is a 22 year old male to female transsexual who is in the process of completing her operative procedures. One evening, Tanish was out with an attractive man at a local bar, and they decided to go back to his place for a night cap. Tanish decided to tell her date that she was in the process of gender transition. Her date was shocked, and he quickly turned to anger, accusing her of lying and shouting that he "wasn't no homo." When Tanish tried to leave, her date threw her down on the sofa and anally raped her. He then passed out on the floor and Tanish escaped. Tanish went directly to the hospital, where a nurse examiner brought her into a room and began asking her questions about her medical history and sexual contact history. Tanish tried to explain that she was an MTF transsexual, but the nurse kept asking her questions about her menstrual cycle and forced vaginal penetration. When the nurse began the physical examination, she saw that Tanish had full male genitalia, began to giggle uncontrollably and quickly left the room. A few minutes later, she returned with another nurse to complete the examination.

HOMOPHOBIA AND LGBTQ YOUTH

Homophobia continues to be a major problem in schools across the United States. According to the National School Climate Survey, 84% of LGBTQ students hear homophobic remarks like "faggot" or "dyke" at school, and 69% of LGB students and 90% of transgender students report feeling unsafe in their schools. Administrators, faculty, and staff are also a part of the scholastic experience, and unfortunately perpetuate homophobia through negative attitudes toward gays and lesbians (75%) and opposing integration of gay and lesbian themes into curricula (85%).[52]

Victimization is a major consequence of homophobia in school settings, and LGBTQ students report experiencing jokes, name calling, vandalism, and physical assault because of their sexual orientation.[53-55] Ueno[56] suggests that sexual minority students sometimes do not belong to a gay/lesbian/bisexual community like their adult counterparts, which puts youth at a disadvantage in terms of resources for homophobia and overall support for their sexuality.

Home life for many LGBTQ youth remains problematic as well. Pilkington and D'Augelli[57] find that 40% of their respondents reported verbal abuse and 10% reported physical assaults from family members. Further, "the family conflict over a youth's sexual orientation or gender identity is a significant factor that leads to homelessness or the need for out-of-home care."[58] Cochran et al[59] find that LGBTQ youth run away from home an average of 12 times, as compared to 7 times for their heterosexual counterparts. LGBTQ youth experience a higher rate of homelessness than their heterosexual counterparts. Although studies are unable to pinpoint the exact number of LGBTQ homeless youth, estimates suggest that 15 to 20% of homeless youth identify as LGBTQ. LGBTQ homeless youth are also exposed to higher levels of physical and sexual abuse from caretakers or family members before becoming homeless.[60] Further, data show that, once homeless, "LGBTQ youth experience higher rates of physical assaults, sexual exploitation, and mental health deterioration than their heterosexual homeless peers."[61]

In addition to victimization and homelessness, suicide, depression, and substance abuse are also likely consequences of homophobia for LGBTQ youth.[62] Serious suicide attempts among LGBTQ youth are at least 4 times as high as the general adolescent population,[63] and this figure may be even higher due to rates of underreporting. Statistics show that LGBTQ teens make more lethal suicide attempts than their heterosexual peers,[64] and young gay men are at the highest risk for suicide.[65] While data does show that the rates of completed suicide are comparable between LGBTQ and heterosexual youth,[66,67] studies clearly demonstrate that lesbian, gay, and bisexual youths are a high-risk group for suicidal behavior.

SPECIAL CIRCUMSTANCES: MORE BARRIERS TO REPORTING

One of the most widely spread myths about the LBGTQ community is that relationship violence does not occur to the extent that it does in heterosexual couples. This is false, and the consequence of such a myth involves perpetuating an environment in which individuals must suffer in silence. The rates of same-sex relationship violence are similar to heterosexual rates, and awareness of same-partner violence is key in dispelling the myth of relationship violence occurring only within a heterosexual context.[27,28]

An example of keeping the "phobia alive" comes from a May 2009 news story that reported that South Carolina passed a Senate bill that would provide resources to teens about dating violence and added an amendment which would prohibit the Department of Education from including mention of same-sex relationships in the materials.[68] South Carolina is currently 1 of 3 states that specifically exclude LGBTQ people from domestic-violence protections.

Another news article from April 2009 described the suicide of an 11-year-old boy who was bullied in school about being gay.[69] Students called him derogatory names, and he hanged himself in the stairwell at his home and left the note for his mother. In a 2007 Gay, Lesbian, and Straight Education Network study, 86% of LGBTQ students said that they had experienced harassment at school during the previous year.[70]

These examples show that myths about same-sex intimate partner violence and victimization are still pervasive and socially sanctioned. Both heterosexual and LGBTQ communities are accountable to make changes, monitor and implement fair treatment for all, and establish policies and procedures to protect every individual. Risk management would support this from a financial liability. The mission statement and vision for a community would also give direction in this area.

CONSIDERATIONS AND INTERVENTIONS

The health care professional should have patient care referrals to organizations, centers, hot lines, internet resources or therapists that deal specifically with the LGBTQ community (See **Table 25-2**). It is imperative that this information be given to the patient in order for the patient to feel safe and that there is someone who understands him or her. One of the reasons violence is tolerated within the LGBTQ community is that many fear the response to reporting same-sex violence will be insensitive and inadequate.[71] Social services or the DV/rape crisis center in the community should also have lists of referrals specifically for LGBTQ individuals that the health care professional at the hospital, clinic, or physician's office can provide in the discharge instructions to the patient. (See **Table 25-3**). Some references and resources are listed at the end of this chapter.

PREVENTION EFFORTS

A new study has looked at risk and sexual coercion and unwanted sex among gay and bisexual men. Analysis identified a vulnerable individual which is addressed in prevention education and awareness. Models of prevention work on strengthening a person's ability to avoid or resist coercion, thereby preventing potential violence. The prevention can be broader for the community or individual when working with primary prevention with this group.[72] Another study looked at ages of men who are at risk for HIV infection based on unprotected sex. Very young gay and bisexual men engaging in unprotected anal sex at rates comparable with those for their older counterparts are very much at risk for HIV. This information supports that interventions must target the younger men and prevention programs should be able to communicate with this

Table 25-2. Suggestions for Professionals Working with LGBTQ Survivors

Sabrina Gentlewarrior, PhD, LICSW, offers specific recommendations via the VAWnet Applied Research Forum to those who work with LGBTQ survivors of sexual violence[1]:

1. Engage in ongoing identification and rectification of attitudes or behaviors predicated in homophobia, biphobia, and/or transphobia.

2. Prioritize the production and dissemination of information focused on LGBTQ survivors of sexual violence in community-based and peer-reviewed venues.

3. Ensure that our agencies have workers and administrators that reflect the social identities of all of those we serve.

4. Commit to developing a knowledge base about LGBTQ individuals that includes:

   a) information about their historical and current experiences of oppression.

   b) knowledge regarding the coming out and identity development processes.

5. Develop and utilize LGBTQ-affirmative practice models. Initial steps toward this goal include:

   a) use of inclusive language verbally and in all written forms and literature.

   b) assessment of all survivors for bias as well as non-bias oriented victimizations.

   c) ability to honor clients' multiple and interconnected social identities and effectively serve clients in view of these identities.

6. Identify or, if needed, create LGBTQ community resources dedicated to offering safe, affirming support on a range of issues relevant to members of these communities.

7. Provide professional development opportunities for area agencies focused on the self awareness, knowledge and skills needed to offer culturally competent services to LGBTQ survivors of sexual violence.

8. Participate in policy and social change work dedicated to providing equity of treatment and acceptance to members of the lesbian, gay, bisexual and transgender communities.

Table 25-3. Actions Health Professionals Must Take

1. Identify the abuse

2. Validate the patients experience; say "I am sorry this has happened to you"

3. Assessment of patient and safety of patient

4. Documentation written and photographic

5. Referrals and reports

younger group through primary prevention as well.[73] Clinics staffed by young men advocates would be a good example of this. This allows for a peer to peer discussion about self esteem and other issues relevant to this age group.

The prevention literature states that motivating individuals to change their lifestyles involves empowering them with the information they need to make choices and develop skills that lead to healthy behaviors. The advice of health care providers has been associated with reductions in morbidity, mortality, risk behaviors, and risk factors, as well as an increase in healthy behaviors. This is a key point for health care providers.[74] While encouraging healthy behaviors and strengthening a potential victim's ability to avoid or resist potential trauma may be viable prevention techniques, several macro-level shifts in expanding cultural definitions of masculinity, heterosexuality, and normative gender/sexual structures are also necessary if the goal is to reduce incidents of intimate partner violence and sexual trauma specific to the LGBTQ population.

Case Study 25-3.

Sally is a 23 year old. She graduated from high school and began working in the textile industry in downtown Los Angeles. She met Lupe and they became friends and moved in together. Sally is a lesbian and Lupe is as well. Their relationship progressed. Several months later arguments began with Lupe yelling and verbally abusing Sally. The violence escalated over the next year. Sally came to work one day with facial injury and was referred to the occupational health nurse. The nurse had been trained in screening for domestic violence. The nurse asked direct questions and Sally told the nurse her partner Lupe had hurt her. The nurse understood Sally did not want this reported as she feared she would lose her job. Referrals were given to the LGBTQ crisis center and a safety plan was discussed by the nurse. The nurse would be a mandated hospital reporter in some states and might have to report this to law enforcement. When law enforcement responded they took the report in a sensitive manner from Sally. Sally went home and reported back to work the next day. This case demonstrates a good example of secondary prevention and what a health care provider can do to help their patients. The nurse identified the facial injuries were from domestic violence in a LGBTQ relationship by asking direct questions. The nurse gave referrals to the LGBTQ crisis center and educated her patient on domestic violence. The nurse also talked with the patient about a safety plan as well as how to handle inquiries from peers at her job. An example of primary prevention by the Occupational Health Nurse would be talking with employees about domestic violence and identification screenings in her annual health checkups with the employees. Tertiary prevention would be the identification and dealing with the outcomes of past violence and abuse.

CONCLUSION

Intimate partner violence and sexual violence are public health issues that affect people of all genders and sexual orientations. Medical personal are especially important in improving the health care of individuals who identify as LGBTQ. Maintaining a non-homophobic position and using gender-neutral terms are essential steps in providing the best care possible to LGBTQ survivors of violence. It is especially important for health care providers to have a positive attitude that demonstrates particular understanding and sensitivity to LGBTQ patients. The best way to dispel myths and counter stereotypes about same-gender partner violence and sexual victimization is to integrate LGBTQ content throughout the entire medical school curriculum. Providing training on gender and sexual minority issues is key in the education of medical providers to improve patient health and overall care of all patients, and those who identify as LGBTQ in particular. If the medical community can consistently demonstrate an inclusive and sensitive attitude while understanding the specific safety and medical concerns for the LGBTQ population, then we move one step closer to providing effective health care and trauma response to all patients, regardless of gender and sexual orientation.

Referrals and Resources

Project RADAR

http://www.vahealth.org/injury/projectradarva/index.htm

A provider-focused initiative to promote the assessment and prevention of intimate partner violence in the health care setting. Through the RADAR initiative, the Division of Injury and Violence Prevention at the Virginia Department of Health seeks to enable Virginia's health care providers to recognize and respond to intimate partner violence (IPV) by providing them access to "best-practice" policies, guidelines, and assessment tools, training programs, and specialty-specific curricula awareness and educational materials information on the latest research/data related to IPV.

The Network for Battered Lesbians and Bisexual Women

617-423-SAFE (hotline in English and Spanish)

This program offers free services in English and Spanish for battered lesbians, bisexual women, and transgender people. These services include a hotline, emergency shelter, and advocacy programs. Located in Boston, Massachusetts.

The Gay Men's Domestic Violence Project

1-800-832-1901

This grassroots, nonprofit organization provides community education and direct services for clients. GMDVP offers shelter, guidance and resources to allow gay, bisexual, and transgender men in crisis to leave violent situations and relationships. Located in Cambridge, Massachusetts.

Lambda Legal "Getting Down to Basics" Tool Kit

1-866-LGBTeen or 212-809-8585 or
download for free at www.lambdalegal.org or www.cwla.org.

This tool kit offers short articles that include definitions, resources, and vignettes about LGBTQ youth in care, caseworkers with LGBTQ clients, attorneys, guardians ad litem, and advocates representing LGBTQ youth, and recommendations for training and education on LGBTQ issues.

Parents, Families, and Friends of Lesbians and Gays (PFLAG)

202-467-8180, www.pflag.org

A national organization that promotes the health and well-being of gay, lesbian, bisexual and transgendered persons, their families and friends. Their web site provides users with information on local chapters, advocacy and support information, and other resources that support the family and friends of gays and lesbians. 1726 M Street, NW, Suite 400, Washington, DC 20036. *info@pflag.org*

The Northwest Network

206-568-7777, 206-517-9670 (TTY), www.nwnetwork.org

Provides support and advocacy for bisexual, transgender, lesbian, and gay survivors of abuse and dating violence. P.O. Box 20398, Seattle, Washington 98102.

National Coalition of Anti-Violence Programs

212-714-1141 (24-hour bi-lingual hotline), 212-714-1134 (TTY), www.avp.org

A coalition of 40 anti-violence organizations that monitor, respond to, and work to end hate, domestic and sexual violence affecting LGBTQ communities. 240 West 35th St., Suite 200, New York, NY 10001.

The Los Angeles Gay and Lesbian Center
323-993-7400, www.laglc.org

The center's wide array of services includes: free HIV/AIDS care and medications for those most in need; housing, food, clothing, and support for homeless LGBT youth; support and advocacy services for LGBT seniors and LGBT-parented families; low-cost counseling and addiction-recovery services; legal services; health education and HIV prevention programs; transgender services; a cultural arts program and much more. McDonald/Wright Building, 1625 N. Schrader Boulevard, Los Angeles, CA 90028-6213.

Internet sites:
http://www.advocate.com/
http://www.youtube.com/watch?v=M-1q0Vk5OXk&feature=fvw
http://www.youtube.com/watch?v=tjg8ha2Zg9o&feature=related
http://www.youtube.com/watch?v=CikZ1p5fFTc&feature=related

Transgender and Intersex-Specific resources:
www.survivorproject.org/ - The Survivor Project
www.gpac.org/ - GenderPac
www.ifge.org/ - International Foundation for Gender Education
www.annelawrence.com/ - Transsexual Women's Resources
www.isna.org/ - Intersex Society of North America
my.execpc.com/~dmmunson/Nov99_1.htm - FORGE Newsletter on DV (Nov1999)

FOUNDATIONS

Gill Foundation
http://www.gillfoundation.org

Aims "...to secure equal opportunity for all people, regardless of sexual orientation or gender identity...by providing grants...strengthening leadership and managerial skills... increasing financial resources...building awareness of the contributions...of diverse sexual orientations and gender identities..."

The Point Foundation
http://www.thepointfoundation.org

"A scholarship lifeline for LGBT students...mentoring program for GLBT students..."

Pride Foundation (Seattle)
http://www.pridefoundation.org/

Funds organizations and scholarships in Alaska, Idaho, Montana, Oregon, and Alaska. In 2009 the Bill & Melinda Gates Foundation gave Pride Foundation a special grant to increase the Queer Youth Initiative which supports youth centers in education, training and coming out for the youth in this community.

Uncommon Legacy Foundation (US)
http://www.uncommonlegacy.org

Offers scholarships and grants; "...a nonprofit foundation dedicated to enhancing the visibility, strength and vitality of the lesbian community...". Site includes list of previous recipients, mostly in the fields of education, civil rights and health, but also cultural studies.

ACADEMIC/PROFESSIONAL/EMPLOYEES

American Association for Italian Studies. AAIS Queer Caucus
http://www.aais.info/queer.html

American College Personnel Associations' Standing Committee on LGBT Awareness
http://www.sclgbta.org/

American Library Association Gay, Lesbian, Bisexual, and Transgendered Round Table. GLBTRT of the ALA.
http://www.ala.org/glbtrt

American Psychological Association. Division 44: Society for the Psychological Study of Lesbian, Gay, and Bisexual Issues
http://www.apadivision44.org/

Association des Medecins Gais (France)
http://www.medecins-gays.org

An association of doctors, specialists, students, psychoanalysts, dentists, physical therapists, psychologists, and sexologists.

Association for Gay, Lesbian, and Bisexual Issues in Counseling
http://www.aglbic.org

A division of the American Counseling Association.

Association of Lesbian and Gay Psychologists Europe
http://www.psychologie.uni-trier.de/projects/ALGP/alghome.html

Federal Globe. Gay, Lesbian, and Bi Employees of the Federal Government (US)
http://www.fedglobe.org

Links to employee groups in federal agencies, state agencies, and the private sector.

Gay and Lesbian Medical Association (GLMA) (US)
http://www.glma.org

Over 2 000 LGBT physicians, medical students and supporters; "combats homophobia in the medical profession and advocates for quality health care for the LGBT community." Online table of contents and abtracts to its journal, Journal of the Gay and Lesbian Medical Association (JGLMA).

Gay, Lesbian, and Straight Education Network GLSEN (U.S.)
http://www.glsen.org

Formerly GLSTN, Gay, Lesbian, and Straight Teachers Network

Gays and Lesbians in Foreign Affairs Agencies USA
http://www.glifaa.org

Represents personnel in the US Dept of State, US Agency for International Development, Foreign Commercial Service, Foreign Agricultural Serve and other foreign affairs agencies of the US Government.

GLARP. Gay and Lesbian Association of Retiring Persons
http://gaylesbianretiring.org/

International Association of Lesbian and Gay Judges
http://home.att.net/~ialgj/

International Association of Lesbian/Gay Pride Coordinators, Inc.
http://www.interpride.org

League at AT&T
http://www.league-att.org

Medical Library Association. Lesbian, Gay, Bisexual and Transgendered Health Sciences Librarians (SIG) (US)
http://lgbt.mlanet.org

Includes full text newsletter and selected resource links.

MediGay (Switzerland)
http://www.bboxbbs.ch/home/medigay/

Physicians and health care professionals; available in English; with health information for gays and lesbians.

National Consortium of Directors of LGBT Resources in Higher Education (US)
http://www.lgbtcampus.org

National Lesbian and Gay Journalists Association (US)
http://www.nlgja.org

National Lesbian and Gay Law Association, affiliate of the American Bar Association
http://www.nlgla.org/

National Organization of Gay and Lesbian Scientists and Technical Professionals (US)
http://www.noglstp.org/

NIST Globe. Gay, Lesbian, or Bisexual Employees. National Institute of Standards and Technology. (US)
http://www.nist.gov/globe

Salutaris. The NIH Gay and Lesbian Employee's Forum. NIHGLEF (US)
http://www.recgov.com/salutaris/index.html

LGBT employees of the National Institutes of Health.

SLA Gay & Lesbian Issues Caucus. Special Libraries Association (US)
http://www.sla.org/caucus/kglic/

The Sociologists' Lesbian, Gay, Bisexual and Transgendered Caucus (US)
http://www.qrd.org/qrd/www/orgs/slgc/

US Department of Justice Pride
http://www.dojpride.org

With links to glbt organizations in other federal agencies.

REFERENCES

1. Gentlewarrior S. *Culturally Competent Service Provisions to Lesbian, Gay, Bisexual and Transgender Survivors of Sexual Violence.* Harrisburg, PA: VAWnet, a project of the National Resource Center on Domestic Violence/Pennsylvania Coalition Against Domestic Violence. Violence Against Women Web site. http://www.vawnet.org. Published September 2009. Accessed December 1, 2009.

2. Kulkin H, Williams J, Borne H, de la Bretonne D, Laurendine J. A review of research on violence in same-gender couples: a resource for clinicians. *J Homosex.* 2007;53(4):71-87.

3. Murray C E, Mobley AK. Empirical research about same-sex intimate partner violence: a methodological review. *J Homosex.* 2009;56:361-386.

4. Spitzer RL. The diagnostic status of homosexuality in DSM-III: a reformulation of the issues. *Am J Psychiatry.* 1981;138:210-215.

5. Troiden RR. *Gay and Lesbian Identity: A Sociological Analysis.* New York, NY: General Hall; 1988.

6. Weston K. *Families We Choose: Lesbians, Gays, Kinship.* New York, NY: Columbia University Press; 1991.

7. Wosick-Correa KR. Identity and community: the social construction of bisexuality in women. In: Stombler M, Baucach DM, et al, eds. *Sex Matters: The Sexuality and Society Reader.* Boston, MA: Allyn and Bacon; 2007:42-52.

8. Kelly GF. *Sexuality Today.* Boston, MA: McGraw Hill; 2008.

9. D'Emilio J. *Sexual Politics, Sexual Communities: The Making of a Homosexual Minority in the United States, 1940-1970.* Chicago: Chicago University Press; 1998.

10. Paul JP. The bisexual identity: an idea without social recognition. *J Homosex.* 1984;9(2-3):45-63.

11. Ault A. Ambiguous identity in an unambiguous sex/gender structure: the case of bisexual women. *Sociol Q.* 1996;37(3):449-463.

12. Klein F. *The Bisexual Option.* New York, NY: Arbor Hourse: 1978.

13. Collins JF. Biracial-bisexual individuals: identity coming of age. *Intl J Sex Gender Stud.* 2000;5(3):221-253.

14. The Gender Education and Advocacy (GEA) Web site. www.gender.org. Accessed December 1, 2009.

15. Chivers M, Bailey JM. Sexual orientation of female-to-male transsexuals: a comparison of homosexual and nonhomosexual types. *Arch Sex Behav.* 2000;29(3):259-278.

16. Doctor R, Fleming JS. Measures of transgender behavior. *Arch Sex Behav.* 2001;30:255-271.

17. Intersex Society of North America (ISNA) Web site. www.isna.org. Accessed September 26, 2010.

18. Blackless M, Charuvastra A, Derryck A, Fausto-Sterling A, Lauzanne K, Lee E. How sexually dimorphic are we? Review and synthesis. *Am J Human Biol.* 2000;12:151-166.

19. Herek GM. The context of anti-gay violence: notes on cultural and psychological heterosexism. *J Interpers Violence.* 1990;5:316-333.

20. Cabaj RP, Stein TS, eds. *Textbook of Homosexuality and Mental Health.* Washington, DC: American Psychiatric Press; 1996.

21. Wright RH II, Cummings NA III, eds. *Destructive Trends in Mental Health: The Well-Intentioned Path to Harm.* New York, NY: Routledge; 2005.

22. Haaga D. Homophobia? *J Soc Behav Pers.* 1991;6:171-172.

23. Fyfe B. "Homophobia" or homosexual bias reconsidered. *Arch Sex Behav.* 1983;12:549-554.

24. Johnson MP, Ferraro KJ. Research on domestic violence in the 1990s: making distinctions. *J Marriage Fam.* 2000;62(4):948-963.

25. Burke LK, Follingstad DR. Violence in lesbian and gay relationships; theory, prevalence, and correlational factors. *Clin Psychol Rev.* 199;19:487-512.

26. Elliot P. Shattering illusions: same-sex domestic violence. *J Gay Lesbian Soc Services.* 1996;4(1):1-8.

27. Brown MJ, Groscup J. Perceptions of same-sex domestic violence among crisis center staff. *J Fam Violence.* 2009;24:87-93.

28. Balsam KF, Rothblum ED, Beauchaine TP. Victimization over the life span: a comparison of lesbian, gay, bisexual, and heterosexual siblings. *J Consult Clin Psychol.* 2005;73:477-487.

29. Merrill GS, Wolfe VA. Battered gay men: an exploration of abuse, help-seeking, and why they stay. *J Homosex.* 2000;39:1-30.

30. Cruz JM, Firestone JM. (1998). Exploring violence and abuse in gay male relationships. *Violence Vict.* 1998;13(2):159-173.

31. Renzetti CM. *Violent Betrayal: Partner Abuse in Lesbian Relationships.* Thousand Oaks, CA: Sage; 1992.

32. Baum RE, Moore K. *Lesbian, Gay, Bisexual and Transgender Domestic Violence in 2001: a Report of the National Coalition of Anti-Violence Programmes.* ncavp.org/common/document_files/Reports/2001ncavpdvrpt.pdf. Published 2002. Accessed July 9, 2013.

33. Klinger RL. Gay violence. *J Gay Lesbian Psychother.* 1995;2(3):119-134.

34. Seelau SM, Seelau EP. Gender-role stereotypes and perceptions of heterosexual, gay and lesbian domestic violence. *J Fam Violence.* 2005;20:363-371.

35. Wise AJ, Bowman SL. Comparison of beginning counselors' responses to lesbian vs. heterosexual partner abuse. *Violence Vict.* 1997;12:127-135.

36. McClaughlyn K. A safe haven on the reservation: protecting women from intimate partner violence. *Office of Minority Health Newsletter: Closing the Gap.* January/February 2002:8-9.

37. Brown LS. Preventing heterosexism and bias in psychotherapy and counseling. In: Rothblum ED, Bond LA, eds. *Preventing Heterosexism and Homophobia.* Thousand Oaks, CA: Sage; 1996: 36-58.

38. Friedman LJ. An examination of attitudes toward gay men and lesbians among Louisiana licensed professional counselors. *Dissertation Abstracts Intl.* 1996;56(10-A):3837.

39. Smith GB. Homophobia and attitudes toward gay men and lesbians by psychiatric nurses. *Arch Psychiatr Nurs.* 1993;7:377–384.

40. Letellier P. Gay and bisexual male domestic violence victimization: challenges to feminist theory and responses to violence. *Violence Vict.* 1994;9(2):95-106.

41. Chan E, Cavacuiti, C. Gay abuse screening protocol (GASP): screening for abuse in gay male relationships. *J Homosex.* 2008;54(4):423-438.

42. McLaughlin E, Rozee P. Knowledge about heterosexual versus lesbian battering among lesbians. *Women and Therapy.* 2001;23(3):39-58.

43. Waldner-Haugrud LK, Gratch LV, Magruder B. Victimization and perpetuation rates of violence in gay and lesbian relationships: gender issues explored. *Violence Vict.* 1997;12:173-184.

44. White BH, Kurpius SER. Effects of victim sex and sexual orientation on perceptions of rape. *Sex Roles.* 2002;46:191-200.

45. Duncan D. Prevalence of sexual assault victimization among heterosexual and gay/lesbian university students. *Psychol Reports.* 1990;66:65-66.

46. McConaghy N, Zamir R. Heterosexual and homosexual coercion, sexual orientation, and sexual roles in medical students. *Arch Sex Behav.* 1995;24(5):289-502.

47. Frank DJ, Harding T, Wosick-Correa K. The global dimensions of rape-law reform: a cross-national study of policy outcomes. *Am Sociol Rev.* 2009;74(2):272-290.

48. Lev AI, Lev S. Sexual assault in the lesbian, gay, bisexual, and transgendered communities. In: Mc Clennen, JC, Gunther J, eds. *A Professional's Guide to Understanding Gay and Lesbian Domestic Violence: Understanding Practice Interventions.* Lewiston, NY: Edwin Mellen; 1999:35-61.

49. Lev AI, Lev SS. Sexual Assault in the Transgender Communities. http://my.execpc.com/~dmmunson/Nov99_7.htm. Published 1999. Accessed March 8, 2009.

50. Courvant D, Cook-Daniels L. Transgender and intersex survivors of domestic violence: defining terms, barriers, and responsibilities. In: National Coalition Against Domestic Violence. Conference Manual. Denver, CO; 1998.

51. Jordan B. Intersex Survivors of Domestic Violence. Healthy Place Web site. http://www.healthyplace.com/gender/inside-intersexuality/intersex-survivors-of-domestic-violence/menu-id-1427/. Published 2007. Accessed 26 September, 2010.

52. Hirschfield S. Moving beyond the safe zone: a staff development approach to anti-heterosexist education. *Fordham Urban Law J.* 2002;29(2):611-26.

53. D'Augelli A. Development implications of victimization of lesbian, gay, and bisexual youths. In: Herek GM, ed. *Stigma and Sexual Orientation: Understanding Prejudice Against Lesbians, Gay Men, and Bisexuals.* Thousand Oaks, CA: Sage; 1998:187-210.

54. Savin-Williams RC. Verbal and physical abuse as stressors in the lives of lesbian, gay male, and bisexual youths: associations with school problems, running away, substance abuse, prostitution, and suicide. *J Couns Clin Psychol.* 1994;62:261-269.

55. Smith GW, Smith D. The ideology of 'fag:' the school experience of gay students. *Sociol Q.* 1998;39:309-335.

56. Ueno K. Sexual orientation and psychological distress in adolescence: examining interpersonal stressors and social support processes. *Soc Psychol Q.* 2005;68(3):258-277.

57. Pilkington N, D'Augelli AR. Victimization of lesbian, gay, and bisexual youth in community settings. *J Community Psychol.* 1995;23:33-56.

58. Ray N. Lesbian, Gay, Bisexual and Transgender Youth: An Epidemic of Homelessness. National Gay and Lesbian Task Force Web site. http://www.thetaskforce.org/reports_and_research/homeless_youth.pdf. Published 2006.

59. Cochran B, Stewart A, Ginzler J, Cauce A. Challenges faced by homeless sexual minorities; comparison of gay, lesbian, and transgender homeless adolescents with their heterosexual counterparts. *Am J Public Health.* 2002;92(5):773-777.

60. Whitbeck L, Chen X, Hoyt D, Tyler K, Johnson K. Mental disorder, subsistence strategies, and victimization among gay, lesbian, and bisexual homeless and runaway adolescents. *J Sex Res.* 2004;41(4):329-342.

61. National Alliance to End Homelessness. www.endhomelessness.org/content/article/detail/2141. Published December 8, 2008.

62. Russell ST, Joyner K. Adolescent sexual orientation and suicide risk: evidence from a national study. *Am J Public Health.* 2001;91:1276-81.

63. Bagley C, Tremblay P. Elevated rates of suicidal behavior in gay, lesbian, and bisexual youth. *Crisis.* 2000;21:111–117.

64. Smith MU, Drake MA. Suicide and homosexual teens: what can biology teachers do to help? *Am Biol Teacher.* 2001;63(3):154-162.

65. Harrison AE. Primary care of lesbian and gay patients: educating ourselves and our students. *Family Med.* 1996;28(1):10-23.

66. McDaniel JS, Purcell D, D'Augelli A. The relationship between sexual orientation and risk for suicide: research findings and future direction for research and prevention. *Suicide Life Threat Behav.* 2001;31:84-105.

67. Spirito A, Esposito-Smythers C. Attempted and completed suicide in adolescence. *Ann Rev Clin Psychol.* 2006;2:237-266.

68. SC gay rights activists to protest date violence bill. *Edge Boston.* May 19, 2009. http://www.edgeboston.com/news////91364/sc_gay_rights_activists_to_protest_date_violence_bill. Accessed August 6, 2013.

69. Simon M. My bullied son's last day on Earth. CNN Web site. http://www.cnn.com/2009/US/04/23/bullying.suicide/. Published April 24, 2009. Accessed August 6, 2013.

70. Kosciw JG, Diaz EM, Gretak EA. The 2007 National School Climate Survey: *The Experiences of Lesbian, Gay, Bisexual and Transgender Youth in Our Nation's Schools.* New York, NY: GLSEN; 2008.

71. Sheridan D. Treating Survivors of intimate partner abuse: forensic identification and documentation. In: Olshaker J, Jackson M, Smock W, eds. *Forensic Emergency Medicine.* 2nd ed. Philadelphia, PA: Lippincott Williams & Wilkins; 2007.

72. Braun V, Terry G, Gavey N, Fenaughty J. Risk and sexual coercion among gay and bisexual men in Aotearoa/New Zealand-key informant accounts. *Cult Health Sex.* 2009;(2):11-24.

73. Waldo CR, McFarland W, Katz MH, MacKellar D, Valleroy LA. Very young gay and bisexual men are at risk for HIV infections: the San Francisco Bay Area Young Men's Survey II. *J Acquir Immune Defic Syndr.* 2000;24(2):168-74.

74. Cohen L, Davis R, Mikkelsen L. Comprehensive prevention: improving health outcomes through practice. *Minority Health Today.* March/April 2000;1:38-41.

Chapter 26

Intimate Partner Violence in the Military Community*

David W. Lloyd, JD
Mary E. Campise, LICSW
Brian C. Ross, JD

Key Points

1. Military culture is both distinct from and part of the broader culture of America's civilian society. Service members and their families are not isolated from social problems in the civilian sector but also experience stressors unique to military life.

2. Military culture is performance based, and rooted in principles of positive socialization and both personal and communal responsibility. Because military programs that support active component families are intended to support military readiness, military commanders are involved in individual and family issues.

3. The unique demographics of the military community (ie, mostly young males) and the stressors associated with combat exposure may increase the likelihood of intimate partner violence.

4. The Department of Defense addresses domestic abuse with a 5-part approach: (1) primary and secondary prevention, (2) advocacy for victims, (3) early intervention and social worker assessment, (4) safety and support for victims, including medical and mental health treatment as appropriate, and (5) action as appropriate to address perpetrators' behavior.

5. Most services to assist victims of intimate partner violence are tied to the victims' eligibility for military benefits and the unique needs of the military. Confidentiality for victims is not absolute.

Introduction

The US military is a unique subculture of American society in a number of ways. First, although it is a subculture it also contains its own subcultures. Some of these are the traditions and behaviors unique to each of the 4 Services in the "active component" (the Army, Navy, Marine Corps, and Air Force) in which their respective Service members take great pride – and which are occasionally viewed with amusement by those of the other Services. There are also longstanding enlisted and officer corps subcultures, but they operate synergistically to complete the military mission.

The branches in the reserve component (Army National Guard, Air National Guard, Army Reserve, Navy Reserve, Marine Corps Reserve, and Air Force Reserve) form an additional subculture in comparison to the active component due to their part-

*The views, opinions, and/or findings contained in this chapter are the authors' own and should not be construed as an official position, policy, or decision of the Department of Defense unless so designated by other documentation.

time status and unique roles. Reserve component personnel are only part of military culture when they train, frequently one weekend a month and 2 weeks per year, and unless and until the President calls them to federal active duty. As a result, the reserve component is excluded from the purview of this chapter. However, over 600 000 members of the reserve component entered into the Service subcultures of the active component when the Department of Defense (DoD) created a "total force" to fight Operation Enduring Freedom (OEF) and Operation Iraqi Freedom (OIF) (the wars in Afghanistan and Iraq, respectively).

UNDERSTANDING THE MILITARY CULTURE

Although people can join and leave the military voluntarily, the Services control the departure of their members—a Service member must complete his/her term of enlistment upon penalty of imprisonment. During the early part of OEF and OIF the military imposed "stop loss," which retained personnel beyond the expiration of their enlistment period. Further, under certain circumstances, personnel who have retired can be recalled to active duty. The Services also may expel Service members from active duty by administrative discharge or by discharge after a court-martial conviction. For an officer, performance may control departure: failure to be promoted at certain steps in the career means that the officer will be separated from the Service.

Second, at the same time that new Service members are assimilating to the military subculture(s), many of them are also simultaneously assimilating to the larger American culture from foreign cultures. New immigrants have enlisted in the US military since at least the Civil War, and since World War II significant numbers of Service members have married those from other nations whom they met while assigned abroad. Federal law[1] permits naturalized citizens and resident aliens to enlist; in 2009, more than 21 000 naturalized citizens and resident aliens were members of the active duty force.[2]

Third, the military culture is performance-based. Service members learn how to perform a military mission: identify the goals and objectives, get trained to achieve them, provide support to other individuals and units to help them achieve related goals and objectives, measure progress in achieving these goals and objectives, be individually accountable for achieving them (or failing to do so), identify lessons learned from this effort, and take corrective action for improvement. Almost every facet of military performance is reviewed via an ***after-action report*** and corrective action may involve individual or unit re-training. Sometimes it results in a poor performance appraisal that affects promotion rather than disciplinary action. This cultural emphasis on corrective action may influence how commanders respond to incidents of intimate partner violence (IPV), especially if the Service member has not had previous behavioral problems and the incident is perceived as minor.

Fourth, military culture is one of positive socialization.[3] Service members and their family members are reminded every day that the values of duty, integrity, and sacrifice on behalf of others, and numerous other values are to be implemented concretely. Every day Service members are shown directly and indirectly that they can succeed and are expected to succeed, and that their career is built upon steppingstones of success. They tend to carry this positive socialization into their personal life and their spouses indirectly learn it also. They believe that they will have strong families and most succeed.

Fifth, military culture is one of both personal and communal responsibility.[3] From the outset, the military seeks to instill in recruits an appreciation for good order and the communal nature of their obligations. From the first day of basic training, Service members learn that military service is not an individual effort; when an individual makes a mistake the superiors take corrective action by punishing the group. A new Service member quickly finds that he is not trying to succeed to save himself from pushups; he's trying to succeed to save his comrades! Leaders emphasize the need for members of the same unit to look out for and assist each other. Military culture encourages the pursuit of group interests over individual interests due to battlefield necessity, but this also influences the response to harmful behavior on the home front. Whether it takes the form of buddies pulling an overly belligerent young Service member from the brink of a bar fight or neighbors intervening to stop domestic violence, the military is far less likely than the civilian world to regard problems as purely individual.

Communal responsibility has both positive and negative effects in terms of preventing IPV. Good and bad behavior reflects on the Service member's unit as well as on the Service member, which reinforces a desire to have good interpersonal relationships. Spouses also embrace the communitarian life. They tend to be heavily involved in military community activities, especially if they live on the installation, such as the chapel, volunteer groups to assist new personnel, and youth programs. One's peers in the military are more involved in dissuading, correcting, or reporting problematic relationships than they would be in civilian culture. However, this can also lead couples, units, and installations to resist assistance from civilian service providers and organizations. For example, soldiers are encouraged to become "Army Strong," which may be interpreted to mean that seeking help is not strong.

The civilian spouses of active duty personnel must learn how to mix both their spouses' military subculture(s) and the larger civilian culture throughout their spouse's military service, perhaps more than their military spouses do. Even if both spouses like the military subculture, the conflicts in the expectations of each subculture can contribute to marital conflict. Civilian spouses of those in the reserve component are far less exposed to the military culture since their lives are wholly in the civilian community until their spouse is mobilized to federal active duty.

Sixth, military culture is quite hierarchical. It emphasize the chains of command in which every Service member, whether enlisted or an officer, reports to a higher leader in a pyramid to the highest military officer of that Service, then through the civilian leadership of the Office of the Secretary of Defense to the President.[3] Each leader has broad autonomy over subordinate Service members to accomplish the military mission and their welfare. Service members and their family members take personal problems that they cannot solve to the lowest level of leadership that should be able to solve them. When they can't be solved at lower levels they take them to leaders higher up the pyramid.

After the draft was ended in the early 1970s, the percentage of Service members who have married rose dramatically to the current level of 57%, so that military culture became more family friendly, leading to the adage, "recruit the single person and retain the family." Most commanders understand that Service members perform better if their families are valued and well cared for. They publicize benefits available to military families and frequently initiate actions that promote family functioning, such as unit picnics and entertainment. The DoD has expanded its long tradition of "taking care of our own" by creating formal policies and programs to support such military families and address their problems.

Finally, unlike other American subcultures the military is formally established under the Constitution and therefore has its own regulations and disciplinary system over Service members to address their behavioral problems. Although these are similar to those in the civilian sector they are not identical to them, creating conflicts that require negotiation between military and civilian leaders to seek resolution, sometimes taking on a quasi-cross-cultural negotiation. Formal agreements between military installations and either state or local agencies are called Memorandums of Understanding (MOUs); formal agreements that assign responsibilities over US personnel assigned to installations in foreign countries are called Status of Forces Agreements (SOFAs).

DEMOGRAPHICS OF THE MILITARY COMMUNITY

Given the unique mission of the Armed Forces, it is not surprising that most Service members are young men (only 14.5% are female[4]) and more than two-thirds (66%) of active duty members are younger than 30, with 43% younger than 25.4 In comparison, women comprise nearly 51% of the total US population and only 19% of adults are 30 or younger.[5] What may be surprising is that Service members are, on average, better educated than their civilian peers; more than 90% of enlisted personnel have high school diplomas and nearly 83% of the officers have a baccalaureate degree.[4] Hispanics are under-represented but African Americans make up a considerably higher proportion of the active duty force than in the civilian population.

Civilian spouses tend to mirror their military spouses demographically. They too are young (almost 24% are under age 25, and 47% are younger than 30) and predominantly female.[4] They are more likely than unaffiliated civilians to have graduated from high school and attended college, but, often owing to the rigors of the military lifestyle, they are 3 times as likely to be out of work. A typical military family moves once every 3 years. In 2010 approximately 15% of military spouses seeking work were unemployed, and 45% were not actively seeking employment.[4] This financial dependence on the Service member makes it difficult for a victim of domestic abuse to leave the relationship.

These demographic differences from the civilian population explain some of the differences between military and civilian prevalence rates for intimate partner violence. Young men commit more violent crimes than any other demographic group, and young married couples are more likely to engage in physical violence than older ones. Younger people are also less likely to report observed domestic violence.

MILITARY LIFE

On military installations, officer and enlisted housing areas are separate. Nearly 60% of military personnel live outside the military installation and, due to the cost of available housing, a large proportion of Service members tend to reside in the same neighborhoods, creating homogeneity in the demographic makeup of whole neighborhoods. The absence of more mature couples and the frequent rotation of personnel in and out of these communities may establish unacceptable norms for marital behavior. Both civilian and military law enforcement personnel are frequently familiar with particular neighborhoods where domestic abuse is over-represented.

Moves are frequent, creating long distances to friends and family. About 15% of military families live abroad and communication to loved ones can be difficult if they are multiple time zones (and frequently the International Date Line) away, particularly for first time parents. Even if the family does not move, the Service member may have an unaccompanied tour or deployment, both of which mean that the Service member's family can be stressed. The spouse may feel socially isolated, especially if he or she is far from home. A young bride from the Midwest may have moved to Korea with her soldier husband. He could soon deploy, leaving her learning about military life while in Korea alone. If he rejoins her and they move to Washington, for a few months before he deploys again, it is understandable if she chooses to end the marriage.

When the Service member returns from an unaccompanied tour or deployment both spouses and any children must readjust, as military parenting is frequently an unpredictable cycle of single parenting to dual parenting to single parenting. Similar adjustments must occur between unmarried couples. The frequency of deployments ("OPTEMPO") for military operations can create stress in the relationship. During the last month before a combat-related deployment the Service member is focused on training and related activities, along with completing a significant amount of paperwork. The couple's communication with each other and with their child(ren) can be affected by their unspoken fear of injury or death. The partner who is left behind may be depressed and have little energy for caring for the child(ren). While there is frequently a honeymoon period after return the couple soon must adjust to the changes that each has made during their separation. For some Service members the relationship and parenting feel less personally rewarding than the excitement they felt in the deployed environment with their buddies, trying to achieve a noble purpose. Then the Service member begins preparing for the next deployment, which the partner may resent. Some Service members have difficulty in their relationships after a deployment due to combat-related depression. Some with posttraumatic stress disorder may even lash out at others with violence, erroneously perceiving a threat to their safety.

Case Study 26-1: Combat Experience and Family Life.

Master Sergeant Joe Gordon is a very proud soldier. He has spent 20 years on active duty in the Army, beginning with his first deployment to Saudi Arabia during the first Gulf War. Joe's friends and colleagues have always appreciated his gregarious sense of humor and laid back demeanor, although he always takes his duties very seriously.

MSG Gordon and his wife, Sally, have been married since the month after they graduated from high school together in 1990. They have 3 children and have lived in Germany, Korea, Hawaii, and Alaska, in addition to Army posts within the continental US. Though the Gordon family was well accustomed to the rigors of military life, his recent deployment to Afghanistan was particularly stressful for all of them. This deployment was particularly difficult—the most stressful of Joe's long career—and casualties were significant. Because of the remote location and sensitive nature of his unit's mission, Joe was able to call home only rarely and could say very little about his activities when he did. While Joe had to endure horrific battles and the loss of several close friends, Sally had to care for their children while having a lot of anxiety about her husband's safety.

Upon his return from deployment, Joe's demeanor had clearly changed. Instead of his former light hearted attitude he was often anxious, reserved, and prone to agitation in public places. Though he'd previously been a very patient man, small irritants began to provoke angry outbursts. During increasingly frequent arguments with Sally, he would scream and curse and direct a torrent of belittling comments her way, which he had rarely done before. During one argument over finances that began with a seemingly insignificant issue, Joe smashed a beer bottle across the kitchen counter, and punched a nearby wall so hard that he both injured his hand and dented the wall. Concerned that his outbursts were becoming violent, Sally took her children to a friend's home and contacted the Family Advocacy Program (FAP) in hope of getting counseling for her husband.

The Family Advocacy Program (FAP) was able to provide counseling and support to Sally and her children, and at her request, couples counseling for Sally and Joe. Because Joe seemed to be suffering from posttraumatic stress disorder, the FAP clinician wanted Joe to be assessed by the behavioral health unit at the local military hospital. Joe was reluctant to go even though he had recommended and in some cases strongly encouraged soldiers in his unit who were depressed after their return from Iraq to seek help. Seeking help was contrary to his self-image as a strong soldier. Sally begged him to follow his own advice: it is a sign of strength to seek help, not a sign of weakness. Reluctantly, Joe made an appointment.

IPV in the Military Community

DoD began a long-term process of improving its response to IPV in the mid 1990s, with several conferences and working groups. In the National Defense Authorization Act for Fiscal Year 2000,[6] Congress authorized a Defense Task Force on Domestic Violence, composed of 12 senior leaders in DoD and 12 civilian experts. In its 3 annual reports the Task Force made nearly 200 recommendations to DoD, the Department of Justice and the Congress. DoD agreed with about 75% of the recommendations pertaining to it, had already implemented some, and has implemented the remainder.

Until 2004, DoD did not have a DoD-wide definition for domestic violence but instead used the narrower definition of *spouse abuse* of the DoD Family Advocacy Program (FAP). This definition did not address IPV between former spouses and between current and former intimate partners.

In 2011 DoD updated the following definitions:

Domestic Abuse: Domestic violence or a pattern of behavior resulting in emotional/psychological abuse, economic control, and/or interference with personal liberty that is directed toward a person who is: a current or former spouse; a person with whom the abuser shares a child in common; or a current or former intimate partner with whom the abuser shares or has shared a common domicile.

Domestic Violence: An offense under the United States Code, the Uniform Code of Military Justice,[8] or State law involving the use, attempted use, or threatened use of force or violence or a violation of a lawful order issued for the protection of a person, who is: a current or former spouse; a person with whom the abuser shares a child in common; or a current or former intimate partner with whom the abuser shares or has shared a common domicile.[9]

The Department of Defense addresses both domestic abuse with a 5-part approach: (1) primary and secondary prevention, (2) advocacy for victims, (3) early intervention and assessment, (4) safety and support for victims, including medical and mental health treatment as appropriate, and (5) action as appropriate to address perpetrators' behavior. DoD also conducts annual reviews of domestic abuse-related fatalities to identify opportunities for prevention.

PREVENTION

FAP sees IPV as one part of the spectrum of violence, of which contributing factors include sexism, sociopathic behavior, mental illness, poor impulse control, greed, racism, political beliefs, religious beliefs, and response to perceived threat. In DoD's experience, while some violence by intimate partners derives from male misogyny, other such violence involves one or more of these other factors, especially mental illness and poor impulse control. Numerous spouses have related that after their spouses have returned from combat operations in Iraq and Afghanistan, such veterans' behavior has changed so that they now escalate arguments into situations in which the risk for violence is elevated. It is likely that combat-related depression has impaired their relationship skills. Similarly, when women in the military community initiate violence against their male intimate partners, FAP personnel believe that some factor other than misogyny is the primary contributing factor.

Prevention of IPV in the military is therefore part of a broad effort to prevent violence, perhaps more than the prevention efforts within the domestic violence field within the civilian sector. DoD's goals in prevention of domestic abuse are broader than raising public awareness of the problem or encouraging victims to report their victimization, and broader than creating a stigma in the military community to discourage such behavior. Prevention in DoD devotes attention to stressors unique to the military, and to coping, communication, and relationship skills that need periodic improvement to prevent situations from erupting into violence.

Under the Constitution the military is expected to maintain *readiness*, ie, to be able to deploy quickly to whatever location is appropriate to perform the tasks assigned to it for the nation's security. *Personnel readiness* means that Service members are physically and mentally fit, trained for their mission responsibilities, and are ready to deploy to perform them. As both the number and roles of women in the force have expanded, the prevention of IPV is increasingly seen as a readiness issue, as a culture that excuses the victimization of women jeopardizes unit cohesion and discipline. Men who regard women as less capable or less deserving of respect are less likely to rely on women performing essential battlefield functions and less likely to accept female leadership. The importance of readiness means that the military has a strong practical interest in correcting inequities based on gender, race, or culture because of their detrimental effect on mission accomplishment. Beyond even mere principle, practical considerations compel action.

Because the military culture values strong and supportive families, chaplaincy programs and family centers on military installations offer classes and counseling on relationships, marriage, and parenting. Family centers and behavioral health clinicians provide classes and individual counseling to improve stress management techniques and to help both Service members and their families cope with the current rapid cycle of preparation for deployment, return from deployment, readjustment, and preparation for the next deployment.

Other programs provide family support to strengthen couple relationships, such as the wide range of services provided by Military OneSource (MOS) that provides information and referral worldwide on a 24/7 basis, through toll-free telephone, email, and a web site.[10] In 2008, the leading 5 issues for which individuals called MOS were couple relationships, stress, emergency financial resources, deployment, and family relationships, especially in reference to children. Balancing work and life, coping with deployment, preparing for deployment, managing stress, and coping with grief and loss were the top 5 reasons individuals accessed the online assistance.[11] Each of the military branches has a similar online resource for military leaders. Three (Navy, Marine Corps, and Air Force) have Leaders Guides for Managing Personnel in Distress that help military leaders learn what actions they may take to both prevent domestic abuse and intervene appropriately, in addition to other situations.

MOS and the Military Family Life Consultant (MFLC) program provide non-medical counseling to couples who want to strengthen their relationships to prevent more serious problems. Service members and their family members are likely to regard such efforts as part of the "we take care of our own" thread in military culture rather than domestic abuse prevention, but these programs nevertheless contribute to reducing risk factors. Installation commanders can request MFLCs during the stressful times before, during, and after deployments to help couples address problems in their relationships.

Another factor that may indirectly contribute to prevention of IPV is the military's culture of controlling the use of violence. Military leaders instruct their forces in the occasions, frequency, intensity, and circumstances of violence the Service members under their command will initiate and continue against the enemy; these rules of engagement are intended to accomplish the military mission without using excessive force unnecessarily or violating the international rules of war.

Control over the use of violence continues to installations outside the theatre of combat operations: they are expected to be violence-free. Access to government weaponry, from artillery to assault rifles, from bombs and grenades to ammunition, is strictly controlled. The only personnel authorized to carry firearms in locations other than rifle ranges and hostile locations are military police and plainclothes investigators. Those who live in government quarters on the installation are required to store personal firearms in special armories, although those living in family housing or in the civilian community are not.

With respect to formal efforts to prevent domestic abuse, FAPs have primary responsibility for public awareness and education efforts. In conducting these campaigns, FAPs are required to "coordinate with local civilian domestic abuse programs and with national and state civilian domestic abuse public awareness and education programs, modifying informational materials as appropriate for the military community."[9] DoD partners in the development of these programs have included the American Bar Association, which created the Teen Dating Violence Prevention and Awareness Toolkit that was mailed to military youth programs and schools, and "Take a Stand" and other public awareness campaigns created by the Family Violence Prevention Fund, now known as Futures Without Violence, and the National Domestic Violence Hotline.

The FAPs at each installation conduct special public awareness activities, centered on October as National Domestic Violence Awareness Month, in conjunction with activities by local civilian organizations. The FAP in the Office of the Secretary of Defense and the Armed Forces Radio and TV Service (AFRTS) creates TV and radio public service announcements in lieu of advertisements during broadcasts of commercial radio and TV shows on military TV and radio at overseas installations. Special public service announcements are aired on the Pentagon Channel and at domestic installations throughout the year that publicize the FAP as a resource for prevention.

Military OneSource is the official web site for program information, policy, and guidance for Service members and their families, leaders, and service providers. Searches can be made by specific populations: troops and families, leaders, or service providers. They can also be made by specific quality of life topic. Service members and their family members can locate the appropriate family service/support center, hospital, chaplain, FAP, victim advocate, domestic abuse community resources, and national and state domestic abuse hotlines.

All medical providers in the military treatment facility receive annual training on the prevention, identification, and reporting options for suspected domestic abuse. In particular, the obstetrics/gynecology, pediatrics, and women's health clinics work closely with the installation FAP to promote prevention initiatives and programs.

In addition to requiring annual training for key personnel and first responders, DoD policy[9] requires ongoing community education and training to all personnel on the dynamics of domestic abuse, DoD and Military Service-specific policy and procedures, common misconceptions associated with domestic abuse, beliefs, attitudes, and cultural issues associated with domestic abuse, and available civilian and military resources. Outreach to family members in community training is strongly encouraged. The primary purpose of this training is to promote community norms that support social action and increase awareness of the role all community members play in preventing and responding to violence in relationships.

Victim Advocacy

By law, DoD is required to provide victim advocates for victims of intimate partner violence.[12] DoD provides victim advocacy to victims of intimate partner violence in the military community but there are some differences that provided in the civilian sector, namely eligibility, safety planning record, the availability of military legal actions and resources for protection and resources, and limits on the confidentiality of communications.[8] Because of these and other differences, civilian domestic violence advocates need additional materials to assist victims whose alleged abuser is in the military.[13]

Eligibility

In DoD, the victim of domestic abuse must be eligible to receive military medical treatment, including eligibility on a fee-paying basis. Those eligible include active duty personnel and their enrolled family members, retirees, and in some locations outside the US, civilian employees and contractors. For a victim of domestic abuse who is a member of the reserve component, or whose alleged abuser is a member of the reserve component, eligibility is limited to situations when the domestic abuse occurred while the Service member has been mobilized to federal active duty status or during inactive duty training. For a victim who does not meet these eligibility requirements (such as the civilian intimate partner of a Service member), the victim advocate offers safety planning services and referral to civilian support services and victim advocacy.

Safety Planning Record

For a domestic abuse victim the advocacy authorized by DoD is similar to that provided in the civilian sector, although the safety plan is recorded on DD Form 2893, Victim Advocate Safety Plan. All victims, including victims who are not eligible for military medical care, are provided with a copy of the initial safety plan. If an eligible victim provides a copy of the safety plan to the victim advocate because the victim will continue to see the advocate, the victim advocate will use it for further discussions of the victim's safety, to change or develop the safety plan more fully, and to record services provided to the victim. DoD victim advocates are expected to review the victim's safety plan with the victim periodically.

Information on Military Administrative and Disciplinary Actions and Other Resources

The victim advocate will discuss with the victim available information and resources, including administrative and disciplinary actions available through the military and legal actions and services in the civilian sector, as well as local military and civilian resources for immediate safety and long-term protection, workplace safety, housing, childcare, clinical resources, medical services, and religious counseling. The victim advocate advises the victim of the impact of domestic abuse on children and offers referrals for assessments of the physical and mental health of involved children.

The domestic abuse victim advocate also provides the victim with basic information about payment for an eligible victim's transportation and shipment of household goods when this is required for the victim's safety and the transitional compensation program, which includes medical and dental benefits and commissary and exchange benefits, available to a family member who was abused by a Service member on active duty. Both of these, unique to the military, are discussed more fully below.

If the victim has made an unrestricted report (defined below), the victim advocate assists the victim in contacting appropriate military and civilian legal offices for personal legal advice and assistance specific to the victim's circumstances or case, including the filing for civilian protective orders (CPOs) and/or military protective orders (MPOs), although the victim advocate is not permitted to provide legal advice. When the incident involves an offense punishable under the Uniform Code of Military Justice (UCMJ), the victim advocate consults and works with the Victim/Witness Liaison assigned from the installation legal office, including accompanying the victim to appointments and civilian and military court proceedings, as appropriate and when requested by the victim.

If the victim has given signed authorization, the domestic abuse victim advocate participates in those portions of FAP meetings in which supportive services (including safety planning) and clinical treatment for the domestic abuse victim, and for any children living in the victim's home, are discussed. The victim advocate promotes a coordinated community response for the prevention of domestic abuse and for intervention. As a systems advocate, the victim advocate promotes a coordinated community response for the prevention of domestic abuse and for intervention when domestic abuse occurs, including an ongoing assessment of the consistency and effectiveness of the domestic abuse victim advocate program at the victim advocate's installation, collaboration with other agencies and activities to improve system response to, and support of, victims.

DoD domestic abuse victim advocates may be DoD employees or contractors, volunteers, or civilians who are part of civilian domestic violence programs who provide services to a nearby military installation through a memorandum of understanding or contract. Because military personnel who deploy to hostile areas do so without accompanying family members, domestic abuse victim advocates need not be deployable. Depending on the Service, domestic abuse victim advocacy and sexual assault victim advocacy may be combined into one program, or they may be separate programs where the installation FAP manager supervises the domestic abuse victim advocates and the sexual assault response coordinator (SARC) supervises the sexual assault victim advocates.

Restricted and Unrestricted Reports

To maintain personnel readiness military commanders thus have a need to know about the day to day health and mental health status of active component Service members much more than do employers in the civilian sector, and to know if they face legal proceedings that may jeopardize their ability to perform their mission.

The military's "need to know" is a cultural difference with special significance with respect to intimate partner violence. If the victim of domestic abuse in the military community discloses the incident to a third party, or if someone witnesses or hears the domestic abuse, or if the alleged offender admits to someone that he/she has committed domestic abuse, the person with knowledge of the intimate partner violence is expected by the military culture to notify military law enforcement or the commander. As a result, active component Service members who are victims of domestic violence have limited confidentiality: the only person in their military community in whom they can confide who has total confidentiality is a chaplain hearing confession or providing spiritual counseling to the victim.

However, the Defense Task Force on Domestic Violence and many civilians advocating that DoD improve its response to domestic abuse and sexual assault urged DoD to reflect on the challenges this lack of confidentiality poses for victims. DoD agreed and has attempted to address this through authorizing a restricted reporting option.[9]

In addition, if the victim is a Service member who at the time of the IPV was engaged in behavior that violates the Uniform Code of Military Justice, such as drinking alcoholic beverages under the legal age, or committing adultery, or "fraternizing" with a service member of a different pay grade within the same command, the victim may be reluctant to report the IPV for fear of being punished by the command for "collateral misconduct" that might be discovered during the investigation.

Case Study 26-2: A Service Member Victim.

Captain Mary Jones, an Air Force nurse, had been assigned at stateside and European medical treatment facilities. In 2009, she was deployed to a forward operating base in Afghanistan, where she provided in-field care for traumatic injuries. Though it was a difficult and often stressful deployment, Capt Jones found it to be a very fulfilling experience.

Upon her return to a duty station at Joint Base Maguire-Dix-Lakehurst in New Jersey, her civilian boyfriend Bob became preoccupied with suspicions that she had cheated on him during her deployment. He began obsessing about Captain Jones' whereabouts, demanding to know where and with whom she is at all times, and even going so far as to follow her in his car. Frequent arguments regularly devolve into screaming matches and 2 recent fights became violent. After the first one a month ago, he shoved her against the wall and locked her inside a bedroom in her off-base apartment. She didn't report the incident at that time. More recently, Bob became enraged after she refused to say where she'd been the previous evening, and punched her hard in the stomach.

Capt Jones made a restricted report to an Air Force domestic abuse victim advocate at the Joint Base and also was assessed medically. Because Bob was not yet divorced from another woman, Capt Jones and the victim advocate were concerned that she might face disciplinary action for adultery (which is a serious offense under the Uniform Code of Military Justice, especially for officers). The challenge for the victim advocate and Capt Jones was how to ensure her safety while Bob was stalking her without jeopardizing her career. If she took the unusual step for an officer of submitting a formal request to command for bachelor officers' quarters on the base it might raise a red flag but if she merely moved to a new apartment in the civilian community it might be both costly and unsuccessful – Bob could follow her car as she exited the base at the end of a duty day. If she disclosed the abuse to seek either a military protective order or a civilian protective order she would run the risk of an investigation discovering her "collateral misconduct" of adultery.

DoD thus created an intermediate step: a ***restricted report*** in which there is no disclosure to military law enforcement or to the commander (**Figure 26-1**). The restricted report may only be made by a victim who chooses restricted reporting (not by the alleged offender or a third person in whom the victim confided) to a domestic abuse victim advocate, or sexual assault victim advocate, or health care provider (including FAP clinical staff), or to a supervisor of the victim advocate or health care provider.

Figure 26-1.

*By filing a restricted report, an IPV victim may receive support from advocates and health care providers without fear of punishment for misconduct related to his or her victimization; however, a victim's report may become unrestricted should he or she seek legal intervention or should mandated exceptions to non-disclosure apply (see **Table 26-1**).*

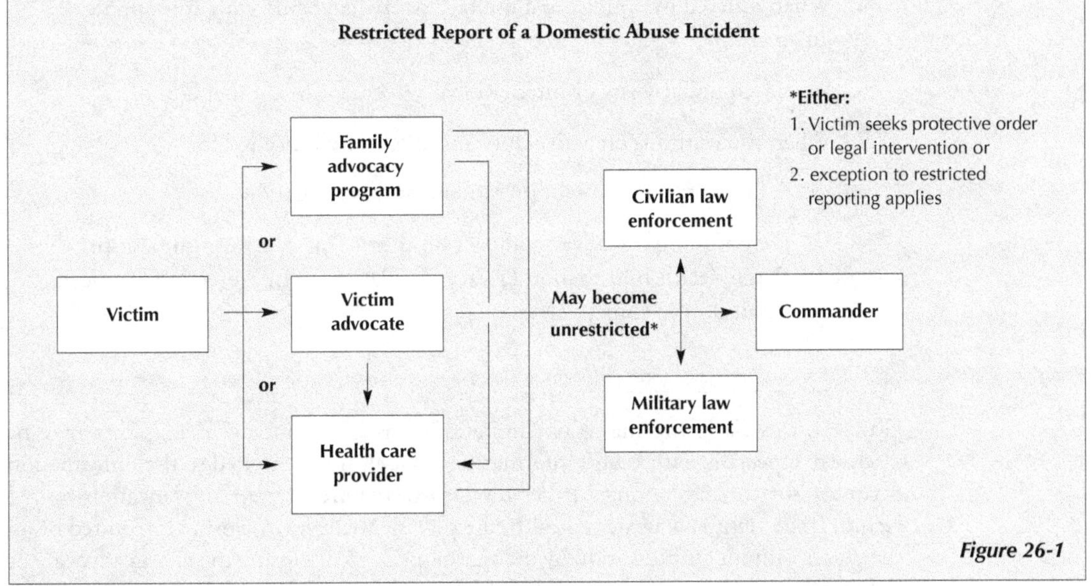

There are sanctions for a victim advocate or health care provider who makes improper disclosure, including discipline under the UCMJ if the victim advocate or health care provider is a Service member, loss of credentials to practice as a victim advocate or health care provider at a military installation, or other adverse or administrative action. One example of such improper disclosure would be the intentional or unintentional disclosure of the IPV to someone in the Service member's chain of command without the victim's authorization. Less frequently, the advocate or health care provider could have disclosed the victim's statements or released copies of notes concerning them to an investigator from a law enforcement agency without the victim's authorization or to an attorney in response to a subpoena that was issued without appropriate jurisdictional authority. If the victim advocate is a Service member, the commander could take such administrative action as writing a negative report for the Service member's personnel file or terminating the person's duty as an advocate. If the victim advocate is a civilian employee the commander could initiate an adverse personnel action; unauthorized disclosure would be grounds for terminating the employment of an advocate who is a contractor.

A restricted report does not provide absolute confidentiality, however. The victim advocate or health care provider or supervisor may disclose the restricted report to military law enforcement or to the command under any of specified conditions (see **Table 26-1**).

Table 26-1. Exceptions to Non-Disclosure of a Restricted Report of Domestic Abuse or Sexual Assault
1. The victim provides a written authorization,
2. If necessary to prevent/lessen a serious and imminent threat to the health or safety of the victim or another,
3. The victim discloses child abuse by the alleged offender or the victim,
4. If needed for supervision of the victim advocate or health care provider,
5. When ordered by a judge to a military or civilian court with appropriate jurisdiction,
6. When required by law or international agreement to another authority,

7. When the victim is on active duty and disclosure is needed for:
   a. A fitness for duty disability retirement determination, or
   b. Determining the adverse impact on the victim's duty assignment per the DoD Health Information Privacy Regulation, with protection for specific details of the abuse.

However, the disclosure may have limitations on the amount of details that may be disclosed, especially with health information.[14] Disclosure is limited to that information necessary for the exception. Further disclosures require written authorization by the victim. If the victim advocate or health care provider believes disclosure is required by an exception without authorization by the victim, prior to disclosure the victim advocate or health care provider must consult with his/her supervisor and the appropriate military legal office, and must make a reasonable effort to provide the victim with advance notice. Whether the report was restricted or unrestricted, the domestic abuse victim advocate or supervisor notifies the command at the next quarterly meeting Family Advocacy Committee of the number of domestic abuse restricted reports received but provides no information that could lead to identification of the victims.

A victim who wishes a commander to issue a Military Protective Order (MPO) cannot make a restricted report. Instead he/she must make an unrestricted report, either to the victim advocate, to a health care provider (including FAP), to military law enforcement, or to the command. If any of these receive an unrestricted report, the others are notified so that appropriate coordination may begin (See **Figure 26-2**).

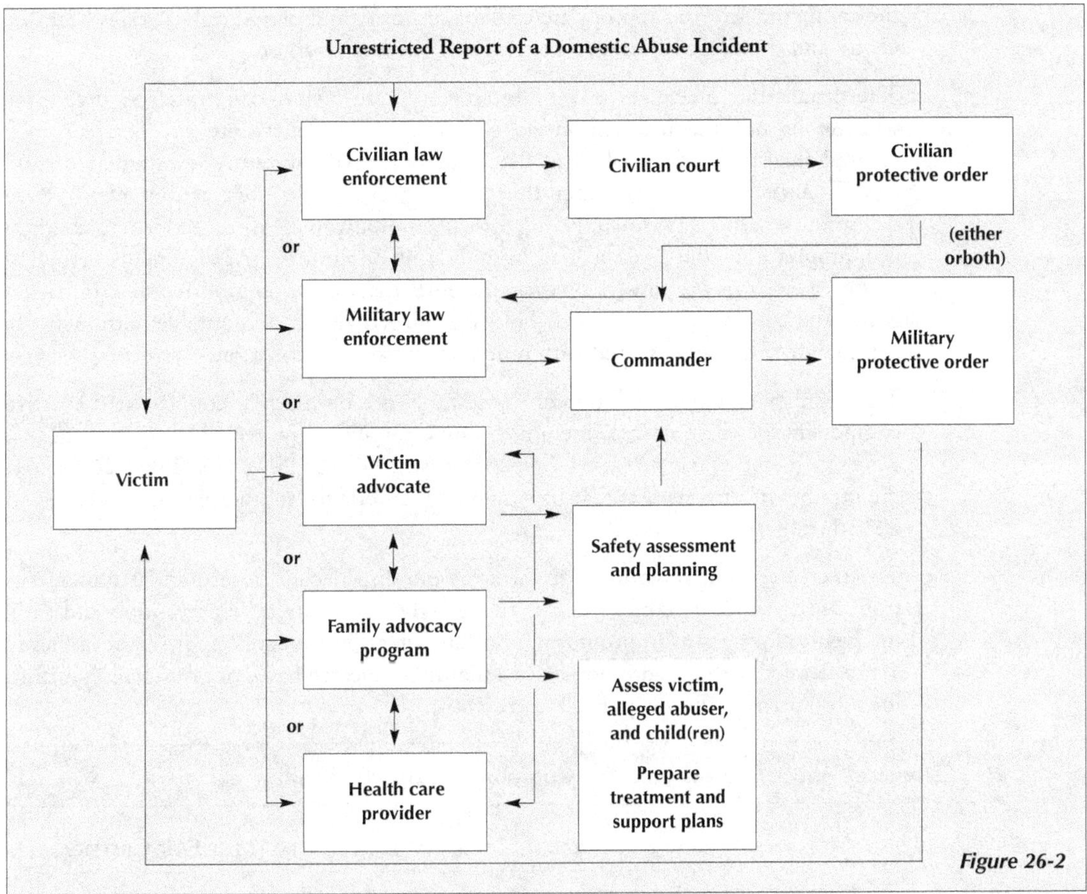

Whether or not the victim has requested a restricted report, the victim should be seen by appropriate medical staff to ascertain whether or not any treatment is appropriate and to document the presence of any evidence. In the case of sexual assault by an intimate partner, a Sexual Assault Forensic Examination (SAFE) "rape kit" is used and the evidence collected is stored in case a victim who made a restricted report later changes his/her mind and wants to make an unrestricted report, at which time the evidence will be turned over to an appropriate law enforcement investigator.

Figure 26-2. *An unrestricted report of IPV filed with civilian or military law enforcement, victim advocates, or health care providers will result in an exchange of information between civilian and military organizations that may lead to a protective order (civilian, military, or both) for the reporting victim. Ideally, the end result is protection for the victim supported by a coordinated effort among civilian and military parties concerned with his or her case.*

Family Advocacy Program

The installation FAP has primary responsibility for ensuring that each reported incident is assessed for risk of further domestic abuse, and for ensuring that victims of domestic abuse are offered a clinical assessment and supportive services on the installation or in the civilian community.[9] The FAP also assesses any children in the family to ascertain whether any child abuse or neglect has occurred, to ascertain the effects of domestic abuse on the child, and to offer appropriate support and treatment to the child.[15]

The FAP also ensures that domestic abusers receive a clinical assessment, or a referral for assessment by civilian providers, and ongoing treatment monitoring. Whether or not the incident involved domestic violence, the FAP risk assessment includes a lethality assessment. If, as a result of the clinical assessment and the commander's disciplinary action or the outcome of civilian criminal proceedings, treatment is appropriate, the FAP either provides it or refers the alleged abuser to a civilian provider. When possible, FAP monitors such treatment and promptly reports violations of treatment rules to the commander or the appropriate civilian authority and periodically assesses both the victim and the alleged abuser to determine the risk of re-abuse.

The installation FAP uses a multidisciplinary case review committee to determine whether or not the incident meets FAP criteria for entry into the Service's FAP Central Registry.[16] Previously, this determination used the terms "substantiated" and "unsubstantiated." Among other things, the Services use their central registries to determine whether a person applying for a position involving direct services to children is appropriate for the position and in evaluating applicants for assignments involving access to nuclear weapons. However, the FAP case review committee determination is not the commander's action to hold the alleged abuser accountable, although the commander may be presented with much of the same information.

The number of reports of spousal domestic abuse by married couples in the active component of the Services, including domestic abuse by a civilian spouse against a Service member, has increased 1.5% between 2001 and 2012 (See **Table 26-2**). Yet, the number of such reports that have met FAP criteria for substantiation has decreased 24% during the same period.

This increase in initial reports with the corresponding decline in substantiated incidents from fiscal year 2001 could indicate the effectiveness of military prevention and early intervention programs in promoting the early identification and reporting of domestic abuse coupled with the adoption of a standardized research based decision tree algorithm for substantiating those reports (**Figure 26-3**).

Table 26-2. Domestic Abuse Reports in Active Component Military Families

		Total		Substantiated (Met FAP Criteria)	
Fiscal Year	Couples	Reports	Rate*	Reports	Rate*
2001	664701	18398	27.7	10967	16.5
2002	682656	17909	26.2	10546	15.4
2003	694527	17072	24.6	9845	14.2
2004	698160	16392	23.5	9434	13.5
2005	702727	15894	22.6	8306	11.8
2006	707895	15399	21.8	7586	10.7
2007	708178	15260	21.5	7257	10.2
2008	718526	15939	22.2	6767	9.4
2009	738067	18208	24.7	7467	10.1
2010	751758	18785	25.0	8411	11.2
2011	753110	19277	25.6	8386	11.1
2012	734308	18671	25.4	8345	11.4

Per 1000 married couples
Source: DoD Family Advocacy Program

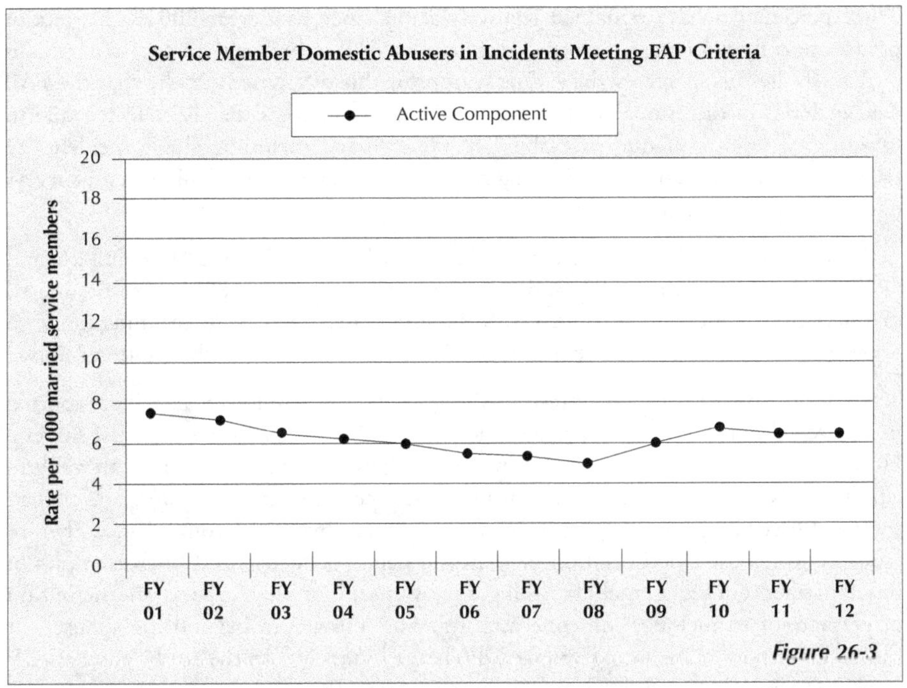

Figure 26-3.
Service member domestic abusers in incidents meeting FAP criteria

In fiscal year 2012, approximately 56% of the substantiated spouse abuse incidents in the active component military community were committed by active duty military personnel of whom 91% were active duty men. The other 39% of substantiated spouse abuse was committed by civilian spouses against their active duty military spouses. Of the active duty abusers in incidents meeting FAP criteria for substantiation, 92% were in the E1-6 pay grades. Within this cluster, E1-3 account for 25% of abusers and the E4-6 account for 67% with the majority in the E4-5 ranks. When the total of substantiated domestic abuse is viewed through the lens of gender, 67% was committed by men and 33% by women (**Figure 26-4**).

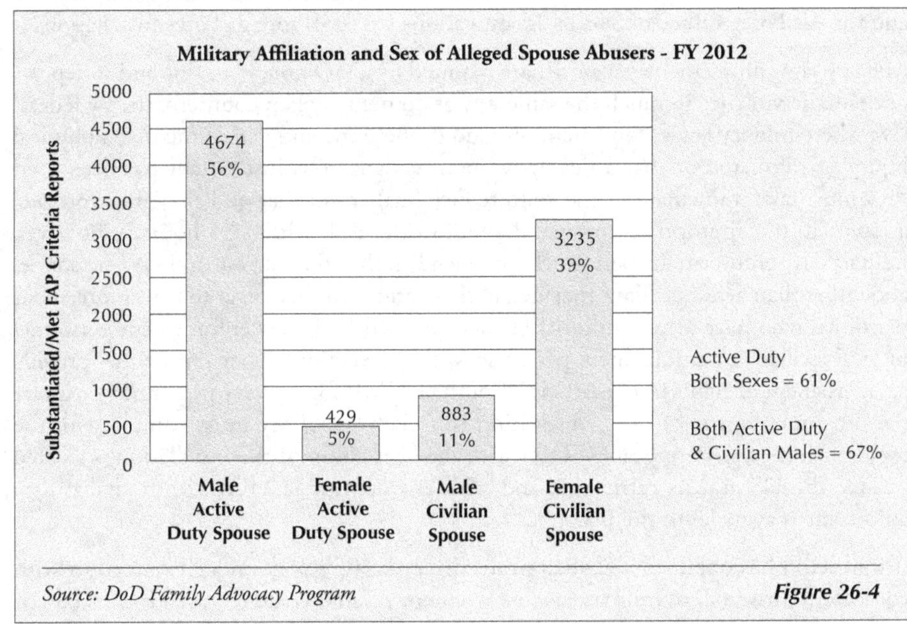

Source: DoD Family Advocacy Program

Figure 26-4

Figure 26-4.
Military affiliation and sex of alleged spouse abusers

These percentages have remained relatively stable since fiscal year 2001. This rate of perpetration by women in reported incidents to FAP is higher than that reported in civilian studies using survey data. One reason for this difference may be that the FAP data includes bi-directional violence among military couples that is collected due to unrestricted reports of domestic abuse in the military, including single incidents of relatively minor abuse or violence[17] that might not be collected in civilian sector surveys of chronic severe violence.

Of all adult spouse abuse victims, about 42% were between the ages of 18 and 24, and 46% were between the ages of 25 and 35. The vast majority (about 85%) of substantiated or "met criteria" incidents involve physical abuse either solely or in combination with other types of abuse. A smaller percentage (about 13%) involves solely emotional abuse.

The rates of spouse abuse in unrestricted reports to FAP are lower than that reported in research about domestic violence in the military that have used confidential surveys. However, this may be due to different methodologies. Unrestricted reports can result in administrative or disciplinary action against a service member abuser, and in a civilian spouse abuser being barred from the base, which are obviously strong disincentives to reporting one's own victimization or that of a neighbor or friend. Other examples of different methodologies include asking survey questions that expand the definition of perpetrator to include "someone important to" the victim beyond the spouse[18] or intimate partner, or including veterans discharged years ago in the study population[19] or using a clinical population of active duty personnel.[20]

MILITARY LAW ENFORCEMENT

Military law enforcement practice is slightly different than that of civilian law enforcement. First responders in the Army are military police (MPs) assigned to the installation's Provost Marshal's Office (PMO). Marine Corps first responders are Marine Corps Police (MCPs) in the Provost Marshal's Office (PMO). In the Navy they are security police (SP). In the Air Force they are security forces. However, serious domestic violence incidents are the responsibility of the installation's detachment of felony-level offense investigators: the Criminal Investigations Command (CIC) for the Army, the Naval Criminal Investigative Service (NCIS) for Navy and Marine Corps installations, and the Air Force Office of Special Investigations (AFOSI) for Air Force installations.

Military law enforcement personnel are required by DoD policy[9] to respond to reports of domestic violence in much the same way as do their civilian counterparts. By federal law, when military law enforcement respond to the scene and determine that a physical injury was inflicted or that a deadly weapon or dangerous instrument has been used they must take immediate measures to reduce further violence and they must provide a report to the appropriate commander and to the FAP within 24 hours.[21] However, military law enforcement personnel apprehend, rather than arrest, military personnel and rather than arrest civilians they detain them and turn them over to law enforcement personnel who have arrest authority (either specified DoD law enforcement personnel or local civilian law enforcement personnel with jurisdiction). They must either provide an advisement of rights under Article 31 of the UCMJ (for military personnel) or under the 5th Amendment of the Constitution (for civilians). They must comply with the requirements of any applicable SOFA with the host nation if the installation is located outside the US and its territories, and with any applicable MOUs with civilian law enforcement agencies in the US.

If the victim has obtained a civilian protective order (CPO) from a civilian court with competent jurisdiction, military law enforcement personnel are required by federal law to take all reasonable measures necessary to ensure that a CPO is registered and given full force and effect.[22] If a CPO has not been registered with the installation but military law enforcement personnel have knowledge of it, it must still be given full force and effect, and they must cooperate with civilian law enforcement agencies to ensure that alleged violations of CPOs are investigated. Moreover, when a commander issues an MPO, the military law enforcement personnel are usually delegated the responsibility to ensure that it is transmitted to their appropriate civilian counterparts to meet the requirements of federal law.[23]

Military law enforcement personnel are required to inform the victim of the availability of local shelter facilities, services offered through FAP, victim advocate and other domestic abuse services, and procedures for obtaining both a CPO and an MPO. If the victim wants to go to a shelter the law enforcement personnel must stand by while the victim gathers personal belongings for the stay at the shelter and they must arrange transport to the shelter if needed.

ROLE OF THE COMMANDER

Unlike a civilian public official, such as a mayor, town manager, county executive, or governor, or a civilian employer, a military commander is accountable for performance of the military mission and for good order and discipline of the personnel under his or her command. Such responsibility is exercised both formally and informally and performance is reviewed at least annually; a superior commander can also remove subordinate commanders at any time from their positions when performance is deemed unsatisfactory. A commander with authority over a military installation (depending on the Service, this may be a commander of a garrison, station, base, or camp who does not have authority over some specific military units assigned there) has such responsibility for civilian employees and contractors and for the family members of military personnel assigned there.

However, the commander's disciplinary authority is limited: it must be related to the military mission. The commander cannot order a Service member to attend a domestic abuse prevention program when the Service member has no prior history of committing abuse. On the other hand, when a Service member has committed domestic abuse the commander may order him to attend clinical treatment, because any legal proceedings (especially criminal proceedings or disciplinary proceedings) would distract the Service member from performing his military mission.

The UCMJ grants the commander administrative, nonjudicial, and judicial authority over an active duty Service member 24 hours per day, 365 days a year wherever the Service member is located. In contrast, the commander of a unit in the reserve component only has authority over the Service member during times of training or when called to active duty. The installation commander's authority over civilians is even more limited: he or she can bar a civilian, including a family member of the Service member, from entry onto the installation or military housing, or can authorize entry but place limits upon the civilian's presence.

Administrative Actions to Protect the Victim

The commander has broad inherent administrative authority to protect a victim of domestic abuse and DoD policy specifies some of the actions that commanders can and should take.[9] If the Service member is the alleged abuser a commander should order the Service member into government quarters rather than require the victim (and any children) to leave military housing. The unit commander, working with the installation commander, should ensure that the victim has made safety plans with a victim advocate or health care provider; in domestic abuse cases the FAP may be involved.

By federal law, commanders located within the US must enforce any CPO that has been issued by a court of appropriate jurisdiction.[22] Usually the unit commander will issue an MPO to match the CPO, but he/she can issue an MPO whether or not a CPO has been issued, and can issue an MPO at locations outside the US where a CPO is not enforceable. In the MPO, the commander can require the Service member to turn in any personal firearms and ammunition, and if the Service member is in military law enforcement and would therefore normally carry a firearm the commander can remove authority to carry such a weapon. By federal law the MPO remains in force until the commander terminates it or issues a replacement order.[24] The commander shall ensure that copies of the CPO are given to appropriate civilian authorities,[23] and may task the installation legal staff with providing copies to the appropriate civilian prosecutor(s) and court(s).

If a spouse of an active duty Service member is a victim of domestic abuse and needs to relocate away from the installation for safety, the commander has authority under the Federal Joint Travel Regulation to pay for the victim's transportation and for shipment of the victim's household goods and a vehicle at government expense, provided that either the victim and alleged abuser have agreed to the division of such goods or that a court with appropriate jurisdiction has divided them.[25]

When the Service member deploys for any length of time, an intimate partner who is the victim of domestic abuse may simply attempt to move away without leaving any information for future contact, while a spouse in the same situation may seek a divorce. Other victims bring their victimization to the attention of the authorities now that the Service member is far away, requesting the commander to issue an MPO to prohibit the Service member from contacting the victim. If a Service member known to be abusive is going to be returned from deployment prior to the scheduled end of the deployment, DoD policy expects the unit commander to notify the commander at the home station in advance of the early return so that safety precautions can be planned and implemented in consultation with FAP.[9] If the Service member is returning upon the regular schedule for return, the commander at the home station is expected to notify the FAP so that there is time to plan coordinated safety measures.

Similarly, if the Service member is undergoing intervention by FAP to address his/her behavior, DoD policy expects the commander to consult with personnel officials to delay or cancel any usual temporary duty assignments or permanent change of station (PCS) orders that would interfere with the completion of the intervention. If such orders cannot be canceled or delayed, the commander is expected to ensure that the FAP coordinates efforts with the gaining installation to ensure continuity of services with the FAP and any others, including the victim advocate, to protect the victim.[8]

Jurisdiction over the Alleged Offender and the Offense

It is a bit more complicated to hold accountable those who have committed domestic violence in the military community than it is in the civilian sector. Such issues as the applicability of the UCMJ to the alleged offender, state or federal jurisdiction over the alleged offense and offender, or even the jurisdiction of a foreign court over the alleged offense and offender are all relevant.

The UCMJ applies to Service members on active duty, to students at U.S. Military Academy (West Point), the Naval Academy, and the Air Force Academy, members in the reserve component during military training, members of the Fleet Reserve and Fleet Marine Corps Reserve, certain retirees, members of the Public Health Service and of the National Oceanic and Atmospheric Administration when assigned to serve with the military, and in time of war others accompanying an armed force in the field, and certain others.[26] However, if an act of domestic violence was committed within the US by a Service member in the reserve component but not during military training or when called to active duty, the UCMJ is not applicable. Similarly, if the act was committed by a civilian family member of an active duty Service member, or by a DoD civilian employee or contractor, the UCMJ is as a general rule inapplicable. In all 4 situations the person may be arrested and charged by civilian authorities for violating the applicable state or federal criminal statute.

The UCMJ does not contain a *punitive article* (equivalent to a crime) for intimate partner violence, domestic abuse, or domestic violence. Depending upon the facts of the incident, an active component Service member alleged to have committed domestic abuse may be charged for failure to obey an order or regulation for failing to support his/her family member.[27] If domestic violence is alleged he or she could be charged under one or more of the appropriate punitive articles for murder, manslaughter, assault, maiming, provoking speeches or gestures (if the victim is also a Service member), damaging military property or non-military property, or stalking.[28-35] The Service member could be charged with a sexual offense (rape, sexual assault, aggravated sexual contact, abusive sexual contact[36]), or sodomy,[37] or for failure to obey an order or regulation because he violated the terms of an MPO or CPO.[38] Other acts of domestic violence that are noncapital offenses under federal or state law, such as communicating a threat, non-accidental discharge of a firearm that endangered another, or kidnapping, may be the basis for a charge under Article 134.[39]

In addition to the military commander's UCMJ disciplinary authority over a Service member in the active component, there may also be civilian jurisdiction over the Service member. If the illegal act was committed outside the installation, the local civilian authorities have jurisdiction to arrest and charge the Service member in the appropriate criminal court. If the act was committed on a part of the installation over which civilian jurisdiction applies, either because such location is within the area for which state jurisdiction is concurrent with federal jurisdiction or because it is within the area of state proprietary jurisdiction, the local civilian authorities also have jurisdiction to arrest and charge the Service member in the appropriate criminal court. Finally, if the act was committed outside the US in a nation for which there was a SOFA, the terms of the SOFA apply. A SOFA might specify that the host nation's courts have priority to try certain crimes committed by US Service members regardless of the nationality of the victim, or that such priority will apply only to some or all crimes committed by US Service members against the host nation's citizens. Conversely, the SOFA might specify that the UCMJ has priority. In 2000 Congress enacted the Military Extraterritorial Jurisdiction Act.[40] This law authorizes a criminal prosecution in US federal court of certain Service members, former Service members, or a person employed by (ie, DoD civilian employees and DoD contractors) or accompanying the military outside the US who committed a crime that would be a felony if committed within federal jurisdiction if the host nation has declined to prosecute. The Service member must not be subject to the UCMJ or must be a co-defendant with at least one person who is not subject to the UCMJ (**Table 26-3**).

As a result of the complexity of jurisdiction over the offense and over the person, DoD policy directs commanders to pursue written Memorandums of Understanding with the civilian agencies likely to become involved in incidents of domestic abuse.[9] These may take the form of a coordinated community response (CCR), such as Jacksonville, Florida. At some locations it is very difficult to create a CCR because military personnel reside in different jurisdictions. Fort Campbell spans an area in both Kentucky and Tennessee

Table 26-3. Summary of Jurisdiction

PERSON ALLEGED TO HAVE VIOLATED A LAW	WITHIN THE 50 STATES					WITHIN U.S. TERRITORIES OR MARITIME JURISDICTION	OUTSIDE U.S.
	WITHIN A MILITARY INSTALLATION/PROPERTY IN AN AREA OF:			WITHIN THE CIVILIAN COMMUNITY			
	EXCLUSIVE FEDERAL JURISDICTION	CONCURRENT FEDERAL AND STATE JURISDICTION	STATE PROPRIETARY JURISDICTION	WITHIN A STATE	ACROSS STATE LINES		
Active Component Service Member	UCMJ[1]	UCMJ	UCMJ	UCMJ	UCMJ	UCMJ	UCMJ or Other Nation's Court[2] or Federal Court[4]
Reserve Component Service Member (NOT during training or federal active duty)	Federal Court[3]	Federal Court[3] or State Court	State Court	State Court	Federal Court[3]	Federal Court[3]	Other Nation's Court or Federal Court[4]
Reserve Component Service Member (during training or federal active duty)	UCMJ	UCMJ	UCMJ	UCMJ	UCMJ	UCMJ	UCMJ or Other Nation's Court[2] or Federal Court[4]
DoD Civilian Employee or Contractor	Federal Court[3]	Federal Court[3] or State Court	State Court	State Court	Federal Court[3]	Federal Court[3]	Other Nation's Court or Federal Court[4]
Family Member of Service Member	Federal Court[3]	Federal Court[3] or State Court	State Court	State Court	Federal Court[3]	Federal Court[3]	Other Nation's Court or Federal Court[4]

[1] *Uniform Code of Military Justice*
[2] *Subject to any applicable Status of Forces Agreement (SOFA)*
[3] *If a crime under Title 18 U.S. Code*
[4] *Subject to applicability of 18 U.S.C. §3261 et seq.*

and personnel live in 5 counties. Personnel assigned to one military installation in the Washington, DC area reside in an area that extends nearly 80 miles north and south, including the District of Columbia, 6 counties in Maryland, and 8 counties in Virginia.

Discretionary Authority to Hold the Alleged Offender Accountable

Under Rule 306(a) of the Rules for Courts-Martial[41] the unit commander is the person who ordinarily disposes of offenses that may be tried by court-martial, which includes all of the offenses in domestic violence and sexual assault. A superior commander may withhold such authority from the subordinate commander in all cases, certain types of cases, or individual cases but if that authority has not been withheld the superior commander may not limit the subordinate commander's discretion. Such restriction of the subordinate commander's discretion is called ***unlawful command influence.*** Thus, a superior commander cannot instruct subordinate commanders that he/she wants all domestic violence assaults and sexual assaults within the command to be referred for court-martials or that he/she wants all of such offenses to be referred to civilian prosecutors who have jurisdiction, nor can he/she coach the subordinate commanders on how they should exercise their discretion in disposing of individual offenses with which they are presented.

The commander is expected to dispose of an allegation in a timely manner, using the lowest appropriate level of discipline. To determine the lowest appropriate level of discipline, the commander balances the factors set forth in the Manual for Courts-Martial discussion of Rule 306(b).

These factors are somewhat similar to those that civilian prosecutors must consider, although a civilian prosecutor isn't faced with considering military exigencies or the effect of the decision on the command. The commander then selects a disposition from among the choices in Rule 306(c): (1) no action (which includes allowing a civilian authority with jurisdiction over the Service member to exert such jurisdiction), (2) administrative action in addition to or instead of other action, (3) nonjudicial punishment, (4) disposition of charges by dismissing them, forwarding them to another commander for disposition, or referring them to a summary, special, or general court-martial, or (5) forwarding the charges to a superior possessing authority to take a form of disposition. The commander thus has broad discretion in holding a Service member who is alleged to have committed domestic violence accountable.

The ***administrative actions*** available to the commander include a wide range of corrective measures such as counseling (including treatment by FAP), admonition, reprimand, exhortation, disapproval, criticism, censure, reproach, rebuke, extra military instruction, or the administrative withholding of privileges, or any combination of these. These are appropriate dispositions for acts of domestic abuse that are not included in the punitive articles under the UCMJ or under state or federal laws as well as for acts that are included.[43] A commander's use of one or more of these measures to hold a Service member accountable for an act of domestic abuse matches other discretionary acts by commanders within military culture, in which Service members regularly undergo training, evaluation, and corrective measures to improve performance.

Administrative actions also include other administrative measures related to efficiency reports, academic reports, and other ratings; rehabilitation and reassignment; career field reclassification; administrative reduction for inefficiency; bar to re-enlistment; personnel reliability program (personnel whose tasks include handling nuclear weapons) reclassification; security classification changes; and pecuniary liability for negligence or misconduct. They also include administrative separation from active duty.

Nonjudicial punishment, authorized by Article 15 of the UCMJ, is a disciplinary measure more serious than administrative action but less serious and stigmatizing than a conviction that might result from referring the offense to a court-martial.[44] However, it is for minor offenses, ordinarily those for which the maximum sentence excludes dishonorable discharge or imprisonment for more than a year; ie, misdemeanors rather than felonies, although other factors may apply.[45] It is therefore not usually appropriate for any offense against an intimate partner other than a simple assault.

It is not uncommon for a commander to cede military disciplinary jurisdiction over the Service member to a civilian authority with jurisdiction so that the civilian authority proceeds with a prosecution. This frequently happens if the civilian authorities have a specific intervention program for those who commit domestic abuse that the Service member could enter through a court diversion program or as a condition of probation. This also occurs frequently in domestic violence situations when the intimate partner victim had no affiliation with DoD (ie, was neither a Service member, nor a family member, nor a DoD employee or contractor). If the civilian court incarcerates the Service member upon a conviction, the commander may charge the Service member with being absent without official leave ("AWOL").[45]

The UCMJ policy that the military commander shall exercise his/her discretion to select the lowest level of appropriate disposition, resulting in the frequent use of administrative corrective actions to address domestic abuse in appropriate cases in lieu of convening a court-martial, contrasts with those civilian jurisdictions with statutes that require criminal prosecutions of domestic violence[46] and with prosecutors' offices that have "no drop" policies in such cases. The civilian justice system's requirement for prosecution would be unlawful command influence if applied in the UCMJ.

Transitional Compensation

The transitional compensation program was enacted by Congress as an incentive for military spouses to report domestic abuse. Sometimes a victim of domestic abuse by a Service member suffered in silence rather than making a report because he/she was financially dependent on the Service member, especially when the couple was living at an installation far from the victim's social supports or outside the US. If the victim dared to make a report and as a result the Service member was administratively discharged from active duty or was convicted upon a court-martial and forfeited all pay and allowances, the victim lost all income from the Service member. The transitional compensation provides an eligible victim of domestic abuse and dependent children with income to be able to start a new life apart from the abuser. There is no counterpart in the civilian sector to the transitional compensation program.

A spouse or former spouse who is the victim of domestic abuse by a Service member on active duty is eligible for transitional compensation if the Service member was (1) convicted by a court-martial for a dependent-abuse offense and pursuant to the sentence the Service member either (a) is separated from active duty or (b) forfeits all pay and allowances, or (2) separated from the Service administratively if the basis includes a dependent-abuse offense. This transitional compensation is available for the victim and any dependent children, based on the rates in effect for dependency and indemnity compensation[47] and the accompanying benefits, are provided up to 36 months after the sentence or separation, depending upon the amount of time remaining in the Service member's enlistment period. The victim forfeits these upon remarriage during that time or upon resuming cohabitation with the abuser.[48] If the victim is entitled under a court order to payments of the Service member's retirement pay (due to annulment, separation, or divorce) the victim must choose between receiving such payments and receiving transitional compensation.[49]

CONCLUSION

The military has several challenges in its ongoing efforts to prevent domestic abuse:

— The Services are concerned about whether domestic abuse is being addressed adequately in the reserve component because they reside in the civilian community. They may not be exposed to the DoD prevention messages and do not come to the attention of FAP for intervention.

— DoD has committed a large amount of effort and funding for family support, thus indirectly preventing domestic abuse, but these programs have not been fully evaluated formally.

— Most civilian prevention programs need significant modification before implementation in the military community. They have little understanding of the impact of military culture on relationships. For example, they may assume that all incidents of domestic abuse will (or should) result in severe military discipline, such as a court-martial. Others are unaware of the restrictions on access to personal information imposed by the Federal Privacy Act.[50]

Because Service members and their families are part of American society, they are not isolated from social problems that also occur in the civilian sector. The Department of Defense first began to address domestic abuse in the mid-1970s programmatically with the FAP and has made great strides since the mid 1990s. Because of the unique military mission and subculture, DoD will continue to address this social problem in a unique manner.

REFERENCES

1. 10 U.S. Code §504(b)

2. Defense Manpower Data Center. Active Duty Citizenship Status Report. September 2009.

3. Soeters JL, Winslow DJ, Weilbull A. Military culture. In: Caforio G, ed. *Handbook of the Sociology of the Military.* New York, NY: Springer; 2006. 237-254.

4. Office of the Deputy Under Secretary of Defense for Military Community and Family Policy. *Demographics 2011: Profile of the Military Community.* Military One Source Web site. http://www.militaryonesource.mil/12038/MOS/Reports/2011_Demographics_Report.pdf. Updated November 2012. Accessed September 10, 2013.

5. US Census Bureau. *Annual Estimates of the Resident Population by Sex and Five-Year Age Groups for the United States: April 1, 2000 to July 1, 2008.* US Census Bureau Web site. http://www.census.gov/popest/data/historical/2000s/vintage_2008/. Accessed September 10, 2013.

6. National Defense Authorization Act for Fiscal Year 2000, P.L. 106-65, §590 *et seq.*

7. 10 U.S. Code §654.

8. 10 U.S. Code, Part II, Chapter 47.

9. Department of Defense Instruction 6400.06. *Domestic Abuse Involving DoD Military and Certain Affiliated Personnel.* http://www.dtic.mil/whs/directives/corres/pdf/640006p.pdf. Published 2007. Updated September 20, 2011. Accessed July 29, 2013.

10. Military OneSource Web site. http://www.militaryonesource.mil.

11. Office of the Deputy Under Secretary of Defense for Military Community and Family Policy. *Report of the 2nd Quadrennial Quality of Life Review.* Arlington, VA: Military OneSource Center; 2009.

12. National Defense Authorization Act for Fiscal Year 1995, P.L. 103-337, §534.

13. Beals J, Erwin PE. *Understanding the Military Response to Domestic Violence: Tools for Civilian Advocates.* Minneapolis, MN: The Battered Women's Justice Project; 2007.

14. DoD Regulation 6025.18-R. *Health Information Privacy Regulation.* Information for the Defense Community Web site. http://www.dtic.mil/whs/directives/corres/pdf/602518r.pdf. Published 2003. Accessed August 12, 2013.

15. DoD Manual 6400.1-M. *Family Advocacy Program Standards and Self-Assessment Tool.* Information for the Defense Community Web site. http://www.dtic.mil/whs/directives/corres/pdf/640001m.pdf.Published 1992. Accessed August 12, 2013.

16. DoD Manual 6400.1-M-1 *Manual for Child Maltreatment and Domestic Abuse Incident Report.* Information for the Defense Community Web site. http://www.dtic.mil/whs/directives/corres/pdf/640001m1.pdf. Published 2005. Accessed August 12, 2013.

17. Forgey M, Badger L. Patterns of intimate partner violence among married women in the military: type, level, directionality and consequences. *J Fam Viol.* 2006;21:369-380.

18. Lutgendorf M, Busch JM, Doherty DA, et al. Prevalence of domestic violence in a pregnant military population. *Obstet Gynecol.* 2009;113:866-872.

19. Teten A, Schumacher J, Bailey S, Kent T. Male-to-female sexual aggression among Iraq, Afghanistan, and Vietnam veterans: co-occurring substance abuse and intimate partner aggression. *J Trauma Stress.* 2009;22:307-311

20. Marshall A, Panuzio J, Taft C. Intimate partner violence among military veterans and active duty servicemen. *Clin Psychol Rev.* 2005;25:862-876.

21. 10 U.S. Code §1058.

22. 10 U.S. Code §1561a.

23. 10 U.S. Code §1567a.

24. 10 U.S. Code §1567.

25. Joint Federal Travel Reg., Vol. 1, Ch 5, Part C, Section 2, U5205, Change 264 U5C2-1, 12/1/08, implementing 37 U.S.C. §406(h)(4).

26. 10 U.S. Code §802, Article 2.

27. 10 U.S. Code §892, Article 92.

28. 10 U.S. Code §918, Article 118.

29. 10 U.S. Code §919, Article 119.

30. 10 U.S. Code §928, Article 128.

31. 10 U.S. Code §924, Article 124.

32. 10 U.S. Code §917, Article 117.

33. 10 U.S. Code §908, Article 108.

34. 10 U.S. Code §909, Article 109.

35. 10 U.S. Code §920a, Article 120a.

36. 10 U.S. Code §920, Article 120.

37. 10 U.S. Code §925, Article 125.

38. 10 U.S. Code §892, Article 92.

39. 10 U.S. Code §934.

40. 18 U.S. Code §3261.

41. Joint Service Committee on Military Justice. *Manual for Courts-Martial United States.* 2012 ed. Rules for Courts-Martial 306(a).

42. Joint Service Committee on Military Justice. *Manual for Courts-Martial United States.* 2012 ed. Rules for Courts-Martial 306(b).

43. Joint Service Committee on Military Justice. *Manual for Courts-Martial United States.* 2012 ed. Rules for Courts-Martial 306(c).

44. Joint Service Committee on Military Justice. *Manual for Courts-Martial United States.* 2012 ed. Part V, Nonjudicial Punishment Procedure 1. General par. g.

45. 10 U.S. Code §886, Article 86

46. Alaska Stat. §18.65.530

47. 38 U.S. Code §1311(a)(1) and (b)

48. Department of Defense Instruction 1342.24. *Transitional Compensation for Abused Dependents.* implementing 10 U.S. Code §§1059 and 1076(e). http://www.dtic.mil/whs/directives/corres/pdf/134224p.pdf. Published 1995. Updated January 16, 1997. Accessed August 7, 2013.

49. 10 U.S. Code §1408.

50. 5 U.S. Code §552a.

Chapter 27

Violence on the Streets: The What, the Who, and the Why of Abuse, Assault & Murder of Sex Workers

C. Gabrielle Salfati, MSc, PhD, C Psychol, F.IA-IP

Key Points

1. The majority of street prostitutes have experienced multiple extreme violent attacks or sexual assaults during their time on the streets.

2. Homicide has been reported as being 1 of the top 2 leading causes of death amongst prostitutes. Serial murder has been suggested to account for a third of prostitute homicides.

3. Violence is committed by a wide variety of people including pimps and intimate partners, but the majority is committed by clients and those pretending to be clients.

4. Most clients are generally non-violent. Violent clients are not typical clients in that they had a much higher level of previous convictions, and overall, those with previous convictions are likely to be repeat offenders.

5. The violence against street prostitutes is part of a much wider ranging cycle of victimization which starts with physical, emotional, and sexual abuse at home and continues with extensive physical and sexual abuse, on and off the job, after entering prostitution. The majority of prostitutes have a drug addiction, which has been shown to increase the risk level for violence.

"In 1994, women in the sex industry were identified as one of three populations most in need of specialized services, primarily as a result of the violence inflicted upon them as a result of their work."[1]

What is the Extent of the Violence Against Sex Workers?

Violence on the Streets

By the very nature of their work, sex workers,* especially those who work on the street, are susceptible to attack. Sex workers who solicit on the streets are more frequently[2] at risk than those who work indoors.[3,4] Regardless of whether or not she‡ works on her own or with others, the actual service for which the sex worker is being paid for will usually

---

*Please note that the current chapter does not look at violence within the sex industry overall. Instead this chapter focuses specifically on violence and abuse experienced by women working in the sex industry on the streets. Terminology may vary from the use of 'prostitute' to 'sex worker' depending on terms used in original sources, but will refer to the same group of women.

‡This chapter will mainly focus on female sex workers.

be between her alone and the client.[5] The service will often take place in a dark, deserted location, and usually in a vehicle, outdoors, in alleyways, industrial units, parks, car or lorry parks, derelict buildings or country areas outside town, or even the client's home.[6] Negotiating for services will often take place through a car window or actually in the car itself. The violence mostly occurs after the street worker and the client have left the soliciting area.[6] Being in an isolated spot therefore, with a client who, more often than not, is a stranger[7] is a potentially dangerous situation for the prostitute. In these situations the street worker is also seen as an easy target for robbery as she will carry her evenings wages on her in cash.[5]

Much of the discussion in the last few years has focused on the risk assessment for violence, on the client and on the transaction as it occurs on the streets. The current chapter aims to summarise and bring in additional aspects of the literature that help to build our understanding of this transaction of violence by fully illustrating the extent of the problem across all aspects of a sex worker's life, spanning their past, their work life, and their current home life, and focusing on the full impact on the sex worker's health.

This chapter will give an overview of the type of violence prostitutes are victims of, and will look at the link between this and the types of people who attack them, and what the nature of the interpersonal transaction is. Risk factors that put prostitutes at greater risk will also be looked at, and will be explained in the light of how this adds to their vulnerability and the overall impact on their health.

VIOLENCE EXPERIENCED BY STREET SEX WORKERS

"About 80% of women in prostitution have been the victim of a rape. It's hard to talk about this because… the experience of prostitution is just like rape. Prostitutes are raped, on the average, eight to ten times per year. They are the most raped class of women in the history of our planet."[8]

Salfati,[9] in a review of the literature on violence against prostitutes and street prostitutes specifically, summarised that studies[10-17] consistently reported that over three quarters of street prostitutes had experienced serious violent attacks during their time on the streets, and that a third had experienced sexual assaults and rapes. Often times these women reported having been attacked numerous times, and often, these attacks were on the extreme end of severity. Brooks-Gordon,[18] in a review of the literature, also shows that this pattern of violence is not culture bound. Other similar findings have been reported in the UK, Scotland, Canada, and Norway,[7,13,19,20] and South Africa, Thailand, Turkey, USA, and Zambia.[17]

When violence is experienced, prostitutes list that the most common reasons for a client to become violent are: disagreements over the time and quality of the services given to the clients; clients try to get their money back; or the clients have been drinking.[6,21,22]

The extent of the vulnerability of street workers however goes even further, with a range of studies highlighting the high risk category street workers are in for becoming a homicide victim. In a comprehensive study, Brewer et al[23] show that between 1998-2000, prostitutes represented 2.7% of female homicide victims in the US. Kinnell[10] in a UK study showed that of 75% of prostitutes who were murdered, 75% were street workers. Being a street prostitute in the US made a woman 18 times more likely to be murdered than non-prostitute women of similar demographics.[24] A UK study concluded that street prostitutes were 12 times more likely to be murdered than the normal rate for women in same age group,[25] and a Canadian study showed that a prostitute on the street was 60-120 times more likely to be murdered than non-prostitute females.[20] This same study also concluded that homicide is one of the top two leading causes of death amongst prostitutes.[20]

WHO OFFENDS AGAINST SEX WORKERS?

THE CLIENT

"Look, men pay for women because he can have whatever and whoever he wants. Lots of men go to prostitutes so they can do things to them that real women would not put up with."[26]

A number of studies have highlighted the key role clients have in the violence perpetrated towards street workers, with 62-81% of the violence being committed by clients.[11,27,28] Similar figures can be seen in homicides (62-64%), and 35% of prostitute homicides can be attributed to having been committed by serial homicide offenders, with approximately one-third of these serial offenders being identified as clients.[23]

In a recent book by Kinnell,[29] the type of clients was analysed in more detail, gleaning an interesting picture that allows an in-depth understanding of the possible issues at play when prostitutes are attacked by clients. Kinnell highlights that attackers are commonly described as 'clients' but when the details of these cases are examined, a high proportion of this violence comes from those who do not actually pay, and since the definition of a client is one who pays for sexual services, these attackers are not clients. This is true even if they may have approached the sex worker as if they were clients, or pretending they were clients, or engaging in initial con-behaviors to suggest they were clients.

Kinnell[29] looked at the suspects in 139 offenses, of which 70% approached the street worker in the guise as a client. About half of these were non-payers. They refused to pay and became violent as soon as payment was requested. About a quarter of these non-payers also robbed the victim. Kinnell concluded that paying for sex may not be the link to violence, instead it is not paying that is.[29] The explosions of anger that erupt when the sex worker insist on payment, Kinnell suggests, indicate that the problem is not that these men believe that paying for sex gives them the right to command women to obey their sexual demands or to inflict violence on them, but they are insulted by the suggestion that they can only get sexual compliance if they pay, that they have the right to 'take' sex from these women and that refusing to pay asserts that right and demonstrates their power.

Salfati et al[5] also reports that in 52% of their sample of prostitute homicide victims, property was stolen from the victim suggesting a link between robbery and violent crime against prostitutes.

In a similar overview of 118 cases where a sex worker was killed, Kinnell[29] observed that of those for whom working method was known, 78% were street workers. The suspect was identified in 94 cases. Of the cases where the information was available, it was assumed that 65% of the offenders approached as a client. This is similar to numbers from Canada[28] and the US.[23] The assumption that offenders approached as clients is based on the belief that the victims were 'at work,' but based on her work on nonfatal attacks, where 30% of attackers did not exhibit any client behaviours even though the victims were at work,[29] Kinnell suggests that the same pattern may be present in murders, although she states that we cannot test this since the victim is deceased, and they may have approached in some other guise or simply attacked the victim.

Demographics

Kinnell[29] also reports that 45% of the suspects were charged with attacks on more than one sex worker. Client suspects were not typical clients in that they had a much higher level of previous convictions, and overall, those with previous convictions were likely to be repeat offenders. These figures are consistent with other studies.[18,23]

According to authors who have looked into the characteristics of offenders[7,30-34] the majority of clients are typically middle-aged, middle-class and married, and likely to be in their mid-thirties.[7,12,35] Indeed, 47.5% of prostitutes regard older men as safer to work with,[35] stating that they will not do business with a client if they look under 30. Salfati et al[5] corroborate this in their study which shows that violence is actually more likely to be committed by younger clients. With regards to the occupational profile of the clients, three-quarters or more are in full time employment.[12,35,36]

Relationship

Most prostitutes would prefer to service clients whom they know, or at least have done business with before. However, Sharpe[35] shows that the majority of clients are not known to the prostitute when they approach them for business. In Ferguson's survey,[37] 45.8% of prostitutes suggested that most of their clients were complete strangers, and 5.6% stated that all of their clients were strangers.

Salfati et al[5] summarises that considering therefore that the average number of clients per day per prostitute ranges from 3 to 7,[7,32,35,37,38] and that an average 'shift' is around 6 hours[37,38] the prostitute is probably having at least 2 to 3 sexual encounters with a complete stranger every 2 to 3 hours of their working day. This has a direct effect on level of risk. As O'Neill and Barberet state,[22] attacks on street prostitutes are more frequent when the client is a stranger than when he is known to the prostitute. They found that most violence against the prostitute was unpredictable and happened suddenly. Violence was also more common when the prostitute was either under the influence of drugs or alcohol.

SERIAL OFFENDERS

"The plan was I wanted to kill as many women I thought were prostitutes as I possibly could. I picked prostitutes as my victims because I hate most prostitutes and I did not want to pay them for sex. I also picked prostitutes as victims because they are easy to pick up without being noticed. I knew they would not be reported missing right away, and might never be reported missing. I picked prostitutes because I thought I could kill as many of them as I wanted without getting caught."[39]

Kinnell[4] stated that the high proportion of attacks ascribed to clients has led to assumptions that a high proportion of clients are violent. However as Brooks-Gordon[18] shows, most clients are non-violent, and the majority of violence is committed by a small proportion of offenders. Based on her study, she therefore concluded that information about attackers suggest that many are serial offenders. Kinnell,[6] in a study of 84 homicides against street workers, also shows the vulnerability of sex workers to serial killers, as do Miller and Jayasundara (D. Linger, personal communication, October 27, 1999).[40] Brewer et al[23] provide an estimate based on their empirical study when they suggest that serial murder accounts for 35% of prostitute homicides, and that all serial offenders were clients. In the nine different samples they surveyed, they also showed that lone perpetrators accounted for most prostitute homicides.

CRIMINAL BACKGROUND

In an analysis of the criminal records of 77 clients stopped by the police for curb-crawling, Brooks-Gordon18 found that 63 had a previous criminal record. Of the 44 cases that were traceable, the age range was 23-66 years, with a mean of 40 years. The mean distance travelled to where they were stopped was 15 miles (however there was no information in the study regarding where these offenders had travelled from). In looking at not the quantity, but the range of offences, the type most frequent across the sample was a previous conviction for violence (21%), followed by theft, handling, and shoplifting (20%). Seven percent had previous convictions for sex offences. Interestingly, Brooks-Gordon followed up these men, and found that 11 of them were re-convicted within 23 months after their arrest for kerb crawling. Of these 11 men, 6 of them were convicted of a violent offence against the person, and one was convicted for a sexual offence. She therefore tentatively concludes that, with keeping in mind the small numbers, the research suggests a link between curb-crawling and more serious crimes committed by only a small number of these men, who are likely to be repeat offenders. Low rates (8%) of previous convictions for violent and sexual offences were also found amongst men apprehended for kerb crawling in Southampton in the UK.[41] Looking at previous convictions of offenders who killed women in different offence groups. Salfati et al[5] report that offenders who kill prostitutes were the least likely to have previous non-violent offences (20%) when compared to offenders who killed non-prostitute women (offenders who killed and sexually assaulted, 41%; offenders who killed but did not sexual assault, 81%). Conversely, offenders who killed prostitutes had significantly more pre-convictions for sexual offences compared to offenders who killed non-prostitute victims (non-sexual and, to a lesser extent, sexual offenders). They also reported that significantly more prostitute homicide offenders (69%) had spent time in prison than offenders who killed non-prostitutes (non-sexual, 27% and sexual, 29%).[5]

In accord with the general literature on violence against prostitutes, a study by Salfati et al[5] shows that in a large proportion (14 out of 19) of offenders who had previous violent convictions, 6 involved a pre-conviction for at least one murder. With figures as high as these they suggest that it is likely that a prostitute will come into contact with clients with violent pre-convictions on a relatively regular basis. Indeed, in one prostitute homicide case in their study, the victim had had sex with a client who had previous convictions for attempted murder and serious sexual assaults on women, in the same night as she was killed by another client who also had previous convictions for attempted murder.

Violent vs. Non-Violent Clients

To understand what clients are the more likely to commit violence against, or kill, a prostitute, it is important to understand this subgroup compared to clients in general, as well as the male population in general, and other men who kill women. A recent NIJ report,[42] looking further at the characteristics of prostitute offenders in the US amongst other issues, looked at the prevalence of clients overall in order to provide a baseline against which we may start to compare the characteristics of clients with the general male population, as well as compare characteristics between violent and non-violent clients. The data included prostitution arrest data from approximately 30 local US jurisdictions, and all 50 states. Analysis was based on men arrested for patronizing a prostitute in several metropolitan communities, and was compared to the General Social Surveys (GSS), a regular national probability sample household survey. Results from these studies estimated that about 2-3% of local male residents in large metropolitan areas in the US patronized local street prostitutes during an observation period of 2-5 years. These figures they report are almost twice as large as those based on self-reports in the GSS. They then compared the clients arrested with men in the general population (as reflected by various social census data), and included a number of characteristics not focused on in previous studies. Clients were more likely to be young men; they were more likely to be Hispanic (hypothesised to be due to the unavailability of non-commercial sexual partners) and, to a lesser degree, black; had substantially less education; were less likely to be married; resided closer to their arrest locations; and drove modestly newer vehicles. In a sub-study focusing on Colorado Springs, they also found that the characteristics of clients of street prostitutes were similar to clients of off-street prostitution.

In a sub-study identified from an extensive national search of media sources, Brewer, Dudek et al[23] and Brewer et al[43] compared clients who assaulted, raped and/or killed prostitute women with clients arrested for patronizing prostitutes in the same jurisdictions and time periods, on observable characteristics easily assessed by police during an investigation. Results showed that violent clients usually picked up their victims in the same areas where police arrested clients for patronizing. Violent clients were similar in age and distance between their residences and victim encounter/arrest locations. Violent clients were less likely to be white, drive cars (as opposed to other motorized vehicles), and have a previous criminal history of miscellaneous other (non-violent, non-property, non-sex, non-patronizing) offences. Men with a criminal history of violent and/or rape offences comprised a pool that included 40% of prostitute killers (47% of serial prostitute killers). In addition, a meaningful proportion of clients arrested for patronizing in 2 jurisdictions had less money in their possession than the price they had agreed to pay for sex or carried weapons at the time of arrest, suggesting a potential for violence in client's interactions with prostitutes. This result is consistent with Kinnell's more recent 2008 study[29] showing that most 'clients' intended non-payment prior to approaching street workers.

Choice of Victim by Violent Clients

"The women I killed were filth – bastard prostitutes who were littering the streets. I was just cleaning up the place a bit."[44]

In another earlier study by Kinnell,[45] on 73 homicides of sex workers, showed that 71% were street workers. Of the 46 cases where a suspect was known, 52% approached their victim as a client. 42% had previous or subsequent convictions for violence, including rape, and homicide both against sex workers, and non sex workers, and against both men and women. Of the (22 out of 35) cases where an offender was identified in Kinnell's study,[6] 49% had previous convictions for homicide or other violent offences. The majority (19 out of 22) of these offenders with previous criminal convictions for violence were clients. Through additional case studies, she further showed that those who kill sex workers do not only target that group, but often targeted non-sex workers, which raises an additional important issue of the consistency in victim target, and reasons for the violence by these men. It also raises the importance of understanding the difference between those men who target only prostitutes and those who target other women (and men). Kinnell[29] shows, in her overview of actual cases, that many people who have attacked and killed sex workers have also committed violence against non-sex workers. Salfati,[46] in her work on serial homicide offenders who target at least one street sex worker, also shows that 58% targeted both sex workers and non-sex workers as part of their series. Salfati et al[5] show that men who assault prostitutes have convictions for assaulting other women as well, which in turn backs up that violence against prostitutes may be considered as part of a continuum of violence against women more generally, and not just against prostitutes specifically.

VIOLENCE BY NON-CLIENTS

"It is unlikely that any occupation or lifestyle exposes a woman to the threat of assault and gratuitous violence as constantly and completely as prostitution."[47]

Clients are not the only group who attack street sex workers, and the violence is not always by strangers. The literature indicates that physical and sexual violence against sex workers is also perpetrated by other people on the streets, police officers, as well as pimps and partners.[14,16,48-51]

Silbert and Pines16 reported that as many as 72% of the rapes reported were unrelated to the prostitute's work, but when the women were identified as prostitutes, the rapes tended to be even more brutal and resulted in more injuries. Miller and Schwartz[15] also showed that 6.6% of their sample had been raped in other contexts on the streets.

Pimps

Research has shown that between 40% and 95% of sex workers involved in street prostitution have pimps.[16,52-54] Silbert and Pines[16] stated that 66% reported being abused by pimps. Similar reports of women being assaulted by their pimps can be found in numerous other studies.[52,55-57]

Faugier and Sargeant[58] record that the Council for Prostitution Alternatives, in Portland, Oregon, reported that of 179 women in their programme who left prostitution in 1990–91, almost half were raped by pimps an average of sixteen times per year. They also calculated that, out of 55 women in their programme, 63% were badly beaten by pimps an average of 58 times a year.

Although runaways without adequate food, clothing, shelter, or other basic needs have been reported to be particularly vulnerable to pimp influence,[56,59-61] adult women become involved with pimps for a variety of reasons, ranging from the emotional to the financial.[16,52,62] Williamson and Cluse-Tolar[54] also state that women who involve themselves with pimps can expect to be subjected to controlling practices and suffer violent treatment that have been described as frequent, pervasive, and brutal.[55,57]

Silbert and Pines[16] document a cycle of victimization which starts with physical, emotional, and sexual abuse at home and continues with extensive physical and sexual abuse, on and off the job, after entering prostitution. Out of the 200 juvenile and adult current and former prostitutes they interviewed, 70% reported that sexual exploitation affected their decision to become a prostitute and 96% started prostitution after running away from home as a result of this abuse. Once on the streets, 70% were victimized both by customers and pimps; they were beaten, robbed, raped, and abused. Similar findings are reported by Hardesty and Greif.[63]

The reason for women's involvement with pimps is complex, as is the relationship between street sex workers and their pimps. Norton-Hawk[53] also shows that if we look at the backgrounds of women controlled by pimps, they endured more problems in their households growing up, experienced sexual activity at earlier ages, ran away significantly earlier, and became involved in routine prostitution at significantly earlier ages. Norton-Hawk goes on to suggest that differences in sexual assault rates and verbal and physical abuse as children are highly suggestive of the vulnerability that would lead these women to be enticed by an older male figure promising love, loyalty, stability, and economic protection, thus highlighting the necessity of identifying these vulnerable girls who leave home early due to dangerous conditions and providing services and support to them.

Norton-Hawk[53] also states that the higher levels of customer violence experienced by women controlled by pimps demonstrate that pimps, contrary to popular belief, do not provide the women with protection from the violence of customers. Instead she suggests that the increased prevalence of violence from customers may be due to the increased risk these women put themselves in. She highlights that drug addiction may make the women targets of more violent customers, who know that they can easily control the women because of their desperate need to avoid drug withdrawal. Also, because pimps demand that the women bring home a certain amount of money each night; these women may work in settings considered more dangerous and expose themselves to more risk in order to avoid violence from the pimps. Norton-Hawk further states that because these women continue suffering the effects of customers' violence but also live in fear of a pimp who takes their earnings, the women need safety plans to escape this control. However, the fear and the violence make safety planning and other life choice decision making difficult.

Drug addiction can also influence the risk level that street workers put themselves in. Faugier and Sargeant[58] and Kinnell[29] specifically highlight how drug addiction affects the vulnerability of street workers, and indicate that drug dealers can become 'new' pimps. Often, intimate partners of prostitutes are also on drugs and may encourage the woman to prostitute to supply his habit.

Stoops[64] states that 98% of street workers are dependent on class A drugs and/or alcohol, a figure that "would be echoed for street sex workers all around the UK." Furthermore, these women are specifically targeted by local dealers. As she summarizes particularly well: "Sex workers are a drug dealer's dream. They've got access to cash, and quickly. They can go out and do a punter or two, go and score, then back again. One woman described it to me as being like a hamster on a wheel – work, score, work, score, work, score, collapse. She didn't have time for eating or bathing."[64]

Violence from Partners, Direct and Indirect

"We usually don't see prostitution as domestic violence because it is just too painful… the carnage: the scale of it, the dailiness of it, the seeming inevitability of it, the torture, the rapes, the murders, the beatings, the despair, the hollowing out of the personality, the near extinguishment of hope commonly suffered by women in prostitution."[65]

Kinnell[29] quotes, in her comprehensive survey of UK cases, that 14% of fatal attacks against sex workers were by partners. El-Bassel et al[66] found that 2 out of 3 sex workers in New York experienced lifetime physical or sexual abuse by either an intimate or a commercial partner.

Karandikar and Próspero[67] investigate experiences of intimate partner violence among sex workers in India. Although a small study based on 9 cases, the case study approach provided in-depth insight into the experiences of these women. Sex workers reported that their intimate partners or husbands had mostly been prior clients. Believing that they would be rescued, the sex workers found themselves in relationships where the partner took full ownership of the woman with total control and decision making power, and made the women continue to work. As with the literature on pimps, a similar pattern can be seen with intimate partner, where, rather than providing safety, the sex workers reported that intimate partners became perpetrators of violence, thus creating a situation of intimate partner violence, which added to the other existing problems that sex workers reported in their work. The common trend was that, in addition to taking advantage of sex workers' vulnerabilities, the intimate partner created additional vulnerabilities to further coerce and control the sex workers. Intimate partners isolated the sex workers from the world outside of the red-light area to prevent escape. They stopped sex workers from having friends and social relationships. The intimate partners kept track of the sex workers' movements and did not let them negotiate their own business (eg, financial, safe sex). Gradually, sex workers lost their independence and confidence in managing their own business. Eventually, the sex workers' intimate partners became their pimps who claimed to manage their business. This transition of an intimate partner becoming a pimp was seen in 5 out of 9 sex workers. The pimps' or intimate partners' coercive demands were almost always followed by threats of physical violence and emotional abuse. Noncompliance by the sex worker was met with physical and/or sexual violence by the intimate partner or pimp. The most common coercive acts by the sex workers' intimate partners were sexual and economic coercion.

In a study aiming to look at the relationship of the sex industry and intimate partner violence, Simmons et al[68] surveyed 2135 female residents of an intimate partner violence shelter regarding their batterer's use of both the sex industry and controlling behaviours in their relationship. Findings indicate that male domestic violence offenders who utilize the sex industry use more controlling behaviours than male domestic violence offenders who do not. As with previous studies highlighted above, this study also shows that this sub-group of offenders consistently shows high levels of aggression, violence, and control.

"There is evidence to show that there are shifting patterns in the way in which prostitution is operating. The trend is away from pimps controlling a number of women and towards 'pimp/partner' relationships. In these circumstances the violence which pimps may use to control their partner is properly classed as domestic violence and those involved in prostitution should be afforded the same protection against the perpetrator as any other victim of domestic violence."[69]

WHY ARE SEX WORKERS TARGETED?

Salfati[5] provides a full review of the literature looking at the reasons why sex workers are targetted. She quotes McKeganey and Barnard[7] who consider the link between violence and sex in the context of prostitution and highlight certain parallels between the position of the female prostitute and that of women generally in our society. They quote Scully[70] who noted the way in which men's justifications for rape are rooted in ideas of the role that society assigns women, and directs 'appropriate' ways that women should act, which excludes overt sexuality. Women who violate this expectation or role, they highlight, are then seen as acceptable and justifiable rape victims. Miller and Schwartz[15] argue that violence against prostitutes is an extreme form of violence against women in general. Themes that emerged from their interview with 16 street prostitutes indicate that there is a large amount of rape and violence perpetrated against these women. They show that people often see prostitutes as "unrapeable" and believe that no harm is done when a prostitute is raped, that prostitutes deserve to be raped, and that all prostitutes are the same. A similar finding was uncovered more recently by Farley et al[26] who showed that the notion that prostitutes are unrapeable was a common belief among the men in their sample. The more accepting men were of prostitution, the more likely they were to also accept cultural myths about rape such as "women say no but they really mean yes" or "a woman who dresses provocatively is asking to be raped." Twenty-seven per cent of their sample of 103 believed that once he pays, the customer is entitled to engage in any act he chooses with the woman he buys (emphasis from source).[26]

Miller and Schwartz[15] explain how these themes of attitudes against prostitutes relates to societal rape myths and how sexual violence in the context of street prostitution illuminates the functions and meanings of violence against women generally in American society. In this way it explains how prostitutes are seen not necessarily as people or individuals that the offender is directly angry with, but rather a category of woman that is objectified. Scully puts it very well: "a man's intent may not be to punish the woman he is raping but to use her because she represents a category to him."[70]

Miller and Schwartz[15] discuss powerful ideologies that define women (and prostitutes) as sexual property. There is a fundamental belief that prostitutes are seen as public property when they give consent to any sexual act through prostitution.[71] Many of the women in their study reported that they felt that the client had purchased their body to use as the client pleased. A striking anecdote that illustrates this point is that it is not uncommon for prostitutes to be picked up by a client who then refuses to pay them. This client would then rape the sex worker, and afterwards pay her. In this scenario they abuse the woman as a mere object and then justify their act of rape by paying the prostitute, and reframe their act as not a rape.

Miller and Jayasundara[40] summarise the work on how society's attitudes and rape myths promote and contribute to violence against prostitutes into a number prevailing attitudes. First is the belief that prostitutes cannot be raped: "The fact that prostitutes are available for sexual negotiation [is interpreted to] mean that they are available for sexual harassment and rape."[72] Second, the belief that no harm was done: "Through a confusion of sex with violence, rape is defined simply as a bad business transaction."[40] Third, the belief that: "Prostitutes deserve violence against them because of their violation of normative expectations of appropriate femininity."[40]

Miller and Jayasundara also show that this objectification of the female prostitute may not always be based on the individual prostitute herself, but be part of a transferred anger from another situation with a prostitute that has been generalised to all prostitutes as a group. They quote Miller and Schwartz's study[15] which noted that women reported being held responsible for the actions of other prostitutes, ie, a client becomes angry with one sex worker, but takes it out on another.

This pervasive bias against prostitutes goes beyond just their victimization as victims-of-crime, but extends to how cases of violence against prostitutes are investigated, cleared and treated within the legal system, all of which goes to feed the original prejudicial attitude against prostitutes.

Miller and Jayasundara[40] discuss in their book how the extent of women's legal protection from sexual violence is shaped by the extent to which they adhere to the standards of this normative femininity. As they state, in the US, this means being white, middle class, and chaste. They go on to suggest that because sex workers fall at the far end of this continuum, some scholars (eg, Miller and Schwartz[15]) have suggested that because the rape of prostitutes generally goes unpunished, that due to this perceived bias, prostitutes do not report crimes that are committed against them.[47] This attitude towards women in general and prostitutes specifically, Miller and Schwartz go on to state, may be a leading reason why violence against prostitutes go uninvestigated and unsolved. They cite the specific example of the Southside Slayer, a serial killer in South Central Los Angeles who targeted mainly African American women working as prostitutes. The police did not bring this series of murders to the attention of the public until 10 women had been killed, and specifically not until white women had been targeted. Moreover, early in the investigation, they quote officers calling these cases "cheap homicides,"[40] and give the example of one officer stating that: "the slayer is doing a better job at cleaning up the streets than we are."[73]

Unfortunately, when areas are cleaned up, the knock-on effect has been suggested to be that prostitutes are displaced to other areas, which they are unfamiliar with, and where they do not have the local information on which clients to avoid due to known previous displays of violence. They are therefore further put at risk of attack.[6]

CONCLUSION: THE HEALTH IMPACT OF VIOLENCE ON THE STREET

"Like combat veterans, women in prostitution suffer from posttraumatic stress disorder (PTSD), a psychological reaction to extreme physical and emotional trauma. Symptoms are acute anxiety, depression, insomnia, irritability, flashbacks, emotional numbing, and being in a state of emotional and physical hyperalertness. Sixty-seven percent of those in prostitution from 5 countries met criteria for a diagnosis of PTSD – a rate similar to that of battered women, rape victims, and state-sponsored torture survivors."[17]

As was highlighted at the start of this chapter, there has been a range of studies highlighting the high risk category street workers are in. They are at risk not only for violence and sexual assault, but also for murder, with some studies showing that homicide is one of the top 2 leading causes of death amongst prostitutes.[20] These figures alone show the very real extreme health implications of life on the streets. But the implications of prostitution on health go beyond that of physical violence, and there is extensive literature documenting that the total cross-sectional life of prostitution causes profound emotional damage.[52,65,74-78] Victims of sexual exploitation and violence before and during prostitution are known to suffer from depression, traumatic stress, dissociative disorders, eating disorders, and other anxiety disorders.[77] The UK's Home Office report on prostitution[69] provides an additional comprehensive list of studies, including authors, samples of groups looked at and key results, that have been done on risk and health factors associated with prostitution as an annex in their report (see Annex C, page 95 of the report) outlining age of entry into prostitution, background of care, runaways and homelessness, and drug use.

In addition to this research which shows the overall health implications of prostitution, Salfati[9] also highlights, based on a thorough overview of the literature, that violence against prostitutes should be considered as part of a continuum of violence against women more generally. As such, it needs to be understood within the larger context of abuse against women across the life course and across situations.

REFERENCES

1. We Can Do Better: Helping Prostituted Women and Girls Make Healthy Choices. Grand Rapids, MI. Nokomis Foundation; 2002.

2. Kinnell H. Violence against sex workers. Response to Church et al. *BMJ*. 2001;322.

3. Benson C. *Violence against female prostitutes* [PhD Thesis]. 1998

4. Kinnell H. Prostitutes' exposure to rape: implications for HIV prevention and for legal reform. Paper presented at: VII Social Aspects of AIDS conference; June 1993; South Bank University, London.

5. Salfati CG, James AR, Ferguson L. Prostitution homicides: a descriptive study. *J Interpers Violence*. 2008;23(4):505-543

6. Kinnell H. Murder made easy: the final solution to prostitution? In: Campbell R, O'Neill M, eds. *Sex Work Now*. Cullompton, Devon: Willan; 2006:141-168.

7. McKeganey N, Barnard M. *Sex Work on the Streets – Prostitutes and their Clients*. Buckingham, UK:: Open University Press; 1996.

8. Hunter SK, Reed KC. Taking the side of bought and sold rape. Speech presented at: National Coalition against Sexual Assault; July 1990; Washington, DC.

9. Salfati CG. Prostitute homicide: an overview of the literature and comparison to sexual and non-sexual female victim homicide. In: Canter D, Ioannou M, Youngs D, eds. *Safer Sex in the City: The Experience and Management of Street Prostitution*. The Psychology, Crime and Law Series. Aldershot, UK: Ashgate; 2009:51-68.

10. Kinnell H. *Violence Against Sex Workers in London: The London Ugly Mugs List*. [Unpublished] October 2000-February 2002.

11. Farley M, Barkan H. Prostitution, violence and post-traumatic stress disorder. *Women & Health*. 1998;27(3):37-49.

12. Benson C, Matthews R. Street prostitution; ten facts in search of a social policy. *Int J Sociology of Law*. 1995;23:395-415.

13. Hoigard C, Finstad L. *Backstreets: Prostitution, Money and Love*. London, UK: Polity; 1993.

14. Miller J. Victimization and resistance among street prostitutes. In: Adler PA, Adler P, eds. *Constructions of Deviance*. 2nd ed. Belmont, CA: Wadsworth; 1997:500-515.

15. Miller J, Schwartz MD. Rape myths and violence against street prostitutes. *Deviant Behavior*. 1995;16:1-23.

16. Silbert MH, Pines AM. Victimization of street prostitutes. *Victimology*. 1982;7:122-133.

17. Farley M, Baral I, Kireman M, Sezgin U. Prostitution in five countries: violence and post-traumatic stress disorder. *Feminism & Psychology*. 1998;8(4):405-426.

18. Brooks-Gordon B. *The Price of Sex: Prostitution, Policy and Society*. Collumpton, UK: Willan Publishing; 2006.

19. Cunnington S. Aspects of violence in prostitution. In: Hopkins J, ed. *Perspectives on Rape and Sexual Assault*. London: Harper and Row; 1984:25-36.

20. Lowman J, Fraser L. Violence against persons who prostitute: the experience in British Columbia. http://mypage.uniserve.ca/~lowman/. Published 1995.

21. Dodd V. Law increases danger, prostitutes say. *The Guardian*. http://www.guardian.co.uk/crime/article/0,,792962,00.html. September 15, 2002.

22. O'Neill M, Barberet R. Victimization and the social organization of prostitution. In: Weitzer R, ed. *Sex for Sale, Prostitution, Pornography, and the Sex Industry*. New York, NY: Routledge; 2000:123-137.

23. Brewer DD, Dudek JA, Potterat JJ, Muth SQ, Roberts JM, Woodhouse DE. Extents, trends, and perpetrators of prostitution related homicide in the United States. *J Forensic Sci*. 2006;51(5):1101-1108.

24. Potterat JJ, Brewer DD, Muth SQ, et al. Mortality in a long-term open cohort of prostitute women. *Am J Epidemiol*. 2004;159(8):778-785.

25. Ward H, Day S, Weber J. Risky business: health and safety in the sex industry over a 9 year period. *Sex Transm Inf*. 1999;75:340-343.

26. Farley M, Bindel J, Golding JM. *Men Who Buy Sex: Who They Buy and What They Know*. Eaves, London. Prostitution Research & Education, San Fransisco; 2009.

27. Church S, Henderson M, Barnard M, Hart G. Violence by clients towards female prostitutes in different work settings; questionnaire survey. *BMJ*. 2001;322:524-525.

28. Lowman J. Violence and the outlaw status of (street) prostitution in Canada. *Violence Against Women*. 2000;6(9):987-1011.

29. Kinnell H. *Violence and Sex Work in Britain*. Cullompton, Devon: Willan Publishing; 2008.

30. James J. Motivations for entrance into prostitution. In: Crites L, ed. *The Female Offender*. Lexington, MA: D.C. Heath; 1976.

31. Kapur P. *The Life and World of Call Girls in India*. New Delhi: Vikas; 1978.

32. McLeod E. *Women Working: Prostitution Now*. London & Canberra: Groom Helm; 1982.

33. Matthews R. Kerb Crawling, prostitution and multi-agency policing. *Police Research Group: Crime Prevention Unit Series, 43*. London: Home Office; 1993.

34. Lever J, Dolnick D. Call girls and street prostitutes. In: Weitzer R, ed. *Sex for Sale: Prostitution, Pornography, and the Sex Industry*. London: Routledge; 2009: 187-204.

35. Sharpe K. *Red Light, Blue Light. Prostitutes, punters and the police.* Aldershot, UK: Ashgate; 1998.

36. Matthews R. Beyond wolfenden? prostitution, politics and the law. In: R Matthews R, Young J, eds. *Confronting Crime.* London: Sage; 1986; 188-215.

37. Ferguson L. *Sex Workers Safety Survey* [videotape]. UK: Channel 4; 2002.

38. May T, Edmunds M, Hough M, Harvey C. Street business: the links between sex and drug markets. *Police Research Series.* 1999; Paper 118.

39. Gary ridgway pleads guilty to green river murders [transcript]. CNN. Cable News Network. November 5, 2003.

40. Miller J, Jayasundara D. Prostitution, the sex industry, and sex tourism. In: Renzetti CM, Edleson JL, Bergen RK, eds. *Sourcebook on Violence Against Women.* Thousand Oaks, CA: Sage Publications; 2001:459-480.

41. Shell Y, Campbell P, Caren I. *It's Not a Game: A Report on Hampshire Constabulary's Anti-Kerb Crawling Initiative.* Hampshire Constabulary; 2001. Cited by: Brooks-Gordon B. *The Price of Sex: Prostitution, Policy and Society.* Collumpton, Devon: Willan Publishing; 2006.

42. Brewer DD, Muth SQ, Roberts JM, Potterat JJ. *Demographic, Biometric and Geographic Comparison of Clients of Prostitutes and Men in the US General Population.* Unpublished Report. Seattle, WA: Interdisciplinary Scientific Research; 2006.

43. Brewer DD, Muth SQ, Dudek JA, Roberts JM, Potterat JJ. *A Comparative Profile of Violent Clients of Prostitute Women.* Unpublished Report. Seattle, WA: Interdisciplinary Scientific Research; 2006.

44. Caputi, J. The ripper repetitions. The Age of Sex Crime. Bowling Green, OH: Bowling Green University Popular Press; 1987:33.

45. Kinnell H. Violence and sex work in Britain. In: Day S, Ward H, eds. *Sex Work, Mobility and Health in Europe.* London: Kegan Paul; 2004.

46. Salfati CG. Prostitutes: Vulnerable or Sexual Targets of Serial Homicide? Paper presented at: Annual American Society of Criminology Conference. Atlanta, GA: November 2007.

47. Fairstein LA. *Sexual Violence: Our War Against Rape.* New York, NY: William Morrow and Company; 1993:171. Cited by: Miller J, Schwartz MD. Rape myths and violence against street prostitutes. *Deviant Behavior.* 1995;16:1.

48. Bracey DH. The juvenile prostitute: victim and offender. *Victimology.* 1983;8:149-162.

49. Maher L. *Sexed Work: Gender, Race, and Resistance in a Brooklyn Drug Market.* New York, NY: Oxford University Press; 1997.

50. Miller J. Gender and power on the streets: street prostitution in the era of crack cocaine. *J Contemporary Ethnography.* 1995;23:427-452.

51. Dalla RA, Xia Y, Kennedy H. You just give them what they want and pray they don't kill you:" street-level sex workers' reports of victimization, personal resources, and coping strategies. *Violence Against Women.* 2003;9(11):1367-1394.

52. Barry K. *The Prostitution of Sexuality.* New York: New York University Press; 1995. Cited by: Faugier J, Sargeant M. Boyfriends, 'pimps' and clients. In: Scambler G, Scambler A, eds. *Rethinking Prostitution: Purchasing Sex in the 1990s.* London: Routledge; 1997.

53. Norton-Hawk M. A comparison of pimp-and non-pimp-controlled women. *Violence Against Women.* 2004;10:189.

54. Williamson C, Cluse-Tolar T. Pimp-controlled prostitution: still an integral part of street life. *Violence Against Women.* 2002;8:1074

55. Giobbe E. A comparison of pimps and batterers. *Mich J Gender Law.* 1993;1(1):33-57.

56. Johnson JJ. *Teen Prostitution.* Danbury, CT: Franklin Watts; 1992.

57. Williamson C. Entrance, maintenance, and exit: the socio-economic influences and cumulative burdens of female street prostitution. *Dissertation Abstracts Int.* 2000;61(2). (UMI No. 9962789)

58. Faugier J, Sargeant M. Boyfriends, "pimps" and clients. In: Scambler G, Scambler A, eds. *Rethinking Prostitution: Purchasing Sex in the 1990s.* London, UK: Routledge; 1997:121-136.

59. Flowers R. *Runaway Kids and Teenage Prostitution: Americas Lost, Abandoned, and Sexually Exploited Children.* Westport, CN: Greenwood Press; 2001.

60. McCormack A, Janus MD, Burgess AW. Runaway youths and sexual victimization: gender differences in an adolescent runaway population. *Child Abuse Negl.* 1986;10(3):387-395.

61. National Center for Missing and Exploited Children. Female juvenile prostitution: problem and response. Arlington, VA: National Center for Missing and Exploited Children; 1992.

62. Holsopple K. Strip clubs according to strippers: exposing workplace sexual violence. In: Hughes D, Roche C, eds. *Making the Harm Visible: Global Sexual Exploitation of Women and Girls, Speaking Out and Providing Services.* Kingston, RI: Coalition Against Trafficking in Women; 1999.

63. Hardesty L, Greif GL. Common themes in a group for female IV drug users who are HIV positive. *J Psychoactive Drugs.* 1994;26(3):289-293.

64. Stoops in interview with David Gilliver for *Drinks and Drugs News.* June 7, 2010.

65. Baldwin, MA. Split at the root: prostitution and feminist discourses of law reform. *Yale J Law Feminism.* 1992;5:47-120. Cited by: Farley M. Prostitution: Factsheet on Human Rights Violations. http://www.prostitutionresearch.com/factsheet. html. Published 2000. Accessed April 10, 2011.

66. El-Bassel N, Witte S. Drug use and physical and sexual abuse of street sex workers in New York City. *Res Sex Work.* 2001;4:31-32.

67. Karandikar S, Próspero M. From client to pimp: male violence against female sex workers. *J Interpers Violence.* 2010;25(2):257-273.

68. Simmons CA, Lehmann P, Collier-Tenison S. Industry to controlling behaviors in violent relationships an exploratory analysis. *Violence Against Women.* 2008;14(4):406-417.

69. Home Office. *Paying the Price: A Consultation Paper on Prostitution.* London, UK: Home Office Communication Directorate; 2004. http://webarchive. nationalarchives.gov.uk/+/http://www.homeoffice.gov.uk/documents/paying_the_ price.pdf?view=Binary. Accessed August 5, 2013.

70. Scully D. *Understanding Sexual Violence: A Study of Convicted Rapists.* Boston, MA: Unwin Hyman; 1990.

71. Rubin G. Thinking sex: notes for a radical theory of the politics of sexuality. In: Vance CS, ed. *Pleasure and Danger: Exploring Female Sexuality.* London: Pandora; 1984:267-319.

72. Hatty SE. Violence against prostitute women: social and legal dilemmas. *Aus J Soc Issues.* 1989;24(4):236. Cited by: Miller J, Jayasundara D. Prostitution, the sex industry, and sex tourism. In: Renzetti CM, Edleson JL, Bergen RK, eds. *Sourcebook on Violence Against Women.* Thousand Oaks, CA: Sage; 2001.

73. Predscod M. Paper presented at: the annual meeting of National Women's Studies Association; June 1990; Akron, OH. Cited by: Miller J, Jayasundara D. Prostitution, the sex industry, and sex tourism. In: Renzetti CM, Edleson JL, Bergen RK, eds. *Sourcebook on Violence Against Women.* Thousand Oaks, CA: Sage; 2001:469.

74. Dworkin A. Prostitution and male supremacy. In: *Life and Death.* New York, NY: Free Press; 1997.

75. Herman J. Introduction: hidden in plain sight: clinical observations on prostitution. In: Farley M, ed. *Prostitution, Trafficking, and Traumatic Stress.* New York, NY: Routledge; 2003:1-13.

76. Hoigard C, Finstad L. *Backstreets: Prostitution, Money and Love.* University Park, PA: Pennsylvania State University Press; 1986.

77. Farley M, Cotton A, Lynne J, et al. Prostitution and trafficking in 9 countries: update on violence and posttraumatic stress disorder. *J Trauma Pract.* 2003;2(3/4):33-74

78. Raymond JG, D'Cunha J, Dzuhayatin SR, Hynes HP, Rodriguez ZR, Santos A. *A Comparative Study of Women Trafficked in the Migration Process.* Amherst, MA: Coalition Against Trafficking in Women; 2002.

Chapter 28

The Co-occurrence of Intimate Partner Violence and Human Immunodeficiency Virus[*]

Rae Spiwak, MSc[1,3]
Jolene Kinley, MA[2]
Jitender Sareen, MD, FRCPC[1,2,3†]
Tracie Afifi PhD[3,1]

[1]*Department of Psychiatry, University of Manitoba*
[2]*Department of Psychology, University of Manitoba*
[3]*Department of Community Health Sciences, University of Manitoba*

Key Points

1. Women and men who have experienced IPV are more likely to report risky health behaviors including current smoking, heavy or binge drinking, and HIV risk behaviors including intravenous drug use and past year unprotected sex. These risky behaviors may increase an individual's chance of acquiring HIV/AIDS.

2. Women's lack of power and knowledge about safe sex practices may limit their ability to protect themselves against HIV, especially in low and middle-income countries. Different degrees of acculturation and changes in gender roles may help to partly explain increased risk of HIV among certain populations.

3. IPV and psychopathology may be linked to decreased immune functioning, which may increase an individual's risk for acquiring HIV/AIDS. The relationship between HIV and psychopathology may be bidirectional with psychopathology leading to HIV through increased risk behaviors and decreased immune functioning, as well as HIV leading to psychopathology due to stress associated with having HIV.

4. IPV and HIV are important and challenging public health concerns. The discussion of prevention and intervention efforts must be tailored to reflect the intersection among IPV and HIV at both the individual and systems level; IPV and HIV affects all genders, all races, and individuals regardless of country of origin. All individuals regardless of risk factors should be routinely offered HIV testing.

5. Although a substantial body of research has focused on the association between IPV and HIV among women, fewer studies have focused on other populations, such as

[*]*This research was supported by funds from the Canadian Institutes of Health Research (CIHR) Institute of Gender and Health (IGH) and Institute of Neurosciences Mental Health and Addictions (INMHA) to PreVAiL (Centre for Research Development in Gender, Mental Health and Violence across the Lifespan)*

[†]*Deceased*

men, gay, lesbian, bisexual, and transgendered individuals. Further research needs to focus on these groups in order to fully understand the relationship between IPV and HIV as well as to develop appropriate interventions.

INTRODUCTION

Intimate partner violence (IPV) and human immunodeficiency virus (HIV) are important public health issues that affect the health of both women and men worldwide. Globally, women have been found to be an increasingly vulnerable group at risk for HIV infection.[1] Gender norms, violence against women, lack of education, and poor financial security each play a role in explaining why gender and HIV are linked.[2] Traditional gender norms support men engaging in relationships with younger women and having more sexual partners, which contribute to women's increased risk of contracting HIV.[2] For women in traditional roles that involve sexual inequality and lack of decision making power, the ability to negotiate safe sex and have access to HIV prevention information is restricted.[3] Similarly, women are more likely to have lower levels of literacy and less knowledge of HIV as compared to men.[2] Although the global HIV epidemic has been linked to violence against women, it is important to recognize that this relationship is complex and impacted by a variety of factors.

The purpose of this chapter is to review the epidemiology and comorbidity of IPV and HIV, including a discussion of potential causal pathways, the relationship between HIV risk behaviors and IPV, the role of psychopathology, and the potential link between IPV and immunity and HIV disease progression. As the literature discussing the relationship between IPV and HIV largely focuses on heterosexual women, a significant proportion of the discourse in this chapter will focus on this demographic; however an examination of this relationship among men, bisexual, gay, lesbian, and transgendered individuals will also be undertaken.

COMORBIDITY OF IPV AND HIV
HISTORY OF IPV

Violence against women in intimate relationships has existed for centuries. English Common law viewed women as the property of their husbands, and as a result it was perfectly acceptable for husbands to beat their wives. In 1782, the "rule of thumb" law was passed which dictated that a husband was allowed to beat his wife, but only providing the rod he used to beat her was no thicker than his thumb.[4] Given that this law existed for approximately another hundred years, it is not surprising that the first article written about IPV was only published in 1971 in the Journal of Marriage and the Family.[5] Following 1971, the discussion around domestic violence or family violence increased and included studies in nursing which began the discussion around battered women syndrome. The study of battered women and the recognition that battering had mental health consequences were important developments in the area of intimate partner violence (see **Figure 28-1**). In 1983, the Centre for Disease Control (CDC) began its focus on the epidemiology of violence. This focus created more awareness of the fact that violence was not a private family matter that occurred behind closed doors with no health consequences; IPV was in fact a public health concern.[5] An important consideration in the history of IPV involves violence against men in heterosexual relationships, as well as gay, lesbian, bisexual, and transgendered individuals in intimate relationships. Many studies of violence in intimate relationships have focused on a male perpetrator and a female victim. Although it is important to discuss the history of IPV in the United Kingdom, the United States, and Canada, it is also important to remember that the history of IPV is different in many countries: in some countries women are still believed to be possessions of their husbands, and to be of lower social status which

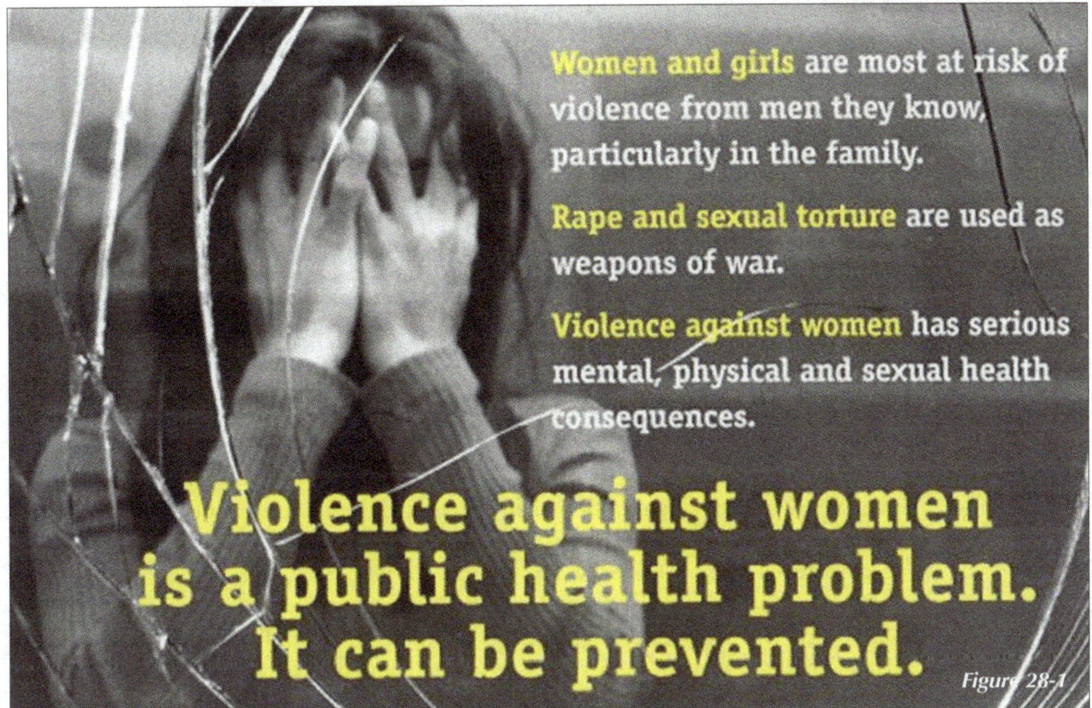

Figure 28-1.
WHO
Advertisement

results in violence.[6] Even in the western world today, IPV is still prevalent and women are fearful in abusive relationships despite awareness of this problem. On the other hand, men in countries like the United States and Canada may fear coming forward as victims of violence at the hands of their male or female partners in these societies.

EPIDEMIOLOGY OF IPV

Intimate partner violence is defined as physical or sexual assault by a romantic or formerly romantic partner.[1] This violence may include patterns of coercion or threats of violence in intimate relationships.[7] A report from the National Institute of Justice indicates that 1 in 6 women have experienced an attempted or completed rape.[8] Tjaden and Thoennes[9] report that in the United States an estimated 1.5 million women experience violence at the hands of their partner every year. Campbell1 reports that the lifetime prevalence of physical violence by male partners over 10 countries ranged from 13% to 62%, and that prevalence of lifetime sexual violence by romantic partners ranged from 6% in Japan to 59% in Ethiopia. Afifi et al[10] found that in the United States, 15.2% of females and 20.3% of males reported experiencing IPV in their current marital relationships. It seems that women from different countries have variable likelihoods of experiencing IPV. For example, African American women report much higher rates of IPV, however this risk difference may be because of differences in disclosure or other demographic or social factors.[11] Campbell[1] also notes that Hispanic American and African American women experience a disproportionate amount of IPV. IPV rates are especially high among women receiving medical care, with 15% currently experiencing violence by their male partners, and a lifetime prevalence of 44%.[12]

Not only is IPV common, it has significant mental and physical health consequences. IPV has been associated with death, traumatic brain injury, chronic pain, disability, and a variety of other health related outcomes such as post-traumatic stress disorder.[13] These relationships have a dose-response pattern in that as duration and severity of IPV increase so do the negative outcomes.[14]

Studies show that femicide, or the murdering of women, is a fatal consequence of IPV.[13] Wadman and Muelleman[15] found that half of femicide victims sought care in an emergency department in the time preceding their murder, and Sharps et al[16] found that almost 70% of victims experienced IPV at the hands of their partner before being killed.

HISTORY OF HIV

In 1981, the disease now known as acquired immunodeficiency syndrome first presented among a small group of homosexual men.[17] A few years later, researchers discovered that this disease was caused by a virus called HIV-type 1,[17] and that this virus decreased immunity allowing other infectious agents which normally would be fought off by the human body to cause infections ending in death.[18] In 1982, it was recognized that AIDS was not a disease only affecting homosexual men, and that both women and heterosexual men were also vulnerable to acquiring the disease.

EPIDEMIOLOGY OF HIV

Since the appearance of AIDS in 1981, millions of people have been infected and died. The World Health Organization estimates that 33.4 million people worldwide were living with HIV in 2008. In 2008, HIV was the leading cause of death among women aged 15 to 44 years.[19] Globally, the number of women that have been infected with AIDS has continued to increase. Additionally, women accounted for more than 80% of new cases of HIV/AIDS cases in 2006.[20] Although all people are at risk for acquiring HIV, some groups of women are more vulnerable than others. Women living in Sub-Saharan Africa appear disproportionately affected by HIV, with women accounting for 60% of HIV prevalence in this region (see **Figure 28-2**).[21]

Figure 28-2.
HIV Prevalence, 2007 (WHO)

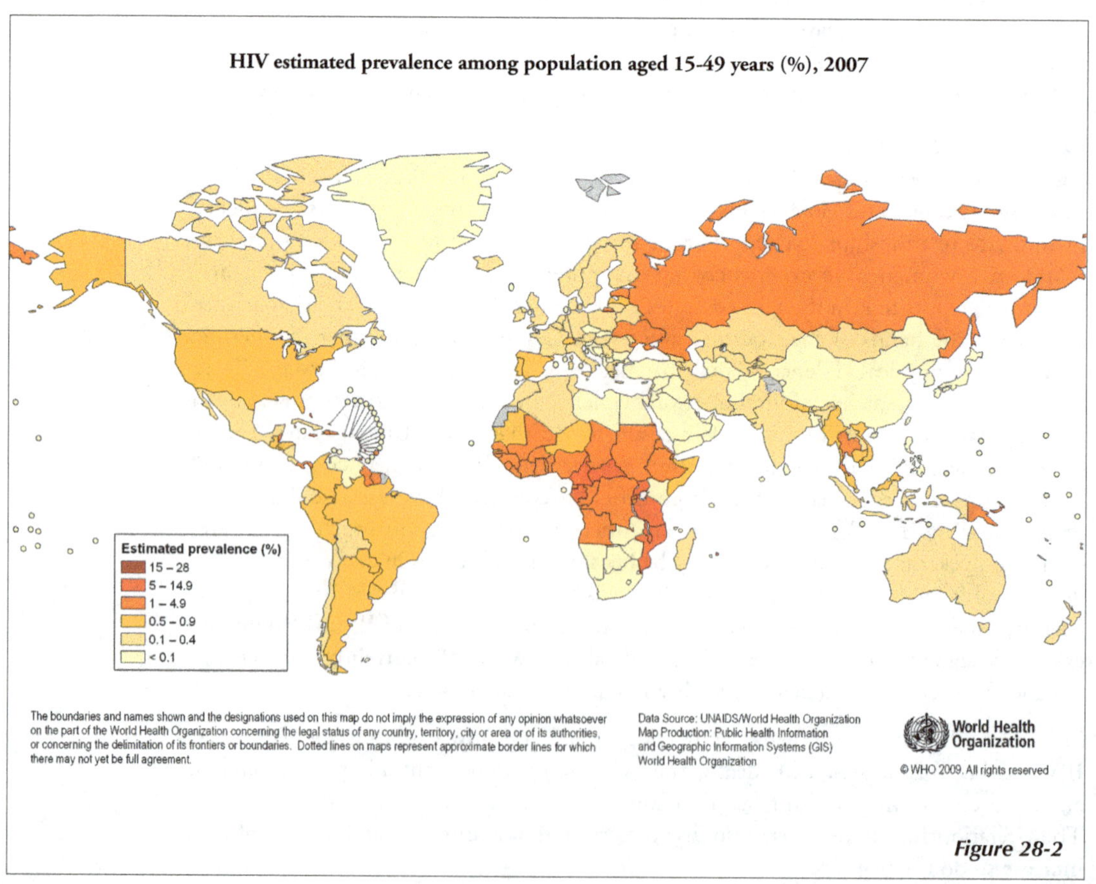

In the United States, women were the fastest growing group of persons with HIV in 2003,[5] but the profile of new infections has greatly changed more recently. New HIV infections have been increasing among men who have sex with men, decreasing among injection drug users, and leveled out among heterosexual individuals (see **Figure 28-3**).[21]

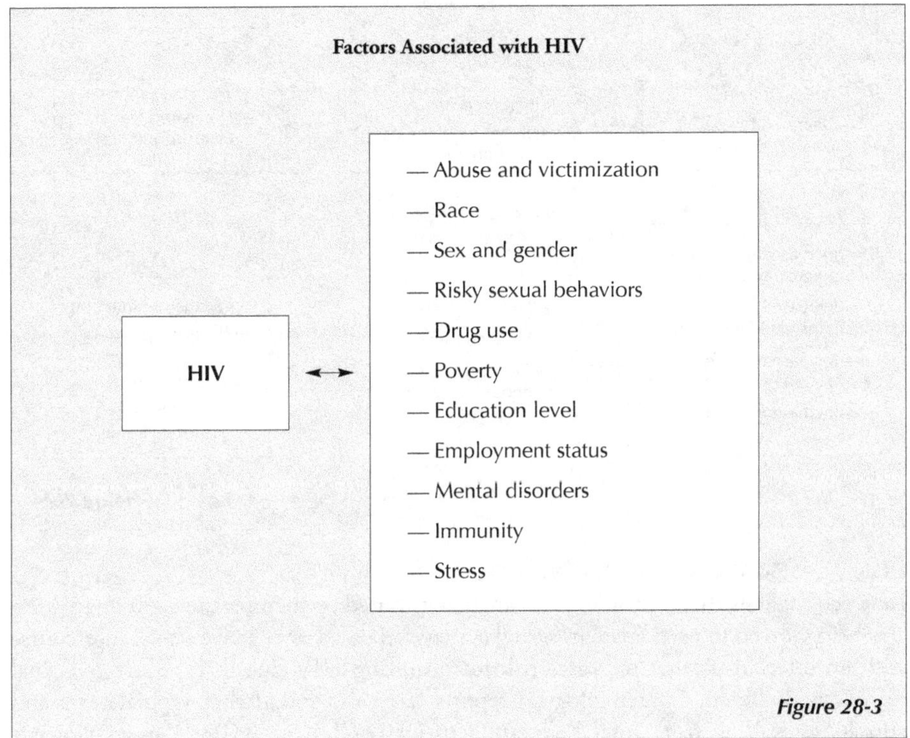

Figure 28-3

Figure 28-3. *Some factors associated with HIV*

Intersectionality Between IPV and HIV

The linkage or intersectionality between IPV and HIV was articulated in the early 2000s with investigations into violence and HIV. Focus on the concurrent experiences of women in abusive relationship and those with HIV infection lead to the rational for linking the vulnerable groups of women. As Gielen et al[11] indicates, subgroups with increased rates of IPV are often the same individuals at risk of HIV; for example, women who are young, of low socioeconomic status, and belong to a minority group. Risk factors for both HIV and IPV include social correlates such as poverty, alcohol and drug use, low education, employment status, and mental disorders.[5] Although there may be similar background factors between individuals with both HIV and IPV, this is a complex relationship.

Causal Pathways

Intimate partner violence has been identified as reducing the ability of a woman to protect and control her reproductive and sexual health.[22] Previous research has begun to identify and formulate causal pathways between IPV and HIV but this area is still far from understood. Although the global HIV epidemic has been linked to IPV, it is important to recognize that like HIV, STI transmission is also a potential outcome of IPV.[23-29] Studies have reported that IPV has been associated with increased risk for chlamydia,[23] cervical cancer and neuroplasia,[24] adolescent pregnancy,[30] alcohol use,[28] and sexually transmitted symptoms such as vaginal irritation and discharge (see **Figure 28-4**).[26]

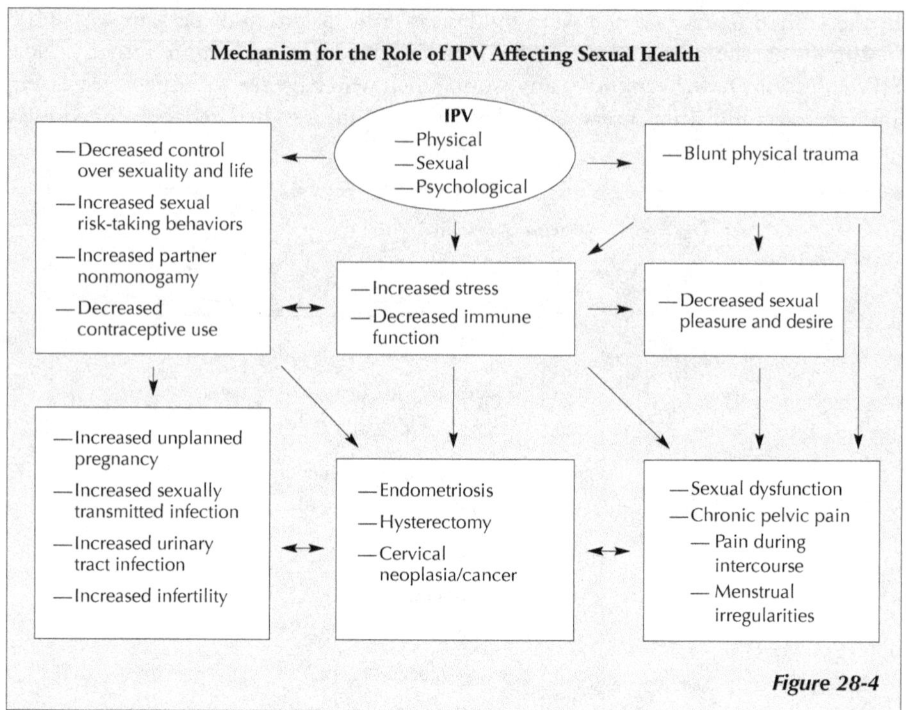

Figure 28-4.
Mechanism for the role of IPV affecting sexual health

FORCED SEX AND CONDOM NEGOTIATION

Research suggests that of women who are being abused by their partners, 40 to 45% are also being forced to participate in sexual activity.[31] Forced or coercive sexual intercourse with an infected partner increases risk for acquiring HIV due to exposure to sexual secretions or blood. Epidemiological reports have also found that vaginal tears and abrasions resulting from forced sex are a major conduit for HIV.[32] Sexual violence among young women and girls is especially dangerous due to immature vaginal tracts that tear easily during sexual intercourse.[33]

Refusal to wear condoms and forced intercourse by abusive partners put women at risk for HIV and STI.[34] Why are men putting women at risk? Men who are abusive have been found to engage in unprotected sexual intercourse and infidelity.[35,36] Decker et al[26] found that multiple mechanisms may be taking place that help to explain the relationship between IPV and HIV, including that women have limited control over sexual relationships with male partners, and that these male partners are more likely to be infected (see **Table 28-1**). The issues of control and increased likelihood of abusive males creates a situation where women are at risk for acquiring HIV. A study looking at the association between men who were perpetrators of IPV and HIV risk behaviors found that violent men reported more lifetime sexual partners, and had experienced physical violence themselves as children.[37] It may be that the intergenerational or cyclic effects of violence may play a role in the intersectionality between IPV and HIV.

With respect to control and power, some research suggests that women who have experienced past abuse may be vulnerable to participating in unprotected sex due to fear of retaliation from new partners 38 and may internalize lack of control from past relationships into the future.[39] This fear and lack of control is not restricted to heterosexual couples; some research shows that lesbian, gay, bisexual, and transgendered individuals are often forced by their partners to have sex, and experience violence as a result of asking partners to practice safe sex.[40] Deceptive condom use among men

---

Table 28-1. Potential Causal Pathways between IPV and HIV

— Forced or coercive sex

— Condom negotiation and refusal to wear condoms

— Engaging in transactional sex

— Intermittent condom use

— Multiple sexual partners

— Partner non-monogamy

— Alcohol and substance abuse

— Child sexual abuse

---

who have sex with men (MSM) have also been found which may indicate that condom negotiation may not always be successful even when agreed upon prior to intercourse.[40]

RISKY BEHAVIORS

As discussed, research has shown that women who were abused by their partners engaged in more risky practices, were less likely to use a condom, and were more likely to have multiple partners. In addition, women's experience of violence has been shown to be linked to the engagement in transactional sex, or sex for resources. In one study, women who had engaged in transactional sex were 1.5 times more likely to have HIV than those women who did not engage in transactional sex.[41] A systematic review of IPV and sexual health examined 51 manuscripts over a 40-year period to help understand the relationship between sexual health and IPV. The review found that women who had experienced partner violence were more likely to be involved with sexual risk taking such as intermittent condom use, multiple sexual partners, and partner non-monogamy.[24]

Other studies have examined the role of alcohol or substance abuse prior to sexual intercourse.[42] In addition to sexual intercourse, a study by Wagner et al[43] found that there was an association between IPV and syringe sharing among young female drug users that may indicate that some women who are victimized engage in non-sexual risky behaviors that increase the likelihood of HIV transmission. Other research has examined the mechanisms between IPV and HIV and have found that sexual risk-taking behaviors such as age at first intercourse and limited condom negotiation are linked to HIV.[44] In addition to risky practices, several studies have found that IPV might have a dose-response relationship when it comes to mental, physical, sexual, and social consequences, meaning that as IPV duration and frequency increase, so do poor health outcomes.[14,45]

In addition to adult IPV, there is a developing body of literature showing that childhood sexual abuse may also be a risk factor for HIV infection. Childhood sexual abuse has been linked to risky behaviors including early age at first voluntary intercourse, unprotected sex, alcohol and substance use, and contracting sexually transmitted diseases.[46,47] Few studies have examined the mechanisms between child sexual abuse and sexually transmitted infections. One of these studies examines the life course model in which early inappropriate sexual scripts are learned in childhood, and these scripts influence future sexual and health behaviors.[48]

In addition to risky behaviors as a precursor to HIV, risky behaviors may also follow HIV. For example, a review by Van Kesteren[49] examined 53 studies that looked at HIV status and risky sexual behavior. Of these 53 studies, 25 were cross-sectional studies of sexual risk behavior among HIV positive men who have sex with men (MSM). Of these 25 studies, more than half supported the idea that HIV positive individuals engaged in unprotected anal intercourse, regardless of the HIV status of their sexual partner.[49] This review concludes that there may be a rise in risky sexual behavior among HIV positive MSM. Other studies have found that HIV positive women also engage in unprotected sex with individuals that are HIV negative or unknown status.[50] Other studies have found that risky drug behaviors such as methamphetamine use may be linked to HIV, and that both alcohol and methamphetamine use is a strong influence in unprotected intercourse among MSM.[51] The link between methamphetamine use and HIV has been recognized as an important area for future research and an important area for which to direct policy.[52]

VIOLENCE AS A CONSEQUENCE OF HIV

Although much discussion has occurred about the relationship between HIV and IPV, violence has also been found to be a consequence of acquiring HIV. Women seeking HIV testing are sometimes afraid to ask for information or testing for HIV.[33] Among those women with HIV, between 16% and 86% choose not to disclose HIV status to partners.[33] Among HIV positive couples, it appears that the association with IPV remains. A study by Deribe[53] found that women's lack of HIV disclosure to their partner was because they feared physical violence. The study found that there was no difference in the proportion of men and women disclosing HIV, but that the barriers and motivators of disclosure did vary by gender. It is important that health services that address IPV and HIV consider the barriers to help seeking in order to target all groups of individuals infected with HIV in order to improve prevention and intervention efforts.

THE ROLE OF CULTURE AND POWER

Women's lack of power as well as knowledge about safe sex practices can limit their ability to protect themselves against HIV infection, and this factor may be especially important in the context of developing countries such as India (see **Figure 28-5**).[54] Silverman and colleagues[55] found that physical violence combined with sexual violence by husbands was associated with an increased prevalence of HIV infection among married Indian

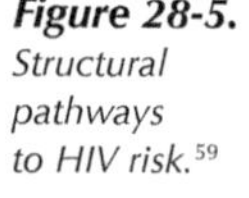

Figure 28-5.
Structural pathways to HIV risk.[59]

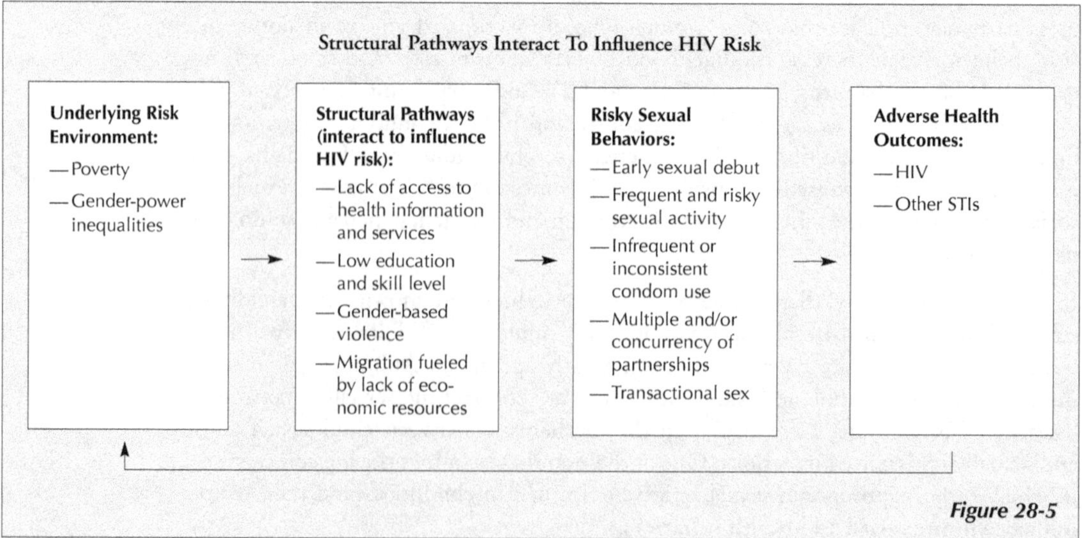

women. Specifically, women who had experienced IPV were nearly 4 times more likely to have HIV as compared to women without IPV. In a cohort study of South African women, Jewkes et al[56] investigated the role of power, IPV, and HIV in this population. The authors found that unequal power and IPV increased the risk of HIV in young South African women and argued that the study provides strong temporal evidence that there is a causal association between IPV and new HIV infection. Although exploring this relationship via a randomized control trial is impossible, the population attributable fractions estimated in this study show that reducing IPV and gender inequity would reduce new HIV infection by 13.9%.[56]

An important consideration in the discussion of power, control, and HIV involves sex workers. A study by Gupta et al[57] investigated the risk of HIV among sex workers in India. This study qualitatively explored the issues of control and power and it was found that lack of control among sex trafficked women and girls increased their risk or vulnerability to HIV via several mechanisms: use of violent rape to initiate sex work; inability to refuse sex; lack of condom use and lack of safe sex negotiation; substance use as a coping mechanism; and poor access to health care.

To understand the mechanisms involved with HIV transmission, research examining the relationship between women's sociodemographic factors, risky sexual behaviors, and HIV is needed. For example, research has investigated the theory of gender and power in understanding of violence and the risk of HIV among sex workers in India.[58] Attention has been placed on using gender and power as a theoretical framework in explaining women's vulnerability to HIV. With respect to the sexual division of power, lack of control over work environments combined with behavioral risk factors such as alcohol abuse and lack of control over condom negotiation creates a situation where women's vulnerability to HIV is increased.[58]

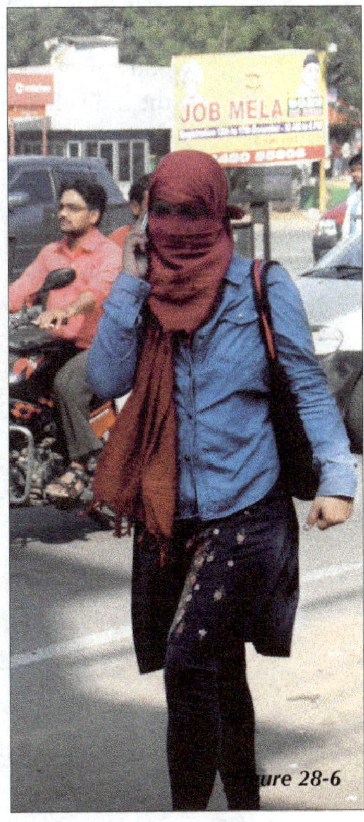

Figure 28-6. The clash between traditional and modern roles in low and middle-income countries may play a part in increasing the incidence of HIV. (Photograph courtesy of Rae Spiwak).

The environment in which sexual negotiation occurs is not only between sex trade workers and their clients but also among married couples.[58] Krishnan[59] states that IPV decreases a woman's ability to: refuse sex with her partner, question her husband's fidelity, and negotiate safe sex. This environment, regardless of the context, is laden with familial and economic complexities that reflect power and sexual norms and roles. Dunkle and colleagues[41] discuss this, and add that the power imbalances inherent in IPV may be further unbalanced when material goods or financial transactions are involved. For example, when a woman accepts material goods she may give up her power in sexual decision-making. The authors also note that men who are likely to give material goods in exchange for intercourse are also more likely to be sexually risky and violent. Although several studies have looked at the association between IPV and HIV in developed and developing countries, further research is needed to examine this relationship in population-based samples, as well as to determine if the mechanisms of transmission differ across different countries and cultures.

Different degrees of acculturation and changes in gender roles may help to partly explain increased risk of HIV among certain populations. For example, the incidence of HIV among Hispanics in the USA has been found to be over 54% higher than whites.[60] The clash between traditional and modern roles also may play a part in increasing the incidence of HIV (see **Figure 28-6**).

For example, some Latina women may be limited in terms of seeking condoms or other resources to protect themselves before marriage, and may have limited power in sexual decision making after marriage.[3] Similarly, married women in India may have very little control over sexual decision-making and therefore have little control over safe sex options.[42] It is clear that culture and context play an important role in understanding the relationship between IPV and HIV. Therefore, an important consideration in intervention programs and future research is to be aware of the role of culture in the relationship between IPV and HIV, as well as to consider national and community contexts.

THE LINK BETWEEN IPV AND OTHER PHYSICAL HEALTH BEHAVIORS

Research has shown that IPV is associated with a number of negative outcomes including risk of death, injury, chronic pain, poor mental health, disability, somatic syndromes, chronic arthritis, migraines, hearing loss, angina, and changes in endocrine and immune functions (see **Table 28-2**).[61] However, the link between IPV and other health behaviors is less clear.[61,62] Breiding et al[61] examined the association between IPV, chronic disease, and other health measures to assess whether both men and women who had a previous history of IPV were at greater risk for poor health outcomes and behaviors. Women and men who reported lifetime IPV were more likely to report risky health behaviors including current smoking, heavy or binge drinking, and HIV risk behaviors including intravenous drug use and past year unprotected sex.[61] In addition, the authors found that those with experience of IPV were also more likely to have joint disease, current asthma, and activity limitations. With respect to health care use, individuals who have previously experienced victimization were found to have not seen a doctor within the past year. The authors report that many of the poor health outcomes were similar for men and women, except for cardiovascular disease where women were at greater risk. Interestingly, the authors note that stress due to IPV may increase the odds of developing poor health or chronic conditions, however it may also be that the individual had poor health or chronic disease prior to the abuse. In this case, stress due to illness may impact the individual, their partner, and may in fact increase the chance of being abused. Bonomi and colleagues[63] also found adverse health effects among women with sexual IPV exposure. Women who had been victimized had lower self-rated health scores (SF-36) as well as more depressive symptoms compared to women with physical IPV exposure. This finding highlights the importance of considering the differences between both sexual and physical IPV and recognizing that each type of IPV may have its own unique risks.

Table 28-2. IPV and Poor Health Outcomes

— Risk of death	— Angina
— Injury	— Change in immune function
— Chronic pain	— Poor mental health
— Disability	— Depression
— Chronic Arthritis	— Post traumatic stress disorder
— Migraines	— Suicidal behavior
— Hearing loss	— Drug and alcohol abuse

IMMUNITY AND DISEASE PROGRESSION

It is well known that there are physical and mental health consequences associated with IPV. Several studies have examined the role of victimization on immunity, and many factors exist to help explain this relationship. Research has shown alterations in immune cell efficacy in individuals who have experienced PTSD due to a variety of traumatic experiences.[64] T-cell function is one measure of immune function which has been examined in the literature. T cells are lymphocytes, which control immune response in the body. Lymphocytes rapidly reproduce to defend the body against antigens. Research has shown that there is a depression of lymphocyte stimulation in situations of chronic stress, therefore examining lymphocytes is a marker for biological stress.[65] A study by Constantino et al[66] found an association between IPV and lower T-cell function; specifically, women who were abused had lower T-cell function. Studies have also found that women with PTSD who were in abusive relationships were more likely to have altered levels of cortisol and dehydroepiandrosterone (DHEA) as compared to women who were not in abusive relationships.[67] Sanchez et al[68] looked at saliva levels to measure immunity among abused women. They found that cessation of physical IPV was the main factor that neutralized HSV-1 and HSV-sIgA levels. In other words, women who were previously abused improved their immune functioning once abuse was eliminated.

In addition to compromised immunofunction, a body of literature supports the idea that HIV disease progression may be impacted by stress. Other studies examine stressful life events and their relationship with HIV. Leserman et al found that faster progression to AIDS was associated with more cumulative stressful life events, depressive symptoms, and less social support.[69] The authors concluded that the probability of getting AIDS was about 2 to 3 times higher among those with higher stress. In a more recent article, the authors found that individuals with more stressful life events and less social support had faster disease progression to AIDS, individuals with more depressive symptoms were more likely to develop AIDS more quickly, and that serum cortisol predicted disease progression.[70] It is clear that chronic depression, stressful events, and trauma may negatively affect HIV disease progression via reduction in CD4 T lymphocytes, and increases in viral load.[70] Further research is needed to fully examine this association, as well as the biological and behavioral factors that may impact immunity, including the order of events. The role of psychopathology on immune functioning and the relationship to HIV will be further discussed later in the chapter.

LINK WITH PSYCHOPATHOLOGY

IPV AND PSYCHOPATHOLOGY

With the stressful and often traumatic nature of IPV, the mental health consequences are important to consider and may influence the risk of HIV. Consistently, IPV has been found to be associated with a wide range of negative mental health outcomes. Severity and duration of IPV is strongly associated with increased mental health problems.[71,72] In 1999, Golding[73] did a meta-analysis examining the literature on these associations and found that although prevalence estimates varied greatly by the sample population, the magnitude of the associations reported between IPV and various mental health problems (depression, PTSD, alcohol abuse/dependence, drug abuse/dependence, and suicidality) were quite consistent across studies. Women with IPV exposure had approximately 4 to 6 times greater odds of experiencing the various mental health outcomes studied.[73] Since this important study was published, a number of other researchers have examined these associations to further clarify the relationship between IPV and psychopathology.

One of the most studied mental health problems associated with IPV is depression or mood disorders.[74-76] The past year prevalence of a mood disorder among women in the general population who experienced IPV was 12% compared to 7% among women who did not experience IPV.[77] With regard to depression, women who were exposed to IPV were 3 times more likely to have depression compared to women without IPV exposure.[74] The relationship between IPV and depression follows a dose-response pattern with increasing frequency, duration, and severity of IPV leading to stronger associations with depressive symptoms.[71,78,79]

Similarly, anxiety is more common among women exposed to IPV compared to women without IPV exposure.[79] Thirty percent of those women who experienced IPV reported a past year anxiety disorder compared to 17% of those not experiencing IPV.[77] The increase in odds of having an anxiety disorder if exposed to IPV ranges from 1.3 to 2.7.[74,77,80] PTSD is one disorder that occurs in response to a specific traumatic event or repeated traumatic events. Due to the traumatic nature of IPV, there may be a unique link between IPV and PTSD with IPV leading directly to PTSD.[81] There appears to be a dose-response relationship with increasing severity of IPV being associated with high levels of PTSD symptoms.[81] Studies have reported that IPV increases the odds of PTSD by up to 6 times,[76] with more conservative estimates of approximately 3 times.[82]

Research suggests that substance abuse is also associated with IPV.[74,77] This relationship exists for any substance abuse,[74,77] alcohol abuse,[71,78] illicit drug use,[80] and tobacco use.[74,76] Substance use problems may be 3 to 6 times more common among those exposed to IPV.[74,77]

There are a number of other mental health problems that are also associated with IPV including general psychological distress,[83] social problems,[74] disruptive disorders (ie, oppositional defiant disorder and intermittent explosive disorder),[77] hostility and somatization,[79] and eating disorders.[80] These findings highlight the wide spreading effects that IPV can have on a woman's functioning in many different areas. Also concerning is the strong association of IPV to suicidal behaviors including ideation,[77,84] attempts,[85] and self-harm.[80] The odds of suicidality may increase as much as 3 to 7 times among women exposed to IPV.[77,84]

With the extent of negative mental health outcomes associated with IPV, it is necessary to examine the cumulative impact that IPV and mental health problems have on society. Vos and colleagues[80] used burden of disease methodology to look at the overall effects that IPV has on women's health. Among women ages 15 to 44, IPV was the greatest risk factor for ill health, accounting for 8% of disease for these women. The next risk factor was illicit drug use, which accounted for only 3.5% of disease for these women. They estimated that of the total disease burden associated with IPV, approximately 73% could be attributed to the high prevalence of depression, anxiety, and suicide among this population.

Although IPV has generally been studied in women, men can also be the victims of IPV. Men's experiences of IPV may be quite different and the mental health consequences are important to examine separately in men. Research findings indicate that IPV is also associated with negative mental health outcomes in men.[77,79,86] However, mental health impairment was more prominent among women victims of IPV compared to men victims of IPV.[77,79,87] Among men who were victims of IPV, externalizing disorders such as substance use or disruptive disorders are particularly common.[77,86,88]

Culture is also important to consider in the relationship between IPV and psychopathology. Different cultures have different norms for relationships and individuals may respond quite differently to an experience based upon expectations. There may also be different mediating and moderating factors within various cultural contexts such as stigmatization, poverty rates, and social support. Although most of the research is from North American, similar associations to psychopathology have been found in Spain,[72] Ethiopia,[84] Australia,[80] South Africa,[88] and India.[89] However, some studies have found differences in the associations in various ethnic groups within the US population. For example, a study of immigrant Latino women found no association between IPV and depression but did find an association with PTSD.[82] The association between IPV and psychopathology may be stronger in white women compared to African American women, likely because of a higher prevalence of psychopathology in non-abused African American women.[90]

Many of the studies have been cross-sectional in nature, making it hard to determine if the stress of IPV leads to increased psychopathology or if certain aspects of psychopathology put individuals at increased risk of being victimized. There has been some evidence to support both hypotheses. IPV has been used to predict later-onset depression, life satisfaction, and functional impairments.[91] Depression has also been used to predict later onset IPV.[92] Another study provides support for both hypotheses but suggests that these pathways may be different for different people.[93] Ehrensaft et al[93] found that psychopathology predicted future IPV to some degree for both males and females, although more so for males, while IPV predicted future psychopathology for females but not males. Perhaps the causal pathways are more complex than the proposed hypotheses. There are many factors that play an important role in understanding the relationship between IPV and psychopathology. The frequency, severity, and duration of the IPV, the gender of the victim, and the cultural context of the relationship are all important to consider when examining these relationships.

HIV AND PSYCHOPATHOLOGY

As with IPV, there has been a great deal of research focusing on associations between HIV and psychopathology. HIV has been linked to depression,[94-96] bipolar disorder,[97] anxiety disorders,[97] PTSD,[98,99] personality disorders,[97] and substance use disorders.[100,101] Comorbidity of HIV, substance use, and another psychiatric disorder are also relatively common with prevalence estimates ranging between 10 and 50%.[100,102,103] However, the prevalence estimates vary depending on the sample population and the instrument used to make diagnoses.[104] When trained clinicians use the MINI for diagnoses, which is considered the "gold standard," 19% of individuals with HIV meet criteria for a current disorder including depression, PTSD, and alcohol abuse or dependence.[104] Suicidality is also quite prevalent in those who are HIV-positive[100] with rates up to 18% higher than in those who are HIV-negative.[105] A large proportion of suicidality is reported to be a response to HIV status.[100] The progressive state of HIV illness may have an impact on psychopathology and suicidality.[100,106] As HIV progresses and becomes symptomatic, rates of depression rise in this population.[94]

Many studies report that the onset of psychopathology generally occurred after a positive test for HIV.[95,105] HIV could lead to psychopathology through the increased stress caused by the illness as well as through the physiological effects that HIV may have in the later stages, such as cognitive decline.[96] HIV is associated with a decrease in social support, fear of disease progression, unemployment, and increased relationship problems.[105] Some suggest that some psychopathology may occur in response to the stigma associated with having HIV, particularly for men in sub-Saharan Africa.[98,107]

However, other data suggests that psychopathology is more likely to precede the onset of HIV with a small percentage of substance use following a positive HIV test to cope with this information.[100] One potential path from psychopathology to HIV is through risky sexual behaviors. Psychopathology is related to unfavorable attitudes towards condom use,[108] engaging in unprotected sex,[108] having multiple sexual partners, and trading sex.109 These findings are not surprising given that some specific disorders include impulsivity and promiscuity in the diagnostic criteria such as borderline personality disorder, antisocial personality disorder, and bipolar disorder.[110] For those with a bipolar disorder, HIV risk behavior is strongly associated with having a recent manic episode.[109] Individuals with low psychopathology also have greater HIV knowledge, less anxiety about contracting HIV, and lower rates of other STIs.[108]

HIV risk behaviors are more common when drug severity is greater.[109] It is quite possible that at least some of the association between psychopathology and risky sexual behaviors is mediated by substance use.[111] The use of some substances (ie, injection drugs) is a direct risk factor for HIV, but substances also reduce inhibitions and can lead to poor decision making.[111] In a psychiatric outpatient population, having a comorbid substance use disorder increases the risk of being HIV-positive 4 or 5 times more than individuals with just 1 psychiatric disorder.[97]

As previously discussed, IPV is associated with decreased immune functioning, as is psychopathology. One of the main indicators of progression from HIV to AIDS is by the reduction in CD4 cells, which fight infection.[112] Longitudinal studies have found that depression predicted lower CD4 counts over 3 months[113] and 6 months.[99] While another, more recent study did not find an association between increased psychopathology and a reduction in CD4 cells.[114] However, this study did not look at changes in CD4 cells but mean number of cells at one time point and did not include stage of HIV in the analyses. It is in the later stages of HIV that new onset depression signals a dropping CD4 count.[115] Depression is also associated with changes in levels of cortisol, which is a hormone released in response to stress, and dehydroepiandrosterone (DHEA), which is a cortisol antagonist.[116]

PTSD does not appear to have the same relationship with CD4 counts among those with HIV in studies with short (ie, 3 to 6 months) follow-ups,[99,117] however one study found that, at a 2-year follow-up, those with PTSD had reduced CD4 counts compared to those without PTSD.[118] PTSD has been linked to a longer duration of infection.[99] There is also some evidence that PTSD may be associated with cortisol levels.[119]

Although psychopathology may have a direct effect on immune system functioning, there may also be an effect on health behaviors such as adherence to treatment that is related to stage of the illness. Psychological distress in general is associated with reduced adherence to medication.[120] One longitudinal study found that comorbid PTSD and depression predicted adherence over a 3-month period.[113] However, another study that was able to separate PTSD and depression found that depression was the only factor that contributed to less adherence to treatment.[121]

The relationship between HIV and psychopathology may be bidirectional with psychopathology leading to HIV through increased risk behaviors and decreased immune functioning, as well as HIV leading to psychopathology due to stress associated with having HIV. The direction of the relationship may depend on the type of psychopathology in question and the population being studied.

The Intersection of IPV, HIV, and Psychopathology

IPV, HIV, and psychopathology commonly co-occur. However there are few studies examining interactions between these variables. For example, the use of alcohol and the experience of sexual IPV both increase the risk of contracting HIV, but if both risk factors are present the risk becomes even greater although no interactions were examined.[122] Similar results are seen when examining psychopathology as the outcome, with HIV and IPV acting as additive risk factors. IPV appears to be a slightly bigger risk factor for psychopathology than HIV alone, however when they are combined the risk for depression increases by 7 times, anxiety by 5 times, suicidal ideation by 4 times, and suicide attempts by over 12 times.[106]

Substance use is a main factor that has been identified as a potential mediator of pathways to HIV. Substance abuse during sex is associated with risky sexual behaviors such as having sex with an intravenous drug user and having a partner who uses substances during sex.[123] IPV is also related to having a partner who engages substance use during sex. However, it was IPV that demonstrated a 6 times greater risk for having an STI as well as having a sexual partner who has sex with sex trade workers, intravenous drug users, and engages in substance use during sex.[123] Cavanaugh and Hansen124 examined substance use as a mediator between PTSD and risky sexual behavior but substance use did not appear to mediate the relationship. Interestingly, the relationship between IPV and substance use may be stronger among women who are HIV-negative compared to those who are HIV-positive.[101]

Depression, substance use, and IPV are additive risk factors for STIs, increasing the odds by up to 19 times; however there do not appear to be interactions between these factors.[125,126] The paths that link these factors may be more complex and require the use of different models. A path analysis found support for psychopathology as a mediator between IPV and health related quality of life and reduced adherence to HIV treatment.[127]

Dutton and colleagues[128] suggest that PTSD may act as a mediator between IPV and negative health outcomes such as HIV through changes the PTSD has in terms of a person's psychology, biology, neurology, and behavior. This claim brings together the findings about IPV and psychopathology being associated to immune functioning, as well as each other, with mixed results. One study examined the levels of cortisol and DHEA and compared women's experience of IPV and psychopathology.[129] Depression and anxiety were each correlated to cortisol levels although PTSD was not. No type of psychopathology was related to DHEA levels. However, IPV was related to higher levels of both cortisol and DHEA and this relationship was not mediated by psychopathology.[129] This study may suggest that there are direct links between IPV and immune functioning that could lead to vulnerability to HIV.

Another way to examine immune functioning is through the ability of a body to neutralize a virus. Garcia-Linares and colleagues[130] examined the ability of women's saliva to neutralize the herpes simplex virus type 1. Women experiencing depression, state anxiety, PTSD, and IPV all had a reduced ability to neutralize the virus. Again, the relationship between IPV and immune functioning was not mediated by psychopathology.

Although these studies have failed to find a mediating effect of psychopathology, there has been some evidence to support this hypothesis. Woods et al[131] presented a bio-psycho-immunological framework to make specific predictions about what type of immune responses will occur for depression and PTSD. The experience of IPV creates a stress response that affects the hypothalamic-pituitary-adrenal (HPA) axis, a major part of the neuroendocrine system.[131] The HPA axis responds within minutes or hours. It is the HPA axis response that leads to the release of cortisol as well as responds to a negative feedback system to reduce the cortisol response. Decreased sensitivity of the HPA axis to the negative feedback system, which is often seen in those with depression, leads to higher levels of cortisol.[119] Conversely, PTSD is associated with an increased sensitivity of the HPA axis to the negative feedback system, leading to lower levels of cortisol.[119] These different reactions have important implications for the functioning of the immune system and will affect the activity of CD4 cells.

There are 2 different subsets of CD4 cells: the Th1 subset, which promotes inflammation and protects against intracellular microbes, and the Th2 subset, which suppress intracellular defense reactions, protects against helminthic parasites, and leads to the production of antibodies.[132] The response of one subtype of CD4 cells will lead to a reduction in the activity of the other type. The shifts seen in depression facilitate reaction from the Th2 subset, which may be associated with vulnerability to infections, allergies, and tumors.[132] In contrast, the shifts seen with PTSD may facilitate reaction from the Th1 subset, leading to vulnerability to autoimmune disorders and chronic pain.[131]

Woods et al[131] examined one type of biomarker (IFN-γ) for immune functioning that is associated with Th1 activity. Women who had experienced IPV as well as those with PTSD reported more chronic pain, as well as increased IFN-γ levels. The relationship between IPV and IFN-γ level was mediated by PTSD symptoms. Depression did not have an effect on IFN-γ level. Women who had both depression and PTSD responded more like women in the PTSD group than the depression group. This study highlights the importance of examining different types of psychopathology as well as comorbidity when examining immune functioning.

The relationship between IPV, psychopathology, and HIV is complex and an accurate understanding of the pathways that link these conditions required attention to important distinctions in terms of type of IPV, type of psychopathology, and the population being studied. **Figure 28-7** shows the possible pathways that exist between IPV, HIV, and psychopathology. The pathways that have some support link IPV to increased psychopathology, risk behaviors, decreased immune functioning, and potentially sexual IPV directly to HIV. Psychopathology has been linked to increased risk behaviors and reduced adherence to HIV treatment, decreased immune functioning, and increased risk for IPV. Risk behaviors and reduced immune functioning increase the risk of contracting HIV. HIV, in turn, can lead to increased psychopathology and risk behaviors.

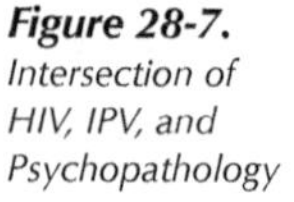

Figure 28-7.
Intersection of HIV, IPV, and Psychopathology

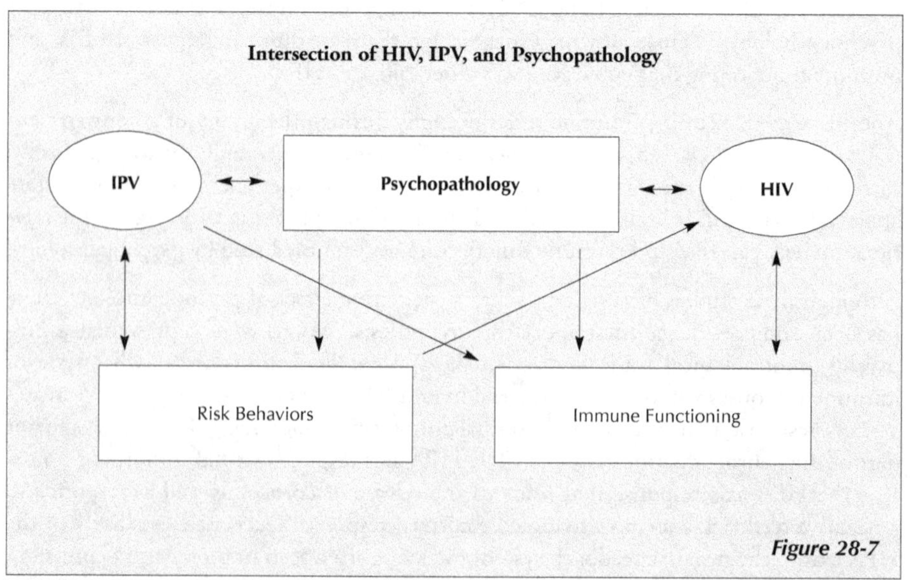

PREVENTION AND INTERVENTION STRATEGIES

IPV and HIV are important and challenging public health concerns. Health care challenges are understandable due to the intersection and overlap of related issues associated with both HIV and IPV. The discussion of prevention and intervention efforts must be tailored to reflect this intersection among IPV and HIV at both the individual and systems level; IPV and HIV affect all genders, all races, and individuals regardless of country of origin. Factors such as the low social status of women, the role of power, and causal pathways are important considerations when designing interventions to target both IPV and HIV. The following section will discuss the following areas associated with prevention and intervention strategies: 1) health care provider interaction; 2) skill building; 3) the level of the individual; and 4) the risk environment.

As the link between violence and HIV become clearer, both HIV and IPV and related factors are being included in prevention and intervention activities at the health provider level. For example, in 2006 the CDC modified violence counseling guidelines to include an option for HIV testing.[133] Although it is important to understand the linkage between IPV and HIV, the presence of risk-based testing is not appropriate, and as such the CDC recommends that all individuals should be routinely offered HIV testing.[134] A study by Rountree and Mulraney[135] focuses on techniques that clinicians and social workers can use to encourage safety among women who have experienced IPV. Patient and health provider contact is an important opportunity to screen and discuss IPV at multiple levels in order to prevent and possibly mitigate some of the negative outcomes associated with HIV. Provider contact is also a time where the encouragement of sexual safety and education can occur by exploring attitudes and beliefs related to sexual history and HIV prevention practices. Patient skill building is an important component of both prevention and intervention programs that can occur along side or independent of health care providers. Screening and effective intervention for IPV can include components of HIV-related services such as prevention programming, counseling and testing, and treatment for HIV.[136]

Individuality is also an important consideration in any prevention or intervention program. Focusing on the level of the individual allows the tailoring of services and prevention efforts. An important point linked to this idea is the lack of consistency as to how women of different races and ethnicities define abuse. Rountree and Mulraney[135] highlight this fact and discuss the importance of clarification around what IPV means to the individual. Similarly, awareness of cultural differences of gender roles has been highlighted as important in helping clinicians to determine a patient's level of HIV risk.[3]

As discussed in this chapter, an important consideration in prevention and intervention programs must include sexual orientation. Individuals of all genders experience IPV differently, and have differing risks of acquiring HIV. Stevens et al[137] found that individuals reporting injection drug use and/or who had experienced childhood sexual abuse were more likely to report IPV. The authors recommend that clinicians working with women who report injection drug use or childhood sexual abuse should be aware of the probability of IPV and include discussions related to of self efficacy, body ownership, and safety. With respect to sexual orientation, the authors found that there were differences in IPV behaviors among heterosexual and gay or lesbian partners with lesbians reporting similar high aggressive IPV behaviors as compared to heterosexual women. This finding highlights the importance of understanding risk factors specific to the individual in order to develop intervention and prevention programs. IPV is not a heterosexual problem or problem that only affects women. The link between IPV and HIV is gendered, and intervention programs need to work to change gender norms and issues of power and control which promote abuse and HIV transmission. Krishnan[59] supports this idea and argues for strategies that target how individual choices impinge on the risk environment, and that interventions that have focused on men and gender norms have demonstrated that gender norms are modifiable. The authors discuss the importance of addressing structural pathways from the risk environment to risk behaviors, and how these strategies must involve the linkage of community, clinicians and practice based groups, as well as researchers. Targeting young boys and men in discussions around power, control, and safe sex, as well as empowering women is an important step in reducing the negative outcomes of a gendered environment.

An important consideration for any intervention not only involves the focus of the intervention and implementation among a group of individuals, but the testing and replication of effective programs and practices. National and jurisdictional policies must be involved to ensure that interventions are not only tailored to meet the needs of individuals, but that they also are evaluated and expanded to increase the number of people who may benefit from their services. Randomized controlled trials that examine the effectiveness of interventions are necessary to determine if these interventions are in fact benefiting vulnerable populations, reducing the risk for IPV and HIV transmission, as well as improving health outcomes among all groups, especially those most vulnerable.

CONCLUSION

The state of the science of IPV and HIV is such that each phenomenon has significant health implications, both individually and combined. Although a substantial body of research has focused on the association between IPV and HIV among women, fewer studies have focused on other populations, such as men, gay, lesbian, bisexual, and transgendered individuals. Further research needs to focus on these groups in order to fully understand the relationship between IPV and HIV as well as to develop appropriate interventions that will prevent and treat this problem. Second, the majority of studies in the field often rely on cross-sectional samples that are methodologically limited. Further research is needed that uses longitudinal designs and randomized trials in order to enhance the conclusions that can be made from such research. Randomized intervention trials would provide empirical support for methods of intervention that hopefully would improve health outcomes for those living with IPV or HIV. Third, more research is needed to help explain the mechanisms involved in the interaction between IPV and HIV, as well as the mediating and temporal effects of certain risk behaviors. This detailed information is needed to create effective intervention and prevention programs, as well as inform health care providers in how to best treat individuals impacted by both IPV and HIV. Fourth, in addition to studies that target the interaction between IPV and HIV, studies are also needed that examine the costs associated with these issues. Understanding the costs of IPV and HIV and associated outcomes are necessary in order to gain support to fuel not only intervention, but also health policy and change.

REFERENCES

1. Campbell JC, Baty ML, Ghandour RM, Stockman JK, Francisco L, Wagman J. The intersection of intimate partner violence against women and HIV/AIDS: a review. *Int J Inj Contr Saf Promot.* 2008;15(4):221-231.

2. WHO. Gender inequalities and HIV. World Health Organization Web site. http://www.who.int/gender/hiv_aids/en/. Published 2013. Accessed July 5, 2013.

3. Weidel JJ, Provencio-Vasquez E, Watson SD, Gonzalez-Guarda R. Cultural considerations for intimate partner violence and HIV risk in Hispanics. *J Assoc Nurses AIDS Care.* 2008;19(4):247-251.

4. Barnett OW, Miller-Perrin CL, Perrin RD. *Family Violence Across the Lifespan.* Thousand Oaks, CA: Sage; 1997.

5. Manfrin-Ledet L, Porche DJ. The state of science: violence and HIV infection in women. *J Assoc Nurses AIDS Care.* 2003;14(6):56-68.

6. Lafta RK. Intimate-partner violence and women's health. *Lancet.* 2008;371(9619): Paper presented at: 1140-1142.

7. Krugg E, Dahlberg L, Mercy J, AZwi, Lozano R. *Violence-A Global Health Approach.* Geneva, Switzerland: World Health Organization; 2002:3-21.

8. Tjaden P, Thoennes N. Extent, Nature, and Consequences of Intimate Partner Violence: Findings from the National Violence Against Women Survey. National Institute of Justice Web site. www.ojp.usdoj.gov/nij/pubs-sum/181867.htm. Published July 2000. Accessed July 5, 2013.

9. Tjaden P, Thoennes N. The role of stalking in domestic violence crime reports generated by the Colorado Springs Police Department. *Violence Vict.* 2000;15(4):427-441.

10. Afifi TO, MacMillan H, Cox BJ, Asmundson GJ, Stein MB, Sareen J. Mental health correlates of intimate partner violence in marital relationships in a nationally representative sample of males and females. *J Interpers Violence.* 2009;24(8):1398-1417.

11. Gielen AC, Ghandour RM, Burke JG, Mahoney P, McDonnell KA, O'Campo P. HIV/AIDS and intimate partner violence: intersecting women's health issues in the United States. *Trauma Violence Abuse.* 2007;8(2):178-198.

12. Thompson RS, Bonomi AE, Anderson M, et al. Intimate partner violence: prevalence, types, and chronicity in adult women. *Am J Prev Med.* 2006;30(6):447-457.

13. Plichta SB. Intimate partner violence and physical health consequences: policy and practice implications. *J Interpers Violence.* 2004;19(11):1296-1323.

14. Bonomi AE, Thompson RS, Anderson M, et al. Intimate partner violence and women's physical, mental, and social functioning. *Am J Prev Med.* 2006;30(6):458-466.

15. Wadman MC, Muelleman RL. Domestic violence homicides: ED use before victimization. *Am J Emerg Med.* 1999;17(7):689-691.

16. Sharps PW, Koziol-McLain J, Campbell J, McFarlane J, Sachs C, Xu X. Health care providers' missed opportunities for preventing femicide. *Prev Med.* 2001;33(5):373-380.

17. CDC. Kaposi's sarcoma and pneumocystis pneumonia among homosexual men. New York and California: CDC; 1981:305-308.

18. Kalichman SC, Williams EA, Cherry C, Belcher L, Nachimson D. Sexual coercion, domestic violence, and negotiating condom use among low-income African American women. *J Womens Health.* 1998;7(3):371-378.

19. WHO. HIV/AIDS programme highlights 2008-2009. Geneva, Switzerland: World Health Organization; 2010.

20. CDC. Extent, nature, and consequences of rape victimization: Findings from the National Violence Against Women Survey. Washington, DC: Centers for Disease Control and Prevention; 2006.

21. WHO. AIDS epidemic update. Geneva: Joint United Nations Programme on HIV/AIDS (UNAIDS) and WHO 2009; 2009.

22. Jewkes R, Sen P, Garcia-Morena C. Sexual Violence. In: WHO, ed. *World Report on Violence and Health*. Geneva: World Health Organization; 2002.

23. Alvarez J, Pavao J, Mack KP, Chow JM, Baumrind N, Kimerling R. Lifetime interpersonal violence and self-reported chlamydia trachomatis diagnosis among California women. *J Womens Health (Larchmt)*. 2009;18(1):57-63.

24. Coker AL. Does physical intimate partner violence affect sexual health? a systematic review. *Trauma Violence Abuse*. 2007;8(2):149-177.

25. Coker AL, Flerx VC, Smith PH, Whitaker DJ, Fadden MK, Williams M. Intimate partner violence incidence and continuation in a primary care screening program. *Am J Epidemiol*. 2007;165(7):821-827.

26. Decker MR, Miller E, Kapur NA, Gupta J, Raj A, Silverman JG. Intimate partner violence and sexually transmitted disease symptoms in a national sample of married Bangladeshi women. *Int J Gynaecol Obstet*. 2008;100(1):18-23.

27. Dude A. Intimate partner violence and increased lifetime risk of sexually transmitted infection among women in Ukraine. *Stud Fam Plann*. 2007;38(2):89-100.

28. Ghebremichael M, Paintsil E, Larsen U. Alcohol abuse, sexual risk behaviors, and sexually transmitted infections in women in Moshi urban district, northern Tanzania. *Sex Transm Dis*. 2009;36(2):102-107.

29. Laughon K. Abused African American women's processes of staying healthy. *West J Nurs Res*. 2007;29(3):365-384; discussion 85-94.

30. Roberts TA, Auinger P, Klein JD. Intimate partner abuse and the reproductive health of sexually active female adolescents. *J Adolesc Health*. 2005;36(5):380-385.

31. Campbell JC, Soeken KL. Women's responses to battering: a test of the model. *Res Nurs Health*. 1999;22(1):49-58.

32. Lichtenstein B. Domestic violence, sexual ownership, and HIV risk in women in the American deep south. *Soc Sci Med*. 2005;60(4):701-714.

33. WHO. Violence Against Women and HIV/AIDS: Critical Intersections. http://www.who.int/hac/techguidance/pht/InfoBulletinIntimatePartnerViolenceFinal.pdf. Published 2004. Accessed June 5, 2013

34. Rowntree M, Mulraney M. HIV/AIDS risk reduction intervention for women who have experienced intimate partner violence. *Clin Soc Work J*. 2010;38:207-216.

35. El-Bassel N, Witte SS, Wada T, Gilbert L, Wallace J. Correlates of partner violence among female street-based sex workers: substance abuse, history of childhood abuse, and HIV risks. *AIDS Patient Care STDS*. 2001;15(1):41-51.

36. Raj A, Cheng DM, Levison R, Meli S, Samet JH. Sex trade, sexual risk, and non-disclosure of HIV serostatus: findings from HIV-infected persons with a history of alcohol problems. *AIDS Behav*. 2006;10(2):149-157.

37. Maman S, Yamanis T, Kouyoumdjian F, Watt M, Mbwambo J. Intimate partner violence and the association with HIV risk behaviors among young men in Dar es Salaam, Tanzania. *J Interpers Violence*. 2010;25(10):1855-1872.

38. Champion JD, Shain RN, Piper J. Minority adolescent women with sexually transmitted diseases and a history of sexual or physical abuse. *Issues Ment Health Nurs*. 2004;25(3):293-316.

39. Amaro H, Raj A. On the margin: power and women's HIV risk reduction strategies. *Sex Roles.* 2000;42(7-8):125-134.

40. Heintz AJ, Melendez RM. Intimate partner violence and HIV/STD risk among lesbian, gay, bisexual, and transgender individuals. *J Interpers Violence.* 2006;21(2):193-208.

41. Dunkle KL, Jewkes RK, Brown HC, Gray GE, McIntryre JA, Harlow SD. Transactional sex among women in Soweto, South Africa: prevalence, risk factors and association with HIV infection. *Soc Sci Med.* 2004;59(8):1581-1592.

42. Silverman JG, Raj A, Mucci LA, Hathaway JE. Dating violence against adolescent girls and associated substance use, unhealthy weight control, sexual risk behavior, pregnancy, and suicidality. *JAMA.* 2001;286(5):572-579.

43. Wagner KD, Brief DJ, Vielhauer MJ, Sussman S, Keane TM, Malow R. The potential for PTSD, substance use, and HIV risk behavior among adolescents exposed to Hurricane Katrina. *Subst Use Misuse.* 2009;44(12):1749-1767.

44. Sareen J, Pagura J, Grant B. Is intimate partner violence associated with HIV infection among women in the United States? *Gen Hosp Psychiatry.* 2009;31(3):274-278.

45. McCauley J, Kern DE, Kolodner K, Derogatis LR, Bass EB. Relation of low-severity violence to women's health. *J Gen Intern Med.* 1998;13(10):687-691.

46. Greenberg JB. Childhood sexual abuse and sexually transmitted diseases in adults: a review of and implications for STD/HIV programmes. *Int J STD AIDS.* 2001;12(12):777-783.

47. Kalichman SC, Gore-Felton C, Benotsch E, Cage M, Rompa D. Trauma symptoms, sexual behaviors, and substance abuse: correlates of childhood sexual abuse and HIV risks among men who have sex with men. *J Child Sex Abus.* 2004;13(1):1-15.

48. Browning CR, Laumann EO. Sexual contact between children and adults: a life course perspective. *Am Sociol Rev.* 1997;62(4):540-560.

49. Van Kesteren NM, Hospers HJ, Kok G. Sexual risk behavior among HIV-positive men who have sex with men: a literature review. *Patient Educ Couns.* 2007;65(1):5-20.

50. Weinhardt LS, Kelly JA, Brondino MJ, et al. HIV transmission risk behavior among men and women living with HIV in 4 cities in the United States. *J Acquir Immune Defic Syndr.* 2004;36(5):1057-1066.

51. Rose VJ, Raymond HF, Kellogg TA, McFarland W. Assessing the feasibility of harm reduction services for MSM: the late night breakfast buffet study. *Harm Reduct J.* 2006;3:29.

52. Degenhardt L, Mathers B, Guarinieri M, et al. Meth/amphetamine use and associated HIV: implications for global policy and public health. *Int J Drug Policy.* Sep 2010;21(5):347-358.

53. Deribe K, Woldemichael K, Wondafrash M, Haile A, Amberbir A. Disclosure experience and associated factors among HIV positive men and women clinical service users in Southwest Ethiopia. *BMC Public Health.* 2008;8:81.

54. Halli SS, Ramesh BM, O'Neil J, Moses S, Blanchard JF. The role of collectives in STI and HIV/AIDS prevention among female sex workers in Karnataka, India. *AIDS Care.* 2006;18(7):739-749.

55. Silverman JG, Decker MR, Saggurti N, Balaiah D, Raj A. Intimate partner violence and HIV infection among married Indian women. *JAMA.* 2008;300(6):703-710.

56. Jewkes RK, Dunkle K, Nduna M, Shai N. Intimate partner violence, relationship power inequity, and incidence of HIV infection in young women in South Africa: a cohort study. *Lancet.* Jul 3 2010;376(9734):41-48.

57. Gupta J, Raj A, Decker MR, Reed E, Silverman JG. HIV vulnerabilities of sex-trafficked Indian women and girls. *Int J Gynaecol Obstet.* 2009;107(1):30-34.

58. Panchanadeswaran S, Johnson SC, Go VF, et al. Using the theory of gender and power to examine experiences of partner violence, sexual negotiation, and risk of HIV/AIDS among economically disadvantaged women in Southern India. *J Aggression Maltreat Trauma.* 2008;15(2):155-178.

59. Krishnan S, Dunbar MS, Minnis AM, Medlin CA, Gerdts CE, Padian NS. Poverty, gender inequities, and women's risk of human immunodeficiency virus/AIDS. *Ann N Y Acad Sci.* 2008;1136:101-110.

60. Straus MA, Smith C. Violence in Hispanic Families in the United States: Incidence Rates and Structural Interpretations. New Brunswick, NJ: Transaction; 1990. Cited in: Weidel JJ, Provencio-Vasquez E, Watson SD, Gonzalez-Guarda R. Cultural considerations for intimate partner violence and HIV risk in Hispanics. *J Assoc Nurses AIDS Care.* 2008;19(4):247-251.

61. Breiding MJ, Black MC, Ryan GW. Chronic disease and health risk behaviors associated with intimate partner violence-18 U.S. states/territories, 2005. *Ann Epidemiol.* 2008;18(7):538-544.

62. Dutton MA. Complexity of women's response to violence: response to Briere and Jordan. *J Interpers Violence.* 2004;19(11):1277-1282.

63. Bonomi AE, Anderson ML, Rivara FP, Thompson RS. Health outcomes in women with physical and sexual intimate partner violence exposure. *J Womens Health (Larchmt).* 2007;16(7):987-997.

64. Woods SJ. Intimate partner violence and post-traumatic stress disorder symptoms in women: what we know and need to know. *J Interpers Violence.* 2005;20(4):394-402.

65. Stein M, Miller AH, Trestman RL. Depression, the immune system, and health and illness. findings in the search of meaning. *Arch Gen Psychiatry.* 1991;48(2):171-177.

66. Constantino RE, Sekula LK, Rabin B, Stone C. Negative life experiences, depression, and immune function in abused and nonabused women. *Biol Res Nurs.* 2000;1(3):190-198.

67. Griffin MG, Resick PA, Yehuda R. Enhanced cortisol suppression following dexamethasone administration in domestic violence survivors. *Am J Psychiatry.* 2005;162(6):1192-1199.

68. Sanchez MM, McCormack K, Grand AP, Fulks R, Graff A, Maestripieri D. Effects of sex and early maternal abuse on adrenocorticotropin hormone and cortisol responses to the corticotropin-releasing hormone challenge during the first 3 years of life in group-living rhesus monkeys. *Dev Psychopathol.* Winter 2010;22(1):45-53.

69. Leserman J, Jackson ED, Petitto JM, et al. Progression to AIDS: the effects of stress, depressive symptoms, and social support. *Psychosom Med.* 1999;61(3):397-406.

70. Leserman J, Pence BW, Whetten K, et al. Relation of lifetime trauma and depressive symptoms to mortality in HIV. *Am J Psychiatry.* 2007;164(11):1707-1713.

71. Bonomi AE, Thompson RS, Anderson M, et al. Intimate partner violence and women's physical, mental, and social functioning. *Am J Prev Med.* 2006;30(6):458-466.

72. Ruiz-Pérez I, Plazaola-Castaño J. Intimate partner violence and mental health consequences in women attending family practice in Spain. *Psychosom Med.* 2005;67:791-797.

73. Golding JM. Intimate partner violence as a risk factor for mental disorders: a meta-analysis. *J Fam Violence.* 1999;14(2):99-132.

74. Bonomi AE, Anderson ML, Reid RJ, Rivara FP, Carrell D, Thompson RS. Medical and psychosocial diagnoses in women with a history of intimate partner violence. *Arch Intern Med.* 2009;169(18):1692-1697.

75. Bonomi AE, Anderson ML, Rivara FP, Thompson RS. Health outcomes in women with physical and sexual intimate partner violence exposure. *J Womens Health (Larchmt).* 2007;16(7):987-997.

76. Rhodes KV, Houry D, Cerulli C, Straus H, Kaslow NJ, McNutt L-A. Intimate partner violence and comorbid mental health conditions among urban male patients. *Ann Fam Med.* 2009;7(1):47-55.

77. Afifi TO, MacMillan H, Cox BJ, Asmundson GJG, Stein MB, Sareen J. Mental health correlates of intimate partner violence in marital relationships in a nationally representative sample of males and females. *J Interpers Violence.* 2009;24:1398-1417.

78. Nicolaidis C, Curry M, McFarland B, Gerrity M. Violence, mental health, and physical symptoms in an academic internal medicine practice. *J Gen Intern Med.* 2004;19(8):819-827.

79. Próspero M. Mental health symptoms among male victims of partner violence. *Am J Mens Health.* 2007;1:269-277.

80. Vos T, Astbury J, Piers LS, et al. Measuring the impact of intimate partner violence on the health of women in Victoria, Australia. *Bull World Health Organ.* 2006;84:729-744.

81. Woods SJ, Hall RJ, Campbell JC, Angott DM. Physical health and posttraumatic stress disorder symptoms in women experiencing intimate partner violence. *J Midwifery Womens Health.* 2008;53(6):528-546.

82. Fedovskiy K, Higgins S, Paranjape A. Intimate partner violence: how does it impact major depressive disorder and post traumatic stress disorder among immigrant Latinas? *J Immigr Minor Health.* 2008;10:45-51.

83. Edwards VJ, Black MC, Dhingra S, McKnight-Eily L, Perry GS. Psychiacal and sexual intimate partner violence and reported serious psychological distress in the 2007 BRFSS. *Int J Public Health.* 2009;54:S37-S42.

84. Tadegge AD. The mental health consequence of intimate partner violence against women in Agaro Town southwest Ethiopia. *Trop Doct.* 2008;38:228-229.

85. Pico-Alfonso MA, Garcia-Linares MI, Celda-Navarro N, Blaso-Ros C, Echeburúa E, Martinez M. The impact of physical, psychological, and sexual intimate male partner violence on women's mental health: depressive symptoms, posttraumatic stress disorder, state anxiety, and suicide. *J Womens Health (Larchmt).* 2006;15(5):599-611.

86. Carbone-López K, Kruttschnitt C, MacMillan R. Patterns of intimate partner violence and their associations with physical health, psychological distress, and substance use. *Public Health Rep.* 2006;121:382-392.

87. Vaeth PAC, Ramisetty-Mikler S, Caetano R. Depression among couples in the United States in the context of intimate partner violence. *J Interpers Violence.* 2010;25(5):771-790.

88. Wong FY, Huang ZJ, a DiGangi J, Thompson EE, Smith BD. Gender differences in intimate partner violence on substance abuse, sexual risks, and depression among a sample of South Africans in Cape Town, South Africa. *AIDS Educ Prev.* 2008;20(1):56-64.

89. Chandra PS, Satyanarayana VA, Carey MP. Women reporting intimate partner violence in India: associations with PTSD and depressive symptoms. *Arch Womens Ment Health.* 2009;12(4):203-209.

90. Ramos BM, Carlson BE, McNutt L-A. Lifetime abuse, mental health, and African American women. *J Fam Violence.* 2004;19(3):153-164.

91. Zlotnick C, Johnson DM, Kohn R. Intimate partner violence and long-term psychosocial functioning in a national sample of American women. *J Interpers Violence.* 2006;21(2):262-275.

92. Lehrer JA, Buka S, Gortmaker S, Shrier LA. Depressive symptomatology as a predictor of exposure to intimate partner violence among US female adolescents and young adults. *Arch Pediatr Adolesc Med.* 2006;160:270-276.

93. Ehrensaft MK, Moffitt TE, Caspi A. Is domestic violence followed by an increased risk of psychiatric disorders among women but not among men? a longitudinal cohort study. *Am J Psychiatry.* 2006;163:885-892.

94. Esposito CA, Steel Z, Gioi TM, Huyen TTN, Tarantola D. The prevalence of depression among men living with HIV infection in Vietnam. *Am J Public Health.* 2009;99(52):S439-S444.

95. Jin H, Atkinson JH, Yu X, et al. Depression and suicidality in HIV/AIDS in China. *J Affect Disord.* 2006;94:269-275.

96. Nakasujia N, Skolasky RL, Musisi S, et al. Depression symptoms and cognitive function among individuals with advanced HIV infection initiating HAART in Uganda. *BMC Psychiatry.* 2010;10:44-50.

97. Beyer JL, Taylor L, Gersing KR, Krishnan KRR. Prevalence of HIV infection in a general psychiatric outpatient population. *Psychosomatics.* 2007;48:31-37.

98. Adewuya AO, Afolabi MO, Ola BA, et al. Post-traumatic stress disorder (PTSD) after stigma related events in HIV infected individuals in Nigeria. *Soc Psychiatry Psychiatr Epidemiol.* 2009;44:761-766.

99. Olley BO, Seedat S, Stein DJ. Persistence of psychiatric disorders in a cohort of HIV/AIDS patients in South Africa: a 6-month follow-up study. *J Psychosom Res.* 2006;61:479-484.

100. Atkinson JH, HIggins JA, Vigil O, et al. Psychiatric context of acute/early HIV infection. The NIMH Multisite Acute Infection Study: IV. *AIDS Behavior.* 2009;13:1061-1067.

101. Burke JG, Thieman LK, Gielen AC, O'Campo PJ, McDonnell KA. Intimate partner violence, substance use, and HIV among low-income women: taking a closer look. *Violence Against Women.* 2005;11:1140-1161.

102. Chander G, Himelhoch S, Moore RD. Substance abuse and psychiatric disorders in HIV-positive patients: epidemiology and impact on antiretroviral therapy. *Drugs.* 2006;66(6):769-789.

103. Palmer NB, Salcedo J, Miller AL, Winiarski M, Arno P. Psychiatric and social barriers to HIV medication adherence in a triply diagnosed methodone population. *AIDS Patient Care STDS.* 2003;17(12):635-644.

104. Myer L, Smit J, Le Roux L, et al. Common mental disorders among HIV-infected individuals in South Africa: prevalence, predictors, and validation of brief psychiatric rating scales. *AIDS Patient Care STDS.* 2008;22(2):147-158.

105. Schlebusch L, Vawda N. HIV-infection as a self-reported risk factor for attempted suicide in South Africa. *Afr J Psychiatry (Johannesbg).* 2010;13:280-283.

106. Gielen AC, McDonnell KA, O'Campo PJ, Burke JG. Suicide risk and mental health indicators: do they differ by abuse and HIV status? *Womens Health Issues.* 2005;15:89-95.

107. Simbayi LC, Kalichman S, Strbel A, Cloete A, Henda N, Mqeketo A. Internalized stigma, discrimination, and depression among men and women living with HIV/AIDS in Cape Town, South Africa. *Soc Sci Med.* 2007;64:1823-1831.

108. McMahon RC, Malow RM, Devieux J, Rosenberg R, Jennings T. HIV risk and history of STDs in MCMI-II psychopathology subgroups of comorbid substance abusers. *Am J Drug Alcohol Abuse.* 2008;34:329-337.

109. Meade CS, Graff FS, Griffin ML, Weiss RD. HIV risk behavior among patients with co-occurring bipolar and substance use disorders: associations with mania and drug abuse. *Drug Alcohol Depend.* 2008;92(1-3):296-300.

110. American Psychiatric Association. *Diagnostic and Statistical Manual of Mental Disorders.* 4th ed. Washington, DC: American Psychiatric Association; 1994.

111. Elkington KS, Bauermeister JA, Zimmerman MA. Psychological distress, substance use, and HIV/STI risk behaviors among youth. *J Youth Adolesc.* 2010;39(5):514-5237.

112. Begtrup JH, Melbye M, Biggar RJ, Goedert JJ, Knudsen K, Anderson PK. Progression to acquired immunodeficiency syndrom is influenced by CD4 T-lymphocyte count and time since serocenversion. *Am J Epidemiol.* 1997;145:629-625.

113. Boarts JM, Sledjeski EM, Bogart LM, Delahanty DL. The differential impact of PTSD and depression on HIV disease markers and adherence to HAART in people living with HIV. *AIDS Behavior.* 2006;10(3):253-261.

114. Vink F, Sullman S, Buck N, Kidd M, Seedat S. Psychopathology, fundamental assumptions and CD-4 T lymphocyte counts in HIV-positive patients. *Afr J Psychiatry (Johannesbg).* 2010;13:267-274.

115. Atkinson JH, Heaton RK, Patterson TL, et al. Two-year prospective study of major depressive disorder in HIV-infected men. *J Affect Disord.* 2008;108(3):225-234.

116. Parker KJ, Schatzberg AF, Lyons DM. Neuroendocrine aspects of hypercortisolsim in major depression. *Norm Behav.* 2003;43(1):60-66.

117. Sledjeski EM, Delahanty DL, Bogart LM. Incidence and impact of posttraumatic stress disorder and comorbid depression on adherence to HAART and CD4+ counts in people living with HIV. *AIDS Patient Care STDS.* 2005;19(11):728-736.

118. Reilly KH, Clark RA, Schmidt N, Benight CC, Kissinger P. The effect of post-traumatic stress disorder on HIV disease progression following hurricane Katrina. *AIDS Care.* 2009;21(10):1298-1305.

119. Yehuda R. Current status of cortisol findings in post-traumatic stress disorder. *Psychiatr Clin North Am.* 2002;25(2):341-368.

120. Adewuya AO, Afolabi MO, Ola BA, et al. The effects of psychological distress on medication adherence in persons with HIV infection in Nigeria. *Psychosomatics.* 2010;51:68-73.

121. Vranceano AM, Safren SA, Lu M, et al. The relationship of post-traumatic stress disorder and depression to antiretroviral medication adjerence in persons with HIV. *AIDS Patient Care STDS.* 2008;22(4):313-321.

122. Zablotska IB, Gray RH, Koenig MA, et al. Alcohol use, intimate partner violence, sexual coercion and HIV among women aged 15-24 in Rakai, Uganda. *AIDS Behavior.* 2009;13:225-233.

123. González-Guarda RM, Peragallo N, Urrutia MT, Vasquez EP, Mitrani VB. HIV risks, substance abuse, and intimate partner violence among Hispanic women and their intimate partners. *J Assoc Nurses AIDS Care.* 2008;19(4):252-266.

124. Cavanaugh CE, Hansen NB, Sullivan TP. HIV sexual risk behavior among low-income women experiencing intimate partner violence: the role of posttraumatic stress disorder. *AIDS Behavior.* 2010;14:318-327.

125. Laughon K, Gielen AC, Campbell JC, Burke J, McDonnell K, O'Campo P. The relationship among sexually transmitted infection, depression, and lifetime vioence in a sample of predominatly African American women. *Res Nurs Health.* 2007;30:413-428.

126. Senn TE, Carey MP, Vanable PA. The intersection of violence, substance use, depression, and STDs: testing a syndemic pattern among patients attending an urban STD clinic. *J Natl Med Assoc.* 2010;102(7):614-620.

127. Pantalone DW, Hessler DM, Simoni JM. Mental health pathways from interpersonal violence to health-related outcomes in HIV-positive sexual minority men. *Consult Clin Psychol.* 2010;78(3):387-397.

128. Dutton MA, Green BL, Kaltman SI, Roesch DM, Zeffiro TA, Krause ED. Intimate partner violence, PTSD, and adverse health outcomes. *J Interpers Violence.* 2006;21(7):955-968.

129. Pico-Alfonso MA, Garcia-Linares MI, Celda-Navarro N, Herbert J, Martinez M. Changes in cortisol and dehydroepiandrosterone in women victims of physical and psychological intimate partner violence. *Biol Psychiatry.* 2004;56:233-240.

130. Garcia-Linares MI, Sanchez-Lorente S, Coe CL, Martinez M. Intimate male partner violence impairs immune control over herpes simplex virus type 1 in physically and psychologically abused women. *Psychosom Med.* 2004;66:965-972.

131. Woods AB, Page GG, O'Campo P, Pugh LC, Ford D, Campbell JC. The mediation effect of posttraumatic stress disorder symptoms on the relationship of intimate partner violence and IFN-γ levels. *Am J Community Psychol.* 2005;36(1/2):159-175.

132. Abbas AK, Lichtman AH. *Basic Immunology.* Philadelphia, PA: WB Saunders; 2001.

133. Tufts KA, Clements PT, Wessell J. When intimate partner violence against women and HIV collide: challenges for health care assessment and intervention. *J Forensic Nurs.* 2010;6(2):66-73.

134. Branson BM, Hunter Hansfield H, Lampe MA, et al. Revised recommendations for HIV testing of adults, adolescents, and pregnant women in health care settings. Center for Disease Control Web site. http://www.cdc.gov/mmwr/preview/mmwrhtml/rr5514a1.htm. Published 2006. Accessed July 5, 2013.

135. Rountree M, Mulraney M. HIV/AIDS risk reduction intervention for women who have experienced intimate partner violence. *Clin Soc Work J.* 2010;38:207-216.

136. Davila YR, Bonilla E, Gonzalez-Ramirez D, Grinslade S, Villarruel AM. Pilot testing HIV and intimate partner violence prevention modules among Spanish-speaking Latinas. *J Assoc Nurses AIDS Care.* 2008;19(3):219-224.

137. Stevens S, Korchmaros JD, Miller D. A comparison of victimization and perpetration of intimate partner violence among drug abusing heterosexual and lesbian women. *J Fam Violence.* 2010;25(7):639-649.

Chapter 29

Intimate Partner Violence in China and the Chinese American Community

Kathy Bell, MS, RN
Cheryl C.D. Hughes, PhD

Key Points

1. The Confucian influence on Chinese culture has resulted in a patriarchal society. Confucianism promotes the family as the most important social unit, with the father as the leader of the family.

2. Accurate statistics on the prevalence of IPV in China are unavailable, as either the research has not been done or it is not accessible to Westerners. However, violence against pregnant women in China is prevalent; as studies have shown between 17.9% and 43% of pregnant Chinese women have experienced abuse. Violence often extends into the postpartum period.

3. Many Chinese women suffer domestic abuse in silence because of China's cultural values. Abused Chinese women often suffer from mental health issues and sexual and reproductive issues due to this abuse. Suicide rates in China are higher for women than for men.

4. Chinese American women also suffer from IPV. Often newly-arrived Chinese wives will be particularly vulnerable as they cannot speak the local language and are often pressured to send money back to China.

5. Protection and support for Chinese women experiencing IPV in China and in the United States is limited, although steps are being made to improve this situation.

Introduction

The epidemic of intimate partner violence (IPV) and its associated traumas affect China's 1.3 billion citizens as it does all the citizens of the world. The People's Republic of China (PRC), covering approximately 3.7 million square miles and divided into 23 main provincial units, is the Earth's 4th largest country. It is located in eastern Asia, bordering the East China Sea, Korea Bay, Yellow Sea, and South China Sea, between North Korea and Vietnam. Bordering countries include Afghanistan, Bhutan, Burma, India, Kazakhstan, North Korea, Kyrgyzstan, Laos, Mongolia, Nepal, Pakistan, Russia, Tajikistan, and Vietnam.[1] The climate is diverse, ranging from tropical in the south to subarctic in the north. The Han Chinese forms the dominant ethnic group in the country, with about 91% of the population. There are at least 18 other ethnic groups that account for the rest of the Chinese peoples. Due to the one-child-per-family policy, China is now one of the fastest aging countries in the world. China is a communist state where the Communist Party holds tight political control. In 1978, the Chinese government embarked on market reforms that opened its economy to the Western world.[2] Though China has become an economic powerhouse that now leads the world in exports, the income gap between its richest and poorest citizens is vast and growing. The total population living in poverty is 2.8% according to PRC statistics, yet poverty rates can be deceptive, as each nation devises its own definition of poverty. PRC rural population figures indicate that 21.5 million people live below the official "absolute poverty" line, which is defined as approximately $90 per year, or less than 25 cents a day; an additional 35.5 million rural people live above that level but below the official "low income" line of approximately $125 per year, a mere 35 cents a day.[1] Even in developing China, these are paltry sums. There are also major differences in the socioeconomic poles between the rural and urban areas, the eastern seaboard and the west, and the north and the south, which includes Hong Kong.

Intimate Partner Violence and Chinese Culture

In order to effectively address the serious issues surrounding China's intimate partner and familial violence, one must have an understanding of what motivates Chinese to commit violence or put up with violence and what sets them apart from anyone else. China has a very old and complex history, and for many years it dominated the world's arts and sciences. Its ancient history still influences the Chinese customs and mores of today. Culture shapes how we view life. It embodies the way we live and helps define what is important to us. It establishes a set of rules and expectations for appropriate behavior. An individual's perception of violence and victims reflects the norms, opportunities, and restrictions of gender that exist within one's sociocultural environment. It is through the family that the individual learns about culture.[3]

There are cultural values that influence family violence. The influence may either be supportive, allowing the population to thrive violence-free or, conversely, add to the occurrence of family violence. Patriarchy within the Chinese culture is almost always mentioned when discussing relationship violence. Much of the blame for family violence has been placed on patriarchal views that devalue women and girls.[4] Male violence displays a patriarchal sense of possessiveness and control.[5] According to Chinese Confucian cultural norms, girls must obey their fathers, wives must obey their husbands, and widows must obey their eldest son. Suffering, endurance, and fatalism in this rigidly hierarchical system are other factors that may influence tolerance for violence within families. Historically, women have been socialized into submissive and subservient roles. In spite of the emphasis on family harmony and conflict avoidance, violence against women is tolerated. It has been suggested that because of the inferior status given women in the society it has been argued that this makes aggression more tolerable.[6] Perseverance is derived from the Confucian tradition of self-control and includes strategies of patience and non-resistance making it unusual for a woman to blatantly resist abuse. Buddhist influences in predestination beliefs are seen within interpersonal and social events.[6] "Face" is another important aspect of Chinese women's tendency to do nothing about domestic violence. "Face" is a set of complex personality constructs including self-esteem, social desirability, need for achievement, social anxiety, and interpersonal relationships.[7] The value of saving face may keep a victim of violence from ever reporting or discussing the event so that humiliation and disgrace are avoided at all costs. It is not uncommon for abused women to be more concerned with their partners and families than with themselves. China's civilization is over 5000 years old. These values and associated family structures did not just appear overnight. In large cities such as Beijing and Shanghai, some of the opportunities such as education and careers that have always been afforded to men are now opening up to women so that the entire society is in a state of flux economically and socially. The more educated and economically self-sufficient women in the newly urbanized China are less likely than their rural, more traditional sisters of old to fatalistically endure the sufferings of family violence. The willingness of these better educated urban women to confront abuse and abusers is opening up space in Chinese society to finally do something about violence toward women.

The World Health Organization cites violence against women as both a consequence and a cause of gender inequality.[8] Chinese gender inequality and violent familial or intimate relationships are rooted in antiquity and grounded in the values of its Confucian, Daoist, and Buddhist past.[9] While Confucianism is more explicitly androcentric, Daoism and Buddhism are less so. The subjugation of women is most often laid at the doorstep of Confucian thought, prevalent almost throughout the Imperial Period (221 BCE-1919 CE) and beyond, with influence even into the present. Indeed, Confucianism was the official ideology of the state from the Han Dynasty (206 BCE-220 CE) on and formed the substance for the imperial examinations by which young men attained entrance into the civil service at varying ranks and levels of administration. Communist China has sought without much success to bring equality to the sexes, for as Mao observed, "Women hold up half the sky." A brief review of Confucian values and ideas and those of Daoism and Buddhism will form the background for understanding Chinese familial and gender relations.

CONFUCIONISM

Confucius (510-479 BCE) lived in the small state of Lu during the Spring and Autumn Period (771-475 BCE) and the Warring States Period (475-403 BCE).[9] His was a time of almost ongoing conflict and war. As a result, Confucius was concerned primarily with political harmony. For Confucius, the family was the most important social unit and the crucible for all other relations. Harmony in the home would lead to social harmony, and social harmony would lead to harmony within the state, because the emperor's moral, beneficial, and benevolent rule was to mirror that of the father within the family. The emperor was to be "father" to all the Chinese people and by Heaven's Mandate held his power only for their benefit. The emperor was to be the embodiment of ren, a word that does not translate easily into English. **Ren** is a verbal expression that literally means "two" and "human," indicating that one is fundamentally a part of a larger whole.[10] The person who embodies ren has achieved a specific social excellence appropriate to specific social relations wherein a person is situated. An excellent son displays the "ren" appropriate to "sonship." Ren is a virtue comprehensive in scope that is to be cultivated by all people according to their specific positions in life.

To promote familial harmony and to nurture ren, Chinese children were taught the 5 constant virtues of benevolence, righteousness, propriety, wisdom, and fidelity. These were the virtues to be developed by everyone, male and female. Confucius believed that men and women were basically good and that self-cultivation of virtue and attention to duty resulted in harmonious relationships, encompassed by the 5 main relationships: ruler-subject, husband-wife, father-son, older brother-younger brother, and friend-friend.[11] Except for the friend-friend relationship, an implied verticality and hierarchy is involved in each of these relationships. The woman Confucian scholar Ban Zhoa (45-116 CE) argued for the education of women parallel to that of men.[11] She reasoned that if the Confucian man became a superior being, one with ren, through self-cultivation and education, so could a woman. Yet even so, in her Lessons for Girls, Ban Zhoa cautioned women "to yield to others; let her put others first, herself last."[11]

Marriage and Divorce

The relationship between husband and wife is viewed in Confucianism as the most important relationship within the family. One Confucian statement reads, "A happy union with wife and children is like the music of lutes and harps.... Thus may you regulate your family and enjoy the delights of wife and children."[12] In theory, a woman was subject to her father and her older brother until her marriage. After marriage she was subject to her husband and his parents. As a widow, she was subject to her in-laws if they were still alive or to her son. In practice, many happy homes existed where respect and affection reigned, but also homes remained where men ruled with an iron fist or the wife even ruled. Some emperors were known to be scandalously under the influence of their wife or mother. Dowager empresses especially could and did wield great power as regents for their infant son emperors. Cixi, the last empress of China, is an excellent case in point. She was referred to as the Dragon Lady.[13]

Because Chinese families are patrilineal, that is, calculated through the man's lineage, and patriarchal, with the highest authority by custom, convention, and law invested in the senior most male, wives left their natal homes to live with their husband's family in either extended family homes or in close proximity to their in-laws. Women essentially had no name or rank; they were accorded the deference due to the wife of a man of a certain rank.

Traditionally marriages were arranged between families with or without the mediation of a marriage broker. There was only one legal wife, though concubinage was very common and recognized by law. Concubinage was as common as marriage, but it involved a lower status for the concubine and her children. An emperor could have hundreds or thousands of women in his harem, but only one empress. According to the Confucian text, The Book of Rites, a wife's main duty was to serve her husband and his family by providing sons to carry on the lineage and to oversee the ancestral rites. Wives, then, were functional and substitutable. A wife may be divorced and sent back to her family for failing to produce an heir.[9]

Divorce was a great humiliation for a woman and was generally uncontestable. Even though Confucius considered marriage a contract that could be broken by either party, most women in unhappy marriages, as a rule, did not seek divorce. However, a husband could divorce his wife for 7 reasons, including the failure to produce a son: she is insubordinate to her in-law parents, she is lewd or vulgar, she is envious and sows discord in the family, she is too loquacious, she becomes ill with a foul disease, or she is known to steal. A wife had only 3 defenses to protect herself from divorce: she has been married so long that she has no natal home to go to, she has already observed full mourning for her parents-in–law, or she entered the family when it was poor and helped it to attain great wealth. Short of divorce, a husband could punish his wife, but not mutilate or kill her without the intervention of a state magistrate. A father could also discipline his children but not to include mutilation or death. Such extreme punishments were supposed to be overseen by the state, but it is not uncommon to find households where ultimate punishments were meted out by the husband or father, as the law was usually lax with such men.

Children

Filial piety was the greatest duty in the Confucian world of traditional China. A father's complaint of unfilial behavior on the part of his son or daughter could be punished by death. Filial piety was expressed in 2 main actions, unquestioning obedience to parents, including the mother, and sacrificial rites to ancestors. Such strictures were incumbent on even adult children. Youths and adult children were to do nothing that would bring shame on the family name. They were brought up to be in awe of the emperor, to love their mother, to love and honor their father, and to revere their ancestors. According to the Confucian Mencius (372-289 BCE), there are 5 unfilial acts: laziness; gambling and drinking; prizing money, goods, wives, or children over one's father; falling to wicked temptations or depravity; and reckless bravery, quarrelling, or fighting. These unfilial acts not only bring shame and disharmony in the family, but they also give rise to disharmony in society and so are unfilial to the emperor as well as to one's father.

Male children were especially valued in Chinese families, and in rural and poor families female infanticide was not uncommon. In families with multiple concubines, the legal wife held the place of honor. If she had no male children, she could be replaced by a subsequent concubine who presented the master with a son. Concubines held a rank below that of the wife, but equal to one another and could only gain rank through their sons. This led to jealousy and discord in families that could, in its most egregious form, result in the murder of male children and their mothers by scheming concubines. Step-parenting was common in traditional families, especially where the husband loved and esteemed his first wife, even though she bore no sons. The son of a concubine could be taken away from her and given to the first wife to rear as her own. The child would call number one wife "mother" and his birth mother "aunty." In the case where concubines were raised to the rank of first wife, her step-mothering of the previous wife's children could be very harsh and even fatal to any sons older than her own. The preference for male children and the favoring of older members of a family also led to older brothers holding tyranny over younger siblings. The current 1-child policy in China has led to such a high abortion rate for female babies that there is a serious gender imbalance in the younger Chinese population. The highest imbalance was reached in 2008 when there were 120.56 baby boys for every 100 girl babies. For 2012 the ratio of Boy to girl babies was 117 to 100.[14]

Yin and Yang

A belief common to Confucianism, Daoism, and Chinese Buddhism that affects the way Chinese think about gender and familial relationships is that of the complementarity of yin and yang. Most people think of yin and yang as binary opposites. Yin is thought of as female, soft, passive, wet, in, diffuse, cold, night, moon, yielding, earth, while yang is considered male, hard, hot, assertive, dry, out, solid, focused, fire, sky, sun. Oppositions between yin and yang are thought to be natural divisions of "just the way things are and how they are supposed to be;" and, therefore, between the spheres of maleness and femaleness, men and women, with men being privileged over women in the hierarchy, there is naturally a division and the unfortunate hierarchy. Rosenlee states, "The concept of male/female whose distinction rests exclusively on biological, sexual differences, in the Confucian tradition, by and large applies to animals, not humans. Gender in the human world signifies strictly social roles and relations. It is through occupying different familial, kinship roles that 'woman' as a gendered being is made."[15] Because the kinship system is hierarchical, so are the relations between men and women. In fact, as can be clearly seen in the symbol, yin and yang are a continuum along which the boundaries may be negotiated. Thus, correctly understood, yin and yang do not indicate conflict and competition, but complementarity. This is an important but perhaps too subtle of a philosophical and ontological difference which nonetheless has worked to the disadvantage of women and children in China.

Women in Daoism and Buddhism

Daoism, even with its emphasis on yin and yang distinctions, is not inherently sexist; rather, it sees women's activities and representations in accordance with five "visions and roles:" female as cosmic mother and as an expression of fertility; women as symbols of the cosmic yin, as the complement to the cosmic yang; women as divine teachers; women mediators of divine communication and divine healing; the female body as the locus for the ingredient to achieve immortality. There are a number of Daoist female deities, such as the Queen Mother of the West, who was worshipped before the rise of Daoism, Queen of Immortals, Mother of the Dao, and the astral Dipper Mother. The primary text of Daoism, the Daode Jing, promotes the virtues of gentleness and receptivity which are seen in the West as feminine virtues. The text itself is gender neutral in the Chinese except for the sixth verse:

The Spirit of the Valley never dies.

They call it wondrous female.

Through the portal of her mystery

Creation ever wells forth.[16]

One role that both Daoism and Buddhism opened up for women was that of a nun, and, with it, its attendant education. Nuns and their monasteries were very important in the rise of Daoism and Buddhism as religions. Rather than withdrawing from the community, nuns contributed to its well-being by virtue of their charity and teaching roles. In addition, they performed various purifications, social rituals, and exorcisms for the benefit of their nearby communities. Monasteries were also havens for divorced or widowed women and orphaned children. As the recipients of largess from the imperial court and the court families, as well as from wealthy merchants and landlords, religious women could exercise a great deal of independence and influence as the founders or abbesses of convents, great and small. In fact, both monasteries for men and women became so rich and powerful that they would be abolished periodically by the emperor and their monks and nuns turned out. Some of the Daoist and Buddhist nuns have become Daoist immortals or Buddhist bodhisattvas, those who through compassion for suffering humanity put off Nirvana to help bring others to Enlightenment. The Tang Empress Wu Zetian (624-705), China's only female monarch, claimed to be a bodhisattva. Chinese nuns have become important role models for the behavior of other women, and remain so today. On the other hand, as an ancillary in the abuse of women, Buddhism may contribute to the wife's role in an abusive marriage by encouraging the idea that through the wheel of birth-death-and-rebirth she ought to accept her karma in this life as punishment for sins in her past life, with the belief that, by fulfilling her duty in this life, she is ensuring herself a better life in her soul's next reincarnation.

INTIMATE PARTNER VIOLENCE IN CHINA TODAY

The People's Republic of China has gone through political, economic, and social changes that have significant impact not only on the daily lives of her citizens but also on their values and worldviews.[17] Since 1979, the PRC government has formulated or amended laws and regulations to increase the protection of women.[17] In 1992 the Law on the Protection of Rights and Interest of Women, which prohibits discrimination against and maltreatment of women, was enacted. In 2001 an amendment to the marriage law included the term "domestic violence" for the first time. In 2001, Xu, Campbell, and Zhu outlined needs for practice, policy, and research, some of which are now being realized.[18] They included:

— Effect policy change in China in term of IPV and women's rights issues, the Chinese society and government's awareness of IPV need to be increased.

— Research about IPV is needed to increase Chinese society's awareness of spousal assault.

— As well as research, public education through mass media and educational courses is essential to increase public awareness of IPV.

— Researchers need to investigate the unique culturally related issues (barriers, risk factors) of IPV among Chinese populations

— Culturally valid instruments with the same operational definitions of IPV are needed to make cross-cultural comparisons of IPV

— Health care providers need to take action to conduct culturally appropriate assessments of IPV and assessments of its mental and physical health ramifications.

Although much had been done to address the rights of women, as recently as 2004 there was little known about the prevalence and extent of spousal violence in China. It has been estimated at 1.8% to 50%, depending on the samples and instruments used.[19] Given the size of the population, it is clear that millions of individuals are affected by violence. Such a wide range in the percentages may be due to the lack of consistency in the definition of violence against women. A 2002 study indicated that a broad definition of violence against women was best predicted by using the infliction of psychological harm as a determining criterion.[17] This same study showed that human service professionals had the greatest agreement in identifying rape, unwanted physical touch, and wife abuse as constituting violence against women, but they did not agree on whether foul language, pornography, and sexual discrimination fit the classification. In 2008, the first court order for the protection of personal safety was issued, prohibiting a husband from beating or humiliating his wife.[20] The All-China Women's Federation reported in 2010 that one-third of Chinese households have experienced domestic abuse. The report described those households as mostly rural, with young families, and where there are low educational levels.[20] However, abuse is not limited to the rural areas, and examples throughout most of the literature on abuse in China reflect abuse of all ages, incomes, educational degrees, and spheres of life. Another possibility for the apparent dearth of information on IPV in China is that although some studies and reports of abuse might have been done, they have not been released or made available to Western researchers.[20] This adds to the confusion about the actual incidence of Chinese IPV.

One reference to males as victims was identified, and it stated that 18% of males reported that they had been hit during their current relationship.[21] Same-sex relationships were not mentioned in sources from the Mao years and there were scattered reports during the reform era that mentioned lesbianism as a reaction to abuse or neglect by men or as a compensatory form of sexual contact in the absence of male sexual partners.[22] No known researchers have turned up data specific to same-sex relationships and partner violence in China.

Intimate Partner Violence during Pregnancy

Risk factors for intimate partner violence in general include young age, poverty, low social status, women's disempowerment, stress in daily life, alcohol consumption, and jealousy.[21] Prior to 2001 there were only 2 Chinese population studies that identified risk factors for IPV.[18] These risk factors included unplanned pregnancy and women with husbands or partners who were unemployed. It is unclear whether the actual incidence of violence against women is on the rise. Assaults have been directed at women in their gendered roles particularly if they married far from home or if they failed to produce male children.[22]

More recent studies concerning violence and pregnancy indicate that the percentage of pregnant women that experience violence in China ranges from 17.9% to 43%, indicating a very vulnerable population, with violence often extending into the postpartum period. A current study by Chan indicated that pregnancy is significantly associated with partner violence against women. However he concluded that the demographic and behavioral characteristics of the male perpetrators accounted for the pregnant partners' odds of experiencing any violence or injury. Age was shown to be a factor, especially if the perpetrator was under the age of 34. Financial problems, defined as indebtedness and receiving social security, put the perpetrators at a higher risk for assaulting their partners. Unemployment was not found to be a risk in this particular study, but males who earned more income were at a higher risk for perpetration. Households no longer commonly have a mother-in-law and daughter-in-law residing together as often.[22] It is however common for a mother-in-law to follow the will of her son by disciplining a wife.[19] In-law conflict in relation to abuse of pregnant women was recently studied for the first time in the Chinese population. Women were more at risk of in-law conflict in situations of chronic illness, debt, and use of alcohol. In-law conflict has a strong association with intimate partner violence in the year preceding pregnancy.[19] From the woman's perspective, Chan found that the low income group is at higher risk of pregnancy violence. The man's use of alcohol, just as in many other studies, also was a factor in IPV occurrence aimed at pregnant Chinese women.

The Effects of IPV on Chinese Women

Until earlier in the 21st century there was little written about the response of women in abusive relationships. Tiwari explained the lacunae as resulting from women's persevering approach to problems. She described it as deriving from the Confucian tradition of self-control, which includes such strategies as self-instruction in patience and non-resistance. Tiwari also explained the Buddhist concept of yuan, or predestination, as a protective function in explaining away negative exchanges. Chinese women's response to abuse is limited to the options available to them. The cultural stigma of abuse keeps many from reporting the abuse. Sexual abuse is less likely to be reported because many women believe it is their duty and obligation to submit to their husbands sexually. Other studies have found that Chinese people are generally reluctant to discuss sexual matters at all because sex is a taboo subject in the Chinese culture.[6]

In the first published study of the resiliency and resourcefulness of Chinese women in the face of abuse, Tiwari explained that the women often use the word ren, which in this usage means "endurance," to describe their way of coping.[6] Examples of ren include actions such as doing what the partner wants, trying to please, suffering in silence, or ignoring the abusive behavior. Ren is a conscious purposeful choice that women use to avoid escalation of violence or to please their partner in the hope that the relationship will improve. Just as in other cultures, Chinese women endure the abuse because of socio-economic realities, issues surrounding shame, views of marriage being forever, and ren. However, there are some women who use ren and yuan in the context of ending a relationship. Instead of enduring the abuse, they re-evaluated their situation. Yuan was referred to as the reason for the failed relationship and these women had no apparent feelings of guilt or self-blame.[6] Wu,[23] in 2005, reported that 11.22% of women who had been beaten did not tell anyone. The first people the women preferred to ask for help were family members (39.4%), then friends (32.3%), the police (5.5%), or the community committee (4%).

Sexual and Reproductive Outcomes

Sexual and reproductive health issues are also of concern. Abortions as a result of interpersonal violence are common. According to Wu's surveys, whose study was the first to attempt to understand the situation of domestic violence (DV) among women seeking abortion, the prevalence of DV among ordinary women ranged between 3.4% and 30%, and its prevalence among woman seeking abortion was 15% to 39.5% higher than that among other women.[23] One of the consequences of sexual abuse is the high rate of unwanted pregnancies, because there is usually a failure to use contraception. Specific to the Chinese women seeking abortion, Wu found that more than one-fourth had experienced violence in their daily lives. Sexual abuse was found to be the most common type of abuse in this study, of the women who experience physical abuse, 45.7% were also sexually abused.[23] Wu concluded that there is tremendous opportunity to identify and respond to abuse by educating health care professionals who are still lacking in relevant knowledge of domestic violence. Wu was able to confirm a 2004 study by Parish, who identified severe hitting as a significant risk factor for self-reported adverse general and sexual health outcomes, including sexual dysfunction, sexual dissatisfaction, and unwanted sex.[23]

Mental Health Outcomes

The expression of mental health symptoms vary widely between Chinese and Western cultures. Depression, for example, is largely unreported in the Chinese culture. With careful evaluation of why this might be, it should be noted that Western evaluation tools are being applied within the Chinese context, and they are not capable of generating the results that would be expected in Western cultures.[24] Somatization of psychological symptoms is commonly associated with Chinese cultures just as in many other cultures.[24] On further inspection, it becomes more evident that this may really be another difference in cultural expression and translation. One study in 2007 specifically addressed depression. Lee discussed how depressive emotions are encoded and inscribed not only in feelings and thoughts, but also in bodily experiences and social contexts. Themes were identified in the course of his study, including the embodied emotional experience. Lee described this phenomenon as a linguistic feature where statements about emotional or psychological disturbances are combined with references to the body, especially the heart. The experiences thus became both emotional and physical for victims.[24]

In an earlier study of Chinese language usage employing body-related expressions, Tung shed some light on this feature.[10] He explained that language reflects the cultural values, beliefs, and world-views of the people using it, and that, for the most part, people are not aware of those meaningful revelations. The Chinese language has a large number of words that can be called "body-related," such as heart (mentioned by Lee[24]), the body, or the hand, without directly referring to these body parts. Tung identified 60 expressions of emotions ranging from anger, anxiety, disgust, distress, fear, grief, guilt, happiness, and vexation that invoke the image of heart.[24] Tung used a number of examples to illustrate this phenomenon. One example is shen fen and means social status. Shen means the body and fen means portion or share. Another example is one's mood, xin jin. The first word means heart and the second is area or territory. Qi is another important concept which means breath, air, energy, life force, or even spirit and fluid. Qi, sometimes Westernized as chi, is central to traditional Chinese Medicine and to the people's conceptualization of life. Depression is conceptualized as a disorder of qi.[24] When these concepts of language can be applied to some of the observations made of the Chinese people, at least a partial understanding can be reached about some of the behaviors observed, such as saving face. The Chinese concept of "body" is the thinking, experiencing, feeling, and intuiting "self" responsible for social and ethical concerns.[10]

Thoughts of sadness or venting anger at another confound the Chinese because of their effect on others and loss of social connections. Sadness and its expression may be interpreted as a sign of weakness and is shameful. Chinese who will complain of the body's ills in the medical clinic, will talk more directly of feelings at home with family members.[24] It is not uncommon for women to have suicidal thoughts as a result of abuse.[6] The All China Women's Federation reported in 2010 that domestic violence is a main contributor to high rates of suicide in women in rural areas.[20] Researchers attribute many of the female rural suicides and attempted suicides to impulsive decisions made in the aftermath of spousal or family conflicts, often involving a physically abusive husband, with the added factor of readily available lethal pesticides.[22] Zhang identified mental disorder and high hopelessness as important risk factors among young Chinese (age 15-34). Another risk factor is the experience of negative life events which ranked third highest in order of importance and included domestic violence. Negative life events coupled with dysfunctional impulsivity, low social support, poor relationships with parents, and the lack of coping skills were found to increase the risk of suicide. Female suicides were more often related to events involving the family than were the suicides of men.[25]

SUPPORT FOR CHINESE WOMEN EXPERIENCING IPV

A woman's real and perceived options for addressing interpersonal violence differ based on her perceived sense of self as a member of a family and community.[26] Her values influence her perceived options in response to violence. Chinese women do not readily turn to domestic violence or other social services.[27] Even when they do, there is a lack of community support services. As recently as 2001 there were no women's shelters in China.[18] Governmental agencies in the form of local Women's Federation are available within the community, however many women have a fear of authority and are unlikely to report to the government.[18] Some regions of China have set up assistance organizations such as women's shelters. These shelters are limited in what they can provide and how the services are delivered. Treatment programs tend to address psychological trauma with an emphasis on returning the victims to good health.[28]

The legal consequences of domestic abuse are guided by China's current marriage law. Legislation clearly prohibits domestic violence and puts forward treatment measures. The system has some aspects that are working to protect women from violence. Mediation is a deeply rooted tradition of settling marital disputes.[28] There is an extensive system of mediation in the country involving 840 000 committees and 5 million mediators who have explored many effective measures and accumulated rich experiences in mediation works. No empirical data has been presented on the effectiveness of such an approach. Mediation will not provide protection to all victims of domestic violence. Hao states that there are improvements that need to be made, especially in the area of personal protection in which the perpetrator should be segregated from the victim.[28] The perpetrator would be prevented from entering an area occupied by his victim. Treatment and prevention work with the abusers will be enhanced by trying to understand men who do harm to their domestic partners.[7]

CHINESE MEN AND INTIMATE PARTNER VIOLENCE

Men are responsible for 90% of domestic violence assaults.[20] Yet, prior to 2007, men had for the most part escaped the attention of the research community.[29] The part that men play in IPV was especially imperceptible to the Chinese because, according to Jin, in Chinese culture, physical punishment is documented as the most common form of punishment.[26] What is common becomes banal. Children learn that violence is a means to get what one wants. Jin's research suggested that accepting attitudes towards marital violence are at least partly rooted in the batterers' early exposure to violence in the family of origin. Much more research will be needed to address unanswered issues, such as why, when being almost equally exposed to violence in the family of origin, some men develop positive attitudes toward violence and others do not.[29]

Chan argued in 2009 that understanding violent men's views of themselves and their actions are necessary starting points for efforts at effective intervention and rehabilitation.[7] Disclosing undesirable behavior is a challenge faced by individuals who work with abusers. Just as the women who are primarily the victims of abuse do not want the family to lose face, the abusers do not want to lose face. Men have a need to save face in the presentation of their views and the disclosure of their problems, and they see help-seeking and disclosure as signs of weakness. Though some men have a sense that violence is socially unacceptable, they still hesitate to admit their actions in order to prevent the loss of face. In Chan's study,[7] men used 3 concepts to avoid loss of face when interacting with interviewers about their abusive behaviors. The first was to show that they were "healthy men," the second was to minimize the violence, and the third was to avoid the responsibility altogether. The healthy man attitude was displayed through their accounts of how honorable and responsible they are. Their violence was diluted through their use of words such as hit, kick, or punch, rather than abuse, thus avoiding making a negative value judgment on their actions. The men avoided responsibility for the abuse by placing the blame on their wives, victimizing themselves, and/or putting the blame on external factors. Chan's men also maintained that their lack of knowledge about abuse demonstrated that they had no other choices but to use violence because they did not know how otherwise to deal with the marital conflict. The men's various excuses make it easier to shift the responsibility away from them and thereby save face.[7]

IPV IN THE CHINESE AMERICAN COMMUNITY

Chinese American women suffer from IPV and other family dysfunctions and traumas as do their PRC sisters. Chinese Americans make up a significant part of the Asian immigrant population in the United States. During the 1800s Chinese men first came to the United States as laborers to help build the railroads that would take the gold-seekers and other pioneers west.[4] Chinese communities became known as "Bachelor societies" and there was a booming vice industry.[30] These men were subjected to racism and discrimination. The Chinese Exclusion Act of 1882 was put into place due to prejudices against these workers. What this did was to prohibit family members and other workers from entering the United States. Historically, Chinese women brought to the United States often came in as sex slaves.[4] In 1930 immigration laws became more flexible and allowed Chinese American men to have their Chinese wives in the US. In 1943 the exclusions acts were repealed and the War Brides Act in 1946 allowed Chinese males who served in the US armed forces during World War II to apply for immigration visas for family members in China.[30] It wasn't until 1965 that Chinese immigrants entered the US as a family unit, mostly from Hong Kong and Taiwan.[4,30] Once US-Chinese diplomatic ties were established more immigrated to the United States. Many of the recently immigrated males went to China to marry and returned with their Chinese wives who brought the uniqueness of their culture with them. The brides faced many pressures, such as an inability to speak English to communicate outside the home, the need to become employed to supplement the low income of their husbands, pressure to have children, and they may have been expected to send money back to family in China.[30] To complicate a wife's responsibilities even more, she faced contradictions in the expectations of her new role as an American wife. Chinese American wives were to be "good" wives and that meant they should be competent but not too independent, adjust to a new environment but not become "Americanized," and be nice but not "pretentious."[30] The brides' expectations were quite the opposite. They expected to live in a spacious house with a yard, own a car, travel around the country freely, make a lot of money to send home to relatives, and eventually sponsor family members for immigrations visas. This led to a lot of the brides becoming socially and economically isolated and confined to an existence that supported violence with very limited options for help. They developed health problems associated with partner violence in individuals of Chinese descent including general and sexual health problems. These are similar to the findings of individuals in other cultures also experiencing violence, however the manner in which those symptoms are expressed may be very different. Generally speaking, mental health issues commonly include depression, low self-esteem, anxiety, posttraumatic stress disorder, and substance abuse.[31] Chinese cultural values emphasize organic causation of psychological problems and inhibition of emotions, while focusing minimally on the mind-body dichotomy and intrapsychic concerns.[28]

Even today, Chinese immigrating to the United States are influenced by the Confucian values of patriarchy, emotional control, obligations, and duties.[4] The definition of spousal abuse by Chinese Americans in a study conducted in 2000 was generally defined as physical and sexual, but not in psychological terms.[4] Older Chinese Americans showed tolerance of spousal violence perpetrated in response to an extramarital affair. Tong, in 1998, argued that the etiological roots of physical, emotional and sexual abuse of partners of Chinese heritage could be found in problems of adaptation, cross-cultural clashes, racist oppression by white America, and a repressive heritage in which Confucian values were distorted into a justification for cruel and autocratic power by a small male minority.[4]

Research on Chinese American spousal abuse is interspersed among the Asian American literature. Chinese American males may worry about the fidelity of the wife and use psychologically abusive tactics such as prohibiting them from working, learning English, calling or contacting their families in China, and holding onto their legal documents, and threatening them with divorce or interference with immigration status.[4] Forced sex and controlling the reproductivity of a woman is another form of dominance.[23] Knowing the extent of the problem of family violence in the Chinese American population is difficult due to the limited research on the specific culture, as Chinese Americans are often lumped together with a rather generalized Asian American culture. Another factor, discussed by Lum in Lee's Handbook of Asian Psychology, is that the possibility of wanting to make family violence invisible ought to be expected, because it is difficult and unpleasant to face, especially if there is uncertainty in what can be done to stop it. The cultural value of accepting one's fate might inadvertently lead to an acceptance of violence.[32] Additionally there is always the issue of bringing private matters out in public that violates the cultural norms concerning face and shame.[30,32]

INTERVENTIONS AND SERVICES FOR CHINESE AND CHINESE AMERICAN VICTIMS OF IPV

To effectively provide services to Asian American women in general, there are both individual and community factors to consider. Individual factors would include things such as a woman's fluency with social services, mobility within the environment, and her ability to speak the language of the majority.[27] Community factors would include offering social services in her first language, the level of privacy within the community that she can expect when seeking assistance, the types of services that she can receive, and the historical relationship between her community and the helping professionals including law enforcement and faith-based organizations. Just as helpline and advocacy programs exist in the United States to assist victims and their children, they also exist in China. A number of cities have set up helplines and hotlines such as "Dial 110" to assist with reporting of domestic violence and women's rights issues. Some rural police stations have special counters for handling cases and complaints of domestic violence.[33]

In order to successfully address both the individual and community aspects of services to women, Yoshioka suggests that researchers and practitioners look to HIV/AIDS research/work of the past as a model.[26] She intimates that, by taking into consideration the intersections of science and personal and political agendas, better interventions will result. In the anti-HIV/AIDS model, complex high risk behaviors such as shared needles and condom use were evaluated. Although needle exchange programs are effective in reducing HIV transmissions, they were not embraced because of sociopolitical concerns. Another example used by Yoshioka[26] is in the preference of some Latina women engaging in the high risk behavior of not using condoms for fear of loss of a relationship. Taking these factors into consideration the researchers then focused on the development of harm reduction models to provide nonjudgmental options to individuals in order to lower their risk level. Applying these and other similar concepts to IPV will put the emphasis on safety rather than leaving a relationship. It is already well known that leaving is not going to happen in most circumstances, notwithstanding the culture or nationality of the woman.

Health care workers including nurses, law enforcement, and social services may well bring those attitudes to the interactions with victims and perpetrators of interpersonal violence. According to the UN Secretary General's database on violence against women in an effort to address the issue of domestic violence, the Programme for the Development of Chinese Women expressly forbids all forms of violence against women, and distributes this duty in the form of goals and objectives among component organizations of government.[33] In addition, police academies have added content about combating domestic violence to basic level training programs. Special courts have been developed for the protection of women and children in a number of grassroots community court facilities. In 2009 more than 8000 Women's Federation workers were participating as people's assessors in the adjudication of cases involving interpersonal violence.[33]

THE ROLE OF NURSES

Engaging health care professionals in the care of patients experiencing violence can be challenging in any country. In 2008, 2 conferences were held on the national level hosted by the Chinese Ministry of Health and the United Nations Population Fund. The focus of these conferences was on pilot projects in medical intervention in sexual violence as well as multi-departmental cooperation on violence against women. The plan was to expand training into local medical institutions. Nurses will have an opportunity to be key players in this venture. Since the 1980s, reforms have been taken within Chinese nursing practice to strengthen it as a profession and improve nursing quality.[34] In 2004 Pang and co-authors published a paper on the definition of Chinese nursing that provided an understanding based on Eastern ideologies rather than Western concepts. The definition that was drafted states: nursing means to understand the dynamic health status of a person to dialectically verify health concerns, and to devise interventions with the goal of assisting the person to master the appropriate health knowledge and skills for the attainment of optimal well-being.[34]

In looking at the literature available to nurses in China it was discovered that there indeed are efforts in the nursing literature to broaden the knowledge of issues related to violence. One noted effort is that all abstracts from 2007 onwards for the Journal of Clinical Nursing have been translated into simplified Chinese by the members of the Chinese Consortium for Higher Nursing Education.[35,36] One example of an article focused on interpersonal violence translated in 2011 is Keeling and Mason's "Postnatal Disclosure of Domestic Violence: Comparison with Disclosure in the First Trimester of Pregnancy." Endeavors such as this will enhance the opportunity for dialogue and understanding of nursing as it is practiced in other parts of the world.

Examples of articles specific to IPV in Chinese nursing journals were found in the Chinese Journal of Practical Nursing and Nanfang Journal of Nursing. Topics include investigation of domestic violence and ADHD in school age children, emergent traumatic patients, and effects of domestic violence on aggressive behaviors of schizophrenic patients.

Conclusion

The emphasis on one's duty and obedience as a wife or child by all of China's major traditional intellectual and religious movements cannot help but contribute to the intimidation and abuse within intimate family settings and gender relations. Rosenlee, in her book Confucianism and Women: A Philosophical Interpretation, sets the stage for the Confucianist relationship of friend to friend to become the new paradigm for gender relationships as an ethical relationship grounded in equality and a mutual seeking of the good for both parties.[15] In this way, harmony in marriages between superior men with ren and superior women with ren would render the Confucian ideal of harmony in society and in the state. Unfortunately, in the meantime, Chinese women find that, while the foot binding of many centuries is now a thing of the past, child brides, concubinage, and female infanticide and abortion are still with them, despite contrary efforts on the part of the government of the People's Republic of China.[22] Women in the rural areas, where they are still largely uneducated and perform important economic activities, are particularly prone to abuse and violence within the home. Women who have moved from the countryside to the large cities of China also find they are disadvantaged in their isolation from familial support. Divorce still carries a stigma for women in their fast-changing social world, yet many are finding themselves in that position and often with children to support. Economic security becomes an enormous problem for women alone or in abusive relationships. Suicide statistics show women in China have a higher rate of suicide than men.[25] Women that commit suicide are often overwhelmingly poor, have little education, and have little social support.

Confucianism, Daoism, and Buddhism have all contributed to the way gender relations and familial and sexual relationships are viewed to the present day. If one were to reflect on the yin-yang diagram, one would realize that it is within a fluid circle representing the entirety of existence; there is no yin without at least a little yang, and no yang without some yin in it. Yin and yang are equal and complementary; nothing is only, or exclusively, one or the other; right or wrong, higher or lower have nothing to do with the relations between the sexes or within families.

References

1. Central Intelligence Agency. The world factbook: China. CIA Web site. https://www.cia.gov/library/publications/the-world-factbook/geos/ch.html. Accessed May 4, 2011

2. Gao L-L, Chan SW-C, You L, Li X. Experiences of postpartum depression among first-time mothers in mainland China. *J Adv Nurs.* 2010;66(2):303-312.

3. Amar AF, Bess R, Stockbridge J. Lessons from families and communities about interpersonal violence, victimization, and seeking help. *J Forensic Nurs.* 2010;6:110-120.

4. Malley-Morrison K, Hines DA. *Family Violence in a Culture Perspective: Defining Understanding and Combating Abuse.* Thousand Oaks, CA: Sage; 2004

5. Wang T, Parish WL, Laumann EO, Luo Y. Partner violence and sexual jealousy in China: a population-based survey. *Violence Against Women.* 2009;15(7):774-798.

6. Tiwari A, Wong M, Ip H. Ren and Yuan: a cultural interpretation of Chinese women's responses to battering. *Can J Nurs Res.* 2011;33(3):63-79.

7. Chan KL. Protection of face and avoidance of responsibility; Chinese men's account of violence against women. *J Soc Work Pract.* 2009;23(1):93-108.

8. World Health Organization. *WHO Multi:country Study on Women's Health and Domestic Violence against Women: Initial Results on Prevalence, Health Outcomes and Women's Responses.* Geneva, Switzerland: World Health Organization; 2005.

9. LaTourette KS. *The Chinese: Their History and Culture.* 4th ed. New York, NY: Macmillan; 1964.

10. Tung MPM. Symbolic meanings of the body in Chinese culture and "somatization." *Cult Med Psychiatry.* 1994;18:483-492.

11. Swann NL, trans. *Pan Chou: Foremost Woman Scholar of China.* New York, NY: Century Co.; 1932.

12. Legge J, trans. *The Confucian Analects: The Great Learning and the Doctrine of the Mean.* New York, NY: Cosimo Classics; 2009

13. Seagrave S. *Dragon Lady: The Life and Legend of the Last Empress of China.* New York, NY: Vintage; 1993.

14. China's gender imbalance alleviated but still grave. China Daily Web site. http://www.chinadaily.com.cn/china/2013 01/22/content_16156659.htm. Published January 22, 2013. Accessed September 10, 2013.

15. Rosenlee LL. *Confucainism and Women: A Philosophical Interpretation.* New York, NY: SUNY Press; 2006.

16. Tzu L. *Tao Te Ching.* Allchin D, trans. Classics of Integrity and they Way Web site. http://my.pclink.com/~allchin/tao/contents.htm. Published 2002. Accessed June 18, 2013.

17. Tang CS, Cheung FM, Chen R, Sun X. Definition of violence against women: a comparative study in Chinese societies of Hong Kong, Taiwan, and the People's Republic of China. *J Interpers Violence.* 2002;17(6):671-688.

18. Xu X, Campbell JC, Zhu F. Intimate partner violence against Chinese women: the past, present, and future. *Trauma Violence Abuse.* 2001;2(4):296-315.

19. Chan KL, Tiwari A, Fong DYT, Leung WC, Brownridge DA, Ho PC. Correlates of in-law conflict and intimate partner violence against Chinese pregnant women in Hong Kong. *J Interpers Violence.* 2009;24(1):97-110.

20. Moxley M. Rights-China: for too many, domestic violence part of family live. Inter Press Service News Agency Web site. http://www.ipsnews.net/2010/10/rights-china-for-too-many-domestic-violence-part-of-family-life/. Published October 5, 2010. Accessed October 12, 2011.

21. Parish WL, Wang T, Laumann EO, Pan S, Luo S. Intimate partner violence in China: national prevalence, risk factors and associated health problems. *Int Fam Plann Perspect.* 2004;30(4):174-181.

22. Hershatter G. State of the field: women in China's long twentieth century. *J Asian Stud.* 2004;63(4):991-1065.

23. Wu J, Guo S, Qu C. Domestic violence against women seeking induced abortion in China. *Contraception.* 2005;72(2):117-121.

24. Lee TS, Kleinman MA, Kleinman A. Rethinking depression: an ethnographic study of the experiences of depression among Chinese. *Harvard Rev Psychiatry.* 2007;15(1):1-8.

25. Zhang J, Ning L, Tu X, Xiao S, Jia C. Risk factors for rural young suicide in China: a case-control study. *J Affective Disord.* 2011;129:244-251.

26. Yoshioka M, Choi DY. Culture and interpersonal violence research: paradigm shift to create a full continuum of domestic violence services. *J Interpers Violence.* 2005;20(4):513-519.

27. Yick AG, Shibusawa T, Agbayani-Siewert P. Partner violence, depression, and practice implications with families of Chinese descent. *J Cult Diversity.* 2003;10(3):96-104.

28. Hao J. Legal countermeasures for domestic violence: from the perspective of family law in China. *Frontiers of Law in China.* 2009;5(2):302-318.

29. Jin X, Eagle M, Yoshioka M. Early exposure to violence in the family of origin and positive attitudes toward marital violence: chinese immigrant male batterers vs. controls. *J Fam Violence.* 2007;22:211-222.

30. Chin K. Out-of-town brides: international marriage and wife abuse among Chinese immigrants. *J Comp Fam Stud.* 1994;25(1):53-69.

31. Fletcher J. The effects of intimate partner violence on health in young adulthood in the United States. *Soc Sci Med.* 2010;70(1):130-135.

32. Lee CL, Zane NWS. *Handbook of Asian American Psychology.* Thousand Oaks, CA: Sage Publications; 1998.

33. http://webapps01.un.org/vawdatabase/countryInd.action?countryId=346. Accessed December 8, 2011.

34. Pang S, Wong T, Wang C, et al. Towards a Chinese definition of nursing. *J Adv Nurs.* 2004;46(6):657-670.

35. Journal of Clinical Nursing Web site. http://www.wiley.com/WileyCDA/Wiley Title/productCd-JOCN.html. Accessed December 12, 2011.

36. Journal of Clinical Nursing in English Summary. The Hong Kong Polytechnic University School of Nursing. http://www.chinesenursing.org/main/resources. php?lang=cn.

P

S

CPSIA information can be obtained
at www.ICGtesting.com
Printed in the USA
LVHW06s0710210918
590894LV00007B/231/P